# Health Unit Coordinating

# Health Unit Coordinating

**Myrna LaFleur-Brooks, RN, BEd, CHUC**
Founding President, National Association of Health Unit Coordinators
Formerly, Director, Health Services Management Program
Gateway Community College
Phoenix, Arizona

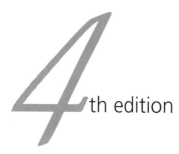

4th edition

**W.B. SAUNDERS COMPANY**
*A Division of Harcourt Brace & Company*
Philadelphia • London • Toronto • Montreal • Sydney • Tokyo

**W.B. SAUNDERS COMPANY**
*A Division of Harcourt Brace & Company*

The Curtis Center
Independence Square West
Philadelphia, Pennsylvania 19106

**Library of Congress Cataloging-in-Publication Data**

LaFleur-Brooks, Myrna.
   Health unit coordinating / Myrna LaFleur-Brooks. — 4th ed.
      p.      cm.
   Includes bibliographical references and index.
   ISBN 0–7216–7186–1
   1. Hospital ward clerks.   2. Medical records.   3. Medicine—
Terminology.   I. Title.
   [DNLM:   1. Personnel, Hospital.   2. Medical Records.   3. Nursing
Records.   WX 159 B873h 1998]
   RA972.55.B76   1998
   651.5′04261—dc21
   DNLM/DLC                                                      97–36857

HEALTH UNIT COORDINATING                                    0–7216–7186–1

Printed in the United States of America

Last digit is the print number:     9    8    7    6    5    4    3    2    1

*To NAHUC,*
*it's leaders and members who have guided the association*
*from its embryo stage to its mature stage,*
*to that of a full-fledged professional association*
*able to meet the obligations of its purpose.*

# CONTRIBUTORS

## ELAINE GILLINGHAM, BS, CHUC

Program Director, Health Unit Coordinator Program, Gateway Community College, Phoenix, Arizona

**Health Unit Coordinating: An Allied Health Career; The Nursing Department; Dietary Orders; Pediatrics**

## IVIE M. HAYES, MSN

Health Sciences Instructor, Gateway Community College, Pediatric RN, Arizona State Hospital, Phoenix, Arizona

**Medication Orders; Recording Vital Signs, Ordering Diets, Supplies, Daily Laboratory Tests, and Filing; Reports, Infection Control, Emergencies and Special Services**

## MAXINE L. PETTI, BS, MS, CM

Certified Instructor ITAA; Adjunct Faculty, Department of Graduate Studies in Counseling, Ottawa University; Phoenix Center, Phoenix, Arizona

**Communication and Interpersonal Skills for the Health Unit Coordinator; Management Techniques for Health Unit Coordinating**

## CECIL D. POWELL, MS

Assistant Professor, Pensacola Junior College, Pensacola, Florida

**The Hospital Environment; Medical/Legal Considerations**

## PATRICIA NOONAN RICE, CHUC

Education Services Instructor, Freeport Health Network, Freeport, Illinois; Interim Co-Director, Education Board, National Associate of Health Unit Coordinators; Former HUC Program Coordinator, Rockford Memorial Hospital, Rockford, Illinois

**Admission, Preoperative, and Postoperative Procedures; Discharge, Transfer, and Postmortem Procedures**

## PATRICIA J. SCHNEIDER, MA

Coordinator, Clinical Medical Assisting Program; Coordinator, Patient Care Technician Program, Phoenix College, Phoenix, Arizona
**Patient Activity, Patient Positioning, and Nursing Observation Orders; Nursing Treatment Orders**

## MONICA MELZER WADSWORTH, BS

Resident Faculty, Gateway Community College, Phoenix, Arizona
**Laboratory Orders; Treatment Orders**

# REVIEWERS

I would like to recognize the following individuals who served as consultants and reviewers during the preparation of the manuscript.

## KAREN CLARK, RN

Staff, Pediatrics Intensive Care Unit, Good Samaritan Regional Medical Center, Phoenix, Arizona

## EDWARD B. DIETRICH, MD

Medical Director, Arizona Heart Institute, Phoenix, Arizona

## M. MAIRATA FRANWICK, BA, CHUC

Health Unit Coordinator Instructor, Mid-State Technical College, Marshfield, Wisconsin

## SHERYL HANEGHAN, RN, CCRN

Director of Critical Care, Columbia Medical Center, Phoenix, Arizona

## ROBERT N. KAPLANIS, BS

Supervisor, Point of Care Services, Good Samaritan Regional Medical Center, Phoenix, Arizona

## JOHN LAMPIGNANO, RT, MEd

Faculty, Gateway Community College, Phoenix, Arizona

## KAREL LEESON, BS, RRT

Instructor, Respiratory Care, Gateway Community College, Phoenix, Arizona

## SUE McKINLEY, RN, BN

Practical Nursing Instructor and Health Unit Coordinator Instructor, Ivy Tech State College, Terre Haute, Indiana

**BONNIE ROILL, RDLD**

Clinical Nutrition Manager, St. Joseph's Hospital and Medical Center, Phoenix, Arizona

**SUSAN TAYLOR, MT**

Supervisor of Laboratory Services, St. Joseph's Hospital and Medical Center, Phoenix, Arizona

**LEROY TROVAR, MT**

Clinical Laboratory, Columbia Medical Center, Phoenix, Arizona

**DONNA VanHORTEN, MS**

Instructor, Nursing Division, Gateway Community College, Phoenix, Arizona

**PETER ZAWICKI, MS, PT**

Program Director, Physical Therapy Assistant Program, Gateway Community College, Phoenix, Arizona

# PREFACE

The fourth edition of *Health Unit Coordinating* reflects the latest changes in health care technology and in unit coordinating practice. This edition also addresses the drastic changes that have occurred and are continuing to occur in health care delivery systems and health care insurance programs. It will continue to be beneficial as a theory textbook in the health unit coordinating curriculum or as a reference book for health unit coordinating practice. The text will be useful in the hospital as a reference on the nursing unit, as a reference for writing unit coordinating practice and procedure, as a reference for building new-employee orientation programs, and as a textbook for cross-training.

## CHAPTER DESIGN

Each chapter begins with chapter objectives and a chapter vocabulary list followed by an abbreviations list. Exercises to learn the abbreviations are included. Once the students have read the objectives, read the vocabulary list, and completed the abbreviation exercises, they are ready to embrace the theory presented in each chapter.

Review questions at the end of each chapter assist the students in evaluating their knowledge of the chapter content. The answers are included in the text to allow the students to evaluate their progress themselves.

## ORGANIZATION

The text is divided into six sections. The material has been carefully chosen so that sections of the text may be used for separate college courses. For example, Section V, Introduction to Anatomic Structures, Medical Terms, and Illness, could be used for a two-credit course on basic human structure. Refer to the *Instructor's Guide* for a complete plan of the text for use in curriculum design. Sections are divided as follows:

### Section I: Orientation to Hospitals, Medical Centers, and Health Care

This section includes the history and current practice of health unit coordinating. A job analysis done in 1988–1989 by the National Association of Health Unit Coordinators is included. An introduction to the health care field and to nursing service and hospital departments is discussed in relation to health unit coordinating. New to the fourth edition is information on health care delivery systems other than the hospital and provider reimbursements. Also included are discussions about communication devices, computers, and telephone etiquette. Voice mail and guidelines for its proper use have been added to the fourth edition.

## Section II: Nonclinical Management of the Nursing Unit

Section II outlines management techniques and communication, interpersonal assertiveness skills for the health unit coordinator, and legal and ethical issues. Because the health unit coordinator constantly interacts with people, "people skills" are vital. Maslow's hierarchy of human needs model is used to study human behavior and is adapted to situations that relate to health unit coordinating. Assertive, nonassertive, and aggressive behavioral styles with examples of conflict and appropriate responses remain in the fourth edition. A communication model is also presented. Real-life hospital situations requiring communication, interpersonal, and assertiveness skills are presented in this section. These situations prepare the student for the hospital environment and allow for lively discussion in the classroom setting. The use of parent, child, and adult ego states to improve communication skills during stressful situations has been added to the fourth edition as well as ethics and "A Patient's Bill of Rights." Managing continuous quality improvement has been included to strengthen the management portion of this section.

## Section III: The Patient's Chart and Transcription of Doctors' Orders

This section deals with the transcription of doctors' orders—the major and most critical function of health unit coordinating. The material presented in this section helps the health unit coordinator to understand doctors' orders, thereby enhancing job performance in the health care setting. The patient's chart and chart forms, trade and generic names of common drugs, and drug uses and dosages are included in this section. Doctors' orders relating to nursing treatment and observation, dietary, laboratory, diagnostic imaging, respiratory care, physical medicine, gastroenterology, and medication are included in this section.

## Section IV: Health Unit Coordinator Procedures

Section IV presents procedures, such as admissions, transfers, and discharges. The fourth edition reflects the changes in procedures required by changes occurring in the health care industry such as direct admissions and organ donations.

## Section V: Introduction to Anatomic Structures, Medical Terms, and Illness

Section V is a complete module on basic human structure and medical terminology designed especially for the health unit coordinator student.

## Section VI: Specialty Services

Specialty services is a new section and provides information for health unit coordinators to prepare for employment in pediatric or psychiatric nursing care units.

## SPECIAL FEATURES

- An *Instructor's Guide* with test questions and suggestions is available for enhancing classroom learning.
- Answers for chapter questions are included at the back of the textbook.
- Assertiveness skills are demonstrated in hospital-related conflict situations especially geared to the health unit coordinator.
- Content is presented in the form of "doctors' orders."
- Tables, lists, and appendices are presented for quick reference and ease of learning. Included are

  Drug categories with trade and generic names
  A comprehensive list of laboratory studies
  Normal laboratory values
  Task analysis for health unit coordinating
  Medical terminology word list
  Abbreviations list
  Vocabulary lists
  Fasting and NPO list for laboratory studies
  A Patient's Bill of Rights
  Common hospital diets

- Highlight boxes are scattered throughout the text. They contain precise organized information that reinforces chapter content or summarizes it in point form.
- Chapters that address doctors' orders include review questions that require the student to convert doctors' orders, as spoken plainly, to written orders as commonly seen on doctors' order sheets using abbreviations and symbols. This learning approach is new to the fourth edition and is intended to further familiarize the student with doctors' orders as they will see them recorded on the patients' charts.

The role of the health unit coordinator is continually expanding, health care technology is rapidly advancing, and the health care delivery systems are constantly evolving. The fourth edition addresses these changes as they affect the health unit coordinating profession.

## EDUCATIONAL PACKAGE

The fourth edition of *Health Unit Coordinating* is now part of a total educational package for health unit coordinating offered by the W. B. Saunders Company. Also available is its companion workbook, the *Skills Practice Manual to Accompany Health Unit Coordinating*. This workbook contains practice exercises for transcribing handwritten doctors' orders. The workbook also includes practice in communication, assembling a chart, and performing unit coordinating skills, such as recording lab values, ordering diets, and recording telephoned doctors' orders. A clinical evaluation section is included. This section is designed to evaluate and record objectively the students' performance during their hospital rotation. Students should take this portion of the workbook with them as they enter their clinical course.

*Certification Review to Accompany Health Unit Coordinating* completes the package. This text is designed to assist the health unit coordinator to prepare for the national certification examination offered each year by the National Association for Health Unit Coordinators.

# ACKNOWLEDGMENTS

Preparing the fourth edition of *Health Unit Coordinating* required the expertise of many since changes in the health care delivery systems and advancement in medical technology demands new knowledge for the health unit coordinator and change in the health unit coordinating practice.

I am grateful for the invaluable expert advice and experience of Elaine Gillingham and Sue McKinley who helped to insure that this was the most up-to-date revision it could be. I would also like to acknowledge the cooperation I received from St. Joseph's Hospital and Medical Center, Good Samaritan Regional Medical Center, Gateway Community College and Phoenix Medical Associates, Columbia Medical Center, Arizona Heart Institute of Phoenix, Arizona who allowed access to their various departments to obtain information to prepare the manuscript.

A special thanks to the following staff of W. B. Saunders, Selma Kaszczuk, Senior Acquisitions Editor, Rachael Kelly, Associate Developmental Editor, and Joan Sinclair, Production Manager for their support and encouragement during the revision of this edition.

# ABOUT THE AUTHOR

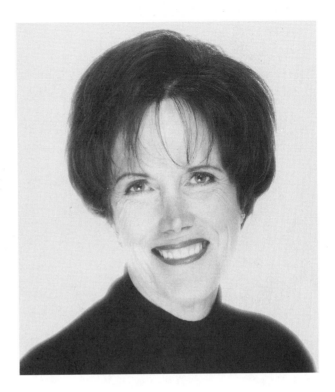

Myrna LaFleur-Brooks received her diploma of nursing from the Grey Nuns Hospital in Regina, Saskatchewan, Canada in 1962 and her Bachelors of Education from Northern Arizona University in 1977. After working as a staff nurse in medical-surgical nursing, she became an instructor then director in Staff Development at Doctor's Hospital in Phoenix. In 1970 she began her 25 year career with Gateway Community College as faculty in the Health Unit Coordinator Program. Frustrated by the lack of textbooks and the lack of recognition of health unit coordinating as a health profession, she and Winnie Starr, Program Director, set out to make changes. They welcomed the offer from W. B. Saunders to write a textbook titled, *Unit Clerking*, published in 1979. Its publication opened networking nationwide which led to the formation of a national association for health unit coordinators. The first organizational meeting was held in Phoenix on August 23, 1980, the date that has since become National Health Unit Coordinator Day, celebrated by unit coordinators and health care facilities alike throughout the nation. The National Association of Health Unit Coordinators (NAHUC), through the dedication of its leaders and members, has brought about the many changes necessary to establish unit coordinating as a health care profession. During her tenure at Gateway Community College, Ms LaFleur-Brooks held positions as director of the health unit coordinating and health services management program and as chair of the health science division. For the past two years she has devoted her time to writing and consulting.

# CONTENTS IN BRIEF

# CONTENTS

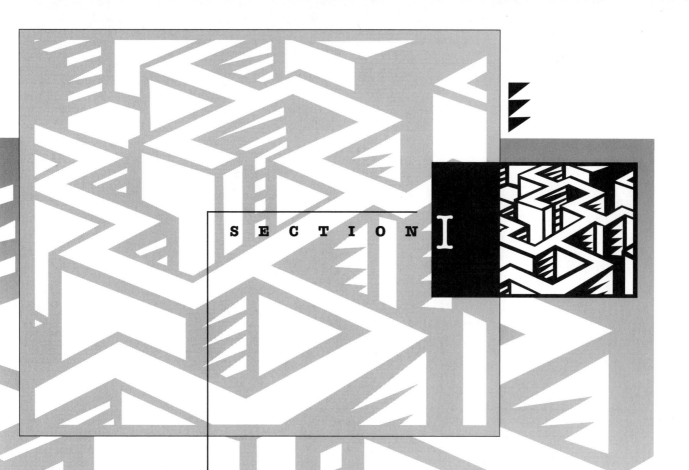

# ORIENTATION TO HOSPITALS, MEDICAL CENTERS, AND HEALTH CARE

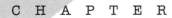

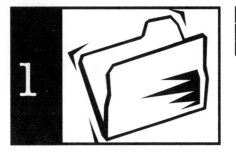

# HEALTH UNIT COORDINATING

## An Allied Health Career

*Upon completion of this chapter, you will be able to:*

1. Define the terms listed in the vocabulary list.
2. Write the meaning of the abbreviations in the abbreviations list.
3. Describe the four stages of evolution of health unit coordinating.
4. Describe three tasks that the health unit coordinator may perform that relate to the nursing staff, to doctors, to other hospital departments, and to visitors.
5. Write the name and purpose of the National Association of Health Unit Coordinators.
6. List the steps of the career ladder for nonclinical practice.

## V O C A B U L A R Y

**Career Ladder** • A pathway of upward mobility

**Certification** • Process of testifying to or endorsing that a person has met certain standards

**Certified Health Unit Coordinator (CHUC)** • A health unit coordinator who has successfully passed the national certification examination sponsored by the National Association of Health Unit Coordinators

**Client** • See definition of patient

**Clinical Tasks** • Tasks performed at the bedside

**Doctor** • A person licensed to practice medicine (used interchangeably with the term *physician* throughout this textbook)

**Doctors' Orders** • The health care a doctor prescribes in writing for a hospitalized patient

**Health Unit Coordinator (HUC)** • The nursing team member who performs the nonclinical patient care tasks for the nursing unit (may also be called unit clerk or unit secretary)

**Hospital Departments** • Divisions within the hospital that specialize in services, such as the dietary department, which plans and prepares meals for patients, employees, and visitors

**Independent Transcription** • The health unit coordinator assumes full responsibility for transcription of doctors' orders; cosignature by the nurse is not required

**Nonclinical Tasks** • Tasks performed away from the bedside

**Nurses' Station** • The desk area of a nursing unit

**Nursing Team** • A group of nursing staff members who care for patients on a nursing unit

**Nursing Unit** • An area within the hospital with equipment and nursing personnel to care for a given number of patients (may also be referred to as a wing, floor, pod, strategic business unit, ward, or station)

**Patient** • A person receiving health care, including preventive, promotion, acute, chronic, and all other services in the continuum of care (used interchangeably with *client* throughout the text)

**Policy Manual** • A handbook with such information as guidelines for practice, hospital regulations, and job descriptions for hospital personnel

**Recertification** • A process for certified health unit coordinators to exhibit continued personal, professional growth and current competency to practice in the field

**Revalidation** • A mandatory process that keeps one's certification in a current status and ensures that records are accurate and complete

**Transcription** • A process used to communicate the doctors' orders to the nursing staff and other hospital departments; requisitions or computers are used

## ABBREVIATIONS

| Abbreviation | Meaning |
| --- | --- |
| CHUC | certified health unit coordinator |
| HUC | health unit coordinator |
| SBU | strategic business unit |
| SHUC | student health unit coordinator |
| Pt | patient |

## EXERCISE 1

Write the abbreviation for each term listed below.

1. certified health unit coordinator          *CHUC*

2. health unit coordinator          *HUC*

3. strategic business unit          *SBU*

4. student health unit coordinator          *SHUC*

5. patient          *Pt*

## EXERCISE 2

Write the meaning of each abbreviation listed below.

1. CHUC          *Certified health Unit Coordinator*

2. HUC          *Health Unit Coordinator*

3. SBU          *Strategic Business Unit*

4. SHUC          *Student Helth Unit Coordinator*

5. Pt          *Patient*

## HEALTH UNIT COORDINATING: AN INTRODUCTION

Whether you are a student beginning an educational program or a health care employee, you have probably experienced difficulty in trying to explain to a relative or a friend what you do or will be doing as a health unit coordinator. Why? Because the public is aware of doctors, nurses, dentists, and possibly a few other health occupations, but most people do not understand the important role of the health unit coordinator in the delivery of health care.

By contrast, understanding of your profession is much different within the health care community. When you share with another health professional that you are a health unit coordinator or that you are studying to become one, the comments are: "It's one of the most important positions on the nursing unit," "we are so disorganized if the unit coordinator is not there," "the unit coordinator creates the attitude for the entire unit," "the unit coordinator sets the pace for the day's work," and "ask the unit coordinator—he or she knows everything."

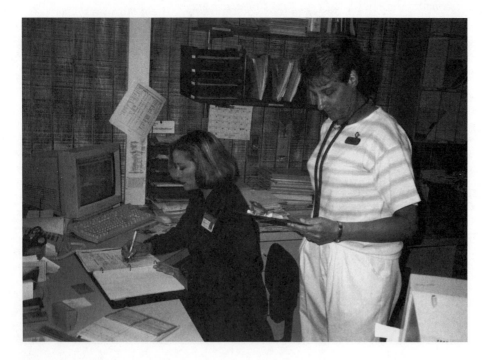

FIGURE 1–1 • The health unit coordinator's work area is the nurses' station.

Comments such as these are heard because the health unit coordinator organizes the activities for the nursing unit and manages its nonclinical functions; therefore, the health unit coordinator can enhance or inhibit the delivery of health care to the patients on the nursing unit.

The overall job is nonclinical in nature. The work area is the nurses' station. In the past, many health unit coordinators wore nursing uniforms to work. Now there is a clear delineation between nonclinical and clinical practice, and health unit coordinators are opting for professional, nonclinical garments such as shown in Figure 1–1.

## History of Health Unit Coordinating

### Hospitals

During World War II hospitals experienced a drastic shortage of registered nurses. To compensate for this shortage, auxiliary personnel were trained on the job to assist the registered nurse. The health unit coordinator was trained to assist the nurse with the nonclinical tasks, whereas the nursing assistant was trained to assist the nurse at the bedside.

Following World War II, the same shortage of nurses did not exist; however, the duties of the nurses were expanding. Advancement in technology was increasing the workload of the doctor, which resulted in the shifting of many tasks, such as taking blood pressure and starting intravenous therapy, to the nursing staff. Federally sponsored health programs required more detailed record keeping; hospitals were becoming larger and more complex; and increasing numbers of specialists were required to carry out the new tests and treatments. The nonclinical

demands of every hospitalized patient increased proportionally; therefore, the need for employing health unit coordinators continued. Today a 500-bed hospital has approximately 150 health unit coordinating positions. The role continues to change and expand.

### Professional Association

Traditionally, health professions have evolved through four stages: on-the-job training, formal education, the formation of a national association, and certification or licensure.

Health unit coordinating is no exception to the tradition. Health unit coordinators were trained on the job for over 20 years. The first record of health unit coordinating is found in an article published in *Modern Hospital* in 1940, which discussed the implementation of health unit coordinating at Montefiore Hospital in Pittsburgh, Pennsylvania. The author, Abraham Oseroff, a hospital administrator, stated that "a new helper was introduced to the nursing unit to take care of the many details of secretarial nature that formerly made demands on the limited time of the nurse." The title of the "new helper" was "floor secretary." Interestingly, the author wrote, ". . . the idea of floor secretary was first met with scepticism, but it proved to be worthwhile from the beginning."

In 1966, one of the first educational programs for health unit coordinating was offered in a vocational school in Minneapolis, Minnesota (Fig. 1–2). An article published in *Nursing Outlook* in 1966 described a research project that led to the implementation of this program. The most popular title for "floor secretary" had become ward or unit clerk. The article's author, Ruth Stryker, recommended that the title be changed to "station coordinator" because

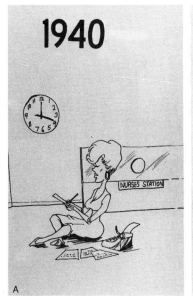
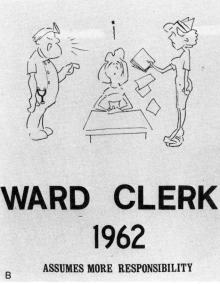
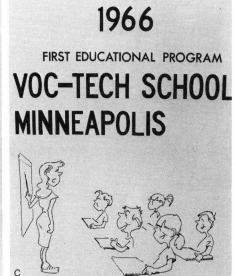

FIGURE 1–2 • History of health unit coordinating. (A) In 1940, health unit coordinating was first introduced as a health care occupation. The first job title was "floor secretary." (B) In 1962, the more common title was "ward clerk." More responsibilities were added to the job. (C) In 1966, the first vocational educational program for health unit coordinating was established.

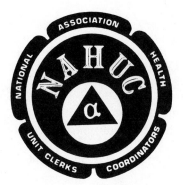

**F I G U R E   1–3** • The logo for the National Association of Health Unit Coordinators. The five outer segments represent doctors, nursing staff, patients, visitors, and hospital departments. The circle connecting the segments is symbolic of the health unit coordinator's role in coordinating the activities of these five groups.

the data showed that the unit clerk "did a great deal of managing in the form of coordinating activities." Ruth Stryker wrote one of the first textbooks for health unit coordinating, *The Hospital Ward Clerk*, which was published by the C. V. Mosby Company in 1970. Today, prior to employment, most health unit coordinators are educated in one of the many community colleges or vocational technical schools nationwide that offer health unit coordinator educational programs.

The occupation of health unit coordinator existed and grew for 40 years without the guidance of a professional association. The purpose of a professional association is to set standards of education and practice by peers to be enforced by peers for the protection of the public. Altruistic in nature, it is designed to enlighten its members and guide the profession to better serve the public. The constitution states the basic laws and principles of the association, and elected officers carry out the purpose listed in the constitution. By 1980, several educational programs were well established across the nation, and the educators in these programs began to discuss the possibility of forming a national association.

The first organizational meeting was held in Phoenix, Arizona, on August 23, 1980. This date has since been pro-

claimed as National Health Unit Coordinating Day by the national association. The 10 founding members represented both education and practice. In attendance were Kathy Jordan, Winnie Starr, Connie Johnston, Estelle Johnson, and Myrna LaFleur from Arizona; Kay Cox from California; Helga Hegge from Minnesota; Jane Pedersen from Wisconsin; Carolyn Hinken from New Mexico; and Velma Kerschner from Texas. During this first meeting the founding members declared the formation of a national association for health coordinators to be called the "National Association of Health Unit Coordinators" (NAHUC) (Fig. 1–3). The founding members recognized the need to update the title and to have a uniform title used nationwide. *Health unit coordinator* was the title chosen. Since *unit clerk* was the most popular title nationwide in 1980, *clerk* was included in the title of the national association with the intent that *clerk* be dropped from the title when *coordinator* became recognized. In 1990, the national association changed its name to the "National Association of Health Unit Coordinators," dropping *clerk* from its name.

At the second organizational meeting, held in San Juan Capistrano, California, the constitution was ratified and the officers were elected. Today, the association has over 3000 members. Standards of practice (see Appendix C), including educational requirements and a code of ethics (see Appendix E), have been adopted. The association has three boards that govern various branches of the association. The Certification Board is responsible for offering the certification exam and maintaining records. The Education Board is responsible for activities related to educational aspects of the profession. The Accreditation Board is responsible for determining and evaluating standards of educational programs nationwide (see NAHUC Membership Information).

---

## FIVE REASONS TO BECOME CERTIFIED

- Increased credibility
- Gain a broader perspective of health unit coordinating (not just your own specialty)
- Increased mobility, geographically and/or vertically
- Peer and public recognition and respect
- Improved self-image

---

## NAHUC MEMBERSHIP INFORMATION

To receive an NAHUC or certification test application:

- Phone:
    Toll-free—1-800-22-NAHUC
    Locally—215-545-1985
- Address: 1211 Locust St.
    Philadelphia, Pennsylvania 19107
- Fax: 215-545-8107
- E-mail: 73764.123@compuserve.com

---

## FIVE REASONS TO BECOME A MEMBER OF NAHUC

- Professional representation
- Format to share ideas and challenges
- National networking
- National directory
- Opportunity to develop leadership skills

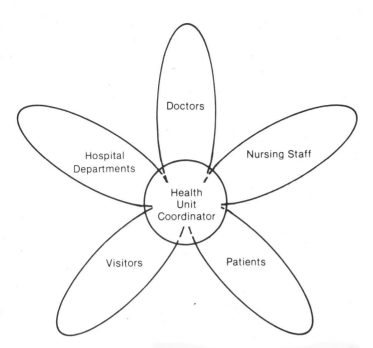

**FIGURE 1–4** • The health unit coordinator coordinates the activities of the doctors, the nursing staff, the hospital departments, the patients, and the visitors for the nursing unit.

The final step in the evolution of a health profession is certification and licensure. The first certification examination was offered by NAHUC in May, 1983. American Guidance Service, a professional testing company, was employed to administer the test. Nearly 5000 took the first exam. The examination now is administered nationwide at testing sites using an electronic system called "EXPRO." Questions are answered on a touch-sensitive computer screen and test results are given immediately upon completion of examination. The goal of every student of health unit coordinating should be to become certified. Passing the national certification examination indicates that you have met a standard of excellence and that you are competent to practice health unit coordinating (see Five Reasons to Become Certified).

For a group to become a profession they must have the following:

■ National association
■ Formal education
■ Certification or licensure
■ Code of ethics
■ Identified body of systematic knowledge and technical skill
■ Members who function with a degree of autonomy and authority under the assumption that they alone have the expertise to make decisions in their area of competence

Formation of the national association and the dedication of health unit coordinators nationwide to developing and implementing the above-mentioned structure and practices has advanced health unit coordinating to the professionalism it deserves.

Students are encouraged to join the NAHUC (see "Five Reasons to Become a Member of NAHUC").

For general information or information on membership or certification testing sites, write to NAHUC, 1211 Locust St., Philadelphia, Pennsylvania, 19107 or call toll free: 888-22-NAHUC; locally: 215-545-1985; fax: 215-545-8107; e-mail: 73764.123@compuserve.com.

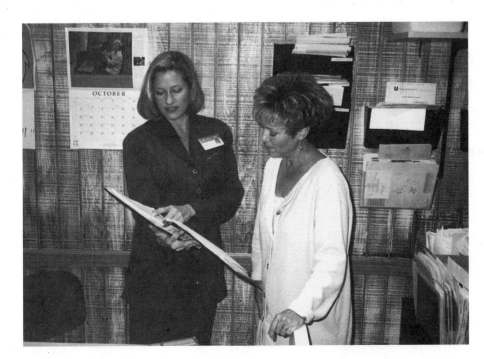

**FIGURE 1–5** • The health unit coordinator is a member of the nursing team and functions under the direction of the nurse manager or unit manager.

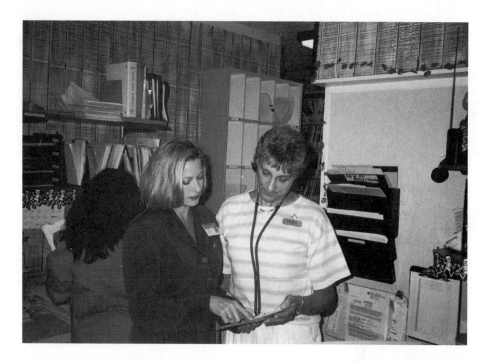

FIGURE 1–6 • The health unit coordinator works closely with the nursing staff.

## HEALTH UNIT COORDINATING TODAY

Although health unit coordinating began as a clerical job to assist the nurse, today it is a position that consists of many responsibilities. These responsibilities include coordinating the activities of the nursing staff, the doctors, the hospital departments, the patients, and the visitors for the nursing unit (Fig. 1–4). Health unit coordinators may also be employed in doctors' offices, clinics, and long-term care facilities assisting the nurse with clerical duties related to the clients' health records.

## The Health Unit Coordinator's Responsibilities

### Responsibility to the Nursing Staff

The health unit coordinator is a member of the nursing team (Fig. 1–5) and functions under the direction of the

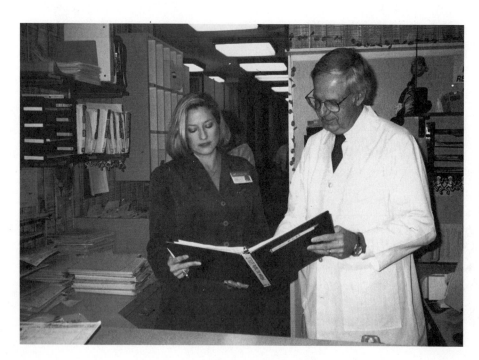

FIGURE 1–7 • The health unit coordinator assists the doctor with obtaining charts and equipment stored in the nursing unit.

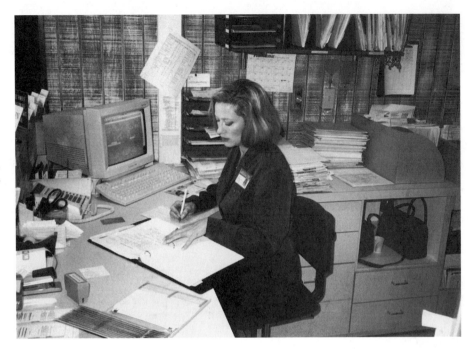

FIGURE 1–8 • A major responsibility of the health unit coordinator is transcribing doctors' orders.

nurse manager or unit manager. Responsibilities include (1) communicating all new doctors' orders to the patient's nurse (Fig. 1–6); (2) maintaining the client's chart; (3) performing the nonclinical tasks for admission, discharge, and transfer of a patient; (4) preparing the client's chart for surgery; and (5) handling all telephone communication for the nursing unit.

## Interaction with the Doctor

The health unit coordinator greets the doctors on their arrival at the nurses' station and assists them, if necessary, to obtain the patients' charts and to procure equipment (such as a stethoscope) for patients' examinations (Fig. 1–7).

Other responsibilities include (1) transcribing the doctors' orders (Fig. 1–8), and (2) placing calls to and receiving calls from the doctors' offices.

## Relationship with Hospital Departments

The health unit coordinator is the communicator between the doctor and nursing personnel and other hospital departments. Responsibilities include (1) scheduling diag-

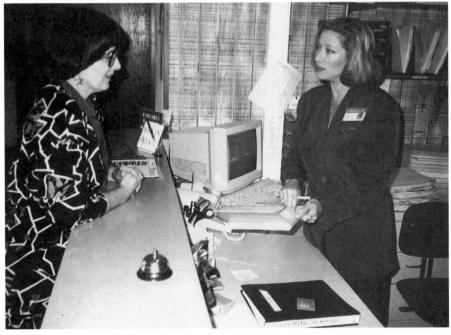

FIGURE 1–9 • The health unit coordinator informs the visitors of visiting hours and of any special precautions needed.

nostic procedures and treatments; (2) requesting services from maintenance and other service departments; (3) working closely with the admitting department to admit, transfer, and discharge patients; and (4) ordering all supplies for the nursing unit ranging from food to paper products and bandages.

### Interaction with the Patient

The health unit coordinator greets new patients when they arrive on the nursing unit and may accompany them to their rooms. By use of the intercom in each patient's room, the health unit coordinator relays patients' requests to the nursing personnel. The health unit coordinator has little bedside contact with the patients.

### Interaction with Hospital Visitors

The health unit coordinator (1) informs visitors of the visiting rules and of any special precautions regarding their visit to a patient's room, (2) receives telephone calls from relatives or friends inquiring about the patient's condition, and (3) is often the first person to handle visitor complaints (Fig. 1–9).

## JOB DESCRIPTION

The tasks that may be performed by the health unit coordinator are many. Appendix D lists health unit coordinator task and knowledge statements compiled from a nationwide research project done between 1988 and 1989 by the National Association of Health Unit Coordinators' Certification Board.

Hospitals outline the responsibilities for each category of employee in a formal written statement called a *job description*. Since health unit coordinating practice varies from hospital to hospital, look at your hospital's job description for health unit coordinating to find out what your responsibilities will be during employment. Job descriptions are a part of the hospital's policy manual, which is located on all nursing units.

Educational programs also outline the competencies or job skills that students are expected to know upon completion of the program. The following is an example of competencies for an educational program.

## ADDITIONAL TRAINING AND RESPONSIBILITIES

The current trend in health care facilities is to crosstrain health care givers to improve and expedite client care. It would be advantagious for the health unit coordinator to be proactive in seeking additional education and training. Client bedside admitting, some health record tasks, staffing, medical transcription, and information processing are examples of responsibilities that some health care facilities

### AN EXAMPLE OF COMPETENCIES FOR AN EDUCATIONAL PROGRAM

**Statement of Competency for Health Unit Coordinator**

Upon completion of the program, the student demonstrated the ability to:

- Demonstrate the health unit coordinator responsibilities and accountability to the nursing personnel, to the medical staff, to other hospital departments, and to the patients and visitors
- Operate the nursing unit communication systems: computer terminal, telephone, intercom, pager, imprinter device, and conveyor system
- Record telephoned doctors' orders, diagnostic test values, vital signs, and census data
- Order daily diets and daily laboratory tests
- File reports on the patients' charts
- Transcribe doctors' orders utilizing basic knowledge of anatomy and physiology, disease processes, medical terminology, and accepted abbreviations (competent to perform this task without the checking and cosignature of the registered nurse)
- Perform the nonclinical tasks for patient admission, transfer, discharge, preoperative and postoperative procedures
- Plan and execute a daily routine for the performance of nonclinical tasks for the nursing unit
- Manage the nonclinical functions of the nursing unit
- Maintain the nursing unit supplies
- Prepare patient consent forms
- Maintain the patients' charts
- Coordinate scheduling of patients' tests and diagnostic procedures
- Transcribe medication orders, utilizing concepts of drug categories, automatic stop dates, automatic cancellations, time scheduling, and routes of administration
- Practice within the professional ethical framework of health unit coordinating
- Schedule radiologic procedures that require patient preparation
- Communicate effectively with patients, visitors, and members of the health care team

are adding to the health unit coordinator position. Surveying health care facilities in the area of desired employment would be beneficial in choosing educational opportunities.

## AN EXAMPLE OF A CAREER LADDER FOR HEALTH UNIT COORDINATORS

### Health Unit Coordinator I

*Education*

- Must be a graduate of a recognized educational program

*Overall Responsibilities*

- Manages the supplies and equipment on a nursing unit
- Manages and performs the nonclinical nursing tasks for a nursing unit
- Manages and performs the receptionist role for a nursing unit
- Uses discretion and protects the confidentiality of patient information
- Sets priorities and organizes the workload on a nursing unit

*Job Duties*

- Performs the telephone communications for the nursing unit
- Transcribes the doctors' orders
- Performs patient admission, transfer, and discharge procedures
- Performs nonclinical preoperative and postoperative procedures
- Operates the nursing unit equipment: imprinter device, pneumatic tube system, intercom system, fax machine, and computer
- Maintains the daily census sheet and census board
- Orders the daily diets
- Requisitions the daily laboratory studies
- Maintains each patient's chart: files patient data in the chart holder, imprints and places standard forms in the chart holder as needed, and records the whereabouts of the chart if it is removed from the nursing unit
- Maintains the central service department supplies on the nursing unit
- Determines the need for and orders unit supplies from the purchasing department
- Maintains an up-to-date bulletin board
- Prepares a weekly utilization report
- Communicates pertinent data and hospital procedure to the patient's visitors
- Assists, as directed, during an emergency situation
- Maintains the doctors' supplies stored on the nursing unit
- Maintains the reference books and the policy/procedure manuals
- Assists doctors and other health personnel as needed at the nurses' station

*Job Relationships*

- Functions under the supervision of the nurse manager

## CAREER LADDER FOR HEALTH UNIT COORDINATING

The *career ladder* is a concept that is becoming popular for nursing personnel in health care facilities. Because of their success, we are beginning to see career ladders for health unit coordinating. The ladder varies among institutions, but essentially represents the pathway of upward mobility for a profession. It illustrates how individuals can advance if they function to the potential commensurate with their knowledge and skill. Refer to the following example of a career ladder for health unit coordinators. Two levels of employment, listing job responsibilities and professional preparation, are included.

## CAREER PATH

More and more, health unit coordinating is becoming recognized as the entry level job in the nonclinical career path. Upon acquiring the education needed, the health unit coordinator can advance to a health unit management position. A health unit manager's position includes performing the following duties for one or more nursing units:

## AN EXAMPLE OF A CAREER LADDER FOR HEALTH UNIT COORDINATORS (Continued)

### Health Unit Coordinator II

*Education*

- Must have 3 years experience and be NAHUC certified

*Job Duties*

- Performs all the functions listed under Health Unit Coordinator I
- Writes telephoned doctors' orders on the doctors' order sheet
- Completes the time schedule for the nursing personnel assigned to the nursing unit
- Supervises Health Unit Coordinator I employees assigned to the nursing unit
- Precepts health unit coordinator students and orients other health personnel to health unit coordinator skills
- Liaison between patient, visitor, and nursing personnel
- Independent transcription

*Job Relationships*

- Functions under the supervision of the nurse manager

- Establishing policies and procedures for the nursing units
- Planning departmental organization
- Hiring, motivating, and supervising health unit coordinators
- Providing staff development programs
- Preparing the nursing unit budget
- Participating in research

The next step of advancement is to health service administration. Figure 1–10 gives an example of career advancement for nonclinical practices.

## SUMMARY

Health unit coordinating is now a recognized health-care profession. Because individuals practicing as health unit coordinators soon realize that they have far-reaching effects on the delivery of care to the patients, job satisfaction is high. The career ladder concept and the introduction of computers into the nursing units have added extra excitement to the field of nonclinical practice.

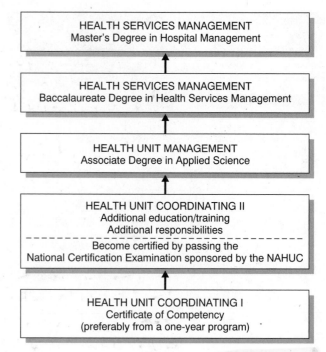

FIGURE 1–10 • Career path for nonclinical practice.

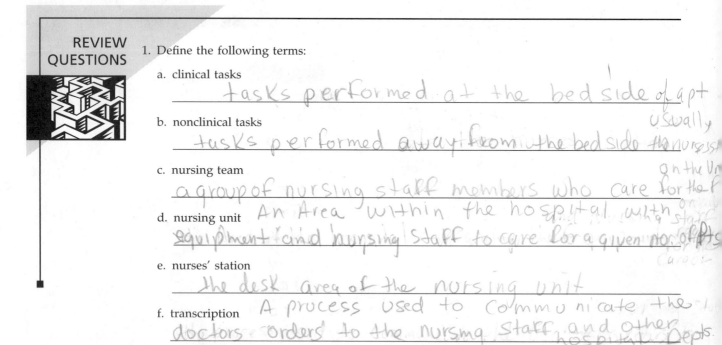

REVIEW QUESTIONS

1. Define the following terms:

   a. clinical tasks

   _tasks performed at the bedside of a pt_

   b. nonclinical tasks

   _tasks performed away from the bedside than nurses usually on the Un_

   c. nursing team

   _a group of nursing staff members who care for the p_

   d. nursing unit   _An Area within the hospital with on staff equipment and nursing staff to care for a given nor of pts cared_

   e. nurses' station

   _the desk area of the nursing unit_

   f. transcription   _A process used to communicate the doctors orders to the nursing staff, and other hospital Depts._

   g. doctors' orders

   _the healthcare a doctor prescribes in writing for a hos_

   h. independent transcription   _A HUC assumes full responsibilit of trascribing the doctors orders not requiring a nurses cosignature_

i. certification

→ certain standards of the HUC proffession

the process of endorsing that a person has met

j. recertification   A process of

the process of continued personal + proffessional growth and continued education on the practice of the HUC field

k. revalidation

mandatory process that keeps a certification current, up to date ensuring accurate + complete records

2. The four stages of evolution of a health profession are listed below. Write the year they began for health unit coordinating, and describe the events surrounding the dates.

a. on-the-job training

1940 during World War II due to a shortage of RNs

b. education   1966 due to a research project a HUC program was developed at a vocational school in Minneapolis, Minn.

c. professional association

40 years of existance + growth without guidance by a professional group led to the first organized meeting in Arizona in 1980 Aug 23 to form national organization

d. certification or licensure   offered by NAHUC in 1983 after a certain standards of practice including education and a code of ethics wer adopted

3. List health unit coordinating tasks that relate to the:

a. nursing personnel

i. Communicating all New Dr's Orders to Pt's Nurse

ii. maintaining clients charts + handling telephone Communication

iii. performing nonclinical tasks for admission, discharge + transfer of patients

b. doctor

i. assist in obtaining patient charts and equipment

ii. transcribing Doctors orders

iii. placing + recieving calls from the Drs office

c. hospital departments

i. Scheduling diagnostic procedures and treatments,

ii. requesting services from other service depts in hospital

iii. ordering all supplies for the nursing unit admit transfer and discharge patients

d. client's relatives and friends

i. Inform on visiting rules and any special precautions concerning pt.

ii. recieve telephone inquiries requarding patient cond.

iii. handle visitor complaints

4. The name of the national association for health unit coordinators is  NAHUC the National Association of Health Unit Coordinators

5. Describe the purpose of a professional association.  to set standards of education and practice by peers to be enforced by peers to protect the public

6. List three reasons to become a member of the National Association of Health Unit Coordinators.

   a. _Professional Representation_

   b. _Format to share Ideas and Challenges_

   c. _Opportunity to develop leadership skills_

7. List three reasons to become certified.

   a. _Increased credibility and self image_

   b. _Increased mobility geographically or personal_

   c. _peer & publics recognition and respect_

8. Becoming a registered nurse is a step on the nonclinical career ladder. (true or false) _false_

9. The steps of the career path for nonclinical practice are:

   a. _Health Unit Coordinating I_

   b. _Health Unit Coordinating II_

   c. _Health Unit Management_

   d. _Health Services management_

## References

*Mosby Medical, Nursing, and Allied Health Dictionary*, 3rd ed. St. Louis, The C. V. Mosby Co., 1990.

*National Association of Health Unit Coordinators, Inc. Hand Book.*

Oseroff, Abraham: In favor of floor secretaries. *The Modern Hospital*, Nov.: 69, 1940.

Rambo, Beverly J.: *Ward Clerk Skills*. New York, McGraw-Hill Book Co., 1978.

Schutt, Rusche R.: A blueprint for ward clerks. *Hospital Progress*, Jan.: 106, 1962.

Stryker, Ruth Perin: Hospital study leads to vocational program. *Nursing Outlook*, Aug.: 43, 1966.

Stryker, Ruth Perin: *The Hospital Ward Clerk*. St. Louis, The C. V. Mosby Co., 1970.

Wilson, Florence A. and Neuhauser, Duncan: *Health Services in the United States*, 2nd ed. Cambridge, MA, Ballinger Publishing Co., 1976.

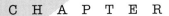

CHAPTER 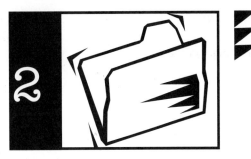 2

# THE NURSING DEPARTMENT

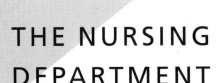

## CHAPTER OBJECTIVES

*Upon completion of this chapter, you will be able to:*

1. Define the terms in the vocabulary list.

2. Write the meaning of the abbreviations in the abbreviations list.

3. List three categories of personnel commonly employed in the nursing service department and briefly describe the role of each personnel category.

4. List 14 kinds of nursing units and briefly describe services provided by each.

5. Describe intensive care units and perioperative services.

6. List two methods of organizing a nursing unit and describe the health unit coordinator's communication line for each.

7. Identify two reasons for restructuring in health care facilities.

## VOCABULARY

**Certified Nursing Assistant** • A health care giver who performs basic nursing tasks and has been certified by passing a required certification examination

**Director of Patient Services** • A registered nurse in charge of nursing services (may be called director of nursing, nursing administrator, or vice president of nursing services)

**Licensed Practical Nurse (Licensed Vocational Nurse)** • A graduate of a 1-year school of nursing who is licensed in the state in which he or she is practicing

**Nurse Manager** • A registered nurse who is in charge of one or more nursing units (may also be called unit manager, clinical manager, or patient care manager)

**Nursing Service Department** • The hospital department responsible for all the nursing care administered to the patients

**Nursing Unit Administration** • A division within the hospital responsible for nonclinical patient care; this system is used in some hospitals

**Patient Care Technician** • A certified nursing assistant trained to do bedside testing and phlebotomy

**Patient Support Associate** • A person who cleans the nursing unit and patient rooms and transports patients as necessary

**Perioperative Services** • A department of the hospital that provides care before (preoperative), during (intraoperative), and after (postoperative) surgery

**Registered Nurse** • A graduate of a 2- to 4-year college-based school of nursing or a 3-year diploma, hospital-based program, who is licensed in the state in which he or she is practicing

**Restructuring** • Reorganization of health care facility labor, supplies, and technology

**Shift Manager** • A registered nurse who is responsible for one or more units during his or her assigned shift (may also be called assistant to director or nursing care manager or assistant nursing care manager)

**Staff Development** • The hospital department responsible for both orientation of new employees and continuing education of employed personnel (may also be called educational services)

**Team Leader** • A registered nurse who is in charge of a nursing team (may also be called pod leader)

## A B B R E V I A T I O N S

| Abbreviation | Meaning |
| --- | --- |
| ATD | assistant to director |
| CCU | coronary care unit |
| CNA | certified nursing assistant |
| DSU | day surgery unit |
| ED | emergency department |
| ER | emergency room |
| Gyn | gynecology |
| ICU | intensive care unit |
| LPN | licensed practical nurse |
| LVN | licensed vocational nurse |
| Med | medical |
| Neuro | neurology |
| OB | obstetrics |
| OR | operating room |
| Ortho | orthopedics |
| PACU | postanesthesia care unit |
| PCT | patient care technician |
| Peds | pediatrics |
| PSA | patient support associate |
| Psych | psychiatry |
| RN | registered nurse |
| RR | recovery room |
| SAD | save a day (admitted on day of surgery) |
| SDS | same-day surgery (admitted on the day of surgery) |
| Surg | surgical |
| SSU | short-stay unit |

## E X E R C I S E 1

Write the correct abbreviation for each term listed below.

1. assistant to director — ATD
2. coronary care unit — CCU
3. intensive care unit — ICU
4. certified nursing assistant — CNA
5. licensed vocational nurse — LVN
6. surgical — Surg
7. obstetrics — OB
8. medical — Med
9. emergency room — ER
10. psychiatry — Psych
11. pediatrics — Peds
12. orthopedics — Ortho
13. gynecology — Gyn
14. neurology — Neuro

15. recovery room — RR
16. registered nurse — RN
17. licensed practical nurse — LPN
18. patient care technician — PCT
19. patient support associate — PSA
20. operating room — OR
21. day surgery unit — DSU
22. emergency department — ED
23. postanesthesia care unit — PACU
24. short-stay unit — SSU
25. save a day (admission) — SAD
26. same-day surgery — SDS

## E X E R C I S E 2

Write the meaning of each abbreviation listed below.

1. Surg — surgical
2. Neuro — neurology
3. LPN — Licenced Practical Nurse
4. LVN — Licenced Vocational Nurse
5. ATD — Assitcount to Director
6. CNA — Certified Nursing Assistant
7. ICU — Intensive Care Unit
8. CCU — Coronary Care Unit
9. ER — Emergency Room
10. Ortho — Orthopedics
11. Gyn — gynecology
12. RN — Registered Nurse
13. OR — operating room
14. RR — recovery room
15. Med — medical
16. DSU — Day surgery Unit
17. OB — obstetrics
18. Peds — pediatrics
19. Psych — psychiatry
20. PCT — patient care tech
21. PACU — post anesthea care Unit

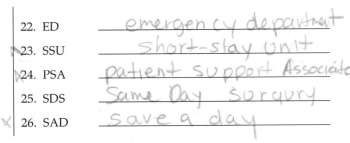

22. ED   *emergency department*
23. SSU   *short-stay unit*
24. PSA   *patient support Associate*
25. SDS   *Same Day surgery*
26. SAD   *save a day*

## NURSING SERVICE ORGANIZATION

Nursing service is responsible for the physical and emotional care of the hospitalized client, for performing nursing treatment, and for coordinating treatment and diagnostic studies performed by other hospital departments. Other responsibilities include patient observation and recording, planning and implementing patient care plans, and patient teaching. As you can see, nursing service is the single largest component of the hospital. Often 50% of all hospital personnel are employed in the nursing service department.

Although the organization of nursing service varies among hospitals, and different titles may be used for the same level of authority, the basic concepts remain the same. Figure 2–1 is a typical nursing service organizational chart. It denotes the titles and the lines of authority within the nursing service organization.

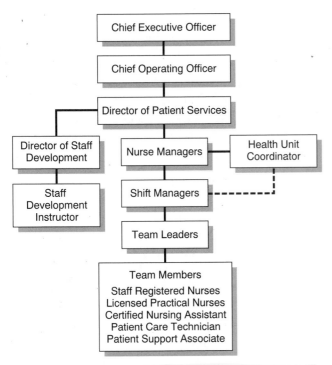

F I G U R E   2–1 • Nursing service organizational chart.

## Nursing Service Administrative Personnel

The **director of patient services**, also called the **vice president of nursing**, is responsible for the overall administration of nursing service. Setting nursing practice standards and staffing are two examples of the responsibilities of the director of nursing. The director of nursing is responsible to the chief executive officer of the health care facility.

The **unit manager** or **clinical manager** assists the director of nursing in carrying out administrative responsibilities. The **unit manager** is responsible to the **director of patient services**.

The **director of staff development** is responsible for the orientation and evaluation of new nursing service employees and for the continuing education of all employed nursing service personnel. He or she is usually responsible to the director of nursing.

## Hospital Nursing Units

As you recall from Chapter 1, the health unit coordinator works at the nurses' station on the nursing unit. The hospital is divided into nursing units according to the type(s) of service(s) provided to the patients.

Many methods are used to name the nursing units within the hospital. Sometimes the units are named according to the service offered, such as pediatrics; or the name may be derived from the floor level and direction of the hospital wing, for example, 4 East.

### Regular Nursing Units

Most nursing units are designed to accommodate 18 to 50 hospitalized patients. A regular nursing unit may provide one of the following services:

**Behavioral Health:** Includes psychiatry (Psych), which is the care of patients hospitalized for treatment of disorders of the mind or having difficulty coping with life situations; may also include programs for treatment of alcohol and drug abuse and programs related to changing destructive behaviors such as eating disorders

**Cardiovascular:** Care of clients who are hospitalized for treatment of diseases of the circulatory system

**Gynecology Surgery (Gyn):** Care of women who are hospitalized for surgery of the female reproductive tract

**Medical (Med):** Care of patients who are hospitalized for medical treatment

**Neurology (Neuro):** Care of clients who are hospitalized for treatment of diseases of the nervous system

**Obstetrics (OB), Labor and Delivery, and Nursery:** Care of mothers before, during, and after labor, and care of newborn infants

**Oncology:** Care of patients who are hospitalized for treatment of cancer

**Orthopedics (Ortho):** Care of patients who are hospitalized for treatment of diseases or fractures of the skeletal system

**Pediatrics (Peds):** Care of children (12 and under) who are hospitalized for medical or surgical treatment

**Rehabilitation (Rehab):** Care of patients who are hospitalized for physical handicaps; usually these patients need long-term treatment and care

**Stepdown Unit:** Care of patients who require more specialized care than that given at regular nursing units, but who do not require intensive care (also called intermediate care or maximum care)

**Surgical (Surg):** Care of patients who are hospitalized for general surgical treatment

**Telemetry:** Care of patients with arrhythmias and other heart problems, whose electrocardiogram readings are monitored at the nurses' station

**Urology:** Care of patients who are hospitalized for treatment of disease of the male reproductive or urinary systems or of the female urinary system

### Intensive Care Units

Another type of nursing unit found in the modern hospital is the **intensive care unit (ICU):** its purpose is to provide constant specialized nursing care to critically ill patients. It is usually designed to accommodate fewer than 10 patients. As the condition of the critically ill patient improves, he or she is transferred to the regular nursing unit for less intense nursing care. The personnel employed in the intensive care units are specially qualified for the type of nursing care offered by the unit.

Intensive care units are identified by the type of nursing care they provide; for example, the **surgical intensive care unit (SICU)** cares for surgical patients, the **medical intensive care unit (MICU)** cares for medical patients, and the **coronary care unit (CCU)** cares for patients with heart disease, the **trauma intensive care unit (TICU)** cares for patients involved in trauma, the **neonatal intensive care unit (NICU)** cares for premature and ill newborns, and the **pediatric intensive care unit (PICU)** cares for pediatric patients.

### Specialty Units

Specialty areas within the hospital that are usually a part of nursing service and employ various categories of nursing personnel are:

**Day Surgery or Outpatient Surgery Unit or Ambulatory Surgery:** Care of patients who are having surgery or examinations but who do not require overnight hospitalization; may be referred to as save a day (SAD) or same-day surgery (SDS)

**Emergency Department:** Care of patients who need emergency treatment; after emergency treatment is administered, the patient is either admitted to the hospital or discharged home, according to his or her medical needs

**Perioperative Services**
  **Operating Room:** Area in the hospital where surgery is performed

**Preoperative Area:** Area in the hospital where clients are prepared for surgery

**Postanesthesia Care Unit or Recovery Room:** Area in the hospital where patients are cared for immediately after surgery until they have recovered from the effects of the anesthesia

## Nursing Unit Personnel

To maintain 24-hour coverage, nursing service personnel are usually scheduled in three shifts, normally divided into: 7:00 AM to 3:30 PM (day shift), 3:00 PM to 11:30 PM (evening shift), and 11:00 PM to 7:30 AM (night shift). Two shifts may also be used. The shifts are then usually 7:00 AM to 7:30 PM and 7:00 PM to 7:30 AM (shifts overlap 1/2 hour to allow communication between personnel).

The **nurse manager** (also called **clinical patient care manager** or **unit manager**) is a registered nurse who is usually responsible for the patients and nursing personnel on his or her unit for 24 hours a day. The nurse manager is responsible to the **director of patient services.** Managerial responsibilities include the planning and coordinating of quality nursing care for patients hospitalized on the unit. Selecting, supervising, scheduling and evaluating personnel employed on the unit are other managerial responsibilities of the nurse manager. The nurse manager works closely with the physicians to coordinate nursing care with the care prescribed by the physician. Usually a registered nurse titled a **shift manager** or **nursing care manager** or **assistant nursing care manager** manages the nursing unit in the absence of the nurse manager on the day shift and on the evening and night shifts.

Nursing personnel other than the health unit coordinator who may be employed on the nursing unit and who function under the supervision of the nurse manager are discussed below. If possible, *read* the job descriptions for these persons in your hospital's policy manual.

The **registered nurse** is a graduate of a 2- to 4-year college-based program or a 3-year hospital-based program and is currently licensed in the state in which he or she is practicing. The RN may give direct patient care or supervise patient care given by others. The registered nurse performs all types of treatments, and it is usually hospital policy that only the RN can perform complex procedures, such as administering intravenous (IV) medication. The RN is also expected to maintain accurate records and to teach the clients, their families, and other team members.

The **licensed practical nurse (LPN)** is in some states called the **licensed vocational nurse.** The licensed practical nurse is a graduate of a 1-year school of nursing and is licensed in the state in which he or she is practicing. The LPN functions under the direction of the RN and gives direct patient care, performs technical skills, such as discontinuing an IV, and administers medication to the patients, as prescribed by the physician.

The **certified nursing assistant (CNA)** either is trained on the job or has completed a short training course (approximately 6 weeks) at a vocational school. Some states require a state examination for the nursing assistant to be certified. Nursing assistants perform bedside tasks, such as bathing and feeding patients. They also perform basic treatments, such as taking vital signs and giving enemas. The certified nursing assistant functions under the supervision of the RN.

The **patient care technician (PCT)** is a certified nursing assistant who has been trained and is competent to also perform bedside testing such as EKGs and to do phlebotomy.

## PATIENT CARE ASSIGNMENT

Since health unit coordinators frequently need to communicate information to the nurse caring for a patient, they need to be aware of the types of patient care assignments used by the nursing unit.

### Team Nursing

A **nursing team** is made up of the team leader, also called **pod leader** (a registered nurse), and team members who may be registered nurses, licensed practical nurses, or nursing assistants. The team leader assigns patients for each team member to care for during a shift. Each team member performs the particular tasks for his or her patients that he or she is qualified to perform. For example, if the doctor orders an IV for a patient assigned to a certified nursing assistant for care, the team leader starts the IV. The team leader is responsible for both the clients and the members of his or her team. A team usually cares for 15 or fewer patients; thus a nursing unit may have one to three teams. Many hospitals use modified forms of the team nursing method.

For team nursing, the health unit coordinator communicates patient information directly to the team leader, who then communicates information to the team members as needed. However, each team may have a "medication nurse," who distributes medication to all the clients on the nursing team. The health unit coordinator then usually communicates all information regarding medication to the medication nurse.

### Total Patient Care

In the **total patient care** method of assignment, a registered nurse or licensed practical nurse gives total care, including medications, to a given number of patients. Total patient care assignment is usually practiced in intensive care units. However, there is a recent trend toward practicing total patient care on the regular nursing units also. **Primary nursing** is a type of total patient care in which one nurse is responsible for planning, implementing, and evaluating the patient's care for a 24-hour period throughout the patient's hospital stay. In the total patient care method, the health unit coordinator communicates patient information directly to the nurse assigned to take care of the patient for the 8- or 12-hour shift.

Each day a patient care assignment sheet is made out indicating the member of the nursing unit team who is to care for each patient. Figure 2–2 shows examples of assignment sheets for the team nursing and total patient care methods of assignment. In the hospital, the assignment sheets are posted on the bulletin board or in another visible area on the nurses' station. To locate the nurse who is caring for a patient, simply refer to the assignment sheet.

### Restructuring of Health Care Facilities

Restructuring (also referred to as reengineering, redesign, or downsizing) has transformed health care dramatically in the 1990s. Two facts that forced these drastic changes are (1) that medical technology is evolving at an enormous pace and (2) that Americans are living longer. Restructuring involves the reorganization of health care facility labor, supplies, and technology to emphasize teamwork and place focus on patient care. Home care, outpatient clinics, surgicenters, and long-term care facilities have reduced the number of hospitalized patients. There is a greater focus on wellness and prevention of illness.

Under restructuring you may see both new health care occupations and changes in existing occupation job descriptions.

Some examples of new occupations include:

**Patient Care Technician (PCT):** Performs EKGs, phlebotomy, and patient care
**Patient Support Associate (PSA):** Responsible for cleaning of nursing units and patient rooms, transportation of patients, and answering patient call lights
**Case Manager:** Discharge teaching and consultant

Some examples of changes in existing occupation job descriptions:

**Registered Nurse (RN):** Patient teaching; assess, plan, evaluate care; perform complicated care and some respiratory therapy when needed
**Health Unit Coordinator (HUC):** Bedside patient admitting, some health record responsibilities, and data entry

The focus is on teamwork, with each unit being self-sufficient and providing a continuum of care and service consistency to patients. In addition to nursing personnel, unit teams may include a respiratory therapist, a physical therapist, a pharmacist, and a patient admitting associate. Personnel and job descriptions may vary depending on unit specialty.

## Assignment Sheet

Unit _____          Date _____          Shift _____

| Lunch | Name | Time | | Dinner | Name | Time |
|-------|------|------|--|--------|------|------|
| _____ | | | | _____ | | |
| _____ | | | | _____ | | |
| _____ | | | | _____ | | |
| _____ | | | | _____ | | |
| _____ | | | | _____ | | |
| _____ | | | | _____ | | |

| Pager Number | Nurse | Room Assignment | Patient Name |
|--------------|-------|-----------------|--------------|
| 15-8354 | | | |
| 15-8356 | | | |
| 15-8358 | | | |
| 15-8360 | | | |
| 15-8362 | | | |
| 15-8364 | | | |
| 15-8366 | | | |

### Instructions

|  |  | Pager | Office |
|--|--|-------|--------|
| 1. Dial pager number | | | |
| 2. You will hear a beep and be asked to enter your phone number | Nurse Manager | 15-0121 | 938-5622 |
| | Shift Manager | 15-8999 | 938-5656 |
| 3. Enter number or extension, | Case Manager | 15-7654 | 938-5677 |
| 4. Enter # key and hang up | Social Worker | 15-3976 | 938-5643 |

A

FIGURE 2–2 • Assignment sheet. (*A*) An example of a total patient care assignment. (*B*) An example of a team nursing assignment. *Illustration continued on opposite page*

## Assignment Sheet

Unit _____      Date _____      Shift _____

| Lunch | Name | Time | | Dinner | Name | Time |
|---|---|---|---|---|---|---|
| ___ | ___ | ___ | | ___ | ___ | ___ |
| ___ | ___ | ___ | | ___ | ___ | ___ |
| ___ | ___ | ___ | | ___ | ___ | ___ |
| ___ | ___ | ___ | | ___ | ___ | ___ |
| ___ | ___ | ___ | | ___ | ___ | ___ |

**Pager Number        Team        Room Assignment        Patient Name**

#1

15-8354 RN _____

Team Members _____
_____
_____
_____

#2

15-8356 RN _____

Team Members _____
_____
_____
_____

#3

15-8358 RN _____

Team Members _____
_____
_____
_____

#4

15-8360 RN _____

Team Members _____
_____
_____
_____

### Instructions

|   |   | Pager | Office |
|---|---|---|---|
| 1. Dial pager number | | | |
| | Nurse Manager | 15-0121 | 938-5622 |
| 2. You will hear a beep and be asked to enter your phone number | Shift Manager | 15-8999 | 938-5656 |
| 3. Enter number or extension, | Case Manager | 15-7654 | 938-5677 |
| 4. Enter # key and hang up | Social Worker | 15-3976 | 938-5643 |

B

FIGURE 2–2 • *Continued*

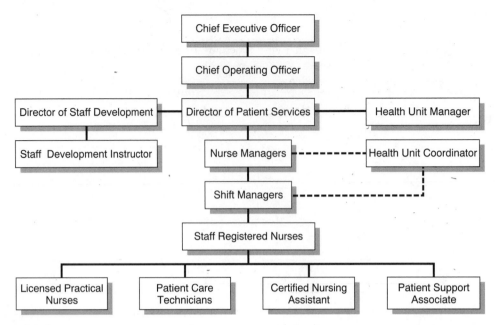

F I G U R E   2–3 • Organizational structure for the nursing service department and nursing unit administration.

## NURSING UNIT ADMINISTRATION

Some hospitals have a division of nursing unit administration that is responsible for nonclinical patient care functions. **Nursing unit administration** is made up of two categories of workers: the health unit coordinator and the health unit manager. We have already discussed the role of the health unit coordinator; however, in nursing unit administration the health unit coordinator is usually supervised by the health unit manager rather than by the nurse manager. The health unit coordinator continues to work very closely with the nursing unit team.

The health unit manager performs supervisory and administrative nonclinical functions, such as budgeting, research, and training new employees, for several nursing units. As mentioned in Chapter 1, health unit management is the second step of the career path for health unit coordinators.

Health unit managers may also be registered nurses or hold degrees in other disciplines. Unit management usually functions under administration (Chapter 3) rather than under the nursing service department. See Figure 2–3 for an organizational chart that includes nursing unit administration.

### HIGHLIGHT

Under restructuring, nursing units have become self-contained, providing a continuum of care and service consistency to patients. Each unit consists of a "team" of health care providers that vary depending on unit specialties. In addition to nursing personnel, unit teams may include a respiratory therapist, a physical therapist, a pharmacist, and a patient admitting associate.

## SUMMARY

Health care delivery is currently undergoing rapid change to keep up with the demands of the marketplace. In fact, by the time this text is published some of this information may be obsolete. It will be your responsibility to keep up and to adapt to the change as it occurs in your place of employment. Currently, many levels of nursing service personnel work together to care for a given number of clients. Although the health unit coordinator does not give direct patient care, his or her performance greatly influences the quality of care delivered by other nursing team members.

**REVIEW QUESTIONS**

1. List three nursing personnel who function under the direction of the nurse manager and briefly describe what each one does.

   a. _shift Manager = manages the nursing unit in the absence of the nurse manager on the day evening + night shifts_

   b. _Registered Nurse - give direct patient care or supervise care given by others perform complex procedures maintain acurate records and teach team members_

   c. _CNA perform bedside tasks, such as bathing an feeding patients basic treatments such as taking vital signs and giving enemas_

2. List 14 different types of services that a nursing unit may provide for the clients

   a. _Cardiovascular_          h. _Pediatrics_

   b. _orthepedic_              i. _Rehabilitation_

   c. _oncology_               j. _step down unit_

   d. _obstetrics_             k. _Medical_

   e. _Neurology_              l. _Surgical_

   f. _Gynecology_             m. _telemetry_

   g. _Behavioral Health_      n. _Urology_

3. Describe the function of nursing unit administration. Briefly describe the duties performed by the health unit manager.

   _the division of nursing unit administration that is responsible for nonclinical patient care function The Health Unit manager supervises the Health Unit coordinator, does budgeting, research, training for new employees for several nursing units, may be an RN_

4. You are working on a nursing unit that uses the total patient care method of assignment. You take a telephone message for a patient to go to the physical therapy department. You should communicate the message to _the nurse assigned to take care of the Pt._

5. You are working on a regular nursing unit that uses the team method of assignment. You are transcribing a doctor's order that states that the client is to be transferred to an intensive care unit. You should communicate this order to _the nursing team Leader (RN)_.

6. Write the meaning of each abbreviation in the following paragraph.

   The patient was brought to the ED _Emergency Dept_ for emergency treatment. He required surgery and went immediately to the OR _Operating Room_. Following the surgery he was sent to the PACU _PostAnesthesiaCareUnit_ until he recovered from the effects of anesthesia. Following PACU care he was admitted to the

ICU _Intensive Care Unit_, where he received concentrated nursing care. The

RN _Registered Nurse_ cared for him while he was in the ICU. As his condition

improved he was transferred to a Surg _Surgical_ nursing unit. Each

day the CNA _Certified Nursing Assistant_ gave him a bath, the LPN _Licensed Practical Nurse_

gave him medication, and the RN started his intravenous therapy and discussed his plans for

discharge. Although the patient was unaware of it, the CHUC _Certified Health Unit Coordinator_

transcribed the orders the doctor wrote for him, ordered his diet, maintained his chart, and

charted his vital signs.

7. Write the type of intensive care unit for each abbreviation:
   a. ICU _Intensive care_
   b. SICU _surgical_
   c. MICU _medical_
   d. CCU _Coronary_
   e. TICU _trauma_
   f. NICU _neonatal_
   g. PICU _pediatric_

8. Describe:
   a. Perioperative services _operating room — where surgury is performed Pre operative — area where clients are prepared for surgery and PACU — Care after surgery_
   b. Emergency department _Care of patient who need emergency treatment either admitted or discharged according to needs_
   c. Day surgery _surgery is performed on patients on an outpatient basis and does not require hospitalization_

9. Why does restructuring occur in health care facilities?
   a. _medical technology is evolving fast_
   b. _Americans are living longer_

## References

Blackburn, Elsa: *Health Unit Coordinator*. Englewood Cliffs, NJ, Prentice-Hall, Inc., 1991.

Wilson, Florence A. and Neuhauser, Duncan: *Health Services in the United States*, 2nd ed. Cambridge, MA, Ballinger Publishing Co., 1982.

Wobbe, Roberta Rambaud: Primary versus team nursing. *Supervisor Nurse*, March: 37, 1978.

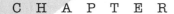

CHAPTER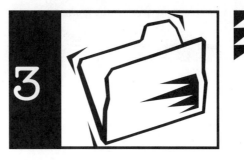

# THE HOSPITAL ENVIRONMENT

## CHAPTER OBJECTIVES

*Upon completion of this chapter, you will be able to:*

1. Define the terms in the vocabulary list.
2. List five functions a hospital may perform.
3. List three ways in which hospitals may be classified.
4. Identify the respective roles of an attending physician and a hospital resident.
5. Identify the title of physicians serving in a specialty.
6. Explain the difference between a doctor of medicine and a doctor of osteopathy.
7. Explain the function of the departments in finance, diagnostic and therapeutic services, additional services, and operational services.
8. Identify the various types of extended care facilities.
9. List the purpose of managed care.
10. Identify three staff models for health maintenance organizations.

## VOCABULARY

**Accreditation** • Recognition that a health care organization has met an official standard

**Attending Physician** • The term applied to a physician who admits and cares for a hospital patient

**Capitation** • A payment method whereby the providers of care receive a set dollar amount regardless of services rendered

**Chief Executive Officer** • The individual in direct charge of a hospital who is responsible to the governing board

**Governing Board** • A group of community citizens at the head of the hospital organizational structure

**Health Maintenance Organization** • An organization that has management responsibility for providing comprehensive health care services on a prepayment basis to voluntarily enrolled persons within a designated population

**Managed Care** • The provision of health care services efficiently to a designated group of members by managing patient access to and across a spectrum of health care settings

**Resident** • A graduate of a medical school who is gaining experience in a hospital

## ABBREVIATIONS

These abbreviations are listed as they are commonly written; however, you may also see some in cap and lower case letters and with or without periods.

| Abbreviation | Meaning |
| --- | --- |
| CEO | chief executive officer |
| COO | chief operating officer |
| DO | doctor of osteopathy |
| DRG | diagnosis-related group |
| ECF | extended care facility |
| HMO | health maintenance organization |
| HO | house officer |
| ICD | International Classification of Diseases |
| IPA | Individual Practice Association |
| JCAHO | Joint Commission on the Accreditation of Healthcare Organizations |
| LTC | long-term care |
| MD | doctor of medicine |
| SNF | Skilled Nursing Facility |

## EXERCISE 1

Write the abbreviation for each term listed below.

1. International Classification of Diseases — *ICD*
2. diagnosis-related group — *DRG*
3. house officer — *HO*
4. chief executive officer — *CEO*
5. doctor of medicine — *MD*
6. health maintenance organization — *HMO*
7. Joint Commission on the Accreditation of Healthcare Organizations — *JCAHO*
8. chief operating officer — *COO*
9. extended care facilities — *ECF*
10. doctor of osteopathy — *DO*
11. individual practice association — *IPA*
12. skilled nursing facility — *SNF*

## EXERCISE 2

Write the meaning of each abbreviation listed below.

1. HO — *house officer*
2. HMO — *health maintenance organization*
3. CEO — *chief executive officer*
4. MD — *Doctor of Medicine*
5. ECF — *Extended Care facility*
6. COO — *Chief operating officer*
7. ICD — *International Classification of Diseases*
8. DO — *Doctor of osteopathy*
9. DRG — *diagnosis-related group*
10. JCAHO — *Joint Commission on the Accreditation of Healthcare*
11. IPA — *Individual Practice Association*
12. SNF — *skilled Nursing facility*

## HISTORY OF HOSPITALS

The history of early Egyptian and Indian civilizations records that crude hospitals were in existence six centuries before Christ. The early Greeks and Romans used their temples to the gods as refuges for the sick.

With the advent of Christianity and the Crusades, *hospitea* were established for pilgrims to rest from their travels. The word *hospital* comes to us originally from the Latin noun *hospes*, which means "guest" or "host." The term *hospice*, which relates to family-centered care for the terminally ill, is also derived from *hospes*.

As Christianity progressed, the care of the sick, although remaining an important part of the work of the church, was moved out of the temples into separate buildings. During the twelfth and thirteenth centuries, there was great hospital growth in England and France. Members of religious orders cared for the needs of the ill. An organizational structure similar to that of the modern hospital began to emerge.

The earliest hospital in what is now the United States served sick soldiers on Manhattan Island in 1663. However, the first established hospitals were founded in Philadelphia in the early eighteenth century.

The development of hospitals continued worldwide as more inventions and discoveries were brought to light. The middle nineteenth and early twentieth centuries were important to hospital growth because during this period the foundations were laid for modern biology, and books on the subject began to be written. The early twentieth century also saw substantial advances in the education of nurses and doctors, and an increase in the number of people being trained for these professions.

And so it has been all through the ages that as people have progressed, they have developed a growing interest in the welfare of their fellow human beings. The hospital of today continues to serve those in need during illness or injury with modern technologies, improved medical knowledge, and compassion.

# HOSPITAL FUNCTIONS

The primary function of the hospital is the care and treatment of the sick. This is true of all hospitals regardless of size. Other functions are the education of physicians and other health care personnel, research, and prevention of disease. Especially in smaller communities, the hospital also serves as a local health center.

Only large hospitals may find it possible to perform all five functions. The functions the hospital performs depend upon many factors, among which are the hospital's location, the population it serves, and the size of the facility.

The care and treatment of the sick or injured necessitate proper accommodations for the patient, with adequate medical and nursing care. Services performed take into account the patient's comfort and safety. The care and treatment of each patient call for a team effort. Each department involved with the patient plays an important role in assisting the patient to return to a better state of health.

Some hospitals maintain schools in various health services, such as radiology, clinical laboratory, and respiratory care, to name a few. Other hospitals provide practical experience for students enrolled in university or community college educational programs in all levels of nursing, diet therapy, hospital administration, health unit coordinating, and other hospital-related fields. A hospital may have a residency program for doctors, and it may also provide additional experiences for medical students.

The type of research carried on in hospitals may depend upon specific services rendered by the hospital. A hospital specializing in the care of cancer patients would do research in cancer, whereas a hospital that specializes in the care of patients with skeletal deformities would perform research in that area.

The trend today is toward the prevention of disease. The hospital may serve as a community health center, providing low-cost or free clinics for detection of symptoms of beginning disease conditions and for immunization programs. Doctors and other health care personnel also provide counseling and instruction in health care.

# HOSPITAL CLASSIFICATIONS

There are many ways of classifying hospitals. The three most common classifications are (1) the type of patient service offered, (2) the ownership of the hospital, and (3) the type of accreditation the hospital has been given.

By "type of service offered" we are referring to the distinction between general hospitals and specialized hospitals. General hospitals—the most common type—render various services for many disease conditions and injuries. Not all general hospitals in a community offer identical services, since it would prove too costly. Specialized hospitals provide services to a particular body part (e.g., an eye hospital), a particular segment of the population (such as a children's hospital), or for a particular type of care (such as a psychiatric or rehabilitation hospital).

The ownership of the hospital is the second type of classification. We know that the federal government maintains hospitals for veterans as well as hospitals for personnel in the Navy and Air Force. The government also provides health services in hospitals for Native Americans. States, counties, and cities are also owners of hospitals. Churches and fraternal organizations may own and control general or specialized hospitals, which are usually nonprofit agencies. Proprietary hospitals operated for profit and owned by a group of individuals or corporations are also in operation.

The hospital of today is often part of a **health care system**. The health care system usually has a "parent" corporation that oversees the other companies within the system. The hospital is one of the subsidiary companies. Subsidiaries are designated either as profit or nonprofit. Each has its own board of directors. Other companies in the system, aside from the hospital, could be a company providing durable medical equipment, another providing home care to the community, another to operate parking facilities or linen services, and so forth. Most health care systems have a component called a **foundation**, whose purpose is to focus on donations and fund-raising activities that benefit the entire system

The third type of hospital classification—by accreditation—refers to recognition that a hospital has met an official standard. For example, a JCAHO-accredited hospital means that the hospital has been surveyed, graded, and approved by the Joint Commission on the Accreditation of Healthcare Organizations. Participation in JCAHO accreditation is voluntary. Several other accrediting agencies also conduct surveys, according to the services provided by the hospital.

The hospital's license to operate is usually granted by the department of health services of the individual state.

# HOSPITAL ORGANIZATION

## Administrative Personnel

The governing board is at the top of the organizational structure of a hospital. The governing board may also be referred to as the *board of trustees* or the *board of directors*. Three of the main responsibilities of the board include establishing policy, providing adequate financing, and overseeing personnel standards. The board is composed of persons from the business and professional communities as well as concerned citizens from all socioeconomic groups. The number of hospital board members varies with the size of the hospital. In hospitals that are part of a health care system, the hospital's governing board is responsible to the board of the parent corporation of the system.

In direct charge of the hospital, responsible to the governing board, is the **chief executive officer (CEO)**. He or she plans for the implementation of policies set forth by

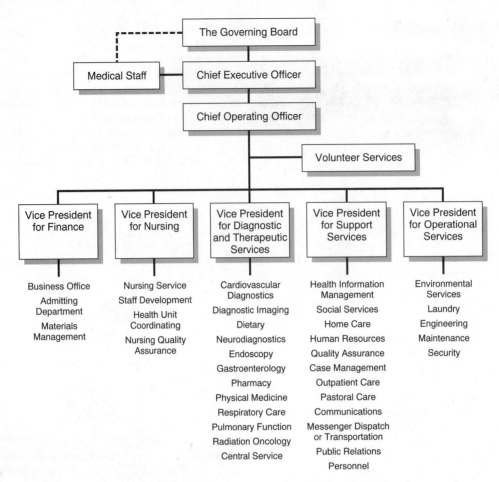

F I G U R E  3–1 • An example of a typical hospital organizational structure.

the governing board. The **chief operating officer (COO)** is responsible for the day-to-day operations of the hospital and reports directly to the CEO. Each service within the hospital is supervised by a vice president or a director. Vice presidents report to the hospital COO (Fig. 3–1).

The board delegates the supervision of the quality of patient care and the conduct of the physicians practicing in the hospital to a committee representative of the medical staff.

## The Medical Staff

Since the health unit coordinator transcribes doctors' orders and acts as the receptionist for the nursing unit, he or she has a great deal of interaction with the medical staff. Therefore, it is helpful for you to know the different roles of the doctors in a hospital.

The hospital governing board has a duty to the community to exercise care in the selection of doctors appointed to the medical staff. A doctor who has submitted his or her credentials to the state medical board and has a license to practice in the state may submit an application for appointment to the staff of a hospital or hospitals.

The physician who has been appointed to the medical staff and sends patients to the hospital for admission is known as the patient's **attending physician**. The attending physician prescribes the care and treatment (doctor's orders) for his or her patients during their hospital stay. A doctor caring for hospital patients may be a doctor of medicine (MD) or a doctor of osteopathy (DO). Identical approved programs of study are pursued by both, but colleges of osteopathic medicine place special emphasis on the relationship of organs and the musculoskeletal system. Structural problems are corrected by manipulation. Attending physicians are not hospital employees and receive no salary from the hospital. However, there may be doctors on the staff (such as the director of medical education, the hospital pathologist, or the director of radiation oncology) who are salaried hospital employees.

Large hospitals may have an educational program for medical school graduates to apply their knowledge in the practice of medicine. The term *intern* is rarely used in reference to the medical school graduate. The term *resident* is applied to all medical school graduates gaining hospital experience. These graduates are frequently referred to as **postgraduate year 1 (PGY-1)** or **first-year resident**. Residents may be referred to as **house staff** or **house officers (HO)**.

Physicians who specialize in a particular aspect of medicine, such as pediatrics, internal medicine, or general surgery, spend 3 to 5 years in a specific residency program. After completing the residency and passing a specific exam, the physician is said to be *board certified*. Often after residency there is a 1- to 2-year fellowship period to gain more familiarity in a specific area, such as cardiology. These practitioners are referred to as **fellows**. Some attending physicians serve as teachers for the hospital residents.

The undergraduate medical student may also be present in the hospital. He or she serves a **clinical clerkship** that allows for limited participation in the hospital's function, such as by performing admission physical examinations and writing the patient's medical history. It is common for these clinical clerks to be designated as **junior clerk** (third year) or **senior clerk** (fourth year).

Many physicians have chosen to practice in special fields and are known by their specialties. It is common to refer to a doctor by his or her specialty, as in the terms *cardiologist, gynecologist,* or *pediatrician.*

In the course of your work at the hospital, you may be required to use medical specialty terms when referring to doctors. The following lists present-day medical specialists.

## HOSPITAL DEPARTMENTS AND SERVICES

As a coordinator for the nursing unit you interact daily with many hospital departments either during the transcription of doctor's orders or when requesting services provided by the department. Therefore, it is important for you to have an overall view of the departments and their functions as they relate to your role as the health unit coordinator.

Below are listed the hospital departments and a brief description of their services. The services are divided into business services, diagnostic and therapeutic services, support services, and operational services.

It is important to remember that not all hospitals have all the departments listed here, nor may the department in your hospital use the same name as we use in this text.

## Business Services

**Business services** deal with the financial aspect of the hospital. The health unit coordinator works closely with the admitting department during the patient's admission to, transfer within, and discharge from the hospital. The health unit coordinator also orders all the unit supplies from the purchasing department.

The **business office** is in charge of patient accounts, budget planning, employee payroll, and payment of bills incurred by the hospital. This office determines the ability of the patient to pay through hospitalization insurance and Medicare or Medicaid. The business office also provides a place for safekeeping of patient valuables. In the area of budget planning, each department and nursing unit is issued a cost-control-center number. For example, the dietary department may be given number 4622. All purchases, maintenance fees, and other expenses must have the cost-control-center number on the request for record-keeping purposes.

The **admitting department**, sometimes called *patient services*, admits new patients to the hospital, transfers patients within the hospital, and discharges patients from the hospital. Upon admission, the admitting department obtains pertinent information from patients or their relatives, witnesses the signing of the admission agreement (see Chapter 19, p. 349) by the patient or his or her representative, and prepares the identification bracelet and imprinter card.

The materials management, or **purchasing department**, is responsible for obtaining all supplies and equipment to be used by hospital departments. Sometimes small hospitals band together to have greater purchasing power and save one another money.

## Diagnostic and Therapeutic Services

The following departments relate to the direct care of the hospitalized patient. During the transcription procedures, the health unit coordinator orders tests, treatments, or supplies from these departments, according to the doctors' orders. The specifics of this process are discussed in the chapters in Section III.

The **cardiovascular diagnostics department** performs tests related to cardiac (heart) and blood vessel function. The diagnostic procedure ordered most frequently is the **electrocardiogram**, which is performed at the patient's bedside. Cardiac catheterization is carried out in the department.

The **central service department** is the distribution area for supplies and equipment used by nursing personnel to perform treatments on patients. Enema kits, dressing trays, bandages, and other supplies used most frequently by the nursing unit personnel may be kept on the nursing unit. Central service department technicians replenish the unit supply daily. Packs of supplies used by the operating and delivery rooms may be processed and sterilized by the central service department personnel.

The **diagnostic imaging department** includes the radiology, nuclear medicine, and ultrasound departments. Diagnostic studies are performed by using x-ray, ultrasound, computed tomography (CT), magnetic resonance imaging (MRI), and radioactive element scanners. A **radiologist**, qualified in the use of x-ray and other imaging devices, is in charge of this department. The **radiographer**, a graduate of a 2- or 4-year educational program, performs many of the technical procedures.

The **dietary department**, which is under the direction of a registered dietitian who is a graduate of a 4-year college program, plans and prepares meals for patients, employees, and visitors. Personnel within the department deliver meals and nourishment to the nursing care units. The

## MEDICAL SPECIALTIES

| Physician's Specialty | Specialty Description |
| --- | --- |
| Allergist | Treats patients who have hypersensitivity to pollens, foods, medications, and other substances |
| Anesthesiologist | Administers drugs or gases to produce loss of consciousness or sensation in the patient; care during surgery and recovery from anesthetic is included |
| Cardiologist | Diagnoses and treats diseases of the heart and blood vessels |
| Dermatologist | Diagnoses and treats disorders of the skin |
| Emergency room physician | Diagnoses and treats patients in trauma and emergency situations |
| Endocrinologist | Diagnoses and treats diseases of the internal glands that secrete hormones |
| Family practitioner | Specializes in primary health care for all family members |
| Gastroenterologist | Diagnoses and treats diseases of the digestive tract |
| Geriatrist | Diagnoses and treats diseases and problems of aging |
| Gynecologist | Diagnoses and treats disorders and diseases of the female reproductive tract |
| Internist | Diagnoses and treats medically diseases and disorders of the internal organs of adults |
| Neonatologist | Diagnoses and treats disorders of the newborn |
| Neurologist | Diagnoses and treats diseases of the nervous system |
| Obstetrician | Cares for women during pregnancy, labor, delivery, and following delivery |
| Oncologist | Diagnoses and treats cancerous conditions |
| Ophthalmologist | Diagnoses and treats diseases and defects of the eye |
| Orthopedist | Diagnoses and treats diseases or fractures of the musculoskeletal system |
| Otolaryngologist | Diagnoses and treats diseases of the ear, nose, and throat |
| Pathologist | Studies cell changes and other alterations of the body caused by disease |
| Pediatrician | Provides preventive care and diagnoses and treats diseases of children |
| Physiatrist | Diagnoses and treats diseases of the neuromusculoskeletal system with physical elements to restore the individual to participation in society |
| Proctologist | Diagnoses and treats diseases of the rectum and anus |
| Psychiatrist | Diagnoses and treats mental illness |
| Radiation oncologist | Treats cancer through the use of radiation |
| Radiologist | Diagnoses and also treats some diseases by using various methods of imaging such as x-ray, ultrasound, radioactive materials, and magnetic resonance |
| Surgeon | Treats diseases and injuries by operative methods; may specialize in a particular area, such as heart, eye, or pediatric surgery |
| Urologist | Diagnoses and treats diseases of the male and female urinary tracts and of the male reproductive system |

dietitian also instructs patients in proper nutrition and in the use of special diets when they are ordered by the doctor. Some hospitals participate in an internship program for college students enrolled in a hospital dietitian curriculum.

The **neurodiagnostics department** performs diagnostic studies of the brain. One study, **electroencephalography**, records the electric impulses of brain waves. An **electroencephalography technician** performs the test. A physician, usually a **neurologist**, interprets the brain wave tracings.

The **endoscopy department** performs diagnostic procedures by using endoscopes. These instruments permit the visual examination of a body cavity or hollow organ, such as the stomach. The studies may be performed by a specialist employed by the hospital or by the patient's attending physician. Registered nurses or licensed practical nurses usually assist the doctors with these procedures.

The **gastroenterology department**, or **GI lab**, performs studies to diagnose disease conditions of the digestive system. Tests are related to problems of the esophagus, stomach, pancreas, gallbladder, and small intestine. A **gastroenterologist**, a doctor with additional education related to disease of the gastrointestinal system, is in charge of the department. A laboratory technologist or registered nurse may assist with these procedures.

The **pathology department**, or **clinical laboratory**, is concerned with diagnostic procedures performed on specimens from the body, such as blood, tissues, urine, stools, sputum, and bone marrow. This department may be separated into several divisions named for the tests or substances to be examined, such as hematology, urinalysis, microbiology, chemistry, and blood bank. Specimens removed during surgery are also examined by the pathologist. Autopsies are performed under the direction of this department. The laboratory functions under the direction

## HOSPITAL DEPARTMENTS

| Department | Service |
|---|---|
| *Business*: | |
| Business office | Patient accounts |
| Admitting | Admission of new patients |
| Purchasing | Obtains supplies and equipment |
| Central services | Storage and distribution of supplies and equipment used for client care |
| | |
| *Diagnostic and therapeutic*: | |
| Cardiovascular diagnostics | Tests related to heart and blood vessels |
| Diagnostic imaging | X-rays, nuclear medicine, and ultrasound studies |
| Dietary | Meals |
| Neurodiagnostics | Studies of the brain |
| Endoscopy | Diagnostic procedures using endoscopes |
| Gastroenterology | Studies related to the digestive system |
| Clinical laboratory | Diagnostic procedures on specimens from the body |
| Pharmacy | Medications |
| Physical medicine | Rehabilitation |
| Respiratory therapy | Treatment related to respiratory function |
| Pulmonary function | Tests to determine lung function |
| | |
| *Diagnostic and therapeutic*: | |
| Radiation oncology | Treatment of cancer growths |
| | |
| *Support services*: | |
| Health information management | Patient records |
| Quality assurance | Quality care |
| Social service | Assistance to patients and families |
| Home care or discharge planning | Transition from hospital to home |
| Outpatient | Services to patients outside the hospital |
| Pastoral care | Spiritual support |
| Patient advocate | Available to patients who have concerns about their care or environment |
| | |
| Communications | Switchboard |
| Transportation | Delivery |
| Public relations | Provides information to the public |
| Volunteer services | A variety of services provided by volunteers |
| | |
| *Operational services*: | |
| Environmental | Housekeeping duties |
| Mechanical | Keeps equipment in working condition |
| Laundry | Maintains linens |
| Human resources | Recruitment, records, and benefits |
| Security | Protection |

of a **pathologist** and employs medical technologists and medical laboratory technicians who have graduated from a recognized school for laboratory personnel.

The **pharmacy** provides the medications used by the patient within the hospital or in the clinics. The pharmacist fills the prescription ordered by the doctor. The pharmacy may also provide lotions and mouthwashes for patient

use. Intravenous solutions to which medications have been added are also prepared in the pharmacy under sterile conditions. A **registered pharmacist** is in charge of the pharmacy.

The **physical medicine department** is composed of several smaller departments related to the rehabilitation of the patient. The physical medicine department is under the direction of a **physiatrist**. **Physical therapy** and **occupational therapy** are the two most common therapeutic areas within the physical medicine department. Small hospitals may have only a physical therapy department. The physical therapy department provides treatment by the use of exercise, massage, heat, light, water, and other methods. **Registered physical therapists** (graduates of a 4-year college program) and **physical therapy technicians** (graduates of a 2-year community college program) carry out the prescribed evaluations and treatments.

The occupational therapy department provides patients with purposeful activities that are designed to evaluate and treat those who are impaired physically, mentally, and developmentally. These activities help prevent deformities, restore function to affected body parts, and preserve morale. **Registered occupational therapists**, graduates of a 4-year college program, are employed in the occupational therapy department.

The **respiratory care department** provides treatment related to respiratory function and assists in maintaining patients on ventilators (breathing machines). The department also administers respiratory physical therapy. The **respiratory care therapist** and the **respiratory care technician**, graduates of 1- to 4-year educational programs, are employed here.

The **pulmonary function department** performs diagnostic tests to determine lung function. **Pulmonary function technicians** or **respiratory care therapists** may perform the tests. In small hospitals, pulmonary function tests may be performed by the respiratory care department.

The **radiation oncology**, or **radiation therapy**, **department** may be a division within the diagnostic imaging department or a separate department. Its primary purpose is to treat cancerous growths. Cobalt beam units and linear accelerators are examples of equipment used in these departments. The **radiation oncologist**, a physician with additional education in the use of radiation for the treatment of disease, is the head of the radiation oncology department.

## Support Services

The following departments are also very important in the concept of caring for all patients' needs. The health unit coordinator interacts with most of the following departments by requesting services for the patients on the nursing unit.

The **health information management department**, also called **health records department**, cares for the patient's record after the patients are discharged from the hospital. Records are stored here and may be retrieved for the doctor if the patient is readmitted. The records may also be used for research. This department is also responsible for coding medical and surgical conditions of patients upon discharge. This coding is related to the system of Medicare reimbursement, involving diagnosis-related groups (DRG), whereby payment is based on the type of illness. Accurate coding of the patient's diagnosis using the International Classification of Disease (ICD) system is a critical function within the department. If coding is not exact, the direct result can be financial loss for the hospital. Medical transcription (not related to transcription as used in the transcription of a doctor's orders) is another service of the health records department that is available to doctors for the dictation of patient's histories, physical examination findings, and so forth. The transcriptionist then prepares typewritten reports from the dictated tapes. The reports are placed on the hospitalized patients' chart.

The **quality assurance department** provides information to various departments within the hospital for the purpose of assisting those departments to provide quality care. Through analysis of actual occurrences and practices against standards set by various departments, quality assurance continuously uses ongoing activities to suggest improvements. Individual departments, such as nursing, may have their own quality assurance component, which coordinates with the hospital-wide quality assurance department. **Risk management** can also be part of the quality assurance manager's responsibilities.

The **social service department** provides services to patients and to their families when emotional and environmental difficulties impede the patient's recovery. The **social worker's** knowledge of the community and of the agencies providing a variety of services aids in lifting emotional and financial burdens caused by the illness. Nursing home and extended care facility placement can also be arranged by this department. The department head holds an advanced degree in social work.

The **home care department** assists patients in preparing for the transition from the hospital to the home. A registered nurse with a public health background usually heads the department. The needs of the patient returning to the home environment are identified. Plans for care by the visiting nurse service (VNS) and rental of needed equipment may be arranged before the patient is discharged. Follow-up studies are also provided for the doctor.

The **outpatient department** or **clinic** provides services to patients outside the hospital. Clinics for various disease conditions, such as diabetes, allergies, and gynecologic problems, may be open weekly. Prenatal care and dental care may also be offered. Visits are usually by appointment. The outpatient area also provides clinical experiences for resident doctors.

The **pastoral care department** provides spiritual support to the patient and family in time of need. There are hospitals that maintain a chaplaincy program for members of the clergy interested in becoming hospital chaplains.

The **communications department** may be called the telephone switchboard in many hospitals. The telephone operators process incoming and outgoing telephone calls and operate the doctor paging system. In emergencies, such as a fire, disaster, or cardiac arrest, communications personnel alert the hospital personnel in code, such as Code 1000 to announce a fire in the hospital. In some hospitals the telephone operator may also serve as an information station for visitors to the hospital.

The **messenger**, **dispatch**, or **transportation department** performs multiple tasks throughout the hospital. Delivery of interdepartmental mail, carrying of specimens to the laboratory, assisting with the discharge or admission of patients, and transporting of patients from one area of the hospital to another are all carried out by personnel of this department.

The **patient advocate** is an individual available for the patient to call from their room if they have a concern or complaint which they feel has not been addressed. The patient may be notified of this resource person on admission to the hospital.

The **public relations department** serves to provide the public with information concerning the hospital's activities. This may be accomplished by means of the community newspaper. Many hospitals publish a weekly, bimonthly, or monthly newspaper for patients and/or employees.

The **volunteer services department** is made up of people from the community. The members of the women's auxiliary or its counterpart, the men's auxiliary, give generously of their time and talents to staff the patient library or gift shop. Many perform tasks for the various hospital departments or on the nursing unit. High school students may also have an auxiliary organization.

## Operational Services

The following services are not related to the direct care of the hospitalized patient but are concerned with the patient's hospital environment. It is the health unit coordinator's task to request services from these departments as needed by the nursing unit.

The main responsibility of **environmental services**, sometimes called the housekeeping department, is to maintain a clean hospital through proper cleaning methods aimed at preventing the spread of infection. Daily cleaning of the hospital is provided by environmental services. Upon the discharge of a patient from the hospital, environmental services is responsible for cleaning the individual patient unit and preparing it for a new admission. Another duty that this department may perform is the changing of draperies and the cubicle curtains around the patient's bed. In some hospitals, environmental services is responsible for the delivery of isolation equipment to the unit. Often it is also charged with the disposition and/or repairing of linen.

The **mechanical services department** of the hospital is responsible for keeping all equipment in working condition. In a large hospital, this department may be divided into various branches, such as engineering, maintenance, and electronic equipment repair. The **engineering division** is concerned with heating, lighting, air conditioning, power systems, water, and sewage. The **maintenance division** is responsible for keeping the hospital and its surroundings, equipment, and furnishings in tip-top condition. Services rendered include painting, maintenance of TVs, carpentry, and pneumatic tube systems repairs. Gardeners and grounds keepers are also members of this department. **Electronic equipment repair** personnel keep operational all equipment that is operated electronically,

such as the machines used to monitor the patient's heart in the coronary care unit.

The **laundry** maintains the linen supply for the hospital. The washing, drying, and storing of linen are the main responsibilities of this department. Laundry personnel may also deliver the linen to the nursing care units. Small hospitals may rent the linen from a commercial laundry service. Other hospitals may join together in ownership of a laundry service, which more economically serves the needs of all.

The **human resources department** organizes recruitment programs, interviews new employees, conducts employee termination interviews, and maintains records for each employee. Employee benefits and retirement records are also the responsibility of the human resource department.

An **employee fitness center** is available in many hospitals to assist employees with their own health maintenance. Some hospitals may have counseling services available to employees to assist them to cope with personal and employment problems.

The **security department** is responsible for protecting the hospital, patients, visitors, and employees. Thefts and disturbances on the premises should be reported to this department.

## OTHER HEALTH CARE DELIVERY SYSTEMS

Health care services are often provided in nonhospital settings. This is particularly true for long-term care. **Extended care facilities (ECF)** provide care for patients who are not acutely ill and cannot be cared for at home. These facilities can provide either skilled or intermediate levels of care. The following facilities are providers of long-term care and provide employment opportunities for health unit coordinators. **Nursing homes** are licensed by the state and may be classified by ownership and accreditation. Nursing homes provide care for those who are so sick or functionally disabled that they require ongoing nursing and support services provided in a formal health care institution. They are generally classified as custodial care; however, another level of nursing home is the **skilled nursing facility (SNF)**, which provides care for those too sick to go home or to a nursing home but who are not so acutely ill that they require the technological and professional intensity of a hospital. Many hospitals also operate an SNF.

**Physical medicine** and **rehabilitation facilities** may also be classified as extended care facilities, although such care may be given not only in an inpatient setting but to outpatients as well. Individuals receiving care in such facilities primarily require special support services in addition to varying levels of nursing care.

Long-term care may also be provided in the home through a **home health agency** such as a Visiting Nurse Association, subdivision of a local state or welfare department, or a department of a local hospital or other health care facility. These agencies provide such services as skilled nursing, rehabilitation (for such problems as speech or language pathology, or for physical or occupational therapy), pharmacy, and medical social work. **Hospice** is another form of care sometimes classified as long-term. It provides palliative and supportive care for terminally ill patients and their families. Emphasis is placed on the control of symptoms and preparation for and support before and after death. The hospice can be free-standing, hospital-based, or home-based. A hospice is really not a type of facility but a new concept of providing health care services where necessary.

Another development in contemporary health care is the emergence of **managed care**. The JCAHO defines managed care as "the provision of health care services efficiently to a designated group of members by managing patient access to and across a spectrum of health care settings." **Managed care systems** are most often associated with **health maintenance organizations (HMOs)**, an organization that has management responsibility for providing comprehensive health care services on a prepayment basis to voluntarily enrolled persons within a designated population. The purpose of managed care (HMOs) is to provide comprehensive services, including preventive measures aimed at retaining good health. In theory, they want to keep people healthier so that the cost of health care is reduced. There are several models of HMOs and each is unique in the way it contracts for the services of physicians.

**Staff model HMO:** A multispecialty group of physicians practicing at a facility that is an HMO and whose physicians are salaried employees

**Group model HMO:** Similar to the staff model, but there is no specific facility called an HMO; physicians contract with the HMO to provide nearly all the services to members

**Individual practice association model (IPA):** The HMO contracts with an association of individual physicians to provide services for members in their private offices; because of their size, physicians are able to contract with large patient populations and still maintain independence (*Restrictions*: Except for emergencies, members must be referred by physicians in the HMO before receiving services outside the facility; failure to do so may result in the HMO not paying for the care)

The area of **case management** is becoming more prominent in today's health care environment. Case managers work in health care facilities to coordinate the patient's care with insurance companies. The case manager's role is to act as an advocate for the patient to most appropriately utilize the benefits and coverage of his or her health policy.

## PROVIDER REIMBURSEMENTS

There are many different ways Americans pay for health care. Some have **private/group-paid health** insurance plans. These plans are often provided through employers and require a copayment and deductible for both inpatient and outpatient care. Premiums are paid periodically through payroll deductions or direct to the insurance carrier. **Blue Cross/Blue Shield** is a nationwide federation of local, not-for-profit insurance organizations that contract with hospitals and other health care providers to pay for health care services provided to their subscribers. **Health maintenance organizations** are a form of health insurance in addition to being a method of delivering health care. **Capitation**, which is a payment method whereby the providers of care receive a set dollar amount (usually per enrollee per month), regardless of the number and type of services enrollees need, is the method most often used by HMOs. There are many types of government plans for reimbursement of health care costs; however, only two will be discussed here. **Medicare** is health insurance for persons over age 65 and has two parts. Part A is hospital insurance and is financed by the federal government after a deductible is paid by the elderly. Part B is primarily for coverage of outpatient care and is financed with premiums paid by the elderly and by federal revenues. **Medicaid** is a medical assistance program designed to meet the needs of low-income people. The program is funded partially by the federal government and partially by the states (and sometimes local governments).

## SUMMARY

You will find that hospitals differ in many aspects. The main variations are in classification, size, and services. The function of the hospital still focuses on the care and treatment of the sick and injured, but emphasis is shifting to the prevention of disease. Knowledge of the hospital, its personnel, and the services that it renders is needed by the health unit coordinator in order to carry out his or her assigned tasks.

**REVIEW QUESTIONS**

1. The primary function of the hospital is ___ _the care and treatment of the sick_

2. Four other functions of a hospital are:
   a. ___ _education of physicians & other health care personel_
   b. ___ _research_
   c. ___ _prevention of disease_
   d. ___ _Serves as a local health center_

3. The doctor who may admit and care for patients in the hospital is known as the patient's ___ _attending Physician_

4. A doctor who is a medical school graduate gaining experience in the hospital is called a ___ _First year resident_

5. An undergraduate medical student allowed limited hospital participation is serving a ___ _clinical clerkship_ ~~considered~~

6. Hospitals may be classified according to:
   a. ___ ~~Bussiness Services~~ _type of patient services offered_
   b. ___ ~~Ownership~~ _ship of the hospital_
   c. ___ ~~services~~ _type of accreditation the hospital has been given._

7. A. Matching
   Match the specialists listed in the left-hand column with their area of expertise by filling in the appropriate letter from the right-hand column. (*Note*: Left-hand column continues on p. 36.)

   | | | |
   |---|---|---|
   | **K** 1. Internist | a. | disorders of the newborn |
   | **N** 2. Cardiologist | b. | treatment of mental disorders |
   | **M** 3. Gynecologist | c. | diseases of ear, nose, and throat |
   | **i** 4. Dermatologist | d. | study of cell changes and other alterations of the body caused by disease |
   | **H** 5. Allergist | e. | treatment of disease by physical elements |
   | **A** 6. Neonatologist | f. | administration of drugs or gases that cause loss of feeling or sensation |
   | **L** 7. Pediatrician | g. | glandular diseases |
   | **b** 8. Psychiatrist | h. | hypersensitivity to foods, pollens, or medicines |
   | **f** 9. Anesthesiologist | i. | diseases of the skin |
   | **C** 10. Otolaryngologist | j. | problems and diseases of the aged |
   | **J** 11. Geriatrist | k. | disease of adults |
   | **g** 12. Endocrinologist | l. | diseases of children |
   | **D** 13. Pathologist | m. | diseases of the female reproductive tract |
   | | n. | heart diseases |

B. Matching
Match the specialists listed in the left-hand column with their area of expertise by filling in the appropriate letter from the right-hand column.

_I_ 1. Surgeon

_g_ 2. Urologist

_J_ 3. Orthopedist

_b_ 4. Neurologist

_L_ 5. Physiatrist

_A_ 6. Radiologist

_c_ 7. Oncologist

_K_ 8. Obstetrician

_f_ 9. Radiation oncologist

_H_ 10. Proctologist

_m_ 11. Ophthalmologist

_D_ 12. Emergency room physician

a. use of x-rays, ultrasound, and radioactive element scanners
b. diseases of the nervous system
c. diagnosis and treatment of cancerous conditions
d. treats trauma patients
e. glandular diseases
f. treatment of cancer by radiation
g. diseases of the male reproductive tract
h. diseases of the rectum
i. use of operative methods
j. diseases of the skeletal system
k. care of pregnant women
l. treatment of disease by use of physical elements
m. eye diseases

8. Name the department in charge of:
   a. patient accounts

   Business Office

   b. transfer, discharge, and admissions

   Admitting department

   c. performing blood, urine, and tissue studies

   Pathology or Clinical Laboratory

   d. diagnostic tests using computed tomography, ultrasound, radioactive element scanners, and radiant energy

   diagnostic Imaging

   e. treatment for cancerous growths

   Radiation Oncology or Radiation Therapy

   f. providing medications for patients

   pharmacy

   g. treatment by use of exercise, heat, and light

   Physical Medicine or Therapy

   h. evaluation, treatment, and preservation of morale by using purposeful activities

   occupational ~~employee fitness center~~ therapy

   i. treatment related to respiratory function

   Respiratory care

   j. food preparation and treatment using foods

   Dietary Dept

   k. diagnosis by use of instruments to view body cavities or hollow organs such as esophagus and bronchi

   ~~Gastro enterology~~ ~~GI lab~~ endoscopy

l.  diagnostic procedures for diseases of the GI tract

Gastro enterology a GI Lab

m. diagnostic studies of the heart

Cardiovascular diagnostics

n.  brain studies

neuro diagnostics

o.  the patient's record on discharge

Health Information management

p.  supplies and equipment for treatment of patients

Purchasing

q.  services to patients outside the hospital

Out patient

r.  providing service for financial and social problems

Social Service

s.  planning the transition from hospital to home

Home care

t.  maintaining a clean hospital

Environmental

u.  supplies and equipment for all hospital departments

~~distribution~~ central service

v.  spiritual services

pastoral care

w. keeping the hospital repaired

Mechanical Services

x.  maintaining the linen supply

Laundry

y.  telephone and paging services

Communications

z.  protecting patients, visitors, employees, and hospital

Security

9. Recognition that a hospital has met an official standard is called JCAHO Accredited

10. The name of the citizen group that is at the head of the hospital's organizational structure is the

Governing Board

11. The individual in direct charge of a hospital who is responsible to the governing board is the

Chief operating officer

12. A doctor of osteopathy differs from a doctor of medicine in that a doctor of osteopathy ____
has a specialty with emphasis on the relationship of organs and the musculoskeletal system

13. Place an X in the space before each extended care facility and an O in the space before each HMO staff model.

_X_ SNF

_O_ IPA

_X_ hospice

_O_ group

_X_ home health care

_X_ rehabilitation

14. Write the purpose of managed care.

*To provide comprehensive services including preventive measures aimed at retaining good health*

## References

Blackburn, Elsa: *Health Unit Coordinator*. Englewood Cliffs, NJ, Prentice-Hall, Inc., 1991.

Sloan, Robert M. and Sloan, Beverly LeBov: *A Guide to Health Facilities*, 2nd ed. St. Louis, The C. V. Mosby Co., 1977.

Urdang, Laurence (ed.): *Mosby's Medical and Nursing Dictionary*, St. Louis, The C. V. Mosby Co., 1983.

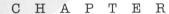

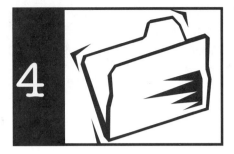

## CHAPTER 4

# COMMUNICATION DEVICES AND THEIR USES

## CHAPTER OBJECTIVES

*Upon completion of this chapter, you will be able to:*

1. Define the terms in the vocabulary list.
2. List six communication devices found in health care facilities and relate the uses of each.
3. List two uses of the telephone "hold" button.
4. List eight rules of telephone etiquette.
5. Describe briefly how to plan to place a telephone call regarding a patient.
6. List six items to be recorded when taking a telephone message and explain why it is important to record messages.
7. List two purposes of an intercom.
8. List two methods of paging within the health care facility and explain the purpose of the paging system.
9. Discuss the health unit coordinator's responsibility in the maintenance of the unit bulletin board.
10. Name two computer components usually located at the nurses' station and describe the function of each.
11. List three uses of the computer located on the nursing unit.
12. List four guidelines for using voice mail.

## VOCABULARY

**Computer** • An electronic machine capable of accepting, processing, and retrieving information

**Copy Machine** • A machine used for making copies of typed or written materials

**Cursor** • A flashing indicator that lets the computer user know the area on the viewing screen that will receive the information

**Doctors' Roster** • Alphabetical listing of names, telephone numbers, and directory telephone numbers of physicians on staff

**Downtime Requisition** • A requisition used to process information when the computer is not available for use

**Dumbwaiter** • A mechanical device for transporting food or supplies from one hospital floor to another

**Fax Machine** • A telecommunication device that transmits copies of written material over a telephone wire from one site to another

**Intercom** • A device used to communicate between the nurses' station and the patient's room on the nursing unit

**Keyboard** • A computer component used to type information into the computer

**Menu** • A list of options that is projected on the viewing screen of the computer

**Pneumatic Tube System** • A system in which air pressure transports tubes carrying supplies, requisitions, or messages from one hospital unit or department to another

*[handwritten margin note:]* # pages, including cover sheet — cover sheet — Who to — who From — Telephone of person send.

**Pocket Pager** • A small electronic device that when activated by dialing a series of telephone numbers delivers a message to the carrier of the pager

**Viewing Screen** • A computer component that displays information; it resembles a television, and it may also be called a monitor, a CRT (cathode-ray tube), or a VDT (video display terminal)

**Voice Paging System** • The system on which the hospital telephone operator delivers a message to a doctor or makes other announcements; the system reaches all hospital areas

## COMMUNICATION DEVICES

In health care facilities, the health care unit coordinator has an opportunity to use many devices to communicate. They will be discussed here so you will have a better understanding of how you will use these devices on the job.

### The Telephone

The telephone is probably the most used communications device at the nurses' station (Fig. 4–1). Because we are so familiar with using the telephone, often we fail to use it in a professional manner in the work place.

At present, we cannot see the person with whom we are conversing via the telephone. Until the time comes that we can see the caller, we must allow our voice to give the caller a word picture, one that is pleasant and eager to receive the call.

How do you feel when you dial a business telephone number and the phone rings many times before it is answered? Have you ever had someone answer the telephone and say, "Will you hold?" and not give you time to answer?

Using an unfriendly voice or being placed on hold by someone using an inconsiderate manner are two of the most common ways to irritate or anger the person who has placed the call. As a representative of the health care facility—one who wishes to foster good public relations—your telephone manners are extremely important.

### Receiving Telephone Calls

#### The Telephone Hold Button

Large hospital units may have many telephone lines. Therefore, it is possible that several phone calls may come into the unit at the same time. The "hold" button allows the health unit coordinator to take care of many calls simultaneously.

If, while you are conversing on one line, a call comes in on a second line, you should excuse yourself from the first caller in order to answer the second line. To do this, ask if you may place the first caller on hold. Refrain from asking the caller to "hold on." Say instead "Do you have time to hold?" or "May I put you on hold?" Having obtained the person's consent, depress the hold button. In the example shown in Figure 4–2, the hold button is on the far right of the bottom row. A blinking light reminds you that there is someone holding. Depress the button on the incoming call, which is indicated by a steady light. After answering the call on the second line, indicate that you have another call waiting and you wish the second caller to hold. Depress the hold button again. Return to the first caller by depressing the proper extension number.

The hold button is also used when you receive a call that requires you to leave the caller, even for a moment, either to locate another person or to obtain information. Never lay the receiver on the desk without using the hold button. Conversation taking place at the nurses' station,

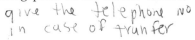
*give the telephone no in case of trunfer*

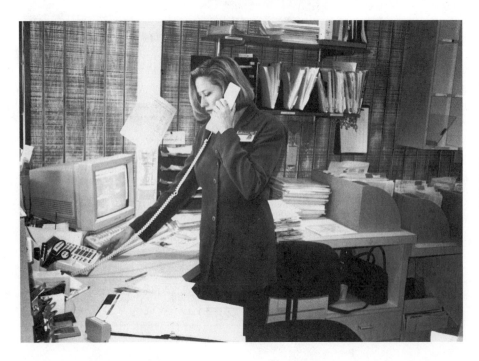

FIGURE 4–1 • The health unit coordinator handles the telephone communication for the nursing unit.

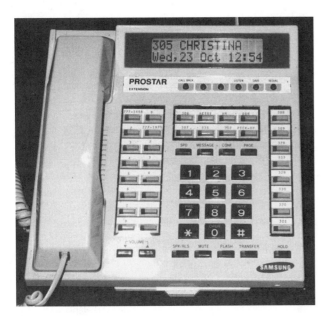

F I G U R E 4–2 • Telephone with several lines and a hold button.

which may be confidential in nature, will filter through to the caller. Use the procedure outlined above to place the caller on hold.

---

**HIGHLIGHT**

Refrain from asking a caller to "hold on" when placing them on hold. Say instead, "May I put you on hold?"

---

■ *Answer the phone promptly.* Answer the phone as quickly as possible—preferably after the second ring. If you are engaged in a conversation at the nurses' station, excuse yourself and answer the phone.

■ *Identify yourself properly.* State the name of the nursing unit, followed by your name and then your status. For example, "B-4, Miss Tracy, Health Unit Coordinator." By stating the unit number first, you assure the caller that he or she has reached the correct number. By identifying yourself and your status, you tell the caller to whom he or she is delivering the message. For example, a doctor calling the nursing unit on a technical matter may wish to speak only with a nurse.

■ *Speak into the telephone.* Do not cover the mouthpiece with your fingers because it may muffle your voice. Keep the mouthpiece uncovered and place your lips about 1¹/₂ inches from the phone receiver.

■ *Give the caller your undivided attention.* You cannot do several things at once and do them well.

■ *Speak distinctly and clearly.* Use a good voice level. Let the tone of your voice convey a smile (Fig. 4–3). Do not answer a phone when you have chewing gum or food in your mouth.

■ *Be courteous at all times.* Do not hesitate to say "please" and "thank you."

■ *When you cannot answer a question,* reply "I will get someone who can answer that question for you." Do not say, "I do not know."

■ *When a call is received for another person who is not close by, always place the caller on hold after getting their permission. When communicating a message concerning a call on hold,* include the name of the caller, the nature of the call, if possible, and which line the call is on. The message may be as follows: "Mr. Barry, Dr. Harrison is on line 1 regarding Mr. Mark's medication order." Do not leave the caller on hold for longer than a minute. Take a message and have the call returned.

F I G U R E 4–3 • Let the tone of your voice communicate with a smile.

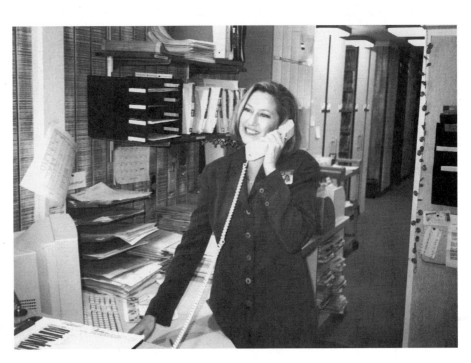

> **TO THE STUDENT**
>
> To practice answering the telephone and placing a caller on hold, complete **Activities 4–1** and **4–2** in the Skills Practice Manual.

> **TO THE STUDENT**
>
> To practice recording messages, complete **Activity 4–5** in the Skills Practice Manual.

## Taking Messages

When taking messages over the telephone or in person, be sure you get all the information needed for the person for whom the call is intended. You must record the following information:

1. Who the message is for
2. The caller's name
3. The date and time of the call
4. The purpose of the call
5. Is a return call expected? If so, the number to call
6. Your name

*[handwritten: repeat back message to clarify]*

Always write the information down. As a student or a newly employed health unit coordinator, gaining the trust and confidence of the nursing team members is important. Putting messages in writing may be the first important step in gaining the confidence of the unit personnel, besides guaranteeing accuracy during the communication process. Always have a pad and pencil or pen near each telephone. Deliver messages promptly. Many health care facilities have special telephone message pads (Fig. 4–4).

To_____

Date_____ Time_____

**WHILE YOU WERE OUT**

M_____

of_____

Phone_____

| Area Code | Number | Extension |
|---|---|---|

| | |
|---|---|
| TELEPHONED | PLEASE CALL |
| CALLED TO SEE YOU | WILL CALL AGAIN |
| WANTS TO SEE YOU | URGENT |
| RETURNED YOUR CALL | |

Message_____

_____

_____

_____

_____

Operator

F I G U R E  4–4 • A pad for telephone messages.

## Placing Telephone Calls

When you are asked to place a call to a doctor or to another department or outside of the health care facility, plan your call. If it concerns a patient, have the patient's chart handy so that you can look for the facts that you may be asked. Also write down the main facts you wish to discuss.

Anyone who asks you to place a call regarding a client should provide you with the patient's name and the reason for the call. You should also write down who requested the call to be made.

Before placing a call for a nurse to a doctor, you should alert the nurse that you are making the call and ask the nurse to stand by if possible to speak with the doctor.

## Voice Mail

Many health care facilities, physician's office, and homes use voice mail to receive incoming calls. Voice mail simply records the callers message. To use voice mail effectively, follow these guidelines.

### Guidelines for Voice Mail

After listening to the recorded greeting and indicated tone:

1. Speak slowly and distinctly so the person listening to the message can hear and understand what you are communicating.
2. If you are leaving a message, include the name of the client or the doctor, give the first and last name, and spell the last name.
3. If the message includes a telephone number or lab values, speak slowly and repeat the numbers twice, allowing time for the listener to record the information.
4. Always leave your name and telephone number, and repeat both twice, so the listener can call you for clarification if necessary.

## Telephone Directories

Many health care facilities publish a **directory of extension numbers** for telephones in the hospital. They are alphabetized and easy to use. Both department numbers and key personnel are listed.

Hospitals using the individual pocket pager may also publish a **directory of pocket pager numbers**.

The **doctors' roster** is another directory frequently used by the health unit coordinator. It contains in alphabetical order the names of the doctors who serve on the staff as attending physicians. It lists their medical specialty, their office telephone number, and the answering service telephone number. When placing a telephone call, select the doctor's number with care, since there are often several doctors listed with the same name. If two doctors have the same first and last names, refer to their specialty to select the correct telephone number.

TO THE STUDENT

To practice placing a telephone call, complete
**Activity 4–3** in the Skills Practice Manual.

**HIGHLIGHT**

Each time you use the telephone for communication,
you are creating an image of your nursing unit for
your customers. Realize this and handle each
telephone conversation with care.

■

## The Unit Intercom

The **intercom** system (Fig. 4–5) is a device used to communicate between the nurses' station and clients' rooms on a nursing unit. The intercom provides a method of taking patients' requests without going to the room. Upon admission, the patient should receive directions for the use of the intercom from a member of the nursing staff. The importance of this step is emphasized by the following story. A little boy admitted to a hospital room was not told about the intercom system. When the health unit coordinator noted that the child had his light on, she turned on the intercom and asked if he needed help. He replied, "Yes, wall."

A buzzer system or light alerts you that someone is signaling on the intercom. The light over the room number on the intercom console designates the caller's room. By pressing the appropriate key you may converse with the patient. Always identify yourself and your location. For example, you may say, "This is Miss Kimberly at the nurses' station, may I help you?" When there are two or more patients in the room, ask the patient to identify himself or herself.

The intercom is also used by the health unit coordinator to locate nursing personnel. To page personnel on the intercom, depress the key that allows for the message to be heard in each of the rooms. A simple message such as "Mr. Darwin to the nurses' station, please," is all that is needed.

The health unit coordinator should be selective in the information to be communicated over the intercom, since some types of messages may prove embarrassing to the patient. For example, do not use the intercom to ask a patient if he or she has had a bowel movement. Also, do not communicate any patient information to a nurse over the intercom, as other patients may hear the message.

## The Pocket Pager

The **pocket pager** may be either voice or digital. The voice **pager** (Fig. 4–6) is a small electronic device used to deliver messages to persons within the hospital. Voice pagers with a longer range may be used to reach persons many miles away from the hospital.

Each person who carries a voice pager is given a pager number, which is similar to the phone number but may have only four or six digits.

Suppose you wish to call Dr. Jordan, who carries a voice pager with the number 13-8049. To call Dr. Jordan, dial 13-8049 on the regular hospital telephone. At the end of a signal, usually a beep, state, "Dr. Jordan, call Bill, 4E, extension 5461." It is important to tell the person you are paging whom to call, where to call, and the extension number. It is extremely frustrating to be paged with a message to call the nursing unit and not be given the telephone extension number of the unit.

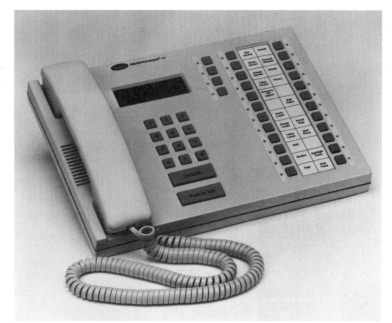

FIGURE 4–5 • A *Responder IV* intercom device. (Courtesy of Rauland-Borg Corporation.)

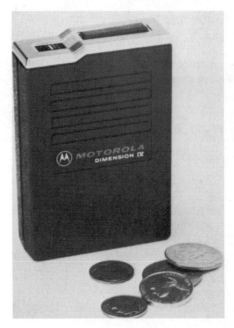

FIGURE 4–6 • A pocket pager. (Courtesy of Motorola Communications and Electronics, Inc.)

Dr. Jordan, who is carrying the voice pager, is alerted by a beeping sound. Your message follows. Dr. Jordan can then go to a telephone and dial the extension number you gave to respond to your call.

A **digital pager** is similar to a voice pager. To contact a person by digital pager, dial the pager number from a touch-tone phone. Listen for a ring followed by a series of beeps. Dial your telephone number followed by the pound sign (#). You hear a series of fast beeps, which indicates a completed page. The number appears on the pager display. The receiver then calls you back for the message.

Key hospital personnel who work in several different areas of the hospital and your instructor during your hospital practice may also carry pocket pagers.

---

### TO THE STUDENT

To practice contacting a person using a digital pager, complete **Activity 4–4** in the Skills Practice Manual.

---

## Copy Machine

Many nursing units have a **copy machine** available for making copies of written or typed communication to be distributed to employees.

## Voice Paging System

The **voice paging system** is another communication system in common use. To locate a doctor with this system, dial the hospital operator. Indicate the name of the doctor who is needed and give the telephone extension number on the unit. The telephone operator announces over this system, which reaches all hospital areas, the name of the doctor needed and the extension number to call.

The voice paging system is also used by the operator to locate a doctor for calls from outside the hospital. The health unit coordinator is frequently asked by doctors to listen for their page, especially when they are in a patient's room. When a page for a doctor is announced, the health unit coordinator may contact the operator for the message and deliver it to the doctor.

## The Pneumatic Tube

The **pneumatic tube** is a system in which air pressure transports tubes carrying supplies, requisitions, or messages from one hospital unit or department to another. These items are placed in a special carrying tube, which is then inserted into the pneumatic tube system. Medications that do not break or spill are transported in this manner. Admission papers and imprinter cards may also reach the unit via pneumatic tube. Do *not* place specimens in the pneumatic tube. When a tube carrying supplies or other items arrives at the nursing unit, it is the health unit coordinator's responsibility to remove the tube from the pneumatic tube system as soon as possible and disperse the items accordingly. You will be instructed in the operation of your hospital's pneumatic tube system during your hospital orientation.

## The Computer

**Computers** have been used in various hospital departments such as the business office for several years. In recent years there has been a trend toward using computers at the nurses' station; this practice allows for quick transmission, updating, and retrieval of information. As a health unit coordinator you will probably use the computer while transcribing doctors' orders and to request diagnostic studies, treatments, medications, and supplies. You may also use it to process information for patient admission, transfer, and discharge or to view stored information. The introduction of the computer to the nurses' station has been an exciting development in the health unit coordinating field since it offers a more efficient and accurate means of processing information.

Health care facilities use many different types of computer systems, and many have developed special programs to suit their needs. On the job you will learn the specifics of how to use your facility's system. We will only discuss a few basic concepts common to all computer systems. Application of computer use for transcription and other health unit coordinating procedures will be introduced in their respective chapters.

Usually three computer components are located at the nurses' station; the keyboard, the viewing screen, and the printer (Fig. 4–7). These may be referred to as a **computer**

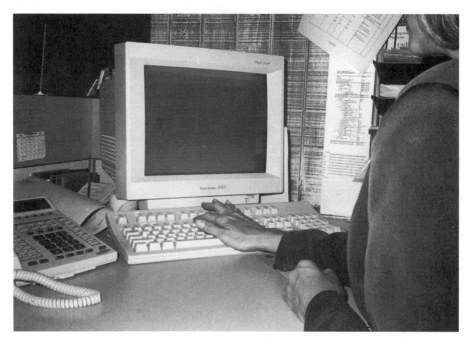

FIGURE 4–7 • A computer terminal.

**terminal**. The keyboard resembles a typewriter, and the keys are depressed in the same way as typewriter keys to feed information into the computer. Typing skills are helpful but not necessary to operate the keyboard. Some computer systems have a light pen or a mouse that may also be used to select information to be fed into the computer (Fig. 4–8). To use the pen, a **menu** is brought up on a screen. The light-sensitive pen is moved across the information to be processed. The mouse is used to move the cursor to the information, then clicked to process whatever is needed.

The **viewing screen** has many names. You may hear it referred to as the monitor, the CRT (cathode-ray tube), or the VDT (video display terminal). The viewing screen re-sembles a television. As you feed information into the computer by using the keyboard, it is seen on the screen. A menu can be brought up on the screen to make a selection of an item or a test to be ordered (Fig. 4–9), or a menu can be recalled for informational purposes only, such as viewing a list of the patients' names and room assignments for your nursing unit.

A flashing indicator called the **cursor** lets the user know the area on the screen that will receive the information. The cursor may be moved to any area on the screen that the user wishes. Most health care facilities computers are connected to a printer. At any given time, the user can give the computer a command to print any of the stored information in requisition form. When the health unit co-

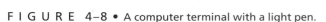

FIGURE 4–8 • A computer terminal with a light pen.

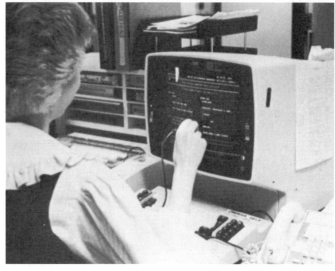

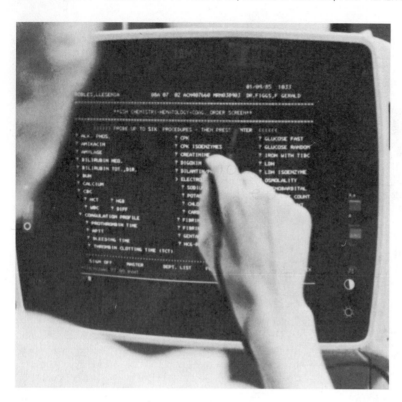

FIGURE 4–9 • A laboratory menu on the computer screen.

ordinator uses the computer to order a client's diet, the diet order prints out on the printer located in the dietary department.

If test results are sent to the unit through the use of the computer, a printer will be located on the unit. The HUC should be alert to printed material being sent via the printer and remove the printed documents as soon as possible.

Many health care facilities now have bedside computers available in each client's room for nursing personnel to record care and treatments performed. These records are generally printed every 24 hours for placement on the clients' chart.

As you can appreciate, the health care facility's computer system contains a great deal of information that is confidential in nature and that must not be tampered with; therefore, a security system is used. Upon employment, you are assigned an identification number or password. Each time you use the computer you gain entry to the system by using your password. Your identification number should never be given to anyone.

There are times when the computer is shut down for servicing or because of mechanical failure. During these times, downtime requisitions are used to process information. When computer function returns, the information processed by the paper method must be fed into the computer.

## The Fax Machine

The **fax machine** is a telecommunication device that transmits copies of written material over a telephone line from one site to another (Fig. 4–10). The fax transmits medical records, diagnostic reports, doctors' orders, and similar documents between departments within the hospital. Some facilities are faxing the pharmacy copy of the doctors' order sheet from the nursing unit to the pharmacy. Using the fax machine expedites the delivery of medication to the patient. It is also used to transmit information from hospitals to other health care facilities or doctors' offices.

To use the fax, insert a sheet of paper containing the information to be transmitted into the machine. Dial the destination number. Push the send button. The document prints on a receiving machine.

## Conveyor Belt or Dumbwaiter

These devices transport supplies or food from one area of the hospital to another. The conveyor belt or **dumbwaiter** is usually placed in a central location in the hospital so that it is convenient to all nursing stations. It is important that the supplies for each unit be removed from the conveyance immediately. If they are not, there may be delay in delivery of supplies to another unit. The health unit coordinator is alerted to remove supplies by a telephone call from the department sending the food or supplies.

## Nursing Unit Boards

Many nursing units have small chalkboards or grease boards in the nurses' station to record important infor-

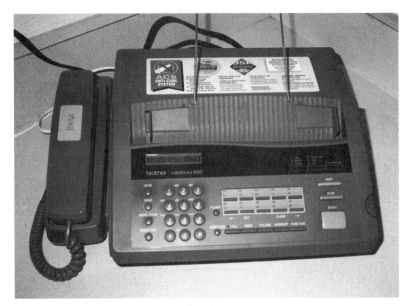

F I G U R E  4–10 • A facsimile (fax) machine.

mation. They may be used to keep track of surgery patients' progress, to record the whereabouts of patients who are off the unit for treatment, to indicate census, or to record patient assignments. Nursing personnel may also indicate on the board that they have left the unit for lunch or dinner.

## The Bulletin Board

The health unit coordinator has the responsibility to maintain the **nursing unit bulletin board**. This responsibility includes posting material in an attractive manner and keeping the posted material current. The material to be posted on the bulletin board may be determined by the nurse manager or may be set forth by administration policy. Bulletins regarding changes that will take place in employment policies, schedules of staff development classes, on-call schedules for resident doctors, and daily nursing assignment sheets are examples of materials posted on the bulletin board.

If no dates are on the bulletin, the health unit coordinator should indicate the date posted. Some notices are very important; in order for the nurse manager to know that all the unit employees have read them, it may be requested that each person initial the notice after reading it. The health unit coordinator should place the initialed notice on the nurse manager's desk when it is removed from the bulletin board. The nurse manager then checks that all personnel have read the notice. A neat board with up-to-date notices prompts unit personnel to read what is posted.

## SUMMARY

Your ability to use the telephone, intercom, and other communications devices efficiently and effectively contributes to the smooth operation of your nursing unit. Accuracy in taking telephone messages and communicating them to the correct person is a must for an efficiently run nursing unit. Using the computer at the nurses' station is an exciting new development for the field of health unit coordinating.

**REVIEW QUESTIONS**

1. Name six communication devices commonly used in the hospital.
   a. _Telephone_
   b. _Intercom_
   c. _Fax machine_
   d. _Computer_
   e. _pocket pager_
   f. _Pneumatic Tube_

2. List eight rules of telephone etiquette.
   a. _answer phone promptly_
   b. _Identify yourself properly_
   c. _speak into the phone_
   d. _give caller your undivided Attention_
   e. _speak distinctively and clearly_
   f. _be courtious at all times_
   g. _ask permission to put on hold_
   h. _dont use I dont know to answer a question_

3. Six items to be recorded when taking a telephone message are:
   a. _who the message is for_
   b. _the callers name_
   c. _the date & time of the call_
   d. _the purpose of the call_
   e. _get number to call if return call expected_
   f. _your name_

4. Define the following:
   a. keyboard
   _the method in which you input data to the computer_ _feed information_
   
   b. menu
   _a pull down screen to select information_
   
   c. cursor
   _Flashing indicator lets the user know the Area on the screen that will recieve the information_
   
   d. viewing screen
   _the place where you see the data and view data_
   
   e. computer
   _a keyboard monitor and viewing screen some times with a printer_
   
   f. pocket pager
   _small electric device used to deliver messages within the hospital may be voice or digital_

g. voice paging system   *used to page the doctor outside the Hospital each person with a voice pager is given a pager number dial on reg phone when a beep is heard then talk into the pager*

h. pneumatic tube system

*air pressure transports tubes carrying supples requisitions or messages from one hospital unit to another.*

i. intercom

*device used to communicate between the nursing station and the client rooms on the nursing unit.*

j. dumbwaiter

*device that transports food and supplies from one area of the hospital to another.*

k. fax

*telecommunication device that transmits copies of written material over a telephone line from one place to another*

5. Two uses of the telephone hold button are:

   a. *when you have another in coming call*

   b. *when you have to leave the caller to locate another person or to obtain information*

6. Briefly describe the plan you would follow to place a telephone call regarding a patient. *where answer the phone as fast as possible say where is the you work gathers from one hundertitle, give them my undivided attention speak clearly and distinctly and be courteous*

7. Two purposes of the intercom are:

   a. *taking patients requests without going to room*

   b. *to locate nursing personnel*

8. Two methods used to page within the hospital are:

   a. *the pocket pager digital or voice*

   b. *the paging system*

9. The purpose of a paging system is *to reach a doctor anywhere inside or outside the hospital*

10. Discuss the health coordinator's responsibility in the maintenance of the unit bulletin board. *to post hospital material and keep it current indicating such as changes in employment policies, schedules of staff development classes, on call schedules for doctors resident and daily nursing assignment sheets the date posted*

11. Below are listed communication devices that you may use as a health unit coordinator.

   a. telephone
   b. unit intercom
   c. pager
   d. fax
   e. pneumatic tube
   f. conveyor belt
   g. computer

In the spaces below, write the letter that is next to the device used to perform each function.

Ex:   _a_   used to place a call to the doctor's office

_E_   used to communicate a laboratory test from the laboratory department to the nursing unit

_D_   used by the student to deliver a message to his or her instructor

_G_   used during transcription to order an x-ray from the diagnostic imaging department

_B_   used to locate a nurse on the nursing unit

_F_   used to send a patient's tray from the dietary department to the nursing unit

12. You answer the telephone on the nursing unit by saying:
    a. "Mrs. Smith, Health Unit Coordinator, may I help you?"
    b. "Pediatrics, Mrs. Smith, Health Unit Coordinator."
    c. "Pediatrics, Smith."
    d. "Pediatrics, Mrs. Smith, may I help you?"
    e. "Pediatrics, Health Unit Coordinator."

13. You have received a telephone call for Jane, the nurse manager, whom you need to locate. You would:
    a. lay the telephone receiver on the desk because it is rude to put a caller on hold.
    b. put the caller on hold.
    c. not put the caller on hold because no one else is in the desk area.
    d. ask the caller's permission, then put the caller on hold.
    e. do none of the above.

14. When you locate Jane, say:
    a. "There is someone on line 1 for you."
    b. "It's Doctor Brown for you."
    c. "Dr. Brown is on line 1."
    d. "Dr. Brown is on line 1. She wants an update on Mrs. White's condition."
    e. None of the above.

15. List three uses of the computer located at the nurses' station.
    a. _transcribing Drs orders_
    b. _request diagnostic studies, medications, supplies, treatment_
    c. _process information for admission, transfer and discharge_

16. When using voice mail, speak fast because you may run out of recording tape. (true or false)

## References

Blondis, Marion Nesbitt and Jackson, Barbara E.: *Nonverbal Communications with Patients*. New York, John Wiley & Sons, 1977.

Cox, Kay: *Being a Health Unit Coordinator*, 2nd ed. Bowie, MD, Robert J. Brady Co., 1984.

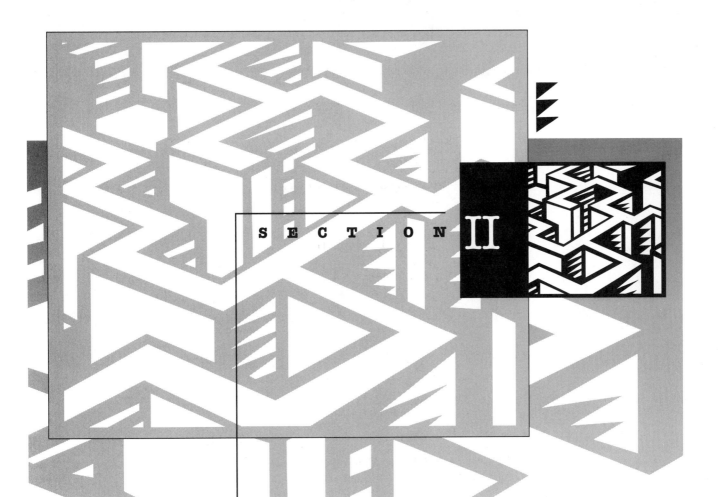

SECTION II

# NONCLINICAL MANAGEMENT OF THE NURSING UNIT

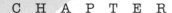

CHAPTER 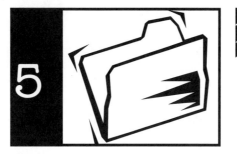 5

# COMMUNICATION AND INTERPERSONAL SKILLS FOR THE HEALTH UNIT COORDINATOR

## CHAPTER OBJECTIVES

*Upon completion of this chapter, you will be able to:*

1. Give instances that exemplify human needs, classify each according to Maslow's hierarchy of human needs, and give appropriate responses to meet the listed needs.

2. List four causes of ineffective communication.

3. List four components of the communication process.

4. Interpret and use the communication model.

5. List eight ways to improve listening skills.

6. List five ways to improve feedback skills.

7. Define the terms in the vocabulary list.

8. List three guidelines to follow to maintain the confidentiality of the contents of a patient's chart.

9. List two responsibilities of the health unit coordinator in maintaining confidentiality of patient information.

10. List six steps to deal with an angry telephone caller.

11. Identify statements as assertive, nonassertive, and aggressive.

12. Respond to situations using assertive skills.

13. Name the three states of mind or personality called "ego states" and describe the pattern of behavior related to each.

14. List the five "driver" messages that interfere with assertive behavior and list the antidotes for each.

## VOCABULARY

**Adult Ego State** • The part of the personality that stores facts and information; used to help protect the inner child part of the personality by interpreting and responding to the environment

**Aggressive** • A behavioral style in which a person attempts to be the dominant force in an interaction

**Antidote** • Anything that counteracts or removes the effects of a poison, disease, or evil; used here to neutralize "driver" messages that put a condition on feeling OK; "I'm OK if I . . . am strong, try hard, hurry up, am perfect, or please me (someone else)"

**Assertive** • A behavioral style in which a person stands up for his or her own rights and feelings without violating the rights and feelings of others

**Autonomously** • Behaving responsibly by choosing the ego states that directly and effectively express feelings, wants, and needs as they occur without discounting self or others

**Broken Record** • Assertive skill, wherein a person repeats his or her stand over and over again

**Child Ego State** • The part of the personality that stores feelings; it is the most potent ego state and when scared enough can immobilize the entire personality if not protected by the parent and/or the adult ego states

**Communication** • The process of transmitting feelings, images, and ideas from the mind of one person to the mind of another person for the purpose of obtaining a response

**Confidentiality** • Keeping secret any private information, either spoken or written

**Discount** • To devalue by ignoring or distorting some aspect of internal or external experience such as the existence, significance, or change possibilities of a problem or one's personal abilities

**Ego States** • Organized systems of thought and feeling that produce patterns of behavior characteristic of the particular ego state active (i.e., parent, adult, and child)

**Esteem Needs** • A person's need for self-respect and for the respect of others

**Feedback** • Response to a message

**Fogging** • Assertive skill in which a person responds to a criticism by making noncommittal statements that cannot be argued against

**Free Information** • The insights to personalities that can be picked up from general conversation

**Love and Belonging Needs** • A person's need to have affectionate relationships with people and to have a place in a group

**Message** • Images, feelings, and ideas transmitted from one person to another

**Negative Assertion** • An assertive skill in which a person verbally accepts the fact that they have made an error without letting it reflect on their worth as a human being

**Negative Inquiry** • An assertive skill in which a person requests further clarification of a criticism in order to get to the real issue

**Nonassertive** • A behavioral style in which a person allows others to dictate her or his self-worth

**Nonverbal Communication** • Communication that is not written or spoken but creates a message between two or more people by use of eye contact, body language, and facial expression

**Parent Ego State** • The part of the personality that stores opinions, beliefs, and values; functions to protect the inner child

**Physiologic Needs** • A person's physical needs, such as the need for food and water

**Receiver** • The person receiving the message

**Sender** • The person transmitting the message

**Visualization** • Creating and using mental thoughts to form images, sounds, and body sensations; used to rehearse successful performances of a skill to reinforce and enhance recall

## INTERPERSONAL BEHAVIOR

To develop effective communication and interpersonal skills, you must first develop an understanding of interpersonal behavior. Interpersonal means between persons. Behavior is how people act, what they say or do. Research indicates that in conversation, a person behaves according to who the other person is and how he or she behaves. An understanding of interpersonal behavior assists us in understanding our own behavior and in understanding the behavior of others.

Although there are several models that may be used to study interpersonal behavior, we have chosen Maslow's hierarchy of needs, developed by the famous psychologist, the late Abraham Maslow. Maslow's human needs model emphasizes that all persons have the same basic needs and that these needs motivate and influence a person's behavior either consciously or unconsciously. The needs are arranged in a pyramid, with the most basic or immediate needs at the bottom of the pyramid and the less critical needs at the top of the pyramid (Fig. 5–1). The lower the need is in the pyramid, the more influence it has on a person's behavior. A person works harder to meet the need for water to drink than to meet the need for self-esteem.

As the lower needs are satisfied to an adequate degree, we become increasingly concerned about satisfying the

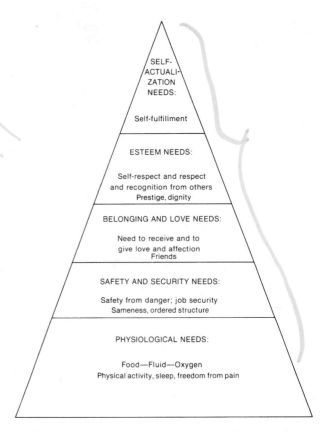

**F I G U R E  5–1** • Maslow's hierarchy of needs.

next or a higher level need. Most people find that all their needs are both partially satisfied and partially unsatisfied at the same time. Unsatisfied needs influence an individual's behavior in terms of motivation, priorities, or action taken. According to Maslow, the average person is satisfied perhaps 85% in his physical needs, 70% in his safety needs, 50% in his love needs, 40% in his self-esteem needs, and 10% in his self-actualization needs.

## Physiologic Needs

Each person needs food, fluids, oxygen, physical activity, sleep, and freedom from pain. These needs are the most basic and the most dominant of all human needs. They are the first to develop in the human organism. The normal adult probably has satisfied his or her physiologic needs.

What about the person who is ill or hospitalized? The illness itself, diagnostic testing, or surgery may interrupt a person's normal eating and drinking habits. Diseases such as emphysema make it impossible for the body to receive the amount of oxygen needed to function normally. Physical activity is decreased upon the patient's admission to the hospital, affecting the body's need for exercise.

---

### EXAMPLE

Bill, a client, has been fasting since midnight for an upper GI. It's now 11:00 AM, the test is completed, and Bill is ready for his breakfast. When he is told by the health unit coordinator that his tray will not arrive from the dietary department until 11:30 AM, Bill becomes angry. Bill's behavior is influenced by his unsatisfied physiologic need.

---

## Safety and Security Needs

Everyone has the need to be sheltered, to be clothed, to feel safe from danger, and to feel secure about his or her job and financial future. Each person has a need for a certain degree of sameness, familiarity, order, structure, and consistency in life. Freedom from fear, anxiety, and chaos are also important.

The normal healthy person probably has met these basic needs; however, illness or hospitalization may interrupt a person's ability to continue to satisfy them. What about the patient who is waiting for test results to learn a diagnosis? The unpredictable course of a lengthy illness? The fear of death? The cost of medical care? The unfamiliarity of hospital routine and medical procedures? As you can see, there are many obstacles that may interfere with meeting the safety and security needs of an ill or hospitalized person.

Hospital employees who are new on the job may feel insecure, and they usually make more mistakes during this stressful time. Rumors about layoffs, true or not, can affect the security needs of employees and often send them scurrying to apply elsewhere for employment.

---

### EXAMPLE

Donna, a client, has just been told by her surgeon that the test results show she has a tumor, possibly malignant. The surgeon has recommended she have surgery as soon as possible. Donna approaches the health unit coordinator and demands that she be able to speak to her family physician immediately. Donna's behavior is motivated by unsatisfied security needs.

---

## Belonging and Love Needs

Once physiologic and safety needs are relatively well met, the need for love and belonging surfaces. Now the person has a desire for affectionate relationships with others and is motivated to belong to or to be a part of a group.

Patients who are hospitalized, especially for a long time, may be cut off from their family, friends, or group.

---

### EXAMPLE

Sarah has been hospitalized for 2 weeks. During this time she has been visited only once by her husband. In an attempt to meet her belonging needs, she has been turning on her call light hourly for minor requests.

---

## Esteem Needs

As a person develops satisfying relationships with others, esteem needs, the need for self-respect and for the respect of others, emerges. Esteem needs may be met by seeking special status within a group, owning a company, learning a skill very well, or developing a talent to be performed for others.

Attainment of self-respect leads to feelings of adequacy, self-confidence, and strength; they result in prestige, recognition, and dignity for the individual.

Hospitalization frequently interferes with the ability to meet esteem needs. Many aspects of hospitalization—hospital gowns, sharing a room with others, siderails on the bed, and being referred to as a room number or a disease instead of by name—serve to depersonalize the patient. Often a patient's past accomplishments and status are overlooked by busy hospital personnel.

---

### EXAMPLE

Tom has been hospitalized for over a week. He is walking past the nurses' station and stops and reads the name tag of the health unit coordinator. "You are Jenny Mason. That's a nice name. You know, since I have been in the hospital no one has called me by my name. I feel like a nobody."

---

## Self-Actualization Needs

Once a person feels basic satisfaction of the first four needs, the next step is for him or her to become "self-actualized." Self-actualization is developing a personality to its full potential. Contentment, self-fulfillment, creativity, originality, independence, and acceptance of other people all characterize the self-actualized person. Self-actualization is growth motivated from within yourself. It is growing and changing because you feel it is important. A self-actualized person has taken steps to make this happen.

### Example of Different Needs in a Conversation

The human needs model can be used to demonstrate interpersonal behavior between health unit coordinators and hospital personnel or between health unit coordinators and patients or visitors.

Health unit coordinator: "Mary is in isolation. You need to put this gown on before you go into her room."

*No dominant need expressed.*

Husband: "Mary is in isolation! what for? I want to know exactly what is going on here."

*Safety need expressed.* The husband is concerned that he may contract what Mary has, and he is concerned about her safety.

Health unit coordinator [defensively]: "Look, if you don't want to wear the gown, don't go in. I don't make the rules here."

*Esteem need expressed.* The health unit coordinator interprets the husband's request for information as an attack on her competence; self-esteem is at stake. Fighting back is used to try to satisfy self-esteem needs.

In this example, if the health unit coordinator had perceived that the husband's question was motivated by *safety* needs, she would have responded with understanding rather than with defensiveness and aggression.

## COMMUNICATION SKILLS

Most of us spend much of our time communicating, but few of us communicate as effectively as we should. Many factors contribute to communication difficulties. For instance, the English language has grown considerably since it was developed, and there are now over 600,000 words in the language. It is impossible to know how many words an individual may have in his or her vocabulary, but it is believed that a high school graduate comprehends 3000 to 5000 words. How does the speaker know which of the 600,000 words are included in the receiver's 5000-word vocabulary? The medical world also has a growing language of its own, which is made up of abbreviations and medical terms. "Remember now, Sidney is NPO." or "Your doctor feels that you may have cholelithiasis, so she

has scheduled you for an ultrasound tomorrow" may have little meaning to those not familiar with the medical terms. Some words have more than one meaning. A *chip* in the computer world has a much different meaning than a *chip* used in a poker game.

Communication is 55% facial expression and eye contact, including the length of glance; 38% vocal qualities, including tone, loudness, firmness, hesitations, and pauses; and 7% verbal, actual words (Fig. 5–2). There is often inconsistency between what a person is saying and how he appears.

"Of course I'm listening to you, Mother," says the 9-year-old as he sits glued to the television set, leaving the mother wondering whether the child is indeed listening to her.

Another major weakness in the communication process is poor listening skills. Often we are thinking of something else while the speaker is talking to us; we are formulating a response or prejudging what is being said.

Daughter: "I have stopped eating breakfast meats."

Mother: "But breakfast is the most important meal of the day, you should not give it up."

Instead of listening to what is being said the mother has prejudged that the daughter is skipping breakfast rather than breakfast meats.

Since the health unit coordinator is the communicator for the nursing unit, effective communication is vital for both job success and proficient operation of the nursing unit.

Communications takes place daily with doctors, nurses, allied health professionals, patients, visitors, and administrators (Fig. 5–3). The health unit coordinator is often the first person seen by the new patient and visitors. The

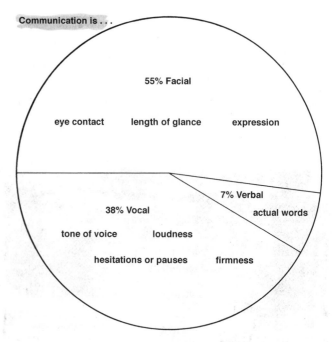

FIGURE 5–2 • Components of communication.

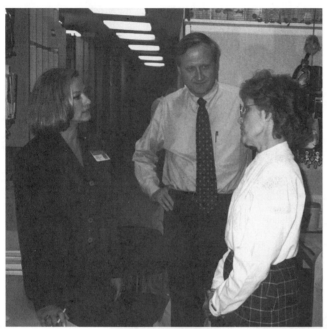

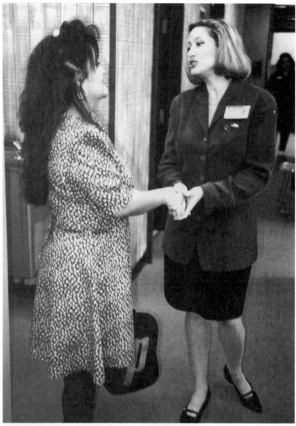

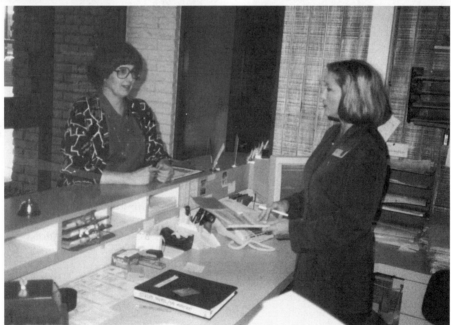

F I G U R E   5–3 • The health unit coordinator is the communicator for the nursing unit. (*A*) Communicating with hospital staff. (*B*) Welcoming a new patient to the unit. (*C*) Informing a visitor.

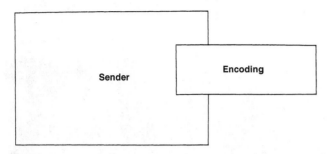

FIGURE 5–4 • The communication process—simple communication.

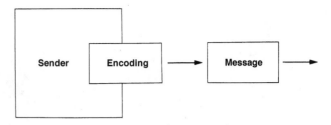

FIGURE 5–5 • The communication process—message sending.

words, gestures, facial expression, and body posture the health unit coordinator uses can be recognized as sounding, looking, and feeling opinionated or supportive, thoughtful or insecure. The tone of voice, the words spoken, and the facial expressions used during the patient's or visitor's initial contact with the nursing unit leave a lasting impression.

## What is Communication?

Communication is the process of transmitting images, feelings, and ideas from the mind of one person to the minds of other persons for the purpose of obtaining a response.

The communication process consists of four components:

**Sender**: The person transmitting the message
**Message**: The images, feelings, and ideas transmitted
**Receiver**: The person receiving the message
**Feedback**: The response to the message

Communication seems like a simple process (Fig. 5–4); however, the act of communicating does not guarantee effective communication has taken place or that the message that was sent was the same as that received. A program was developed for the computer to translate one language into another. The computer translated the English phrase "out of sight, out of mind," into Russian and translated it back into English as "invisible idiot."

## Communication Model

A model is a representation of a process; a map, for instance. We will use a model to take a closer look at the

communication process, to identify why so many of us communicate poorly, and to find ways to improve our communication with others.

### Sender

The sender must translate mental images, feelings, and ideas into symbols in order to communicate them to the receiver. The process is called **encoding**. Encoding involves the sender deciding whether to send the message in verbal symbols or in nonverbal symbols. What are the right words to use so the receiver will understand the message? Different words are used if you are speaking to a child, to an adult, or to another health care professional. Nonverbal symbols, such as facial expressions, may be used to communicate the message. Encoding occurs each time we communicate. A poor choice of words or an inconsistency between verbal and nonverbal messages may result in unsuccessful communication.

### Message

Once the idea, feeling, or image is encoded, it is sent to the receiver. This step of the communication process is called the **message** (Fig. 5–5).

### Receiver

As the message reaches the receiver, he or she must decode the verbal and nonverbal symbols to determine the meaning of the message and transfer it back into images, feelings, or ideas. Unsuccessful decoding can be caused by inconsistency in the verbal and nonverbal symbols from the sender (Fig. 5–6).

"Of course I love you," said harshly may be difficult to decode correctly.

Lifestyle, age, cultural background, environment, and poor listening habits are other reasons for incorrect decoding.

In successful communication the ideas, feelings, and images of the sender match those of the receiver (Fig. 5–7).

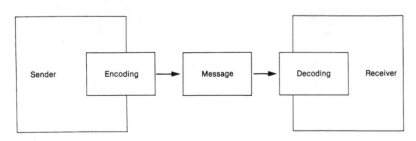

FIGURE 5–6 • The communication process—receiving the message.

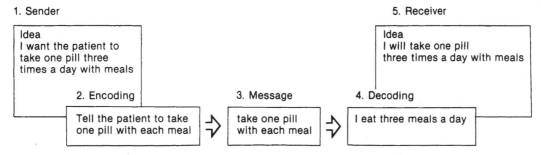

**F I G U R E 5–7** • An example of successful communication.

In unsuccessful communication, errors occur in encoding or in decoding the message (Fig. 5–8).

## LISTENING SKILLS

Listening is something we have done all our lives, but most of us have had little or no training in how to do it effectively. We take it for granted. Many of us think of communication as the sender giving us a message, but for successful communication the sender and the receiver must both actively participate in the communication process. Active participation for the receiver requires effective listening skills.

### Ways to Improve Listening Skills

1. *Stop talking.* The first step toward improving listening skills is to stop talking. The maxim that we have two ears and one mouth may indicate that we need to listen twice as much as we speak.
2. *Teach yourself to concentrate.* The average person speaks between 100 and 200 words a minute. The listener can process up to 400 words a minute. Often we find ourselves passively listening to the speaker, not listening for meaning in the message, and therefore missing important cues or even words. "We cannot send you any help" has a much different meaning from "We cannot send you any help *right now.*"
3. *Take time to listen.* When someone talks to you, stop what you are doing and look at the speaker. Listen for

the meaning of the words and for the nonverbal symbols. "I wish I were dead" spoken by an elderly patient may mean "I'm lonely."

4. *Listen with your eyes.* Look into the eyes of the sender. What are they saying? A visitor standing at the desk saying, "My mother is not back from surgery yet" may really be saying "I'm frightened, she has been in surgery so long there must be complications."
5. *Listen to what is being said, not only how it is being said.* Avoid being distracted by a lisp, by how fast the sender is talking, or by what the sender is wearing. Concentrate on the verbal and nonverbal communication symbols used by the sender.
6. *Suspend judgment.* Often we react emotionally to what is said or what we think is being said. We prejudge what the speaker is saying and unconsciously tune out ideas or beliefs that do not match our own.
7. *Do not interrupt the speaker.* Interrupting the speaker or finishing the sentence discourages the sender and breaks down communication. To break this habit, try apologizing each time you interrupt the sender.
8. *Remove distractions.* Noise, a ringing telephone, and conversations of others are types of distractions that interfere with effective listening.

## FEEDBACK

Feedback, the response to the message sent, is the final component to the communication process. Effective communication is virtually impossible without it. Feedback tells the sender how much of the message was under-

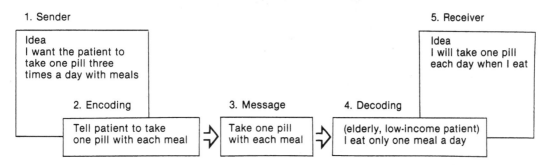

**F I G U R E 5–8** • An example of unsuccessful communication.

stood, indicates whether the receiver agrees or disagrees with the message, and helps the sender correct confusing or vague language.

Feedback can be as simple as a nod, it may be an answer to a question, or it may be used to encourage further communication and to assist the sender in developing ideas or sharing feelings.

## Improving Feedback Skills

1. *Use paraphrasing* (repeat the message to the sender in your own words). Phrases like "Let me see if I have this right . . ." and "This is what you want . . ." are acceptable as lines leading into paraphrasing.

   *For example*: "Let me repeat that to you. For the dressing change tomorrow you want a dressing tray, size 7 gloves, and three packages of 4 × 4's."

2. *Repeat the last word or words of the message* (to allow the speaker to more fully develop the thought). Be careful not to parrot the whole message or the speaker may respond with "That's what I just said."

   Patient: "I'm not sure I want to have the myelogram."

   Health unit coordinator: "Myelogram?"

   Patient: "Yes, I'm scheduled for one this afternoon, and frankly I'm scared stiff. My neighbor had one . . . ."

3. *Use descriptive rather than evaluative feedback.* "Oh, so you are going to develop 31 flavors of popcorn" is better than "I think it is a ridiculous idea."

4. *Use specific rather than general feedback.* "Your idea has merit" is more meaningful than "You are so bright."

5. *Use constructive feedback rather than destructive feedback.* Do not use feedback that makes a person feel worse.

6. *Give feedback that is helpful to the sender.* The response, "Don't worry" to someone who is frightened that they have cancer is of no help. Feedback encouraging the person to expound on their fears would be much more helpful to the person.

## STEPS TO DEAL WITH AN ANGRY TELEPHONE CALLER

At times the health unit coordinator is confronted with an angry or disgruntled telephone caller. Following the few helpful steps outlined below will assist you in handling the situation effectively.

1. When answering the telephone *always identify yourself by nursing unit, name, and status* (Fig. 5–9). Doing this puts you on a more personal level with the caller. Also, callers may become even more upset if they need to ask questions to determine who they are talking to.

2. *Avoid putting the person on hold.* You may be tempted to do this to transfer the call to the nurse manager.

3. *Listen to what the caller is saying.* Do not become defensive. Keep in mind that the caller is not really angry with you.

4. *Write down what the caller is saying.* The notes may come in handy, and they help you control your own anger.

5. *Acknowledge the anger.* Use phrases such as, "I hear you are angry." or "I'd be angry also . . . ."

6. *Do not allow the caller to become abusive.* Say, "I feel you are becoming abusive; call me back in a few minutes," or something similar.

document angry calls

Explain reason for holding

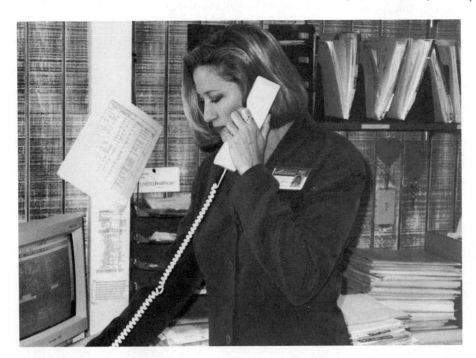

F I G U R E   5–9 • When answering the telephone, always identify yourself by nursing unit, name, and status.

# CONFIDENTIALITY

The health unit coordinator has access to a great deal of confidential information. By the very nature of your job, you are exposed to information that is considered confidential, such as surgical procedures, diagnostic results, and other medical reports. This information must be treated with absolute confidentiality—that is, secrecy—by all health personnel.

As a health unit coordinator you have two responsibilities in maintaining the confidentiality of patient information: one is to not verbally repeat confidential information, and the other is to control the patient's chart in a manner that maintains confidentiality of the contents.

Below are basic guidelines for you to follow to help you establish discipline regarding confidentiality of patient information.

## Self

- *Do not discuss patient information* (other than what is necessary to care for the patient). All patient information is confidential. Some information, such as homosexuality or infection with a sexually transmitted disease, is so confidential that treating it as such is obvious to all; however, other information, such as the patient's age, weight, or test results, may be harder to identify as being confidential material. *Remember*: Never discuss any patient information except when necessary for treatment reasons.
- *Conduct conversations with other health personnel outside of the hearing distance of the patients and visitors.* Never converse about patient information in the hallways, cafeteria, or away from the hospital. Be aware of the identity of others who are at the nurses' station during discussions about patients: often overheard bits of information may be misconstrued by patients or visitors and result in unnecessary apprehension on the part of the patient concerned. Also, factual medical information overheard by the patient in this manner can produce unnecessary worry, anxiety, or even panic in a patient.
- *Do not discuss medical treatment with the patient or relatives* (unless specifically instructed to do so by the doctor or the nurse).
- *Do not discuss general patient information.* Often hospital personnel, other patients, visitors, or your own friends, relatives, or neighbors may ask you questions regarding a specific patient (especially if the patient should happen to be a celebrity) out of curiosity. Politely refuse to give out the information, then quickly change the discussion to another subject.
- *Do not discuss hospital incidents away from the nursing unit.* Discussing code arrest procedures, unexpected death, and so forth with persons other than health professionals or within hearing distance of others may instill in them fear and apprehension regarding health care; this may even cause them to put off seeking necessary health treatment at some future time.

- *Refer all telephone calls from reporters, police personnel, legal agencies, and so forth to the nurse manager.*
- *If in doubt about the authenticity of a telephone caller, ask for necessary information and return the call after you have had time to confirm the identify of the caller.*

## The Chart

- *Follow the hospital policy for duplicating portions of the patient's chart.* Duplication of the patient's chart forms is usually controlled by the health records department of the hospital.
- *Control access to the patient's chart.* Only authorized persons, such as doctors and hospital personnel, should have access to the chart. Always know the status of the person using the chart at the nurses' station. Do not give a chart to someone on request because he or she "looks like a doctor." Should relatives or friends of a patient request to see the chart, do not give it to them under any circumstances.
- *Control transportation of the patient's chart.* Never send the patient's chart to another department through the pneumatic tube system. Do not give patients their chart to hold while they are being transported from one area of the hospital to another.

# ASSERTIVENESS FOR HEALTH UNIT COORDINATORS

Have you ever said yes to a request but really wanted to say no, or left a conversation wishing you had "stood up for yourself"? If your answer is yes, then you responded in a **nonassertive behavior style**.

Have you ever allowed a situation to get out of control, then "blew up" and later wished you had handled the situation better? If your answer is yes, then you responded in an **aggressive behavioral style**.

A third type of response is an **assertive behavior style** in which an individual expresses her or his wants and desires in an honest and appropriate way, while respecting other people's rights.

As a health unit coordinator, you may have to ask patients or visitors to change their behavior to conform to safety regulations and hospital rules or to allow for the comfort of others. For example, you may have to ask a patient's relative not to smoke in the hospital, or you may have to ask a patient to turn down the television volume at the request of the patient's roommate. Asking another person to change his or her behavior can provoke a defensive reaction. Knowing you have a choice of behavior styles and choosing the right way to handle a given situation assists you in communicating more effectively.

Also, as a health unit coordinator, you engage in unlimited encounters during the day that can lead to conflict. Using assertiveness, the art of expressing yourself clearly

## A BILL OF ASSERTIVE RIGHTS

- You have the right to judge your own behavior, thoughts, and emotions, and to take the responsibility for their initiation and consequences upon yourself.
- You have the right to offer no reasons or excuses for justifying your behavior.
- You have the right to judge if you are responsible for finding solutions to other people's problems.
- You have the right to change your mind.
- You have the right to make mistakes—and be responsible for them.
- You have the right to say, "I don't know."
- You have the right to be independent of the goodwill of others before coping with them.
- You have the right to be illogical in making decisions.
- You have the right to say, "I don't understand."
- You have the right to say, "I don't care."

YOU HAVE THE RIGHT TO SAY NO, WITHOUT FEELING GUILTY

From Smith, Manual J.: *When I Say No, I Feel Guilty*. New York, Bantam Books, 1975, with permission.

and concisely, being able to clarify when necessary, and being able to explain and communicate in an open, honest manner, enables you to cope more effectively with problems and conflicts as they arise.

## Behavioral Styles

### Nonassertive Behavioral Style

A nonassertive response is typically self-denying and does not express true feelings. The person does not stand up for his or her rights and allows others to choose for him or her. Because of inadequate behavior the individual feels hurt and anxious.

A nonassertive health unit coordinator may have strong opinions about things going on at the nurses' station but keeps these feelings to himself or herself.

### EXAMPLE

Kim feels that she is scheduled to work more holidays and 12-hour shifts than the other health unit coordinators on the unit. Instead of saying anything to the nurse manager, she is upset every time she looks at the new work schedule.

A nonassertive choice avoids conflict; therefore, feelings of frustration or anger are not expressed to the person responsible.

### EXAMPLE

Robert spent 15 minutes in the unit lounge complaining to coworkers about how Betsy, a nurse, is condescending toward him and makes disparaging remarks in conversations with him. She expects him to leave what he is working on to run special errands for her. He is angry and frustrated but refuses to talk to her directly about these problems.

A nonassertive approach to requesting behavior change is to use general or apologetic statements, or to use words that minimize the message. This low-key approach allows others to easily ignore the request.

### EXAMPLE

Two visitors were relaxing in a visitors' lounge near the nursing station. They both lit cigarettes. A "no-smoking" sign is posted nearby. Mary approaches the visitors and says, "I'm sorry, but I have to ask a little favor, this is not my rule, but smoking is not allowed here."

### Aggressive Behavioral Style

An aggressive response is typically self-enhancing at the expense of others. The person may express feelings but hurts others in the process. Verbal attacks, disparaging remarks, and manipulation indicate aggressive behavior.

An aggressive health unit coordinator uses "you" statements, often followed by personal judgments. Using "you" statements provokes more defensiveness than using "I" statements.

### EXAMPLE

Kim feels she is scheduled to work more holidays and 12-hour shifts than the other health unit coordinators. An aggressive Kim may approach the nurse manager and say, "You are simply unfair, and you don't care about me. I have to work more than the others."

Statements that use *always* and *never* are often part of aggressive communications.

EXAMPLE

Robert is upset with the nurse, Betsy, because she expects him to leave what he is doing to run errands for her. Robert responds aggressively, "You *always* expect me to stop my work for you; you think what you want is so important and you *never* think about anyone else."

An aggressive health unit coordinator uses demands instead of requests. Demanding does not elicit another's cooperation and generates defensiveness. Disparaging remarks also cause the receiver to feel humiliated.

EXAMPLE

An aggressive unit coordinator asks the visitors to stop smoking by saying, "Put out your cigarettes, you can't smoke here. Can't you see the 'no-smoking' sign?"

## Assertive Behavioral Style

An assertive response includes standing up for your rights without violating the rights of others. Assertive behavior is self-enhancing but not at the expense of others. It involves open, honest communication, and being able to express needs, expectations, and feelings. Being assertive also means being able both to accept compliments with ease and to admit errors. It also means taking responsibility for your actions. It is common for a person to assert themselves verbally only after frustration builds. At that point it is too late to communicate assertively, and an aggressive response is used instead. It is useful to use assertiveness in all interactions before frustration builds. It is easy for the beginner to confuse assertive behavior with aggressive behavior. To distinguish the difference, remember that with assertive behavior the rights of another are not violated.

An assertive health unit coordinator is able to use clear, direct, nonapologetic expressions of feelings and expectations. Descriptive rather than judgmental criticisms and "I" rather than "you" statements are used.

EXAMPLE

Kim, as an assertive health unit coordinator, chooses to talk to the nurse manager about her feelings. "I feel that I am working more holidays and more 12-hour shifts than the other health unit coordinators. I had to work both Christmas and Easter this year, and last pay period I had to work four 12-hour shifts. I would like to share working the holidays equally with the others. The 12-hour shifts do not work well with my family life; however, if others also do not like the 12-hour shifts I am willing to work my fair share of them."

An assertive health unit coordinator uses concise statements and specific behavioral descriptions.

EXAMPLE

Robert is assertive in dealing with Betsy, and he chooses to talk to her. He begins with using an "I statement," then describes the incident in which he felt Betsy was condescending. "I felt you were condescending toward me when you said 'even you should be able to see I needed your help'." He also mentions the specific remark she made that he found disparaging. Depending on the discussion that follows, it may also be appropriate for him to ask Betsy for a behavior change. Robert also describes an incident in which Betsy asked him to interrupt his work to run errands for her. He describes how he could be more productive if he was allowed to do the task for her when it was convenient to his work schedule.

An assertive health unit coordinator uses requests instead of demands and personalizes statements of concern.

EXAMPLE

An assertive Mary approaches the visitors and says, "I would like you to stop smoking in this area. I can understand your desire to have a cigarette at this time. You can smoke in a designated area in the cafeteria."

Assertiveness is based upon the belief that each individual has the same fundamental human rights; therefore, the doctor is not better than the health unit coordinator or the teacher is not better than the students. In becoming assertive do not focus on changing your personality, but rather on changing your behavior in specific situations. It is highly unlikely that anyone is always assertive; however, once assertiveness is learned, it can be one of your behavioral choices.

Table 5-1 compares nonassertive, aggressive, and assertive behavioral styles.

EXERCISE 1

Identify the behavioral style of each of the following statements by writing AG for aggressive, AS for assertive, and NA for nonassertive in the spaces provided.

1. _AS_ "I would like to have Monday off."

2. _AG_ "You should know how to order diets, you have been here long enough."

3. _NA_ "I'm sorry, I'm so forgetful, I won't let it happen again."

4. _NA_ "I would kind of like to go on my break now."

| TABLE 5–1 | COMPARISON OF NONASSERTIVE, AGGRESSIVE, AND ASSERTIVE BEHAVIORAL STYLES | | |
|---|---|---|---|
| Components | Nonassertive | Aggressive | Assertive |
| Rights | Does not stand up for rights | Stands up for rights but violates the rights of others | Stands up for rights without violating rights of others |
| Choice | Allows others to choose (to avoid conflict) | Chooses for others | Chooses for self |
| Belief | You're OK, I'm not OK; lose/win | I'm OK, you're not OK; win/lose | I'm OK, you're OK; win/win |
| Responsibility | Others responsible for behavior     Blame themselves for poor results; may blame others for feelings | Responsible for others' behavior     Blames others for poor results     Feelings aren't important | Responsible for own behavior     Assumes responsibility for own errors; assumes responsibility for feelings |
| Traits | Self-denying, apologetic, timid, emotionally dishonest, difficult to say "no," guilty, whining, "poor me" | Dominates, humiliates, sarcasm     Self-enhancing at the expense of others, opinionated | Expresses feelings, feels about self, candid, diplomatic, listens, eye contact |
| Goals | Does not achieve goals | Achieves goals at the expense of others | May achieve goals |
| Word choices | Minimizing words such as     "I'm sorry"     "I believe"     "I think"     "Little," "sort of"     General instead of specific statements; statement disguised as questions | "You statements"     Always/never statements     Demands instead of requests | "I understand . . ."     "I feel . . ."     "I apologize. . ."     Neutral language     Concise statements |
| Body language | Lack of eye contact; slumping, downtrodden posture; words and nonverbal messages that don't match | "Looking-through-you" eye contact; tense, impatient posture | Erect, relaxed posture; eye contact; verbal and nonverbal messages match |

5. __AS__ "The next NAHUC chapter meeting is tomorrow at 6:00 PM. I am going, would you like to go with me?"

6. __AG__ "I know nothing about it. You were here yesterday, you should know."

7. __AS__ "I would like to finish transcribing this set of orders before I take this specimen to the lab."

8. __NA__ "I wish somebody else around here would answer the phone once in a while."

9. __AG__ "Your chart is right here, Dr. James; I would think you could find it on your own."

10. __AS__ "I apologize, I did not order the liver scan. I will order it immediately."

11. __NS__ "You are always late, you never care that I have to stay over and cover for you."

12. __NA__ "I really hate to ask you this, and you don't have to do it, but would you work for me on Saturday?"

13. __AS__ "May I help you find your chart, Dr. McLean?"

14. __AG__ "I don't know what the nurse manager thinks I am, a machine or something. We need more help around here."

15. __AS__ "Mrs. Smith, I would like you to turn your light off so Mrs. Jones can rest."

16. __NA__ "Mary, I would like to switch days off with you."

## Evaluating Your Assertiveness

Table 5–2 is an assertive inventory developed by Alberti and Emmons (1978, p. 40). These authors state that the inventory "provides a list of questions which should be useful in increasing your awareness of your own behavior in situations which call for assertiveness. The inventory is not a standardized psychological test. There are no right answers. The only 'score' is your own evaluation of how you measure up to what you would like to be able to do."

Take time now to respond to the questions in the inventory.

## Assertiveness Skills

The goal of using assertiveness in communication is to arrive at an "I win, you win" conclusion; in other words, a workable compromise. A workable compromise is dealing with a conflict in such a way that the solution is satisfactory to all involved parties.

Four assertiveness skills that may be used to reach a workable compromise are broken record, fogging, negative assertion, and negative inquiry.

| **T A B L E  5-2**  | **THE ASSERTIVENESS INVENTORY** |

The following questions will be helpful in assessing your assertiveness. Be honest with your responses. All you have to do is draw a circle around the number that describes you best. For some questions, the assertive end of the scale is at 0, for others at 3. Key: 0 means *no* or *never*; 1 means *somewhat* or *sometimes*; 2 means *usually* or *a good deal*; and 3 means *practically always* or *entirely*.

1. When a person is highly unfair, do you call it to attention?  0  1  (2)  3

2. Do you find it difficult to make decisions?  0  1  2  (3)

3. Are you openly critical of others' ideas, opinions, behavior?  0  (1)  2  3

4. Do you speak out in protest when someone takes your place in line?  0  (1)  2  3

5. Do you often avoid people or situations for fear of embarrassment?  (0)  1  2  3

6. Do you usually have confidence in your own judgment?  0  (1)  2  3

7. Do you insist that your spouse or roommate take on a fair share of household chores?  (0)  1  2  3

8. Are you prone to "fly off the handle?"  0  (1)  2  3

9. When a salesperson makes an effort, do you find it hard to say "No" even though the merchandise is not really what you want?  0  1  2  (3)

10. When a latecomer is waited on before you are, do you call attention to the situation?  0  (1)  2  3

11. Are you reluctant to speak up in a discussion or debate?  0  (1)  2  3

12. If a person has borrowed money (or a book, garment, thing of value) and is overdue in returning it, do you mention it?  (0)  1  2  3

13. Do you continue to pursue an argument after the other person has had enough?  0  (1)  2  3

14. Do you generally express what you feel?  0  (1)  2  3

15. Are you disturbed if someone watches you at work?  0  (1)  2  3

16. If someone keeps kicking or bumping your chair in a movie or a lecture, do you ask the person to stop?  0  1  (2)  3

17. Do you find it difficult to keep eye contact when talking to another person?  0  (1)  2  3

18. In a good restaurant, when your meal is improperly prepared or served, do you ask the waiter/waitress to correct the situation?  (0)  1  2  3

19. When you discover merchandise is faulty, do you return it for an adjustment?  0  (1)  2  3

20. Do you show your anger by name-calling or obscenities?  0  (1)  2  3

21. Do you try to be a wallflower or a piece of the furniture in social situations?  0  (1)  2  3

22. Do you insist that your property manager (mechanic, repairman, etc.) make repairs, adjustments or replacements which are his/her responsibility?  0  1  2  (3)

23. Do you often step in and make decisions for others?  (0)  1  2  3

24. Are you able to express love and affection openly?  0  1  (2)  3

25. Are you able to ask your friends for small favors or help?  (0)  1  2  3

26. Do you think you always have the right answer?  (0)  1  2  3

27. When you differ with a person you respect, are you able to speak up for your own viewpoint?  0  1  2  (3)

28. Are you able to refuse unreasonable requests made by friends?  (0)  1  2  3

29. Do you have difficulty complimenting or praising others?  0  1  2  (3)

30. If you are disturbed by someone smoking near you, can you say so?  0  (1)  2  3

31. Do you shout or use bullying tactics to get others to do as you wish?  0  (1)  2  3

32. Do you finish other people's sentences for them?  0  (1)  2  3

33. Do you get into physical fights with others, especially with strangers?  (0)  1  2  3

34. At family meals, do you control the conversation?  (0)  1  2  3

35. When you meet a stranger, are you first to introduce yourself and begin a conversation?  (0)  1  2  3

From *Your Perfect Right: A Guide to Assertive Living*, 7th ed. © 1995 by Robert E. Alberti and Michael L. Emmons. Reproduced for Myrna La Fleur-Brooks by permission of Impact Publishers, Inc., P.O. Box 1094. San Luis Obispo, CA 93406, with permission. Further reproduction prohibited.

## Broken Record

The broken record is an assertiveness skill that allows you to say no over and over again without raising your voice or getting irritated or angry. You must be persistent and not give reasons, excuses, or explanations for not doing what the other person wants you to do. By doing this you can ignore manipulative traps and argumentive baiting.

> **E X A M P L E**
>
> Jane: "Let's go to lunch."
>
> Sue: "Thanks for asking; however, *I can't go, I just started a new diet.*"
>
> Jane: "So what! You start a new diet every week. It has never stopped you from going before."
>
> Sue: "Well, thanks anyway, but *I just started a new diet, I can't go to lunch.*"
>
> Jane: "Well you don't have to eat anything fattening."
>
> Sue: "Thanks anyway. *I can't go. I just started a new diet.*"

## Fogging

Fogging is an assertiveness skill that allows you to accept manipulative criticism and anxiety-producing statements by offering no resistance and by using a noncommittal reply, calmly acknowledging that there may be some truth in what the critic is saying, yet retaining the right to remain your own judge. When you use fogging, it is hard for the other person to see exactly what you are saying.

### EXAMPLE

John: "You are really a slow worker!"

Bill: "*I can see it may appear that I am a slow worker; however, I have only been here a month. I will speed up once I know the procedures better.*"

## Negative Assertion

Negative assertion is an assertiveness skill that allows you to accept your errors and faults without becoming defensive or resorting to anger. It is a technique of admitting errors without affecting your worth as a human being. It includes not using self-depreciation, such as "that was so stupid of me."

### EXAMPLE

Dr. Smith: "You didn't order the CBC on Mr. Jones yesterday."

Sue: "*You're right. I did not order it, I apologize. Should I order it today?*"

## Negative Inquiry

Negative inquiry is an assertiveness skill that allows you to actively prompt criticism in order to use the information, or if manipulative, to exhaust it. By doing this you obtain clarification about the criticism and hopefully bring out possible hidden issues that may really be the point.

### EXAMPLE

Nurse manager: "Your work is getting sloppy, if you want to stay on this unit you will have to change."

Unit coordinator: "*You say my work is sloppy. What is it about my work that is sloppy?*"

### EXERCISE 2

Practice writing verbal responses to the situations described below. Use the behavioral style indicated.

1. A coworker comes in at 3:00 PM and finds that the diet sheets were not completed for the entire unit. She throws the clipboard down in front of you and storms off. It was not your job to complete the diet sheets.

*Assertive:*

*I'm sorry your so angry. but completing the diet sheets are not part of my job. If you Like I have time I could help you out by doing them for you when I'm not busy.*

*Nonassertive:*

*I'll try to do them later if I have time. so don't get angry at me.*

*Aggressive:*

*Its too bad that they were not compleated but its not my job and I'm not going to do it for you*

2. You have been asked to float to the pediatric unit. You work on orthopedics. When you arrive on Peds, a nurse says to you: "It would really be nice to get someone who knows what he's doing."

*Nonassertive:*

*I think I'm qualified for the job and I hope I can live up to your expectations*

*Assertive (use negative inquiry):*

*You think you need some one who knows what their doing? Well, I think I'm the one your looking for.*

*Aggressive:*

*I know exactly what I'm doing. so don't worry about it.*

3. You forgot to order a CBC yesterday while transcribing Mr. Jones' orders. When the error was discovered by the nurse manager she said, "You didn't order the CBC on Mr. Jones yesterday!"

*Aggressive:*

I just forgot anybody can make a mistake I'll order it when I have time.

*Nonassertive:*

I'm sorry, I'm so stupid. It won't happen again. ~~can it~~ ~~still~~ order Is it too late to order it.

*Assertive (use negative assertion):*

Your right, I did not order it, I apologize. Should I order it today?

4. A local celebrity is a patient on your unit. The doctor has left strict instructions that only relatives can visit the patient and for only short periods. A visitor has just approached the nursing station. He claims he is the local celebrity's manager and must see the patient about some financial matters today.

*Nonaggressive:*

I really don't think you can see mr so & so, he's only supposed to see relatives so ~~I don't~~ you really can't go in.

*Aggressive:*

Mr. ~~So & So~~ The ~~doctor~~ has given me express orders not to let anyone but relatives visit mr so & so. at this time you will have to come back when he's feeling better.

*Assertive (use broken record):*

You can't go in to see mr so & so, Im

sorry but only relatives can see Mr so & so you really can't see him today.

5. Your immediate supervisor has just told you that your work is simply sloppy and to improve it or else.

*Assertive (use negative inquiry):*

You think my work is sloppy what is it about my work that you think is so sloppy that I can't improve on.

*Nonassertive:*

I didn't realize my work was so sloppy I'll try really hard to improve so I don't lose my job.

*Aggressive:*

What is your definition of sloppy. Whats sloppy to you might not be sloppy to me. What are you going to do fire me if I don't Improve

6. It is 9:00 AM, and Dr. Jones has asked you to please locate the CBC results he ordered yesterday on Mr. Smith. You call the lab, and you cannot immediately locate them. When you tell this to Dr. Jones he responds angrily, "What in the hell is going on here? Can't anybody do anything right on this unit?"

*Nonassertive:* Im sorry Dr. I don't know what happened but your right Dr. nobody can do anything right around here, it seems. ~~and~~

*Aggressive:* How do I know whats going on don't get mad at me It's not my fault

_____

_____

*Assertive* (use fogging):

> I can see that your angry but I think that we'll be able to find the missing lab test lets hope it doesn't happen again

## How To Improve Performance Of Communication Skills Under Stressful Situations

All of the communication skills mentioned so far are excellent techniques and work well. They will become easier for you the more you practice. Practice until they become second nature. Rehearse at home or with your friends until you feel comfortable using all of the assertive skills presented in this section. The importance of rehearsal is emphasized in the following story. A young man with a violin case in his arms rushed up out of a subway entrance in New York City and hurried to a man sitting on a nearby park bench and said, "Pardon me sir, can you tell me how to get to Carnegie Hall?" The man replied, "Practice, practice, practice!"

Two ways to increase the effectiveness of your practice of the new skills is to use **visualization** and verbal repetition of assertive statements. Visualization is the process of creating a scene in your mind, using your senses to see and hear yourself doing the behavior, and to imagine the way the body feels as you successfully carry out the skill you are practicing. People vary in their ability to visualize, but even if at first the scene is hazy continue to rehearse and the mental rehearsal will significantly reinforce your mastery of these useful communication techniques.

Even with mastery of the assertive skills, producing assertive behavior in stressful situations will depend on your ability to call upon the correct part of your personality at the time the skills are needed. Eric Berne, the originator of a theory of personality called transactional analysis, described the personality as having three parts or **ego states**: the **parent**, the **adult**, and the **child** (1973). When we are in stressful situations, there is a tendency to communicate from the child or parent ego states. In these situations, if one uses the child ego state, where feelings are stored, there will be a tendency to be nonassertive. Using the parent ego state under stress, where opinions are stored, may result in aggressive behavior. The adult ego state is the best part of the personality to use under stress because it contains *thoughts* about information (Kahler, 1978) and is uncontaminated by prejudice or fear.

When the adult is active, the person will respond to the environment based on learnings and experience recorded in the adult "computer." The adult looks at the world objectively and uses the facts recorded there to decide how to act. Adult ego state data banks are continuously updated with new information. A person communicating from an uncontaminated adult ego state is willing to change opinions in the presence of new information and is capable of using the communication techniques presented in this chapter.

Under stress you will often have to make a conscious effort to activate your adult to choose the most appropriate response for the situation at hand. Here's how to do it. Stand or sit up straight, with your head level and hands to sides, palms facing out to the front, and take a deep breath. These are the postures and gestures of the adult ego state and assuming the postures helps activate it. Next, think about what you will say and do. Recall the visualization of yourself successfully performing the desired behavior, then *do it*.

Use the adult to get your work done and to deal with stressful situations. Don't send a child (your child ego state in this case) to do an adult's job.

## Why is the "Adult" Sometimes Not Called Upon

As has been pointed out, it is necessary to stay in the "adult" ego state to successfully deal with work problems. Taibi Kahler (1978) says that in everyday communication most people respond in an automatic overlearned fashion based on messages they continually received as children. These responses, as you will see, are often ineffective in the daily work situation.

Kahler called these automatic responses "**drivers**," and he identified five of them. They are to "hurry up," "be perfect," "please me (someone else)," "try hard," and "be strong." "Drivers" are so common that most people exhibit one or two predominately but use all of them from time to time. He says people can function less automatically and more **autonomously** by recognizing driver messages and replacing them with adult messages. The adult message functions as an **antidote**.

Remember that when carrying out instructions of a driver we are using the child ego state rather than the adult ego state, which is the one we have to activate to call up assertive techniques. Not only are assertive techniques unavailable to us while unconsciously responding to these internal drivers, a further problem with drivers is that they are dysfunctional for living in a real world. They don't work. Some examples of common effects of driver behaviors follow.

_____

"Hurry up" behavior results in making mistakes and skipping important activities, and ends up taking more time in the long run.

EXAMPLE

While hurrying to complete orders on the chart, an important preoperative instruction for a diabetic patient is missed and surgery must be canceled.

Adult antidote: **It's OK to give things the time they take.**

"**Be perfect**" behavior stands in the way of making progress by delaying any action until things are done perfectly.

EXAMPLE

You have just enough time to file lab reports on about five charts but want to be perfect and do all lab filing at once. Nothing gets done and filing piles up.

Adult antidote: **It's OK to be imperfect** (and do part of the job.)

The person doing a "**please me**" driver does not use assertive behavior because by attempting to please someone else he or she does not say "no," and usually ends up pleasing no one.

EXAMPLE

Two doctors make stat requests for you to order emergency equipment. You want to please them both and do not assertively ask them to clarify among themselves which has priority. You attempt to do both and pick the less important of the two and are also delayed. Both doctors are displeased.

Adult antidote: **Please yourself** (i.e., in most situations use *your* best judgment about the best thing to do). In this situation, that would be to get clear by asking them to decide and tell you which is needed first.

"**Try hard**" messages invite a person to *try* rather than *do* things.

EXAMPLE

Your supervisor instructs you to try to clean up your work area. That's what you do—you try and try but don't get the job done.

Adult antidote: **Do it.**

"**Be strong**" drivers cause people to discount their needs and feelings. They fail to use stress management techniques to reduce the effects of stress in their lives because they do not acknowledge needs and feelings.

EXAMPLE

You have lost sleep for months replaying hostile remarks made by your supervisor. Using alcohol is the way you eventually get to sleep. You have pains in your stomach but feel you are being weak and ought to be able to "be strong" and take it.

Adult antidote: **It's OK to have needs and feelings and take care of yourself.** Write out a script for dealing with the situation and have an assertive conversation with your supervisor to comment on the process between the two of you. If this is unwise in your work situation, design another script for dealing with the situation and have an assertive conversation with *yourself*. You may decide to learn stress management if you stay, or you may decide to get a different job.

EXERCISE 3

Assume the adult ego state position and practice visualization by imagining yourself successfully performing the assertive responses you listed in Exercise 2. Practice visualizing your assertive response to:

1. The "A coworker comes in at 3:00 PM" example
2. The "You have been asked to float to the pediatric unit" example
3. The "You forgot to order a CBC yesterday" example
4. The "A local celebrity is a patient on your unit" example
5. The "Your immediate supervisor has just told you that your work is simply sloppy" example
6. The "It is 9:00 AM, and Dr. Jones has asked you" example

## SUMMARY

In your role as the communicator for the nursing unit, the importance of using assertive communication and interpersonal skills cannot be overstated. Following the guidelines for practicing confidentiality is also a must to protect the rights of the patients.

**REVIEW QUESTIONS**

1. List in order the first four levels of Maslow's hierarchy of human needs, starting with the most basic.

   a. _Physiological needs_

   b. _Safety and security Needs_

   c. _belonging and love_

   d. _esteem needs_

2. Below are listed instances of human needs. Identify each need as belonging to one of the four levels of Maslow's hierarchy of human needs that you listed above. Write the alphabetical letter preceding the level in the space provided to indicate your answer.

   a. _A_ the need for oxygen

   b. _A_ the need for shelter

   c. _B_ the need to be safe from danger

   d. _C_ the need to be loved

   e. _D_ the need for respect

   f. _D_ the need to feel self-confident

   g. _D_ the need for self-respect

   h. _C_ the need to belong

   i. _A_ the need for exercise

   j. _C_ the need for the feeling of security

   k. _B_ the need for uniformity

   l. _A_ the need for food

   m. _B_ the need to be free from the fear of death

   n. _C_ the need to be accepted by others

   o. _A_ the need for water

   p. _B_ the need for special status

3. Write an example of a behavior situation that exemplifies each of the first four needs outlined by Maslow.

   a. _a baby cries in the middle of the night it either is hungry or needs its diaper changed - physiological needs_

   b. _your parents are separating they don't tell you until you ask "wheres daddy you feel insecure and think its your fault_

   c. _your getting married and you own rite over 200 people only ½ of them show up because most of your supposed friends_

   _Went to the Company Picnic. You feel unloved._

   d. _you have just graduated with a bachelor of Science degree after 5 gruelling years of work. Every one is so proud of you and you feel good about yourself._

4. Describe how the health unit coordinator may practice confidentiality in the following situations.

a. You are having dinner in the cafeteria with several other health workers. A famous television star was admitted to your unit yesterday. The talk turns to the patient. You are asked "Is she really only 35?" . . . "What is her diagnosis?" . . . and other personal questions. What is your response?

_I really cannot divulge any discuss anything about Mr. So & So. It's the hospital Rules. Let's talk about something else._

b. You are working at the nurses' station and you notice a patient's wife approaching your desk. At the same time, two other members of the hospital staff, unaware of the wife's presence, begin talking about her husband's condition. What do you do?

_give them the hint by calling out to the woman by her name and steering her away from ear shot._

c. A patient approaches you at the nurses' station and says, "My roommate hasn't eaten anything today. I'm really worried about her. What is she in the hospital for?" How do you answer?

_I wouldn't worry Mrs so & so, your roomate is getting the best possible care she can get. If she wants to tell you what she's in for I'm sure she will but_

_I'm not able to divulge you that Information_

d. A telephone caller says that he is a reporter from the local newspaper and wants to know if a car accident victim was admitted to your nursing unit. What do you tell him?

_That you have no Idea, and if you did you wouldn't be able to give out any information its hospital policy_

e. You answer the telephone on the nursing unit. The caller states that he is a relative of the patient and asks for personal patient information. The patient is hospitalized for a gunshot wound received during a fight. You are somewhat doubtful about the identity of the caller. How do you handle the situation? _Tell him you can't give out information_

_over the Phone & Ask him his name and number and tell him you will give it to the patient and when he's able he will call him back._

f. You are riding home on the bus after work. Another hospital employee sits down beside you and states, "That was quite a code you had on your unit today. What all happened anyway." How do you respond?

_Tell her that you can't discuss it with her and that she should know you can't break confidentiality_

g. You are out in your yard and your neighbor stops to chat with you. During the conversation, your neighbor tells you her friend is in the hospital on the same nursing unit on which you work. The neighbor asks you what is wrong with her friend and how long she will be in the hospital. What do you tell her?

_I'm not allowed to discuss a patient outside of the hospital to anyone except relatives may know about the patient_

5. Define the following terms:

a. sender: _the person transmitting the message_

b. message: _Images feelings and Ideas transmitted_

c. receiver: _the person recieving the message_

d. feedback: _response to the message_

e encoding: _translating the images feeling and Ideas Into symbols In order to communicate_

f. decoding: _determining the meaning of the message_

6. Two health unit coordinator responsibilities for maintaining confidentiality of patient information are:

a. _not to repeatedly repeat confidential information_

b. _Control the patient chart in a manner that maintains confidentiality of the contents_

7. Three guidelines to follow to maintain confidentiality of the contents of a patient's chart are:

a. _Prohibit hospital patient from duplicating portions of the patients chart_

b. _Control Access to the patients chart_

c. _control tranportation of the chart_

8. Four components of the communication process are:

a. _Sender_

b. _Message_

c. _Reciever_

d. _Feedback_

9. Using the communication model, demonstrate a successful communication process and an unsuccessful communication process. Identify at which step of the process the errors occurred.

   a. Successful communication:

   _____

   _____

   _____

   _____

   b. Unsuccessful communication:

   _____

   _____

   _____

   _____

10. List two common errors in encoding a message.

    a. _____ poor choice of words to use _____

    _____

    b. _____ inconsistency between verbal and non verbal messages _____

11. List two common errors in decoding a message.

    a. _____ Inconsistency in the verbal and non verbal symbols from the sender. _____

    b. _____ Life style, age, cultural background, environment and poor listening habits. _____

12. Evaluate your own listening skills. Identify areas that need improvement and record methods you could use for improvement.

    _____ I tend to interrupt some times and I should teach myself to concentrate I could apologize and check myself before I interrupt. Sometimes I have to listen more closely so I know what being said _____

13. Evaluate your feedback skills. Discuss how your feedback can improve the communication process.

    _____ I could use paraphrasing by repeating the message to the sender in my own words _____

    _____

    _____

    _____

14. Practice identifying the types of human needs listed below. Read each sentence, then write in the space provided the need expressed. Record an appropriate response.

*Situation 1:*

   Patient: "I just can't believe I am having exploratory surgery tomorrow. I hope it's not cancer."

Need expressed: _assurance - safety + security_

Appropriate feedback:
_Why would you think you have cancer do you want to talk about your feelings._

*Situation 2:*

   Patient: "Tell the nurse I need something for this pain right away."

Need expressed: _physiological_

Appropriate feedback:
_~~your nurse~~ your nurse I will page your nurse and tell her your in pain._

*Situation 3:*

   Health unit coordinator: "They have asked me to run for office in our local chapter of NAHUC. I said I would."

Need expressed: _esteem_

Appropriate feedback:
_I think its wonderful that they chose you for nurse and hope by you make it._

*Situation 4:*

   Patient: "When you get to be my age you won't have many friends who are able to visit you when you are in the hospital."

Need expressed: _Belonging + Love needs_

Appropriate feedback:
_____

_____

*Situation 5:*

   Health unit coordinator: "I made such a mess out of running that meeting, I feel like a complete idiot."

Need expressed: _esteem_

Appropriate feedback:
_I don't think it was as bad as you think. practice makes perfect_

*Situation 6*:

    Child: "You are not going to stick *me* with that needle."

Need expressed: _____

Appropriate feedback:

_____

_____


*Situation 7*:

    Nurse: "I really like my job, but somehow it isn't enough. I might start looking for something else to do."

Need expressed: _____

Appropriate feedback:

_____

_____


*Situation 8*:

    Patient: "Just a minute, are you saying that I didn't have the watch with me when I came into the hospital?"

Need expressed: _____

Appropriate feedback:

_____

_____


15. Describe a time when you felt satisfied and happy.

_____

_____

_____

What need was being satisfied?

_____


16. Describe a time when you felt unsatisfied and unhappy.

_____

_____

_____

What need was not being satisfied?

_____

17. The three main parts of the personality are called ego states. Name them and list the corresponding pattern of behavior expressed by each:

| | Ego State | Pattern of Behavior |
|---|---|---|
| a. | *Parent* | *projects Inner, opinions beliefs Values child* |
| b. | *child* | *stores feeling + emotions projects inner child* |
| c. | *Adult* | *stores facts + Information* |

18. A visitor, Mrs. Jones, rushes up to the unit and asks to speak to Dr. White about her father who had been admitted to the unit for observation after a "dizzy spell." Mrs. Jones is obviously agitated, has a frightened look on her face, and says to Dr. White, "Doctor, What has happened to my father? Is he going to die? What are you going to do for him?"

Dr. White responds, "Now, Mrs. Jones, settle down, there is no use getting everyone upset. Control yourself, I'm very busy right now!" The doctor walks down the hall.

Mr. Smith, the health unit coordinator, says to Mrs. Jones, "Mrs. Jones, the nurse in charge, Ms. West, has spoken to the admitting physician and knows the status of your father's condition. She is coming down the hall now and I will ask her to speak to you."

Identify the ego state each person was using in this scenario:

a. Mrs. Jones *child*

b. Dr. White *Parent*

c. Ms. Smith *Adult*

19. List the five "driver" behaviors and their antidotes.

| | Driver | Antidote |
|---|---|---|
| a. | *hurry up* | *give things the time they take* |
| b. | *be perfect* | *its okay to be imperfect* |
| c. | *please somone else* | *Please yourself* |
| d. | *try hard* | *do it* |
| e. | *be strong* | *you have needs and feelings too take care of yourself* |

## References

Alberti, Robert E. and Emmons, Michael L.: *Your Perfect Right*, 3rd ed. San Luis Obispo, CA, Impact Publishers, 1978.

Allaire, Barbara and McNeil, Robert: *Teaching Patient Relations in Hospitals*. Chicago, American Hospital Publishing, Inc., 1983.

Berne, Eric: *What Do You Say After You Say Hello?* New York, Bantam Books, published by arrangement with Grove Press, 1973.

Bower, S. A. and Bower, G.: *Asserting Yourself*. Reading, MA, Addison-Wesley, 1976.

Gerrard, Brian A. et al: *Interpersonal Skills for Health Professionals*. Reston, VA, Reston Publishing Company, Inc., 1980.

Kahler, Taibi: *Transactional Analysis Revisited*. Little Rock, AR, Human Development Publications, 1978.

King, Mark, et al: *Irresistible Communication*. Philadelphia, W. B. Saunders Co., 1983.

Masterson, John T. et al: *Speech Communication Theory and Practice*. New York, Holt, Rinehart and Winston, 1983.

Purtilo, Ruth and Haddad, Amy: *Health Professional and Patient Interaction*, 5th ed. Philadelphia, W. B. Saunders Co., 1996.

Weaver, Richard L., II: *Understanding Interpersonal Communication*. Glenview, Scott Foresman and Company, 1978.

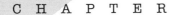
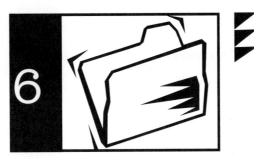

# MEDICAL/LEGAL
# CONSIDERATIONS

## CHAPTER OBJECTIVES

*Upon completion of this chapter, you will be able to:*

1. Define the terms in the vocabulary list.

2. Identify the legal elements necessary to prove a claim of medical malpractice.

3. Explain what the standard of care is for a health unit coordinator.

4. Identify two preventive measures that you can take to minimize the risk of malpractice within your own practice.

5. List two purposes of "A Patient's Bill of Rights."

6. Identify the basic principles involved in medical ethics and their application in health unit coordinating.

## VOCABULARY

**Accountability** • Being answerable to someone for something you have done

**Damages** • Monetary compensation awarded by a court for an injury caused by the act of another

**Defendant** • The person against whom a civil or criminal action is brought

**Deposition** • Pretrial statement of a witness under oath, taken in question-and-answer form as it would be in court, with opportunity given to the adversary to be present to cross-examine

**Ethics** • A term for the study of how we make judgments in regard to right and wrong

**Evidence** • All the means by which any alleged matter of fact, the truth of which is submitted to investigation at trial, is established or disproved; evidence includes the testimony of witnesses, introduction of records, documents, exhibits, objects, or any other substantiating matter offered for the purpose of inducing belief in the party's contention by the judge or jury

**Expert Witness** • A witness having special knowledge of the subject about which he or she is to testify; the knowledge must generally be such as is not normally possessed by the average person

**Informed Consent** • A doctrine that states that before a patient is asked to consent to a risky or invasive diagnostic or treatment procedure he or she is entitled to receive certain information: (1) a description of the procedure, (2) any alternatives to it and their risks, (3) the risks of death or serious bodily disability from the procedure, (4) the probable results of the procedure, including any problems of recuperation and time of recuperation anticipated, and (5) anything else that is generally disclosed to patients asked to consent to the procedure

**Liability** • The condition of being responsible either for damages resulting from an injurious act or from discharging an obligation or debt

**Medical Malpractice** • Professional negligence of a health care professional; failure to meet a professional standard of care resulting in harm to another, for example, failure to provide "good and accepted medical care"

**Negligence** • Failure to satisfactorily perform one's legal duty, such that another person incurs some injury

**Plaintiff** • The person who brings a lawsuit against another

**Respondeat Superior** • (Latin) "Let the master answer." Legal doctrine that imposes liability upon the employer. *Note:* The employee is also liable for his own actions

**Standard of Care** • The legal duty one owes to another according to the circumstances of a particular case; it is the care that a reasonable and prudent person would have exercised in the given situation

**Statute** • A law passed by the legislature and signed by the governor at the state level and the president at the federal level

**Statute of Limitations** • The time within which a plaintiff must bring a civil suit; the limit varies depending upon the type of suit, and it is set by the various state legislatures

**Tort** • A wrong against another person or his property that is not a crime but for which the law provides a remedy

## BACKGROUND INFORMATION

The law is derived from three sources: (1) the constitution—both federal and state constitutions; (2) statutes—written laws drawn up by the legislature; and (3) common law—a case-by-case determination by a judge of what is fair under a given set of facts. Laws are subject to change, but common law is especially changeable because each case presented to a judge is different. Judges look to cases that have been decided previously for guidance on how to rule in a particular situation. However, a judge is free to interpret the law where no precedent exists or to interpret against precedent. Most medical negligence or medical malpractice law is derived from common law. That means that medical negligence law, like other forms of common law, is constantly in a state of change.

The role of the health unit coordinator has expanded broadly in the last 5 years. You are now recognized as an essential member of the health care team. Incidental to this greater recognition and expanding responsibility comes increased accountability. There is a liability dimension to accountability. The health unit coordinator may be held legally responsible for judgments exercised and actions taken in the course of practice.

## STANDARD OF CARE

While working as a health unit coordinator, you are responsible for performing at the level of competence of other health unit coordinators who work under circumstances similar to your own. This responsibility is your legal duty as a health care professional and is the **standard of care** to which you will be held. If you do not carry out this duty and a patient is injured as a result, you have been negligent of your duty and you may be held liable for your actions.

The standard of care is established by **expert witness** testimony. An expert is a person who is trained in your profession and who testifies at trial as to what a reasonably prudent health unit coordinator would have done under the circumstances in question. Evidence of the standard of care may also be found in textbooks, standards from your professional organization, and medical journals, the *Physicians' Desk Reference*, policy and procedure manuals, or standards of the Joint Commission on the Accreditation of Healthcare organizations. This means that you must keep up with the current practices in your profession, read current literature, be familiar with hospital policies and procedures affecting your job, and know your job description and the duties it details.

The standard of care for which you are responsible becomes higher with your increased experience and education. Your actions will be compared with those of a reasonably prudent health unit coordinator with the same experience and education under the same circumstances.

## NEGLIGENCE

*Negligence* is a legal term that means that someone did not satisfactorily perform his or her legal duty, and another person was injured in some way because of it. This breach of duty can occur when something is done that shouldn't be or when something should be done but isn't. Either way, the person responsible for the duty is liable for whatever injury is suffered by the innocent party.

For instance, one of your duties as a health unit coordinator is to transcribe doctors' orders accurately and promptly. If you are negligent in doing so—that is, you don't transcribe the orders properly or don't transcribe them at all—you may be responsible for a patient's injury that results from your negligence.

## LIABILITY

Legally, each of you is responsible for your own acts. When those acts are negligent and are done in the course and scope of your employment as a health unit coordinator, they have special ramifications.

As a hospital employee, the hospital is also **liable** for your negligence on the job because of the legal doctrine *respondeat superior* (which means, "let the master respond"). This means that you *and* the hospital are held responsible for your negligent acts on the job. Remember that the hospital is liable for your actions only when they occur within the course and scope of your employment. If the negligent act is a result of conduct outside the scope of your employment—in other words, outside your job description—you *alone* are held responsible.

The *respondeat superior* doctrine does not take away your personal liability but instead creates an additional party for the injured person to hold responsible for the damage he or she has incurred.

## CONSENTS

As a health unit coordinator, you may be requested to witness a signature of a person consenting to a procedure or surgery. The reason a consent is signed is to document that the person signing has been informed of the risks and characteristics of the procedure and understands them. This is called an **informed consent** and is a mandatory prerequisite for any invasive procedure or surgery.

Your job as a witness to a signature is to verify that the person signing is actually the person whose signature they sign and to make a judgment as to whether it appears that the person is competent to sign a binding, legal document. Competency is a determination you make by the way the patient appears to you. For instance, are they alert and coherent, or under the influence of alcohol or drugs? If you suspect that someone is not competent to sign a consent, check with your supervisor prior to witnessing the consent.

Sometimes an emergency situation may arise in which it is medically inadvisable to wait until a consent form can be signed. This is a medical judgment and is an exception to the mandatory rule. There are some additional special consent situations that may arise during a patient's hospitalization. These may involve an AMA (leaving the hospital against medical advice), a sterilization consent, or a telephone consent. Check your hospital's policy and procedure manual to see if any further precautions are necessary to witness these special consents prior to doing so. For instance, your hospital may require that both husband *and* wife sign a consent for a sterilization procedure or that only nurses witness a telephone consent or that a doctor be notified before witnessing the signing of an AMA document.

## DOCUMENTS

The medical record and chart are permanent legal documents that are the property of the hospital. Everything that is put into the chart is part of the permanent record. That is why everything must be written in ink, and no erasures are allowed. Be specific, accurate, and current in recording the patient's medical record. Be sure that all documentation in a patient's record is legible.

Because the medical record is the legal record of the patient's medical course, you must treat it with the same special care and confidentiality you would other legal documents. No one who is not authorized may read charts or have access to them, nor are medical personnel allowed to read charts randomly for curiosity or non–health-care-related reasons. This protection of the legal record is part of your duty as a health unit coordinator.

## ETHICS

Ethics is that part of philosophy that deals with judgments of what is right or wrong in given situations. Each health care profession has a code of ethics that essentially is derived from a set of basic principles that define our concepts of right or wrong.

## Principles of Medical Ethics

### Autonomy

This principle means that an individual is free to choose and implement one's own decisions. From this basic principle, we have derived the rule involved in informed consent. The American Hospital Association issued a policy titled "A Patient's Bill of Rights" (see below) with the ex-

### A PATIENT'S BILL OF RIGHTS

1. The patient has the right to considerate and respectful care.
2. A patient has the right to obtain from his doctor complete current information concerning his diagnosis, treatment, and prognosis in terms the patient can understand.
3. The patient has the right to receive from his physician information necessary to give informed consent prior to the start of any procedure and/or treatment.
4. The patient has the right to refuse treatment to the extent permitted by law and to be informed of the medical consequences of his actions.
5. The patient has the right to every consideration of his privacy regarding his medical care. Those not directly involved in the patient's care must have the patient's permission to be present during case discussions.
6. The patient has the right to expect that all communications and records pertaining to his care should be treated as confidential.
7. The patient has the right to expect that within its capacity a hospital must make reasonable response to the request of a patient for services.
8. The patient has the right to obtain information as to any relationship of his hospital to other health care and educational institutions insofar as his care is concerned. The patient has the right to obtain information as to the existence of any professional relationship among individuals, by name, who are treating him.
9. The patient has the right to be informed of any human experiments affecting his care and to refuse to participate in such research programs.
10. The patient has the right to expect reasonable continuity of care including care after discharge.
11. The patient has the right to examine and receive an explanation of his hospital bill.
12. The patient has the right to know what hospital rules and regulations apply to his conduct as a patient.

pectation that observance of these rights will result in more effective patient care and greater satisfaction for the patient, the patient's physician, and the health care organization. This bill of rights states that a patient has the right to refuse treatment to the extent permitted by law and be informed of the medical consequences of his actions. The right does not judge the quality of a decision by a patient to refuse treatment, only that the patient has the right to make the decision. This is the process of autonomy at work.

### Veracity

The principle of veracity requires both the health professional and the patient to tell the truth. The health professional must disclose the truth so that the patient can practice autonomy and the patient must be truthful so that appropriate care can be given. Although there are situations where health professionals may feel justified in lying to a patient to avoid some greater harm, other alternatives must be sought. Lying will almost always harm patient autonomy and cause the potential loss of provider credibility.

### Beneficence

This is the principle that any action a health professional may take will benefit the patient. This principle creates an ethical dilemma for clinical practitioners more so than health unit coordinators. The dilemma arises due to the advanced technology available to practitioners today. In cases where a patient is maintained on life support machines and is in a coma or vegetative state, is it of benefit to maintain the patient on the machines?

### Nonmaleficence

This principle, which comes from the Hippocratic oath, means that a health professional will never inflict harm on the patient. Although similar to the principle of beneficence, it differs in that beneficence indicates a positive action promoting the good. In nonmaleficence, the principle is to refrain from inflicting harm. Health unit coordinators should always be aware of the seriousness of transcribing doctors' orders, since an error may result in harm to the patient.

### Confidentiality

Principle 2 of the National Association of Health Unit Coordinators Code of Ethics (Chapter 1, Table 1–2) and the American Hospital Association's "A Patients' Bill of Rights" outline the individual's right to privacy in health care. Health unit coordinators who breach the confidentiality of a patient's medical record have not only violated ethical standards, but may well have violated the law.

Ethical issues and legal issues often become intertwined in the health care context. An ethical dilemma is a situation that presents a conflicting moral claim, a situation that

is at odds with your personal system of values. Sometimes conflicts can occur between what is legal and what is ethical. For example, assume you are working in a gynecology clinic and a patient comes in for an abortion. You may believe that abortions should not be performed and are unethical. However, abortions are legal in our country.

To deal with these situations as a health unit coordinator, you must learn to examine your values and be aware of how they affect your work. All health care professionals must learn methods of reasoning through ethical dilemmas rather than reacting to them emotionally. The issues that may arise and cause conflict are usually situations involving the privacy rights of patients or unprofessional conduct of a fellow health care worker.

In any of the potential problem areas you may run into as a health unit coordinator, you must apply your good judgment, honesty, and reasoning to come up with a moral and ethical way to resolve the conflict.

## What Can You Do?

Here are some tips to avoid legal problems while working as a health unit coordinator:

- *Know your job description.* Don't engage in activities outside your job description.
- *Keep current with your employing agency's policy and procedures.* If you believe the policies and procedures are outdated, bring them to your employer's attention, and see that they are revised.
- *Keep current in your practice.* If you are called upon to do something you are not qualified to do, get help and find out how. Remember, a standard of care can be set by medical literature and periodicals. Continued education is a must for all health care workers. Needless to say, make sure you have the proper training before you assume any position.
- *Don't assume anything.* Question orders, policies, and procedures that don't seem appropriate. Don't do something unless you are sure you know how to do it. Ask questions; it is your biggest safeguard.
- *Do not undertake to perform nursing tasks even as favors.*
- *Be aware of the relationships with patients.* Patients who truly feel you care and have tried to help them to the best of your abilities are less likely to see a lawyer if a problem arises.

## SUMMARY

The modern health care professional is called upon to exercise professional judgment in many complex situations. Through understanding your legal duty and ethical responsibility, you will be able to legally and morally fulfill your professional obligations.

**REVIEW QUESTIONS**

I. Match the terms in column I with the phrases in column II.

EXERCISE 1

**Column I**

a. _9_ accountability

b. _7_ defendant

c. _1_ ethics

d. _6_ expert witness

e. _4_ statute

f. _3_ tort

**Column II**

1. judgments of right or wrong
2. answerable for what you have done
3. a wrong, which is not a crime
4. a law
5. a person against whom action is brought
6. a witness having special knowledge
7. a person who brings a lawsuit against another
8. professional negligence
9. responsible for damage resulting from an injurious act

EXERCISE 2

a. _5_ statute of limitations

b. _9_ damages

c. _6_ *respondeat superior*

d. _2_ deposition

e. _4_ medical malpractice

f. _7_ standard of care

g. _1_ evidence

h. _3_ informed consent

1. testimony of a witness
2. pretrial statement of a witness under oath
3. information a patient is entitled to before consenting to an invasive treatment
4. failure to provide "good and accepted medical care"
5. time within which a plaintiff must bring a suit
6. "let the master answer"
7. care that a reasonable and prudent person would have given in a similar situation
8. values, rules of conduct
9. monetary compensation

II. Indicate whether each statement is true or false.

1. T **(F)** You, as a practicing health unit coordinator, are not held legally responsible for your errors in transcription because you are not licensed.

2. T **(F)** A health unit coordinator cannot witness a signature of a patient consenting to a surgical procedure.

3. T **(F)** It is acceptable procedure to allow all medical personnel to read patients' charts, since they understand the confidential nature of their contents.

4. **(T)** (F) It is acceptable to help nurses with their tasks as long as the nurse provides close supervision and assumes responsibility for what you do.

5. **(T)** F You are transcribing an order which reads "M.S. 30 mg q4h prn pain." A call should be placed to the doctor who wrote the order for clarification prior to transcribing it.

III. For each of the following, identify the universal principle of medical ethics that is being applied.

1. The health unit coordinator safeguards the patient's right to privacy by judiciously protecting confidential information.

   Principle involved: _____ confidentiality _____

2. The health unit coordinator maintains competence in health unit coordinating.

   Principle involved: _____ standard of care _____

3. The health unit coordinator provides services with respect for the patient's right to be informed about his or her medical care.

Principle involved: ___Informed consent    Autonomy___

4. The health unit coordinator reports unethical or illegal professional activities that may harm the patient.

Principle involved: ___Ethics___

5. The health unit coordinator participates in the profession's efforts to protect patients from misinformation.

Principle involved: ___Non maliticence___

IV. Write the two purposes of "A Patient's Bill of Rights."

1. ___More effective patient care___

2. ___Greater satisfaction for the patient___

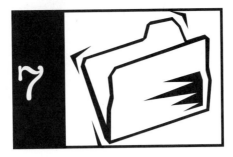

# CHAPTER 7

# MANAGEMENT TECHNIQUES FOR HEALTH UNIT COORDINATING

## CHAPTER OBJECTIVES

*Upon completion of this chapter, you will be able to:*

1. Define the terms in the vocabulary list.
2. List five areas of management.
3. Briefly discuss the management responsibilities for the nursing unit supplies and equipment.
4. Discuss the purpose of the patient activity sheet and identify seven types of information that may be recorded on it.
5. Briefly discuss a method for recording the whereabouts of patients and patients' charts and discuss why it is necessary to keep a record of this information.
6. List three management responsibilities concerning visitors on the nursing unit.
7. List three steps to follow when dealing with visitors' complaints.
8. List six items that should be within reaching distance of the health unit coordinator's desk area.
9. Given a situation in which there are several tasks to be completed, determine their order of priority.
10. List eight time-management tips.
11. Given situations that require practice of the management techniques included in this chapter, describe the appropriate behavior for each situation.
12. List the seven quality tools and define their use.

## VOCABULARY

**Change-of-Shift Report** • The communication process between shifts, in which the nursing personnel who are going "off duty" report patient care and treatment to the nursing personnel who are coming "on duty"

**Continuous Quality Improvement (CQI)** • The practice of continuously improving quality at every level of every department of every function of the health care organization

**Cycle Time Reduction** • Shortening the time it takes to complete a process; usually involves eliminating steps in a process

**Health Care Services** • All services delivered by the organization that involve professional clinical/medical judgment, including those delivered to patients and those delivered to the community

**Internal Customer** • Someone inside your organization who receives work or service from you (e.g., nursing, medical, or other administrative sections)

**Memory Sheet** • A written record of unfinished tasks

**Patient Activity Sheet** • A written record of the patients' activities

**Patient Care Support Services** • Services that support the organization's delivery of health care services to patients

**Patient Health Care Services** • Health care services provided directly to the patient for the purpose of prevention, maintenance, health promotion, screening, diagnosis, treatment/therapy, rehabilitation, or recovery

**Process** • Steps taken to complete a function that is part of a production or service outcome

**Process Simplification** • Actions taken to improve the steps for doing a function by removing unnecessary steps, doing them differently (i.e., better, shorter, faster)

**Staff** • All people who contribute to the delivery of the organization's services

**Stakeholders** • When referring to the organization's customers, these are the customers other than the patient; they could include the patient's family, the community, the insurer/third-party payer, employers, health care providers, and students

**Standard Supply List** • A written record of the amount of each item that the nursing unit should stock to last between ordering dates

**Supply Needs Sheet** • A sheet of paper used by all the nursing unit personnel to jot down items that need reordering

**Unit Log Book** • A record book or notebook used to write down unit information to pass on to other shifts, keep a record of significant events, or to record materials loaded out

## INTRODUCTION

Webster's defines *to manage* as "to control or guide." The health unit coordinator who learns to "manage or guide" certain facets within his or her job is able to enjoy the full potential of health unit coordinating.

In order to implement the management techniques discussed in this chapter, you must first understand the philosophy of your health care facility, and second, know and understand the health unit coordinating job description for your nursing unit. Upon employment, study these areas carefully.

Although the health unit coordinator position does not include the direct management of people, how the health unit coordinator manages certain aspects of the job indirectly affects the other nursing unit personnel and the clients.

Management can be divided into four areas:

1. Management of the nursing unit supplies and equipment
2. Management of the activities at the nurses' station
3. Management related to the performance of tasks
4. Management of time

## MANAGEMENT OF THE NURSING UNIT SUPPLIES AND EQUIPMENT

Your responsibility for the control of the equipment and supplies for the nursing unit will vary greatly among hospitals. However, this function definitely falls in the nonclinical category of tasks and may very well be part of your job description.

Proper management of the nursing unit supplies and equipment greatly enhances the delivery of patient care. Improper management, on the other hand, can result in minor annoyances, such as the doctor discovering that the batteries are burned out when attempting to use the unit's ophthalmoscope to examine a patient's eyes. Serious hindrances in the delivery of health care can also occur, such as failure to locate the emergency equipment during a code alert. Management of the nursing unit supplies and equipment takes you into all areas of the nursing unit. Besides the nurses' station and the patients' rooms, the nursing unit may also include the following areas:

**Kitchen:** Used to store food items and to prepare beverages and snacks for the patients.
**Linen Room:** Used to store linens.
**Lounge Area:** Used by the nursing unit personnel for conferences, coffee breaks, and other activities.
**Medication Room:** Used to store medications and used by the nurse to prepare medications for administration.
**Utility Room:** Used for the storage and care of equipment and supplies. Some hospitals have two utility rooms. One is referred to as a *contaminated* or *dirty utility room*, an area where used equipment is stored until "pick up" by the supply department where it is cleaned, sterilized, and repackaged for distribution to wards and clinics. The other storage room is a *clean utility room*, an area where unused supplies and equipment are stored.
**Waiting Room:** Used as a visiting area for the patients' relatives and friends.

## Management Responsibilities Related to Supplies and Equipment

### The Nursing Unit Supplies

Ordering of the nursing unit supplies is discussed in Chapter 21. The health unit coordinator's management responsibilities for supplies relate to the amount of supplies needed and their location on the nursing unit.

Only the needed amount of supplies should be maintained on the nursing unit. Overstocking may result in waste, since some items become outdated and are no longer useful. Understocking may result in a waste of both time and energy; in the long run this may be costly. We suggest that you maintain a **standard supply list** (Fig. 7–1)—a computerized or written record of the amount of each item that the nursing unit currently needs to last until the next supply order date. To determine and order the amount of supplies needed, simply compare the amount on the standard supply list with the amount of the item on the shelf and requisition the difference. Keep in mind that the standard supply for many items changes, and therefore you must update your standard supply list accordingly.

Standard Supply List

Top Shelf

| | |
|---|---|
| Nurses' admission record forms | 2 pkgs |
| Graphic record forms | 3 pkgs |
| Nurses' discharge planning forms | 2 pkgs |
| Laboratory report forms | 1 pkg |

Middle Shelf

| | |
|---|---|
| Diabetic record forms | 2 pkgs |
| Vital sign record forms | 3 pkgs |
| Surgery consent forms | 1 pkg |
| Consent for HIV testing forms | 1 pkg |

Lower Shelf

| | |
|---|---|
| Computer paper | 4 boxes |
| Computer labels | 2 boxes |
| Computer ribbons | 1 box |

FIGURE 7–1 • A standard supply list.

7-6-00

Supply Needs List

paper clips
medicine cards
paper cups
stool spec cups
I.V LABELS
pencils

FIGURE 7–2 • A supply needs list.

We also suggest that you maintain a **supply needs list** on the nursing unit bulletin board and instruct all the nursing unit personnel to record supplies that are running low (Fig. 7–2). Use the list as a reference for items needed when ordering supplies for the nursing unit.

Efficient placement of the supplies on the nursing unit facilitates the delivery of nursing care. Are the supplies stored in a convenient location? Are the frequently used items placed in the most accessible area? Is it easy for you to place the storeroom items on the shelf? You should discuss ideas for a more efficient location of the supplies on the nursing unit with your nurse manager.

### The Equipment Stored at the Nurses' Station

Each nursing unit has **standard equipment—flashlights, stethoscopes, ophthalmoscopes**, and so on—that is used by the doctors and nurses to examine patients. Check this equipment for working order near the beginning of your shift. If the flashlights or ophthalmoscopes need new bulbs or batteries, make sure these are replaced before the equipment is used. When the doctors and nurses are finished with the equipment, make sure it is returned to its proper storage place.

The **computer terminals** used to transfer information are used mostly by the health unit coordinator; however, at times this equipment is used by all nursing unit personnel. Since overall management of their use is the health unit coordinator's responsibility, follow your organization's computer management policies and procedures for maintenance and repair. Check computer printer ribbons and ink cartridges frequently to see that the print is clear and dark enough to read. Since ink cartridges contain hazardous materials, follow your organization's procedure for their disposal.

Updating the computer information about patients must be done at the same time any patient transaction occurs. Out-of-date computer information may result in dangerous errors (e.g., ordering duplicated medication).

**Pneumatic tube systems** are also used to transport information. The directions for the use of the tube system should be posted near the tube and be easy to understand. This is vital information, especially for students and new employees. Even small errors, such as inserting a tube in the pneumatic tube system the wrong way, can interfere with the functioning of the system throughout the hospital.

Check the **imprinter device** frequently to see that it is reproducing letters clearly, and obtain maintenance and repair as required. The patients' imprinter cards are filed in an imprinter card holder. Each holder may have spaces for 10 to 20 cards. It is important for the user to file the card in the holder immediately after use and to file it in the correct space. Clear identification on the imprinter card holder makes it easier for the user to file the imprinter card correctly. Incorrect filing of a patient's imprinter card may result in serious errors, such as imprinting the wrong patient's name on requisitions for diagnostic studies.

### The Nursing Unit Reference Materials

A small library of **textbooks**, such as the *Physicians' Desk Reference* and the hospital formulary, as well as manuals relating to the hospital itself, such as the policy manual

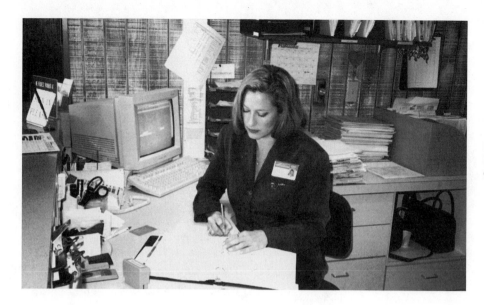

FIGURE 7–3 • Using a unit log book is useful in preserving organizational materials between shifts.

and procedure manual, are kept on the nursing unit. Make sure the textbooks are returned to the unit after use. If your unit is very busy you may want to use a sign-out system as a memory jogger for important reference material. A **unit log book** (Fig. 7–3) may be useful for signing out reference material. However, a log is even more useful for preserving organizational information between shifts. Doing what you can to keep your coworkers informed helps tie the work group together as a team. Keep the hospital manuals up to date by inserting revised material and discarding the outdated material. Keep the doctor's roster (see Chapter 4) current by writing any changes in existing data and by inserting the names and information of new staff members.

*Note*: When using the doctor's roster, locate the telephone number by checking the doctor's *specialty and/or address* along with the doctor's name. Often two doctors may have the same name; if the telephone number is not selected with care, the *wrong* doctor may be called.

### The Nursing Unit Equipment

General *nursing unit equipment* includes *furniture, electrical fixtures, bathroom equipment*, and so forth. As you know from everyday living, equipment needs maintenance, and the old saying "prevention is easier than cure" applies here. Ideas for more efficient location of supplies offer an improvement opportunity and should be discussed with your nurse manager. Most hospital units have equipment lists that show when items are due for replacement. It is useful to be aware of these replacement lists. A piece of equipment requiring frequent repair may need to be replaced sooner than its expected replacement date. Another piece of equipment may be operating very well and not need replacement. You can contribute to the smooth operation of your unit by informing the nurse manager of these situations. Preventive management of the nursing unit equipment requires that the health unit coordinator make rounds of the entire unit (kitchen, utility rooms, pa-

tient rooms, waiting room, linen room, and nurses' lounge) perhaps once or twice a week to check on the functioning of equipment located in these areas. Leaky faucets, frayed electrical cords, and broken hinges are a few examples of the things to look for. Make a list of all the items that need to be checked on your nursing unit. Then, as you make rounds, check each item on the list for its working order. Make a note of the items that need repair. Also, instruct nursing unit staff to note needed repairs in the unit log book. Request equipment repair from the maintenance department.

Preventive management does not take care of all the maintenance needs for the nursing unit equipment. Burned-out electric light bulbs, an overflowing toilet, and other unpredictable problems need immediate attention. For immediate repair service, notify the maintenance department by telephone or pocket pager, and complete the appropriate requisition.

### Patient Rental Equipment

**Reusable equipment** used by the individual patient such as suction machines and traction equipment is usually rented by the patient on a daily basis. When the doctor discontinues the treatment that requires the rental equipment, nursing personnel usually transfer the equipment to the utility room, where it is stored, before it is returned to the proper department. It is the management responsibility of the health unit coordinator to see that the equipment is returned to the proper department promptly and that the daily charges to the patient are discontinued at this time. Patients often bring electrical equipment, such as shavers or hair dryers, into the hospital. It may be hospital policy to have the maintenance department check such equipment for safety prior to their use by the patient.

### The Nursing Unit Emergency Equipment

**Emergency equipment** and supplies include emergency drugs, throat suction, resuscitation equipment, fire extinguishers, and fire doors. Because of the nature of emergency equipment, it must be checked both daily and immediately after use and be restored as soon as possible to be readied for future emergencies.

The health unit coordinator must know what emergency equipment and supplies are stored on the nursing unit and where they are located. Know the operation as well as the location of the unit fire extinguisher. What are the emergency procedures for your unit? Know the signal codes and procedures for fire, behavioral alarms, and evacuation procedures.

What are the procedures for dealing with a hazardous materials spill? Although you may not be directly responsible, knowing the procedures allows you to support timely and safe removal of hazardous materials. During a crisis, the hospital personnel often approach the nurses' station and ask the health unit coordinator to locate emergency equipment and initiate emergency procedures.

Ignorance of the location of nursing unit emergency equipment may cause a delay in the delivery of emergency treatment and result in serious consequences to the patient.

## MANAGEMENT OF THE ACTIVITIES AT THE NURSES' STATION

In Chapter 1 we said that the health unit coordinator through his or her communication responsibilities coordinates the activities of the doctor, the nursing staff, the other hospital departments, the patients, and the visitors to the nursing unit. Good management techniques are necessary to coordinate these activities effectively. The individuals providing **health care services** are your **internal customers** and are dependent on you for information they need to provide clinical and medical **patient health services**.

The scope of the health unit coordinator's responsibilities has increased and broadened with the advent of **continuous quality improvement (CQI)** efforts. As a result of CQI **process simplification** and **cycle time reduction** projects, more hospitals admit patients directly to the nursing units, bypassing admitting departments, and thus increasing the health unit coordinator's responsibilities for admissions.

The health unit coordinator's awareness must broaden to include knowledge about the expectations of a large number of health care **stakeholders**. In continuous quality improvement literature, stakeholders are identified as other people who are concerned with the quality of health care delivery including patients' families, the employer, insurers, health care providers, students, and the community. These groups have an interest or stake in the outcomes of health care services.

## Management Responsibilities Related to Activities at the Nurses' Station

### Patient Activity and Information

The most efficient method for tracking patients and their activities is to use a **patient activity sheet**. Prepare the patient activity sheet at the beginning of each shift from the Kardex forms or from the change-of-shift report. List all the patients' names and room numbers. Record by each patient's name the planned activities that relate to health unit coordinating, such as scheduled diagnostic procedures, surgeries, planned discharges, transfers, and so forth. Also, record the time of the activity, if known (Fig. 7–4).

Record other data that you may use during the shift, such as (1) no phone calls to the patient's room, (2) no code arrest procedure to be initiated, (3) no visitors allowed, (4) do not release information about the patient, and (5) the patient is in an isolation room.

Tape the patient activity sheet onto the surface area of your desk. During the shift, update the information as changes occur.

### Clients and Clients' Charts that Leave the Unit

If the client leaves the nursing unit—for surgery, for a diagnostic study, to visit the cafeteria with a relative, or for one of numerous other reasons—record the time the client leaves the nursing unit and the destination beside the patient's name on the patient activity sheet. When the patient returns to the nursing unit, draw a line through the recording. Use the same procedure to keep track of *clients' charts* that are temporarily off the nursing unit. Much time is lost by trying to locate charts for doctors, nurses, and other professionals. Chart tracking is *essential* for the efficient use of time for all those involved.

Increasingly, patient-centered nursing units are being designed so that diagnostic technicians come to the patient on the unit whenever possible. This practice is more convenient for the patient and also reduces the number of times the chart is off the unit.

Health personnel, doctors, and visitors are constantly asking the health unit coordinator the whereabouts of clients and/or the clients' charts. By maintaining the patient activity sheet, you can find the answer at a glance. Many nursing units average 25 to 30 patients, and so it would be impossible to mentally log the whereabouts of each patient.

| TO THE STUDENT |
|---|

To practice preparing a patient activity sheet, complete **Activity 7–1** in the Skills Practice Manual.

### Visitors

As a health unit coordinator you probably have more contact with the visitors than any of the other nursing unit

PATIENT ACTIVITY SHEET

| 301 | Breath Les | home to-day |
| 302 | Katt Kitty | Surg 11ª   x ray report not on chart |
| 303 | Pickens Slim | |
| 304 | Bee Mae | NPO for IVP to-day x-ray at 9 |
| 305 | Honey Mai | no visitors |
| 306 | Net Claw | home to-day |
| 307 | Ibowl Iris | 11ª Chart to PT |
| 308 | Christmas Mary | Isolation |
| 309 | Nerve Lotta | telephone blocked no calls to room |
| 310-1 | Soforthe Anne | do not give out information |
| 310-2 | Soo Ah | 1ªº to Caf c̄ Mother |
| 311-1 | Bugg June | Surg 9ª 8³⁰ to surg returned 12:30 |
| 311-2 | Kynde Bee | BE to-day |
| 312-1 | Cider Ida | PT at 1ª to-day |
| 312-2 | Saynt Joanne | no code |

FIGURE 7–4 • A patient activity sheet.

personnel, since visitors usually stop at the nurses' station for information or some other type of communication regarding the patient's hospitalization. As a visitor approaches the nurses' station, immediately stop what you are doing and provide assistance. At this moment, you represent the entire nursing unit, and the manner in which you respond to the visitor helps shape his or her attitude about the care the patient is receiving and about the hospital as a whole.

It is your management responsibility to (1) communicate pertinent information to visitors, (2) respond to visitors' questions and requests, and (3) initially handle visitors' complaints.

Communicate pertinent information to the visitor, such as the time for visiting hours, what items may or may not be taken into the client's room, isolation restrictions, the number of visitors allowed in the room at one time, and so forth. Refer to the policy manual for the visitor regulations practiced at your hospital.

The visitor may ask the health unit coordinator such questions as: "May I take the client to the cafeteria?" "May the patient have a milkshake?" "When can the patient go home?" Many questions may be answered by checking the patient's Kardex form or by referring to the nursing unit policy or procedure manual. However, if you are in doubt about the answer, check with the nurse.

*Never discuss aspects of the patient's medical condition with the patient's visitors* (Fig. 7–5). Refer all of these questions to the doctor or nurse. *If you do not know* the answer to a

question or feel the question should be referred to the nurse, respond to the visitor by saying, "*I'll have the nurse discuss this with you,*" or something similar, rather than saying, "I don't know" or "I'm not allowed to give out that information."

The health unit coordinator is often confronted by visitors' complaints, some justified and some unjustified. Visitors, especially the relatives of a critically ill patient, are under a great deal of stress. The uncertainty of the course of the illness, unfamiliarity with the hospital routine, and many other factors contribute to their feelings of uneasiness and insecurity. Also, they are often dealing with emotions, such as guilt and anger. Often these feelings are expressed in the form of complaints regarding the patient's care. How you respond to the visitor's initial remarks may make the difference between the problem's being solved at the nursing unit level and having the problem mushroom up through the nursing administration to the chief executive officer.

Below are three steps to follow when dealing with visitor complaints.

1. *Listen carefully and attentively to what the person is saying* (Fig. 7–6). If the person's voice is raised, or is angry in tone, remember that the hostility is not being directed to you personally. It is important for you to understand that the person is upset and that to listen carefully to what he or she is saying is the first step toward dealing with a challenging situation.

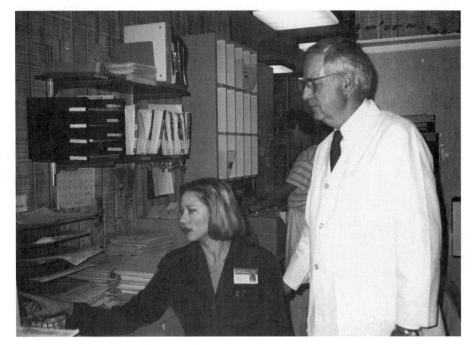

**FIGURE 7–5** • Never discuss aspects of the patients medical condition with the patient's visitors. Refer the questions to the doctor or nurse.

2. *Ask pertinent objective questions and gather as many facts as possible.* Demonstrate a caring attitude when gathering information. Whether the complaint is justified or not is not important at this time.

3. *Respond to the complaint accordingly.* Respond verbally with such phrases as "I understand what you are telling me" or "I understand how you feel." Do not respond defensively with statements such as "I wasn't here yesterday" or "That's not my job." If the complaint needs the attention of the nurse, say, "Please wait here, I will get the nurse to talk with you about this matter." If visitors appear even the least bit anxious or angry, refer them to the nurse immediately, since time often exaggerates a situation out of proportion (Fig. 7–7). You may wish to acknowledge the anger by saying "I can see you're angry" or something similar prior to referring the person to the nurse. Doing this demonstrates a caring attitude.

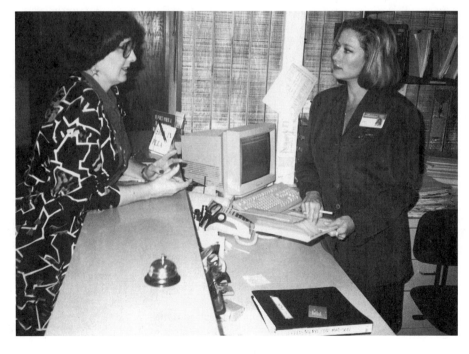

**FIGURE 7–6** • When dealing with the visitor's complaints, listen carefully and attentively to what the person is saying.

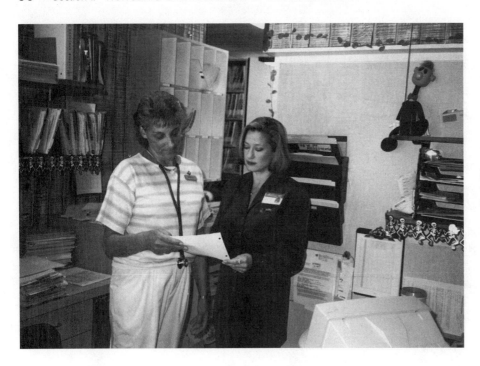

FIGURE 7–7 • You may need to refer visitor complaints to the nurse.

## Organization of the Nurses' Station

A well-organized and neat nurses' station gives the appearance of a well-run nursing unit. First use this list to check your working area at the nurses' station.

■ Is the counter space large enough?
■ Are the requisition and other frequently used forms stored within reaching distance?
■ Is the imprinter device close to you so you do not have to get up to use it?
■ Can you reach the charts?
■ Can you reach the telephone?
■ Is the doctor's roster kept within reaching distance?
■ Are people constantly leaning over you to obtain items that could be stored elsewhere?
■ Is the computer terminal located where it is easy to use?
■ Be sure to position a tower CPU conveniently so that you do not have to bend awkwardly to change disks if the tower is placed on the floor.
■ Adjust your chair so that you sit straight yet in a relaxed position with a backrest supporting the small of your back and your feet flat on the floor.
■ Adjust your chair back to a slightly backward position and extend your legs out slightly so there are no sharp angles that cause pressure to be placed on your hip or knee joints as you work.
■ Your wrists should be straight as you type with forearms level and elbows close to your body.
■ Use a computer wrist pad only to rest.
■ Keep the top of your computer terminal at or slightly below eye level.
■ Position the terminal so that you must look slightly downward to look at the middle of the screen.
■ Take frequent ministretches of shoulders, arms, hands, and legs.

■ Shift your weight in your chair frequently.
■ These small breaks in position help avoid neuromuscular strain and alleviate the tension of job stress (Fig. 7–8).

## A Special Note About Computers

Is the computer positioned conveniently, so that you can work in a natural and relaxed position? Again, are the items you need within easy reach? Most likely you will only use a terminal connected to a centralized data processing system. However, if you use a personal computer for word processing and spreadsheets as well as the terminal to the main data bank, what is the shape of the computer processing unit (CPU)? Is the CPU a desktop or a tower model? If you have ideas for the rearrangement of the items that you constantly use, which would save you time and energy, discuss the matter with your peers and with the nurse manager.

Frequently take the time to stand back and observe the nurses' station area. Is it cluttered and unorganized in appearance? If so, take a moment to restore all items to their original places. Return charts to the chart rack.

### LOCATE THE FOLLOWING ITEMS WITHIN YOUR REACHING DISTANCE OF YOUR WORK AREA

- Forms
- Imprinter device
- Charts
- Telephone
- Doctor's roster
- Computer terminal

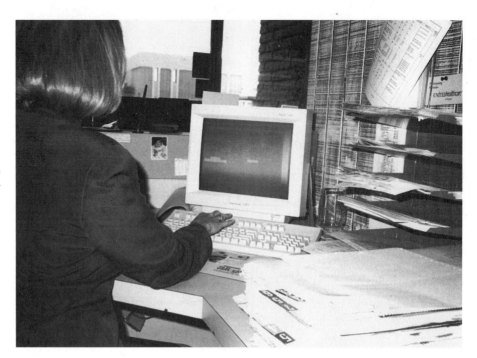

F I G U R E 7–8 • Proper body positioning when using a computer terminal.

## MANAGEMENT RELATED TO THE PERFORMANCE OF HEALTH UNIT COORDINATOR TASKS

### Putting Tasks in Order by Priority

As a health unit coordinator you will often experience situations in which there are several tasks to be performed at the same time. Management involves being able to determine which task takes priority over another. Awareness and experience are necessary to develop skill in determining priorities.

It is impossible to be arbitrary about which task must be completed first, since this varies according to the demands of the total situation. However, the following guidelines may help the beginning health unit coordinator to decide which tasks to perform first.

1. Transcribing stat orders usually takes priority over all other tasks.
2. Communicating a telephoned message for a patient to go to surgery must be done at once, since the patient is medicated for the surgery; the surgeon, the anesthesiologist, and the nursing personnel are waiting; and the operating room is readied for use.
3. Performing the routine tasks at the scheduled times takes priority over performing other tasks (see Fig. 7–10).
4. Answering the telephone usually takes priority over all other activities.
5. Calling the stat laboratory reports to the doctor takes priority over all other tasks.
6. Transcribing the discharge orders takes priority over other orders (except stat orders), so that the clerical work can be processed by the time the patient is ready to leave the hospital.

### Using a Memory Sheet

Keep a list of all the tasks that you are unable to complete momentarily on a **memory sheet** (Fig. 7–9). A memory sheet is simply a sheet of paper on which to record unfinished tasks. You often need to communicate information that is not urgent in nature to a member of the nursing team.

---

E X A M P L E

You receive a telephone message for Mary to call the pharmacy at her convenience. Rather than waste time trying to locate Mary, record this information on the memory sheet. When she returns to the nurses' station, communicate the message to her. Draw a line through the message on the memory sheet to indicate you have communicated the message.

---

E X A M P L E

You need to call the doctor's office and you are unable to complete the call because the line is busy. Record the task on the memory sheet, along with the doctor's telephone number and other pertinent data so that you will have it available when you are able to place the call. When you complete the call, cross it off on the memory sheet.

---

During an 8- or 12-hour shift there are countless items to record on your memory sheet. Near the end of your

3-16-00    Memory Sheet

Call consultation to Dr L Seamer for Ms Joan
Bryce 318-1 re pain in chest requested by
Dr F. Lesser
Call maintenance to check leaking tap in 322 bathroom
Tell Francis to call home when she has a
chance
Recopy harder form for Mr George 338-2
Pick up pm snacks.
~~Get forms xeroxed~~
Jane to go to nursing office sometime today

F I G U R E 7–9 • A memory sheet.

shift, check that all the items listed have been completed and take care of any that remain.

# MANAGEMENT OF YOUR TIME

The ability to manage your time may be the single most important factor toward successful health unit coordinating. However, it is not easy to learn how to effectively use your time. Experience, awareness, flexibility, and motivation are all necessary to achieve the goal of using your time to its full potential.

William Rochti in *Leadership in the Office* (1963) tells a story that superbly demonstrates how the day tends to "go" when there is no plan for managing time.

A farmer told his wife, "I'll plow the south 40 tomorrow." The next morning he went out to lubricate the tractor. But he needed oil; so he went to the shop to get it. On the way he noticed that the pigs hadn't been fed. He started for the bin to get them some feed, but some sacks there reminded him that the potatoes needed sprouting. He walked over toward the potato bin. En route, he spotted the woodpile and remembered that he'd promised to carry some wood to the house. But he had to chop it first, and he'd left his ax behind the chicken coop. As he went for the ax, he met his wife, feeding the chickens. With surprise she asked, "Have you finished the south 40 already?" "Finished!" the farmer bellowed. "I haven't even started."

Like the farmer, the health unit coordinator engaged in one part of his or her job is constantly seeing other tasks that need to be done. Knowing how to plan your day to make the best use of your time helps you avoid the pitfalls of the farmer.

## How to Make the Best Use of Your Time

- *Plan for rush periods.* Take time at the beginning of each day to prepare for anticipated rush periods. For example, since it is always busy in the morning while the doctors are making rounds, allow time to assist the doctors in locating their charts and other items they may need. If several surgery patients are scheduled for your unit, you can anticipate a rush in the afternoon when they arrive on the unit from the PACU; or if there are several empty beds on the nursing unit in the morning when you arrive on duty, you can anticipate a rush during the admitting time in the afternoon.
- *Plan a schedule for the routine health unit coordinator tasks.* Health unit coordinating includes the daily repetition of the performance of the routine tasks covered in Chapter 21. Make a plan for a given day by scheduling the routine tasks to be done at the time of day that produces the best outcome. Figure 7–10 gives an example of a schedule for routine tasks. Plan to perform the regular tasks, such as transcribing doctors' orders, placing telephone calls, and so forth, according to demand between the scheduled routine tasks. Follow your plan to make changes as you discover ways to improve the use of your time.
- *Group activities.* Save time by grouping activities together, such as delivering specimens to the laboratory on your way to lunch or checking the patient's charts for the need for new forms at the same time you file reports.
- *Delegate tasks to volunteers.* Discuss with your nurse manager which of your tasks may be delegated to the volunteer(s) in your unit. Filing records on the chart is

Time Schedule For Routine Health Unit Coordinating Tasks

7:00    Change of shift report
7:30    Check surgery charts
8:00
8:30    Record TPR's
9:00    Order dietary supplies
9:30    Order lunch diets
10:00 -10:15    Morning break
10:30
11:00
11:30    Lunch
12:00
12:30
1:00    Order supplies from the Purchasing Department on Mondays
1:30    Order evening diets
2:00    Order daily laboratory tests
2:30    Afternoon break
3:00    File records and recheck all charts for doctor's orders that may have been missed

F I G U R E  7–10 • A time schedule for routine health unit coordinating tasks.

a time-consuming task that can usually be performed by volunteer workers. Work out a plan to have a volunteer assist you each day at the times that are most helpful to you. Remember that volunteer workers volunteer because they want to work.

■ *Complete one task before beginning another.* This is not always possible because a stat order always takes precedence over whatever else you are doing. However, apply this principle as consistently as possible. Complete transcribing the set of doctors' orders you are working on before going on break or to lunch.

■ *Avoid unnecessary conversation.* Often there are many other health professionals within the nurses' station, and thus it is very easy to be drawn into unnecessary conversation. Be aware of this and avoid when possible.

■ *Know your job and perform your job.* A nursing unit is made up of many people working together to perform the overall function of caring for the patients. In order for effective functioning of the nursing unit, each person must first know his or her job description and, second, perform the tasks outlined in the job description. It is important that you stay within the boundaries of the job and not drift over into performing the tasks assigned to other health personnel.

For example, on a busy day it may seem appropriate for you to "help out" the nursing staff by feeding a patient, passing out food trays, and so forth. We *caution you against this practice* for two reasons. One, *you are not educationally prepared to perform clinical tasks;* and two, you are thereby *leaving your own tasks unattended.* Your greatest contribution to the function of the nursing unit as a whole is to know your job and to perform your job to the best of your ability. If asked by other health personnel to perform tasks that are part of *their* job description, politely refuse to do so.

■ *Take the breaks assigned to you.* Often on a busy day the immediate solution to getting the job done may appear to be to skip lunch, coffee breaks, or both. Don't be tempted to do so. Often a few minutes away from the pressure allows you to recoup and return to handle the situation with renewed vigor and speed.

## MANAGING CONTINUOUS QUALITY IMPROVEMENT

Most health care organizations engage in some form of quality improvement. Continuous quality improvement is a requirement for accreditation by the Joint Commission on the Accreditation of Healthcare Organizations (JCAHO), a department of the American Hospital Asso-

### TOOLS TO MANAGE INFORMATION

- Standard supply list and supply needs list
- Written direction on using the pneumatic tube system
- Unit log book
- Patient activity sheet
- Memory sheet

Review these tools as you begin your employment. Implement any of the "tools to manage information" that will assist you in organizing information for your nursing unit.

ciation; many hospitals seek to attain this level of certification.

Since the 1970s, there have been many approaches to quality improvement. Whether or not you are familiar with a particular approach, remember that the quality movement is not static, but dynamic, and therefore a process of continual change. While one approach or another may become passé as a separate program, quality improvement is expected to remain embedded in the normal operating procedures of modern organizations. Despite continual changes of approach, the fundamental tenets of good practice are retained and fine tuned to be responsive to economic and political changes such as health care reform and downsizing. Old principles work but must be applied in light of current management practices.

A major force in maintaining the quality movement in this country is the national Malcolm Baldridge Quality Award managed by the United States Department of Commerce. The Department of Commerce now has a pilot program to develop a health care award similar to the one granted in business and industrial areas. The health care pilot maintains the seven major criteria that are used to rate an applicant's level of quality in business, but has appropriate changes in content to fit the health care field. Many businesses use the Malcolm Baldridge seven criteria guidelines for continuously improving quality. The criteria contain "areas to address" that are often the responsibility of the senior executive and health care staff. However, many items listed can be directly related to work processes at the nursing unit level. The "areas to address" provide a useful overview of what to emphasize in your quality improvement efforts as the health unit coordinator. For example, criteria 1, "leadership," addresses how the organization focuses on the patient, other stakeholders and how work processes are reviewed and improved.

Today most states have some form of quality award and more states are developing a separate category for the health care quality awards.

How does this translate to the health unit coordinator? Quality improvement will remain an important part of your work. Learn the language of quality. The quality movement is global because continuous quality improvement results in better quality products and service. Competition to provide the best product and service has increased worldwide. Find out who has the "best practices" in health unit coordinating and put those methods to work in your unit whenever you can.

In Europe the newest set of requirements has environmental impact standards that include scores that rate a business's impact on the total community. Health care standards will increasingly address a delivery of health care that supports a healthy community. Just as we have moved toward holistic health practices, the designers of health care are leading us toward a holistic delivery of health care services. The total community will be concerned with how health care is delivered by your organization. As health unit coordinator you have an important role in how efficiently and effectively that service is provided in your area.

**Patient care support services** are, with increasing frequency, being designed to integrate well with clinical services. Patient care support services are services that are not delivered directly to the patient but which support the organization's delivery of health care services to the patient. Such support services might include housekeeping services, paging services, escort services, medical records, and transcription services.

Understanding the process for transporting patients to surgery or rehabilitation helps the health unit coordinator design and continuously improve performance so there is a rapid, accurate, and smooth flow of information to the clinical services. These patient care support service requirements usually depend significantly upon the requirements of many internal customers.

## Quality Improvement Strategies

Learn how to identify gaps between the actual service provided and the ideal service that could be provided. For example, count how many charts have errors or omissions when the chart goes to your internal customer. Is all the lab work on the chart before surgery or does the surgical team have to take time to look it up on a computer in the operating suite? Could you have printed off a lab value? Count the errors or omission (actual) then work with your internal customers to remove them (ideal).

Here are some additional questions you will want to answer and act upon. Do your internal customers agree with your definition of your service to them? What's most important to them? Where do they think your service could be improved? Have you provided a method for them to communicate their needs to you? Have you asked your internal customers if they are willing to work with you to improve your service to them?

Learn to use the basic quality tools (Fig. 7–11). They are:

Brainstorming
Process flow chart
Fishbone chart

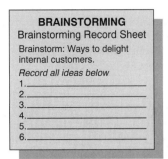

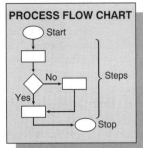

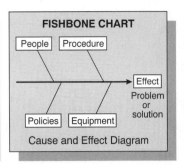

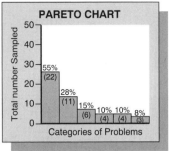

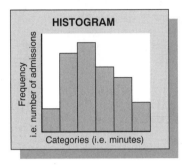

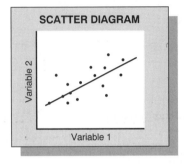

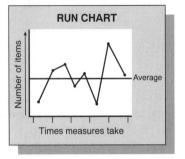

F I G U R E  7–11 • The seven basic quality tools.

Pareto chart
Histogram
Correlation chart (or scatter diagram)
Run chart

## Definitions

- *Brainstorming* is a structured group activity that allows 3 to 10 people to tap into the creativity of the group to identify new ideas. Typically in quality improvement, the technique is used to identify probable causes and possible solutions of quality problems.
- *Process flow chart* is a diagram of steps in a process used to help visualize the steps.
- The *fishbone chart* (also called the "cause-and-effect diagram") is used to organize brainstorming information about the probable causes of an effect. The same technique is used to look for what causes either a solution (a good effect) or a problem (bad effect).
- The *Pareto chart* is a form of a bar chart that is used to show in descending order the most frequently occurring item or event to the least occurring item or event. A final bar of small numbers of events is stacked to the far right and is labeled "others" and contains a combination of items considered trivial. Caution! Sometimes the "trivial few" contains a very important cause of an effect (problem).
- A *histogram* is a chart that displays how often differences occur in some type of measure in a process. It reveals the amount of variation a process has within it.
- The *correlation or scatter diagram* is used to determine if there is a possible relationship between changes in two sets of data. Often used after a cause-and-effect diagram to find out if a suspected relationship between a cause

and an "effect" can be visually plotted and statistically confirmed.
- The *run chart* is used to study the data obtained by plotting process performance measures to look for trends over a particular period of time.

## Using the Histogram

A complete explanation of all of the quality tools is beyond the scope of this chapter; however, an example of how one tool might be used will demonstrate how the tools can further one's understanding of a work process.

A histogram, for example, would be useful if you wanted to improve the process for completing a patient admission.

Generally, the time to complete a patient admission is expected to vary normally. Some admissions go smoothly, are uncomplicated, and don't take much time. Some are about average (whatever is average for your unit) and still others take longer. This process, like most processes, is expected to vary "normally." That is, when admission times values are plotted according to the rule for drawing histograms the shape of the chart should resemble a bell curve (Fig. 7–12). With a little special training quality improvement teams learn to analyze their histograms for clues about whether they have a "common cause" of delayed admissions built into their process with the hump consistently to one side or whether they have several "special causes." The histograms gives a picture of a process that is easier to interpret than columns of figures on a page.

Another way of describing a normal process is to say it is a "stable" process. You want a process to work as dependably as, for instance, a well-operating soda machine. You put your quarters in and—click, click, click—out

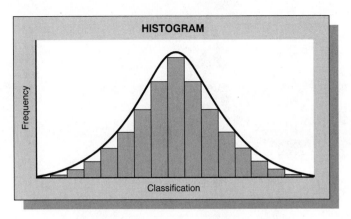

**F I G U R E  7–12** • Normal bell curve.

comes a soda, a stable process. But what if the vending machine company wanted to improve the time it took to get quarters through and a soda out of the machine. (Customer feedback in crowded locations complained the machines took too long.) The engineers or improvement team would experiment only on vending machines that had "stable" processes. If a machine tended to let quarters stick in a chute, that machine would have to be fixed before it could be experimented with as part of the improvement project.

W. Edward Deming, who is credited with the quality transformation taking place in this country, would say you have found a "special cause" of a quality problem and removed it (fixed the sticking quarters), but you are right back where you were before the problem occurred. Fixing "special causes" needs to be done, but it is not *quality improvement*. Dr. Deming says working only on "special causes" is "putting out fires" and tells this story, which he attributes to Dr. Joseph M. Juran, another quality leader.

---

You are in a hotel. You hear someone yell "Fire!" You run for the fire extinguisher and pull the fire alarm. We all get out. Extinguishing the fire does not improve the hotel. That is not improvement of quality. That is putting out fires (Walton, 1986).

Similarly, for the delayed admissions example discussed above, you would need to remove "special causes" of delays. That is, those causes that occur when the computers are down, in "flu" season, or because of tardiness of certain employees. Whatever is not a designed part of the admission process is removed before making significant changes in the methods for doing the process. As Dr. Deming pointed out over and over, you need a stable process to begin a process improvement. If process measures are all over the charts you will not be able to tell if what you did made a real improvement that will stay improved; in other words, whether you can "hold the gain." That's why the quality tools are worth learning. They save you from wasting time "tinkering" with a process without making lasting improvement.

## SUMMARY

To meet the challenge of management requires more effort and motivation on the part of the health unit coordinator than just "getting the job done"; however, the effort and motivation are rewarding. Job success is self-made. We hope you take the step beyond "getting the job done" and employ the management techniques necessary to develop your career to its potential.

Use of these techniques, as already mentioned in Chapter 5, depends on which part of your personality is being used when you are under time pressures. We said in that chapter that for the purpose of simplicity Eric Berne referred to the parts of the personality as parent, adult, and child. Information about time management skills is best retrieved by getting into the adult part of your personality.

When under stress, take a deep breath and resist the impulse to listen to old parental "driver" messages described by Kahler (1978). "Drivers" urge you to "hurry up," "try hard," "please me (someone else)," "be perfect," or "be strong." When you respond to these messages you do so from your child part not the adult. The adult part of your personality is the part you need to recall time management information and successfully use that knowledge.

**REVIEW QUESTIONS**

1. List four areas of management.

   a. nursing unit supplies and equipment
   b. activities at the nurses station
   c. related to the performance of tasks
   d. of time

2. Briefly discuss your management responsibilities for:

   a. nursing unit supplies maintain a standart supply list that relates to supplys needed and Location

   b. equipment stores at the nurses' station check eguipment each day for working order. Return used equipment to proper place. Manage the use of Pnuematic Tube and Imprinter device

   c. nursing unit reference material make sure text books are returned. keep policy manual, procedure manual, doctors roster upto date

   d. nursing unit equipment not applicable

   e. the patient's rental equipment make sure equiptment is returned to proper place as soon as possible and daily charge discontinued

   f. nursing unit emergency equipment know that you have all your emergency equiptment and where it is located

3. You are preparing the patient activity sheet for the day. Indicate, by a check mark, which of the following pieces of information relates to health unit coordinating and should be recorded on the patient activity sheet.

   a. enema today ✓✓
   b. home this AM ✓
   c. surgery at 10 AM for cholecystectomy ✓
   d. continuous IV ✓
   e. limit visitors ✓
   f. reverse isolation ✓
   g. regular diet

   h. cath prn ✓
   i. do not give out patient information ✓
   j. BE today ✓
   k. CBC ✓
   l. EEG today ✓
   m. no code ✓

4. Discuss how you may keep a record of which patients and which of the patients' charts are temporarily away from the nursing unit.

record on the patients Activity sheet
the patients away from the unit when
they left and when they return cross
off by drawing a line through it when they return

5. Why is it necessary to keep a written record of the whereabouts of each patient and patient chart?

to have information available to give (to the doctors,)
nurses and visiters about the patients
whereabouts and their chart.

6. List three management responsibilities concerning visitors.

a. Communicate Information to visitors
b. respond to visitors questions or complaints
c. Initially handle complaints

7. List three steps to follow when dealing with visitor complaints.

a. listen carefully
b. respond accordingly
c. ask pertinent questions

8. A convenient immediate working environment is necessary for you to make the best use of your time. List five items that should be placed within your reaching distance.

a. forms+requisitions
b. doctors roster
c. computer terminal
d. telephone
e. imprinter device

9. You have just arrived on the nursing unit and you are ready to begin the day. The following tasks need to be done. Indicate the order in which you would perform the tasks by numbering them in the spaces provided.

3 two discharge orders must be processed

6 a patient requests a newspaper

1 the telephone is ringing

5 a doctor has placed an order for a chest x-ray

2 the surgical patients' charts must be checked to see that the necessary reports are included in preparation for surgery

4 two tubes have just arrived in the pneumatic tube system

10. List eight steps you may follow to make the best use of your time.

a. plan for rush periods
b. plan a schedule for tasks

c. _group activities_

d. _delegate tasks to volunteers_

e. _complete one task before starting another_

f. _avoid unnecessary conversation_

g. _Know and perform your job_

h. _take breaks assigned to you_

11. Define the following terms:

a. standard supply list _a written record of amount of each item that the unit should stock to last till reorder date_

b. patient activity sheet _a written record of the patients on the units activities for the day_

c. memory sheet _a record of unfinished tasks_

d. unit log book _a record or note book to write down unit imformation to pass on to other shifts_

12. Decribe how you would respond to the following situations:

a. Mrs. Robert Frances, whose husband has been hospitalized for 3 weeks with a cerebral hemorrhage, walks up to the nurses' station and in a loud angry voice states, "No one is taking care of my Robert. When I came in today his lunch tray was just sitting there, cold, and no one was feeding him, and his bed is wet."

_acknowledge her anger / show empathy, ask her husbands name and room number and that you will communicate mrs francis's message to the nurse taking care of her husband._

b. The visiting hours for your hospital state that children may visit the patients only on weekends. A female visitor with a small child and a baby asks you what room Mr. Blair is in. It is Tuesday afternoon.

_Explain to her about the visiting hours and tell her what room Mr Blair is in. If their is a volunteer on duty maybe you could get the volunteer to watch the children while mom visits Mr Blair_

c. The patient, Mr. Christine in Room 365-1, complains to you that the other patient in his room has six people visiting him at this time and he finds this very upsetting.

_Listen to Mr Christine and understand that this is to much for him. Go to his room and ask them if they will rotate their visiting with the patient to 2 people at a time. Because to many people are upseting to the other patient in the room_

d. You have been employed for a month on a very busy surgical nursing unit. The imprinter device and patient imprinter cards are located so far from your working area that each time you need to use them, you must get up from your chair and walk to where they are located.

*Figure out a good place to relocate this device so its more accessable to you, then discuss this relocation with your nurse manager*

e. It is a very busy day, the beds are all full, and two nursing personnel called in sick and were unable to be replaced. At the moment you are all "caught up" with your tasks. A nurse approaches you and asks, "Would you please feed Mr. Turley for me? His room is close to the nurses' station so you will be able to hear the telephone ring."

*you say sorry you can't leave the desk your not trained for clinical tasks and its not part of your job discription.*

13. It is 8:30 AM, the routine time for placing reports on the patients' charts. Several other tasks also need attention. They are:

a. stat order for packed cells
b. six other charts with orders on them (no stat orders)
c. the doctor has requested that you track down an x-ray report
d. a visitor is waiting to ask you a question
e. you need to communicate a message to the nurse that surgery is ready for Mr. Pat Jerri.

At this moment a volunteer arrives on the nursing unit and says, "I'm ready to help."
Explain how you would handle this situation:

*tell the volunteer and visitor that you will be with them in a moment, communicate the message to the nurse, assist the visitor, ask the volunteer to place reports on charts, notify lab for stat orders & complete requisition, locate x-ray report, transcribe other doctor's orders*

14. List the seven quality tools and their uses.

| Tool | Used |
| --- | --- |
| a. *brainstorming* | *identify new ideas* |
| b. *flow chart* | *visualization of steps of process* |
| c. *fishbone chart* | *organize information causes of* |
| d. *pareto chart* | *show in descending order frequency to least* |
| e. *histogram* | *shows amount of variation item requested over* |
| f. *correlation chart* | *relationship in changes of two sets of data* |
| g. *run chart* | *trends in plotted data* |

## References

George, Claude S.: *Supervision in Action: The Art of Managing Others*. Reston, VA, Reston Publishing Co., 1977.

Kahler, Taibi: *Transactional Analysis Revisited*. Little Rock, AR, Human Development Publications, 1978.

NEC Technologies, Inc.: *Ready Multimedia Computers User's Guide, Setting Up A Healthy Work Environment*. Boxborough, ME, 1996.

Scott, Dru: *How To Put More Time In Your Life*. New York, The New American Library, Signet Books, 1980.

Walton, Mary: *The Deming Management Method*. New York, Putnam Publishing Group, 1986.

## Suggested Reading

Brassard, Michael and Ritter, Diane: *The Memory Jogger II*. Melthuen, MA, Goal/QPC, 1994.

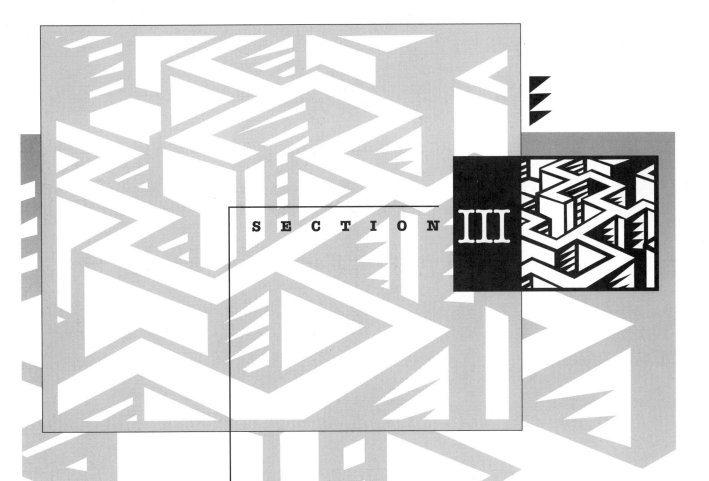

# THE PATIENT'S CHART AND TRANSCRIPTION OF DOCTORS' ORDERS

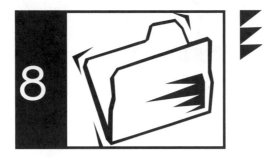

CHAPTER **8**

# THE PATIENT'S CHART

*Upon completion of this chapter, you will be able to:*

1. Define the terms in the vocabulary list.
2. Write the meaning of the abbreviations in the abbreviations list.
3. List six purposes of a patient's chart.
4. List four guidelines to be followed by all personnel when writing on a patient's chart.
5. Name the eight standard chart forms and describe the purpose of each form.
6. Explain how to maintain the confidentiality of the patient's chart.
7. List eight health unit coordinator duties in the maintenance of a patient's chart.
8. List four guidelines to follow in the preparation of a consent form.
9. Describe the methods for correcting an imprinting error and a written entry error on a chart form.
10. Read and write military clock times.

**V O C A B U L A R Y**

**Admission Packet** • A preassembled packet of chart forms to be used on the admission of a client to the nursing unit

**Identification Labels** • Preprinted labels containing individual patient information used in place of imprinter card to identify patient records

**Imprinter** • A device used for printing information on chart forms and requisitions

**Imprinter Card** • A plastic card containing individual patient information, used to identify the patient's records

**Inpatient** • A patient who has been admitted to a health care facility at least overnight for treatment and care

**Name Alert** • A method of alerting staff when two or more patients with the same last name are located on a nursing unit

**Old Record** • The patient's record from previous admissions; this is stored in the health records department

**Outpatient** • A patient receiving care by a health care facility but not admitted to or staying overnight

**"Split" or Thinned Chart** • Portions of the patient's current chart that are removed from the chart holder when the chart becomes too large

**Standard Chart Forms** • Chart forms used on all patients' charts

**Stuffing Charts** • Placing extra blank forms in all the patients charts on a nursing unit to prepare for the next day's recordings

**Supplemental Chart Forms** • Chart forms used only when specific conditions of the patient call for their use

## ABBREVIATIONS

*Note*: These abbreviations are listed as they are commonly written; however, you may also see some in cap and lower case letters and with or without periods.

| Abbreviation | Meaning |
| --- | --- |
| C of A | conditions of admission (form) |
| H&P | history and physical |
| Hx | history |
| ID labels | identification labels |
| MAR | medication administration record |
| NKA | no known allergies |

## EXERCISE 1

Write the abbreviation for each term listed below.

1. history — *H X*

2. no known allergies — *N K A*

3. conditions of admission — *C or A*

4. identification labels — *ID Labels*

5. history and physical — *H & P*

6. medication administration record — *M A R*

## EXERCISE 2

Write the meaning of each abbreviation listed below.

1. C of A — *Conditions of Admission*

2. ID labels — *Identification Labels*

3. H&P — *History & Physical*

4. MAR — *Medication Admin Record*

5. NKA — *no Known Alergies*

6. Hx — *History*

## PURPOSE OF A PATIENT'S CHART

The patient's chart serves many purposes, but as a health unit coordinator you will see the chart used mainly as a *means of communication between the doctor and the hospital staff.*

The chart is also used for planning patient care, for research, and for educational purposes. As a legal document, the chart protects the patient, the doctor, the staff, and the hospital or health care facility. Careful notations by the doctors and personnel provide a written record of the patient's illness, care, treatment, and the outcomes from the hospitalization. If the patient is readmitted to the hospital or health care facility, the chart may be retrieved from the health records department for review of past illnesses and treatment.

## THE CHART AS A LEGAL DOCUMENT

When a client is discharged, his or her chart is sent to the health records department. The health records department personnel analyze and check the chart for completeness. The chart is indexed and stored where it is available for retrieval as needed. The length of time the record must be stored depends upon the laws of the state. The record may serve as evidence in a court of law. As a legal document, it must be maintained in an acceptable manner.

All persons writing on the chart follow the same guidelines. As a health unit coordinator, you have minor charting tasks, but since you are responsible for the chart, you should learn the following basic rules:

■ *All chart form entries must be made in ink.* This is to ensure permanence of the record. Black ink is preferred by many health care facilities because it produces a clearer picture when the record is microfilmed or reproduced on a copier.

■ *The written entries on the chart forms must be legible and accurate.* Entries may be either in script or printed. Diagnostic reports, history and physical examination reports, and surgery reports are usually typewritten.

■ *Recorded entries on the chart may not be obliterated or erased.* The method for correcting errors is outlined later on in this chapter.

■ *All written entries on the chart forms must include the date and time the entry is made.*

■ *Abbreviations may be used according to the health care facility's list of "approved abbreviations."*

### HIGHLIGHT

Purposes of a Patient's Chart
- Means of communication
- Planning patient care
- Research
- Educational purposes
- Legal document
- Written record of illness, care, treatment, and outcomes

## Military Time

Time may be noted on the chart in the traditional method (such as 1:45 PM) or according to military time in which the day has 24 hours and each hour has its own name. In military time 1:45 PM is 1345. If the traditional time is used, include AM or PM, since entries are made on the chart 24

| TABLE 8-1 | STANDARD AND MILITARY TIME COMPARISONS | | |
|---|---|---|---|
| Standard Time | Military Time | Standard Time | Military Time |
| 12:15 AM | 0015 | 1:00 PM | 1300 |
| 12:30 AM | 0030 | 1:15 PM | 1315 |
| 12:45 AM | 0045 | 1:30 PM | 1330 |
| 1:00 AM | 0100 | 1:45 PM | 1345 |
| 2:00 AM | 0200 | 2:00 PM | 1400 |
| 3:00 AM | 0300 | 3:00 PM | 1500 |
| 4:00 AM | 0400 | 4:00 PM | 1600 |
| 5:00 AM | 0500 | 5:00 PM | 1700 |
| 6:00 AM | 0600 | 6:00 PM | 1800 |
| 7:00 AM | 0700 | 7:00 PM | 1900 |
| 8:00 AM | 0800 | 8:00 PM | 2000 |
| 9:00 AM | 0900 | 9:00 PM | 2100 |
| 10:00 AM | 1000 | 10:00 PM | 2200 |
| 11:00 AM | 1100 | 11:00 PM | 2300 |
| 12:00 noon | 1200 | 12:00 midnight | 2400 |

hours of the day. Military time is recorded as follows: The hours after midnight are recorded as 0100, 0200, and so forth. Twelve noon is recorded as 1200 and the hours that follow are arrived at by adding the hours after noon to 1200. Thus, 1:00 PM is 1300, 2 PM is 1400, and so forth. See Table 8–1 for a comparison of standard and military times. The use of military method eliminates confusion because hours are not repeated and AM or PM is unnecessary (Fig. 8–1).

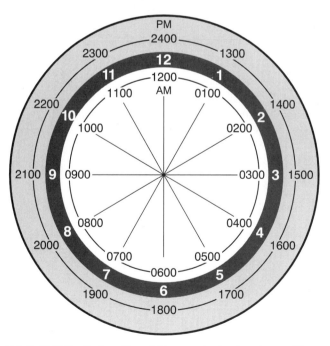

FIGURE 8–1 • The 24-hour clock showing military time.

**TO THE STUDENT**

To practice converting traditional time to military time, complete **Activity 8–1** in the Skills Practice Manual.

## THE CHART IS CONFIDENTIAL

Any information provided by the client to the health care facility and the medical staff is confidential. It was given to assist the doctor in making a diagnosis. The symptomatic history of the present illness, the past medical history, and facts concerning living habits and life style are recorded. Since this information is privileged, it must not be included in casual conversation by hospital personnel in the employee lounge, cafeteria, coffee shop, or any other area outside of the nursing unit. Many health care facilities consider a breach of confidentiality grounds for immediate dismissal.

Some of the information on the chart may be released to companies that carry the patient's health care insurance. This does not violate the rule of confidentiality. Each patient upon admission gives a written permission for release of information in this manner.

As custodian of all patient records on the unit, the health unit coordinator can further serve to maintain confidentiality by requiring all individuals who wish access to the records to identify themselves. Do not be afraid to ask the name and position of anyone you do not know.

Some clients may ask to see the information on their chart. Although the chart is the physical property of the hospital, the information contained within the chart is, in many states, considered the property of the patient and must, according to state law, be made available to the patient upon appropriate request, unless there are specific contraindications. To ensure compliance with state laws and hospital policies, the medical/legal expert in the health records department and the patient's doctor should be consulted when a patient asks to see his or her record.

**HIGHLIGHT**

To maintain confidentiality of patient records, the health unit coordinator must know the identification of all individuals who request access to the patient's chart on the nursing unit.

## THE CHART HOLDER

The forms that constitute the client's chart are kept together in a *chart holder*. The holder may open from the bottom, or it may be a notebook that opens from the side or the bottom (Fig. 8–2).

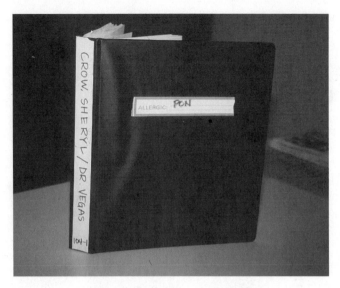

FIGURE 8–2 • A chart holder.

The chart forms in the holder are sectioned off by dividers placed in the chart according to the sequence set forth by the health care facility (Fig. 8–3).

The charts are identified for each patient by a label containing the patient's name and the doctor's name (Fig. 8–4). The room and bed number also appear on the outside of the chart holder. Many health care facilities use colored tape on the outside of the chart to assist the doctors in identifying their patients' charts. The chart holders are often used to alert the hospital staff of special situations. For example, "name alert," a piece of red tape with "name alert" recorded on it, may be placed on the chart holder to remind staff that more than one patient with the same last name is housed on the unit. Or NINP is often recorded on the chart holder to remind the staff that no information or no publication is to be issued on a particular patient.

## THE CHART RACK

The charts are placed in a chart rack when they are not in use. Each slot on the rack holds one patient's chart. The slots are labeled with the room and bed numbers, usually numbered in the same sequence as the rooms on the unit. There are many types of chart racks on the market (Fig. 8–5).

## THE IMPRINTER AND IMPRINTER CARD

When a patient is admitted to the health care facility, an **imprinter card** is prepared in the admitting department. This card, usually plastic, is used to imprint the patient's chart forms and the requisitions needed to obtain services.

Information on the imprinter card consists of the patient's name, sex, age, health records number, account number, and attending physician's name. Other information may be included depending upon the hospital (Fig. 8–6).

The imprinter card must be placed in an imprinting device (either manually operated or automatic) to transfer the information from the card onto the chart forms and requisitions. Many types of imprinting devices are in use by health care facilities. Your instructor will explain the use of the **imprinter** in your facility (Fig. 8–7).

A recent trend is to print a packet of identification labels on the computer when the patient is admitted. Information on the identification labels may include the client's name, age, sex, health record number, room number, admission date, and attending physician's name. These identification labels are kept on the unit in the patient's chart and are used to label chart forms and requisitions, thus eliminating the need for a unit printer.

## STANDARD CHART FORMS

**Standard chart forms** are those that are commonly used on all patient's charts. There are usually 11 forms that are considered "standard":

## 1. Face Sheet or Information Form

The **face sheet** or **information form** (Fig. 8–8) contains information about the patient, such as name, address, telephone number, name of employer, the admission diagnosis, health care insurance policy information, and next of kin. In most health care facilities, the form originates in the admitting department and is then sent to the unit to be placed in the patient's chart. Some facilities may include it in the patient's chart when it is assembled on the unit. Several copies are made and some are distributed to other hospital departments and some copies remain in the client's chart holder to be taken by the attending physician and by consulting physicians to be used for billing purposes. The health unit coordinator uses the face sheet to find information when calling the family or when calling consulting physicians.

## 2. Admission Agreement Form

The **admission agreement form** (Fig. 8–9) is signed by the patient in the admitting department and then sent to the unit to be placed in the patient's chart. The form sets forth the general service the hospital will provide.

## 3. Physicians' Order Form

The **physicians' order form**, or **doctors' order sheet** (Fig. 8–10), which is usually placed at the beginning of the

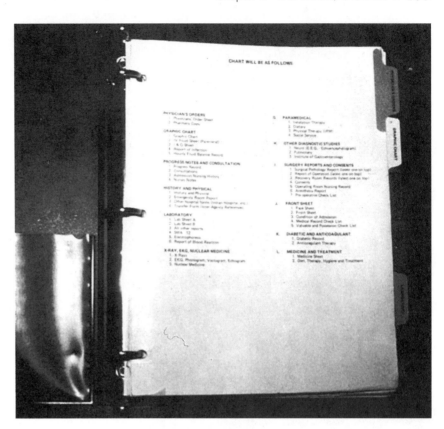

FIGURE 8–3 • A patient's chart with dividers.

chart for the doctor's convenience, is the form on which the doctor requests the care and treatment procedures for the patient. All orders must be dated and signed by the physician giving the order. This form may be in duplicate or triplicate, and may be printed on specially treated paper to eliminate the need for carbon paper. A duplicate of the original physicians' order form may be sent to the pharmacy (commonly called the *pharmacy* or *direct copy*) to order the patient's medications. The direct copy helps to eliminate any drug errors that may occur in the transcription process. If a third copy is produced, it is used by nursing personnel.

## 4. Physicians' Progress Record

The **progress record** is a form on which the physician records the patient's progress during the period of hospital-

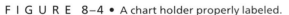

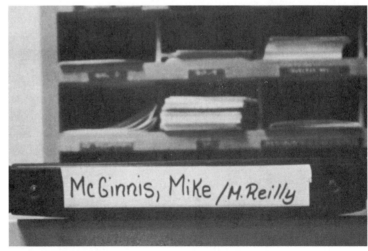

FIGURE 8–4 • A chart holder properly labeled.

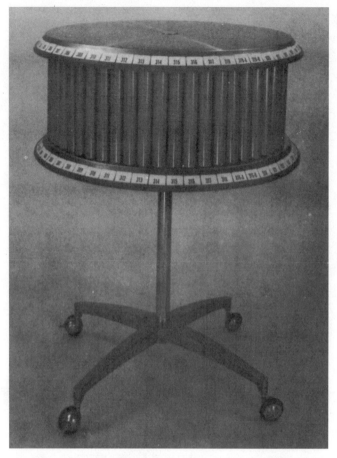

FIGURE 8–5 • Chart rack. (Courtesy of Acme Visible Records, Inc.)

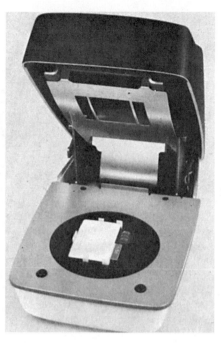

FIGURE 8–7 • Imprinting device. (Courtesy of Addressograph Multigraph Corp.)

may adopt one form on which physicians document orders along with progress notes (Fig. 8–11).

## 5. History and Physical Form

The **history and physical form** (Fig. 8–12) is used to record the medical history and the present symptomatic history of the patient. A review of all body systems or physical assessment of the patient is also recorded. The attending physician or resident may write on this form. The history and physical (H&P) report may be handwritten in ink, or, the physician may dictate the report, which is typed by a medical transcriptionist, and then the report will appear on the chart in typewritten form (Fig. 8–13).

ization. The medical staff rules and regulations as well as the patient's condition dictate the interval allowed between notations. In facilities in which this form is used strictly by the doctors, it may be written upon by the attending physician, residents, and consultants. Hospitals

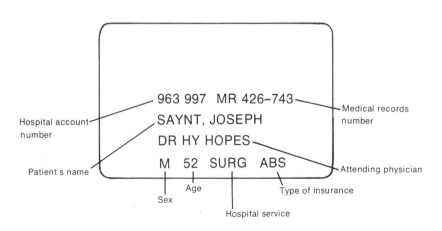

Hospital account number

Patient's name

963 997   MR 426–743

SAYNT, JOSEPH

DR HY HOPES

M   52   SURG   ABS

Medical records number

Sex

Age

Hospital service

Type of insurance

Attending physician

FIGURE 8–6 • Imprinter card.

| 1 | PATIENT HOSP.NO.(M.R.#) 987-654 | INFO STATUS | | | | | | ACCOUNT NO. (BUS. OFF.) 123-456 |
|---|---|---|---|---|---|---|---|---|

| 2 | PATIENT NAME  LAST: Andrews | FIRST: Iver | MIDDLE: S. | ADM. DATE MO. 8 / DAY 7 / YR. XX | ADM. TIME 1345 | HOW BROUGHT TO HOSPITAL Amb. |

| 3 | PATIENT'S CURRENT ADDRESS  STREET, P.O. BOX, APT. NO. 701 East Danish Lane | CITY Carpenterville, AZ | STATE | ZIP CODE 85013 | TELEPHONE NO. 246-XXXX |

| 4 | PATIENT'S PERMANENT ADDRESS  STREET, P.O. BOX, APT. NO. Same | CITY | STATE | ZIP CODE | TELEPHONE NO. |

| 5 | SEX 1. MALE  2. FEMALE [1] | MARITAL STATUS 1. SINGLE  4. DIVORCED  2. MARRIED 5. WIDOWED  3. SEPARATED [5] | RACE 1. WHITE  4. ORIENTAL  2. BLACK  5. OTHER  3. INDIAN [1] | RELIGION 3. PROTESTANT  1. CATHOLIC 4. OTHER  2. JEWISH 5. LDS [3] | AREA OF RESIDENCE |

| 6 | BIRTHDATE 10/6/XX | AGE 69 | PLACE OF BIRTH N.J. | MAIDEN NAME | SOC. SEC. NO./MEDICARE NO. 151-18-XXXX |

| 7 | PATIENT'S OCCUPATION Retired | UNION & LOCAL NO. | PATIENT'S EMPLOYER | ADDRESS | TELEPHONE NO. |

| 8 | PREVIOUSLY TREATED HERE? ☒ YES ☐ NO  NAME USED: Same | | | PREV. ADM. DATE | MO. DA. YR. 2/3/XX | PREV. ADMISSION 1. INPATIENT 2. OUTPATIENT [1] | IF NEWBORN, MOTHER'S HOSP. NO. |

| 9 | UNIT A5 | ROOM NO. | ACCOM. CODES | 1. PRI  3. NURSERY  5. ICU  7. CCU  2. SEMI  4. PREMIE  6. RCU  8. VIP | ROOM RATE [2] | PAY STATUS | CLASS OF ADMISSION 1. EMERGENCY  3. URGENT  2. ELECTIVE  4. OTHER [3] |

| 10 | ADMITTING DIAGNOSIS  Cerebrovascular accident |

| 11 | PHYSICIAN NAME I.M. Human | PHYSICIAN NO. 432 | ADM. SERVICE Med. | INFORMATION OBTAINED FROM: daughter |

| 12 | SPOUSE OR NEAREST RELATIVE (NEXT OF KIN) Kay Ellis | RELATIONSHIP daugh | ADDRESS 301 West Restful Dr. Phoenix | TELEPHONE NO. 258-XXXX |

| 13 | SECOND RELATIVE OR FRIEND Marie Darrow | RELATIONSHIP sister | ADDRESS 12 Center St. Danstown, CA | TELEPHONE NO. 837-XXXX |

| 14 | RESPONSIBLE PARTY NAME Self | | RELATIONSHIP | SOC. SEC. NO. |

| 15 | RESP. PARTY ADDRESS  STREET  P.O. BOX  APT. NO. | CITY | STATE | ZIP CODE | TELEPHONE NO. |

| 16 | RESP. PARTY OCCUPATION | NO. YRS. IN THIS EMPLOY | RESP. PARTY EMPLOYER | ADDRESS | TELEPHONE NO. |

| 17 | LENGTH OF TIME IN ARIZ. 10 yrs. | 1. OWN HOME 2. RENT HOME [1] | TYPE OF HOME Single | BANK NAME & BRANCH Desert National - Camelhead | 1. SAVINGS 2. CHECKING [1] |

| 18 | CREDIT REFERENCES | 1. NAME Deep River S&L | ADDRESS 9832 N. LasVegas Pl. Phoenix | TELEPHONE NO. 943-XXXX |
| 19 | | 2. NAME Yucca Federal | ADDRESS 1903 W. Bottletree Ave. Phoenix | TELEPHONE NO. 246-XXXX |

| 20 | INDUSTRIAL INJURY | DATE: MO. DA. YR. | CLAIM NO. | EMPLOYER'S NAME AND ADDRESS AT TIME OF INJURY |

| 21 | BLUE CROSS | NAME OF PLAN | GROUP NO. | IDENTIFICATION | EFFECTIVE DATE MO. DA. YR. | CITY | STATE |

| 22 | CHAMPUS DATA | PATIENT'S ID NO. | CARD EFFECTIVE MO. DA. YR. | CARD EXPIRES MO. DA. YR. | PATIENT OR SPONSORS BRANCH OF SERVICE | SERVICE CARD NO. |
| 23 | | SPONSORS NAME | | RANK-SERVICE NO. | DUTY STATION |

| 24 | OTHER INSURANCE (INC. BLOOD BANK & BLUE SHIELD) | INS. CO. NO. 1000 | COMPANY NAME Desert State | POLICY HOLDER NAME Iver Andrews | POLICY NO. A657483 | DATE ISSUED MO. DA. YR. 2/17/XX | CITY | STATE AZ |
| 25 | | INS. CO. NO. | COMPANY NAME | POLICY HOLDER NAME | POLICY NO. | DATE ISSUED MO. DA. YR. | CITY | STATE |

| 26 | NAME OF HEALTH FACILITY DISCHARGED FROM WITHIN LAST 60 DAYS None | | ADDRESS |

| 27 | OTHER INFO. | V. A. ☐ | COORDINATION OF BENEFITS ☐ | INTERVIEWED BY G. Talker | TYPED BY W.K.S. |

| 28 | REMARKS: |

FIGURE 8–8 • Face sheet or information form.

## 6. Nurses' Notes and Activity Flowsheet

Flowsheets are standard chart forms utilized by the nurse and auxiliary personnel to record bath, VS, activities, and other information about bedside care. The form may be found on a clipboard at the foot of the patient's bed or outside of the room at the door until the patient is discharged. The nurse records his or her observations of the patient on the **nurses' notes and activity flowsheet** (Fig. 8–14). Entries must be signed by the nurse making the entry and usually include the first name, last name, and professional status (RN, LPN). These notes relate to the patient's behavior and reaction to treatment and other care ordered by the physician. The form serves as the written communication between the doctor and the nursing staff.

# CONDITIONS OF ADMISSION / MEDICAL TREATMENT AGREEMENT

1. **GENERAL DUTY NURSING:** Hospital provides only general nursing care.  If the patient needs special or private nursing, it must be arranged by the patient or physician treating the patient.

2. **CONSENT TO TREATMENT:**  The patient is under the control of the attending physician and the undersigned consents to x-ray examinations, laboratory procedures, anesthesia, medical and surgical treatment or hospital services rendered under the general and special instructions of the physician.  Many of the physicians of medicine furnishing services to the patient, including radiologists, pathologists, anesthesiologists are independent contractors and are not employees of the hospital.  Patient or the undersigned consents to treatment being rendered by these and other physicians.

3. **RELEASE OF INFORMATION:**  The hospital may disclose all or any part of the patient's medical record and or hospital charges (Including information regarding alcohol or drug abuse, psychiatric illness or communicable disease related information including HIV related information) to any person or corporation which is or may be liable or under contract to the hospital for reimbursement on this admission and/or hospital service, including but not limited to, hospital/medical service companies, insurance companies, worker's compensation carriers, welfare funds, governmental agencies and/or any health care provider for continued patient care.  The hospital may also disclose on an anonymous basis any information concerning my case which is necessary or appropriate for the advancement of medical science, medical education, medical research, for the collection of statistical data or pursuant to State or Federal law, statute or regulation.

4. **PERSONAL PROPERTY:**  The hospital has a safe in which to keep MONEY/VALUABLES.  The hospital is not responsible for any loss or damage to personal property not deposited in the safe.  The hospital specifically will not be responsible for loss or damage to glasses, dentures, hearing aids, contact lenses and prosthetic devices.

5. **PRICE QUOTES:**  I understand that any price quotations given may not include physicians' fees or services and are based on averages which may vary significantly from actual charges based on physician practice patterns, secondary or tertiary medical conditions and professional interpretations of a physician's order(s).

6. **PHYSICIAN BILLS:**  Your attending/consulting physicians may be billing you separately from the hospital.  These physicians may or may not participate with the same insurance plans as the hospital which may result in reduced reimbursement from your insurance company for physician fees.

7. **TEACHING PROGRAMS:**  The Hospital participates in programs for training of health care personnel.  Some services may be provided to the patient by persons in training under the supervision and instruction of physicians or hospital employees.  These persons may also observe care given to the patient by physicians and hospital employees.  Photos or video tapes may be made of surgical procedures by physicians or hospital personnel.

8. **FINANCIAL AGREEMENT:**  I agree that in return for the services provided to the patient by the hospital or other health care providers, I will pay the account of the patient, or prior to discharge or make financial arrangements satisfactory to the hospital or any other providers for payment.  If an account is sent to an attorney for collection, I agree to pay reasonable attorney's fees and collection expenses.  The amount of the attorney's fee shall be established by the Court and not by a jury in any court action.  A delinquent account may be charged interest at the legal rate.  I request that payment of any authorized Medicare benefits be made on my behalf, I assign the benefits payable for physician services to the physician or organization furnishing the services or authorize such physician or organization to submit a claim to Medicare for payment.  If any signer is entitled to benefits of any type under any policy of Insurance insuring the patient, or any other party liable to the patient, that benefit is hereby assigned to hospital or to the provider group rendering service, for application to patient's bill.  **HOWEVER, IT IS UNDERSTOOD THAT THE UNDERSIGNED AND THE PATIENT ARE PRIMARILY RESPONSIBLE FOR PAYMENT OF THE PATIENT'S BILL.  EMERGENCY CARE WILL BE PROVIDED WITHOUT REGARD TO THE ABILITY TO PAY.**

**I HAVE READ AND UNDERSTAND THESE CONDITIONS AND I HAVE RECEIVED A COPY.  I AM THE PATIENT OR AM AUTHORIZED TO ACT ON BEHALF OF THE PATIENT TO SIGN THIS AGREEMENT.**

| Witness | (circle one)  Patient  Parent  Authorized Party | Date |

**I HAVE PREVIOUSLY EXECUTED:**

| **POWER OF ATTORNEY FOR HEALTH CARE** | YES | NO | (CIRCLE ONE) |
| **LIVING WILL** | YES | NO | (CIRCLE ONE) |

**POWER OF ATTORNEY FOR HEALTH CARE UNDER A.R.S. 14-5501:**                    I appoint

| Name | Address | Phone # |

as my agent to act in all matters relating to health care, including full power to give or refuse consent to all medical, surgical and hospital care.  This power of attorney shall become effective upon my disability or incapacity or when there is uncertainty whether I am dead or alive and shall have the same effect as if I were alive, competent and able to act for myself.

| Witness | Patient |
| | *(Two witnesses required unless notarized)* |
| Witness | |

COPY 1 - Chart
COPY 2 - Billing
COPY 3 - Patient

MR-684 3/95

**CONDITIONS OF ADMISSION / MEDICAL TREATMENT AGREEMENT**

F I G U R E  8–9 • Admission agreement form.

SAINT, JOSEPH          MR 426-743
10/31/1939  M  57          963997
08/05/96  HOPES, HY

| Date Ordered | |
|---|---|
| 6-10-XX | Admitting diagnosis: acute exacerbation COPD, bronchitis, asthma, abd pain NKA VS q4h w/a I & O Reg NAS diet aminophylline 500 mg/500 cc D5W TRA 35 cc/hr O₂ 3L NP SMA, CBC, UA, EKG  CXR Lasix 40 mg po now then 40 mg po qam Theo level in am K-Dur ī lab BID          Dr Hy Hopes |

Authorization is given for dispensing non-proprietary name unless checked here. ☐

**PHYSICIAN'S ORDERS**

F I G U R E   8–10 • Physicians' order form or doctors' order sheet.

DATE

6/10/xx This 55 yr. old ♀ had rheumatic fever as a child and reports she has a damaged pulmonary valve. She experiences shortness of breath when running but not when doing regular activities. She has cardiac irregularities but takes no regular heart meds. She has had 1–2 episodes of CHF – treated as needed. She was a smoker until 6 wks ago.

She has had general and epidural anesthesia. Preop antibiotics have not been ordered. Physical status II for general anesthesia. She is allergic to tape

Dr. David Smith

6/10/xx Patient tolerated general anesthesia well and was awake when taken to RR.
Dr. David Smith

10/12/xx Complains of N&V. Percocet DC. Changed to Tylenol #3
Dr. Evan Span

FIGURE 8–11 • Physicians' progress record.

Nursing students as well as RNs, LPNs, and in some facilities, nursing assistants may record on this form. Black ink is preferred for all shifts because colored ink, especially red and green, does not photocopy or microfilm well. Some health care facilities use a checklist to take the place of some written nurses' notes.

## 7. The Nurses' Admission Record

In facilities utilizing bedside computer charting, the need for nurses' notes, activity flowsheets, and nurses' admission records, and graphic records may be eliminated. Information is entered into the computer and printed

Physician: _____

Registration/Medical Record Number: _____

| **HISTORY** | **PHYSICAL EXAMINATION** |

**HISTORY**

Present Illness: _____
_____
_____
_____
_____
_____

Past History: _____
_____
_____
_____
_____

Present Medications: _____
_____
_____
_____
_____
_____

Allergies: _____
_____
_____
_____
_____
_____

Diagnosis/Impression: _____
_____
_____
_____
_____

**PHYSICAL EXAMINATION**

General Appearance:   Normal ☐   Abnormal ☐
_____

Head/ENT:   Normal ☐   Abnormal ☐
_____

Heart:   Normal ☐   Abnormal ☐
_____

Lungs:   Normal ☐   Abnormal ☐
_____

Abdomen:   Normal ☐   Abnormal ☐
_____

Genitalia:   Normal ☐   Abnormal ☐
_____

Extremities:   Normal ☐   Abnormal ☐
_____

Breast:   Normal ☐   Abnormal ☐
_____

Focused Examination: _____
_____
_____
_____

Signature: _____ M.D.

F I G U R E   8–12 • History and physical form.

Patient Number:        765 466
Patient Name  Marcia Clerk
Physician Name          Joan  Simone

### HISTORY AND PHYSICAL EXAMINATION

Patient is a 56 year-old female admitted with the chief complaint of severe upper cervical spine pain   The patient has rheumatoid spondylitis and has a fusion of most of the cervical spine, but the upper two vertebra still have motion in their joints, and the patient is experiencing considerable pain because of the progressive arthritis at this level.

PAST HISTORY:  Reveals the patient to have some elevated blood pressure problems. She is currently taking Hygroton, aspirin and Indocin.  Patient has had as appendectomy, hysterectomy and a bilateral salpingo-oophorectomy.

REVIEW OF SYSTEMS:  No auditory or visual symptoms
CARDIORESPIRATORY:  No orthopnea, dyspnea, hemoptysis.
G.I. TRACT:  No weight gain, weight loss ., or change in bowel habits
G.U. TRACT:  No pyuria, dysuria or frequency
NEUROMUSCULAR:        See Present complaints.

PHYSICAL EXAMINATION:  A somewhat frail female in no acute distress.  Patient walks about room with neck flexed.  She is unable to extend neck.

CHEST:  Expansion is limited.  The lungs are clear to auscultation.  Heart tones are regular.  No murmurs.  No cardiomegaly.

ABDOMEN:  Soft.  LKS not palpable.

BACK:  Marked limitations of lumbodorsal motion.  No paraspinous muscle spasm noted.

EXTREMITY:  The patient has limitations of right shoulder motion and active and passive motion causes her significant discomfort, and crepitation is noted.  The neurovascular status of all extremities is intact.

*Joan Simone*

Joan Simone, D. O.

F I G U R E  8–13 • A typewritten history and physical form.

once every 24 hours for placement on the patient's chart. The **nurses' admission record** (Fig. 8–15) usually precedes or leads into the nurses' notes. Printed questions on the form are answered by the patient upon his or her admission to the nursing unit. A member of the nursing care team also compiles a short nursing history from the patient or family member regarding the patient's daily living activities, present illness, and medications the patient is taking. Also recorded on the nurses' admission history form are the patient's vital signs, height, weight, and any allergies to food or medications. The health unit coordinator later records the vital signs and allergies on the appropriate form. It is practice in some facilities to use red ink to note the patient's allergies.

DATE  6-20-XY

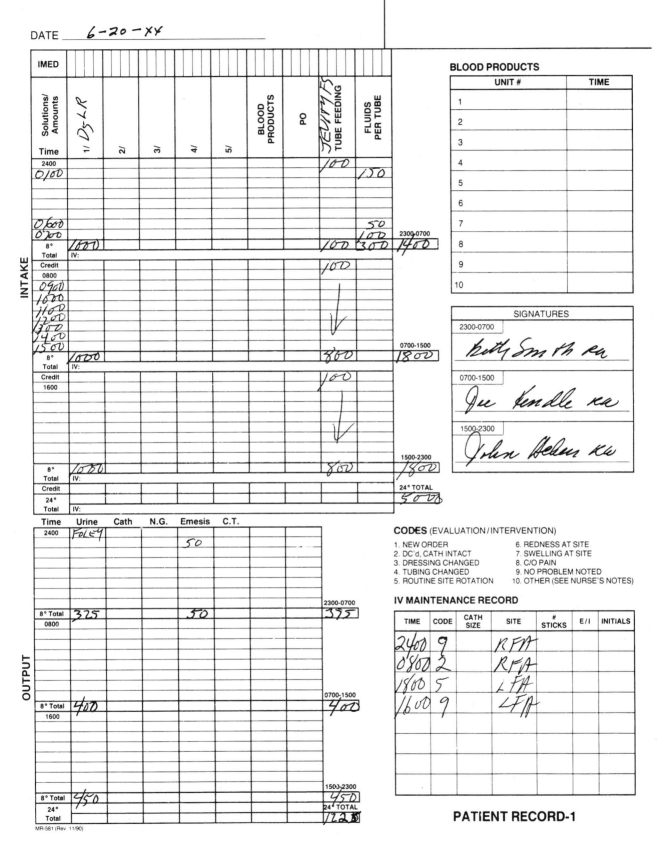

**BLOOD PRODUCTS**

| | UNIT # | TIME |
|---|---|---|
| 1 | | |
| 2 | | |
| 3 | | |
| 4 | | |
| 5 | | |
| 6 | | |
| 7 | | |
| 8 | | |
| 9 | | |
| 10 | | |

| SIGNATURES | |
|---|---|
| 2300-0700 | Betty Smith RN |
| 0700-1500 | Sue Kendle RN |
| 1500-2300 | John Helen RN |

**CODES** (EVALUATION/INTERVENTION)

1. NEW ORDER  
2. DC'd, CATH INTACT  
3. DRESSING CHANGED  
4. TUBING CHANGED  
5. ROUTINE SITE ROTATION  
6. REDNESS AT SITE  
7. SWELLING AT SITE  
8. C/O PAIN  
9. NO PROBLEM NOTED  
10. OTHER (SEE NURSE'S NOTES)

**IV MAINTENANCE RECORD**

| TIME | CODE | CATH SIZE | SITE | # STICKS | E/I | INITIALS |
|---|---|---|---|---|---|---|
| 2400 | 9 | | RFA | | | |
| 0800 | 2 | | RFA | | | |
| 1800 | 5 | | LFA | | | |
| 1600 | 9 | | LFA | | | |
| | | | | | | |
| | | | | | | |
| | | | | | | |
| | | | | | | |

**PATIENT RECORD-1**

MR-581 (Rev. 11/90)

FIGURE 8–14 • Nurses' notes and activity flowsheet. *Illustration continued on following page*

117

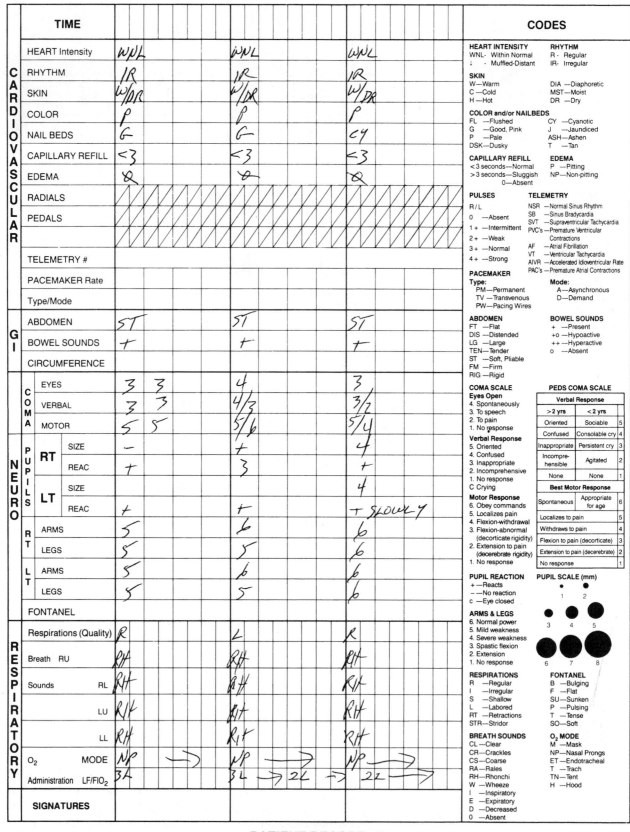

| | TIME | | | | | | | | | | |
|---|---|---|---|---|---|---|---|---|---|---|---|
| **C A R D I O V A S C U L A R** | HEART Intensity | WNL | | | WNL | | | WNL | | | |
| | RHYTHM | IR | | | IR | | | IR | | | |
| | SKIN | W/DR | | | W/DR | | | W/DR | | | |
| | COLOR | P | | | P | | | P | | | |
| | NAIL BEDS | G | | | G | | | CY | | | |
| | CAPILLARY REFILL | <3 | | | <3 | | | <3 | | | |
| | EDEMA | 0 | | | 0 | | | 0 | | | |
| | RADIALS | | | | | | | | | | |
| | PEDALS | | | | | | | | | | |
| | TELEMETRY # | | | | | | | | | | |
| | PACEMAKER Rate | | | | | | | | | | |
| | Type/Mode | | | | | | | | | | |
| **G I** | ABDOMEN | ST | | | ST | | | ST | | | |
| | BOWEL SOUNDS | + | | | + | | | + | | | |
| | CIRCUMFERENCE | | | | | | | | | | |
| **N E U R O** — C O M A | EYES | 3 | 3 | | 4 | | | 3 | | | |
| | VERBAL | 3 | 3 | | 4/3 | | | 3/2 | | | |
| | MOTOR | 5 | 5 | | 5/6 | | | 5/4 | | | |
| PUPILS RT | SIZE | — | | | + | | | 4 | | | |
| | REAC | + | | | 3 | | | + | | | |
| PUPILS LT | SIZE | | | | | | | 4 | | | |
| | REAC | + | | | + | | | + SLOWLY | | | |
| RT | ARMS | 5 | | | 6 | | | 6 | | | |
| | LEGS | 5 | | | 5 | | | 6 | | | |
| LT | ARMS | 5 | | | 6 | | | 6 | | | |
| | LEGS | 5 | | | 5 | | | 6 | | | |
| | FONTANEL | | | | | | | | | | |
| **R E S P I R A T O R Y** | Respirations (Quality) | R | | | L | | | R | | | |
| | Breath RU | RH | | | RH | | | RH | | | |
| | Sounds RL | RH | | | RH | | | RH | | | |
| | LU | RH | | | RH | | | RH | | | |
| | LL | RH | | | RH | | | RH | | | |
| | O₂ MODE | NP → | | | NP → | | | NP → | | | |
| | Administration LF/FIO₂ | 3L | | | 3L → 2L | | | 2L | | | |
| | SIGNATURES | | | | | | | | | | |

**CODES**

**HEART INTENSITY**
WNL- Within Normal
↓ - Muffled-Distant

**RHYTHM**
R - Regular
IR- Irregular

**SKIN**
W—Warm
C —Cold
H —Hot
DIA —Diaphoretic
MST—Moist
DR —Dry

**COLOR and/or NAILBEDS**
FL —Flushed
G —Good, Pink
P —Pale
DSK—Dusky
CY —Cyanotic
J —Jaundiced
ASH—Ashen
T —Tan

**CAPILLARY REFILL**
<3 seconds—Normal
>3 seconds—Sluggish
0—Absent

**EDEMA**
P —Pitting
NP—Non-pitting

**PULSES**
R/L
0 —Absent
1 + —Intermittent
2 + —Weak
3 + —Normal
4 + —Strong

**TELEMETRY**
NSR —Normal Sinus Rhythm
SB —Sinus Bradycardia
SVT —Supraventricular Tachycardia
PVC's —Premature Ventricular Contractions
AF —Atrial Fibrillation
VT —Ventricular Tachycardia
AIVR —Accelerated Idioventricular Rate
PAC's —Premature Atrial Contractions

**PACEMAKER**
Type:
PM —Permanent
TV —Transvenous
PW—Pacing Wires
Mode:
A—Asynchronous
D—Demand

**ABDOMEN**
FT —Flat
DIS —Distended
LG —Large
TEN—Tender
ST —Soft, Pliable
FM —Firm
RIG —Rigid

**BOWEL SOUNDS**
+ —Present
+o —Hypoactive
++ —Hyperactive
o —Absent

**COMA SCALE**
Eyes Open
4. Spontaneously
3. To speech
2. To pain
1. No response
Verbal Response
5. Oriented
4. Confused
3. Inappropriate
2. Incomprehensive
1. No response
C Crying
Motor Response
6. Obey commands
5. Localizes pain
4. Flexion-withdrawal
3. Flexion-abnormal (decorticate rigidity)
2. Extension to pain (decerebrate rigidity)
1. No response

**PEDS COMA SCALE**

| Verbal Response | | |
|---|---|---|
| >2 yrs | <2 yrs | |
| Oriented | Sociable | 5 |
| Confused | Consolable cry | 4 |
| Inappropriate | Persistent cry | 3 |
| Incomprehensible | Agitated | 2 |
| None | None | 1 |

| Best Motor Response | | |
|---|---|---|
| Spontaneous | Appropriate for age | 6 |
| Localizes to pain | | 5 |
| Withdraws to pain | | 4 |
| Flexion to pain (decorticate) | | 3 |
| Extension to pain (decerebrate) | | 2 |
| No response | | 1 |

**PUPIL REACTION**
+ —Reacts
– —No reaction
c —Eye closed

**PUPIL SCALE (mm)**

**ARMS & LEGS**
6. Normal power
5. Mild weakness
4. Severe weakness
3. Spastic flexion
2. Extension
1. No response

**RESPIRATIONS**
R —Regular
I —Irregular
S —Shallow
L —Labored
RT —Retractions
STR—Stridor

**FONTANEL**
B —Bulging
F —Flat
SU—Sunken
P —Pulsing
T —Tense
SO—Soft

**BREATH SOUNDS**
CL —Clear
CR—Crackles
CS—Coarse
RA—Rales
RH—Rhonchi
W —Wheeze
I —Inspiratory
E —Expiratory
D —Decreased
0 —Absent

**O₂ MODE**
M —Mask
NP—Nasal Prongs
ET—Endotracheal
T —Trach
TN—Tent
H —Hood

**PATIENT RECORD - 2**

FIGURE 8–14 • Continued

DATE ___6 – 20 x4___

| PATIENT CARE | 2400 | 0100 | 0200 | 0300 | 0400 | 0500 | 0600 | 0700 | 0800 | 0900 | 1000 | 1100 | 1200 | 1300 | 1400 | 1500 | 1600 | 1700 | 1800 | 1900 | 2000 | 2100 | 2200 | 2300 | CODES |
|---|---|---|---|---|---|---|---|---|---|---|---|---|---|---|---|---|---|---|---|---|---|---|---|---|---|
| ISOLATION | BF ———→ | | | | | | | | BF ———→ | | | | | | | | BF ———→ | | | | | | | | |
| TURN | c̄ ASSIST | | | | | | | | c̄ assist | | | | | | | | c̄ ASSIST | | | | | | | | |
| BATH | | | | | | | | | C BB | | | | | | | | | | | | | | | | |
| ORAL/TRACH CARE | | | | | | | | | ✓ | | | | | | | | | | | | | | | | |
| PERI/FOLEY CARE | | | | | | | | | ✓ | | | | | | | | | | | | | | | | |
| ACTIVITY | B ———→ | | | | | | | | B | C | C | B | B | B | B | B ———→ | | C | ———→ | B | | | | | |
| BACK CARE | | | | | | | | | ✓ | | | | | | | | | | | | | | | | |
| LINEN CHANGE | | | | | | | | | ✓ | | | | | | | | | | | | | | | | |
| ↑ SIDERAILS | ↑↑ | | | | | | | | X2 | | | | | | | | ↑X2 | | | | | | | | |
| | | | | | | | | | | | | | | | | | | | | | | | | | |
| DIET/APPETITE (% or cc's) | JEVITY FS | | | | | | | | JEVITY FS | | | | | | | | JEVITY FS | | | | | | | | |
| EQUIPMENT | KANGAROO PUMP-TELE | | | | | | | | K PUMP TELE | | | | | | | | K PUMP -TELE | | | | | | | | |
| GI TUBE — Placement Checked | | | | | | | | | ✓ | | | | ✓ | | | | ✓ | | ✓ | | | | | | |
| GI TUBE — Tube type/ Suction | FLEX FLOW | | | | | | | | Flexiflow | | | | | | | | FLEXI FLOW | | | | | | | | |
| STOOL — Hematest, Color, Char. | | | | | | | | | | | | | | | | | | | | | | | | | |
| STOOL — Method of Output | | | | | | | | | ✓ | | | | | | | | ✓ | | | | | | | | |
| STOOL — Amt. Description | | | | | | | | | Lg gn solid | | | | | | | | LG GN LIQ/SEMI SOLID | | | | | | | | |
| STOOL — Hematest | | | | | | | | | | | | | | | | | | | | | | | | | |
| URINE — Catheter | | | | | | | | | | | | | | | | | | | | | | | | | |
| URINE — Method of Output | FOLEY | | | | | | | | foley | | | | | | | | FOLEY | | | | | | | | |
| URINE — Specific Gravity Color, Char. | AMBER c̄ CLOTS | | | | | | | | amber c̄ clots | | | | | | | | AMBER c̄ CLOTS | | | | | | | | |
| RESP — Rx Chest Pt. | | | | | | | | | SUN QID | | | | | | | | | | | | | | | | |
| RESP — Suctioned | | | | | | | | | X2 | | | | | | | | X2 | | | | | | | | |
| RESP — Secretions ET (color, type, amt.) Oral | NON PROD LOOSE COUGH | | | | | | | | occ prod cough | | | | | | | | PROD COUGH | | | | | | | | |
| TESTS/PROC — Specimen Sent | | | | | | | | | | | | | | | | sputum sent | | | | | | | | | |
| TESTS/PROC — Procedures | | | | | | | | | | | | | | | | | | | | | | | | | |
| TESTS/PROC — Tests/X-rays | | | | | | | | | PORTABLE CHEST | | | | | | | | | | | | | | | | |
| DRAINS — Site Location | | | | | | | | | | | | | | | | | | | | | | | | | |
| DRAINS — Dressing Change | | | | | | | | | | | | | | | | | | | | | | | | | |
| WOUND — Site: location/ condition | | | | | | | | | | | | | | | | | | | | | | | | | |
| WOUND — Dressing Change | | | | | | | | | | | | | | | | | | | | | | | | | |
| FLAPS/GRAFTS | | | | | | | | | | | | | | | | | | | | | | | | | |
| SIGNATURES | | | | | | | | | | | | | | | | | | | | | | | | | |

CODES

ISOLATION
AFB—Respiratory
BF —Blood & Body Fluids

TURN
R—Right
L —Left
B—Back

BATH
C —Complete
P —Partial
PA—Partial/Assist
S —Shower
SA—Shower/Assist
T —Tub Bath
TA—Tub Assist

ACTIVITY
BRPA
B —Bedrest
A—AROM
P—PROM
H —Held
PR —Playroom
BRP —Bathroom Privileges
BRPA—with assist
BSC —Bedside Commode
BSCA—with assist
C —Chair (Self)
CA —with assist
DA —Dangle/ Assist
W —Walking
WA —Walking/ assist
S —Sleeping

RESTRAINTS
WRIST: left/right
ANKLE: left/right
BW —Both Wrists
BA —Both Ankles
P —Posey
CC —Cadillac Chair
CCA —with assist 2-3-4

DIET
FT—Fed Totally
FP—Fed Partially
TF—Tube Fed

EQUIPMENT
IM —IMED
OX—Oximeter
KP —Kangaroo Pump
AM—Apnea Monitor
HO—Hypothermia Blanket
HP—Hyperthermia Blanket
A —Airshields Warmer
IS —Isolette
K —K-Pad

STOOL/METHOD
T—Toilet
D—Dilly
I —Incontinent

URINE/METHOD
Catheter
Size/Date of insertion
D —Diaper
BP—Bedpan
I —Incontinent

PERI/FOLEY CARE
P—Peri
F—Foley

DRAINAGE
CL—Clear
BL—Bloody
S —Serous
SS—Serosanguinous
T —Tan

**PATIENT RECORD - 3**

F I G U R E 8–14 • *Continued*

119

DATE ___6-20 XX___

| NOTIFICATION | TIME | NURSING CONCERNS | RESPONSE TIME/ACTION TAKEN | INIT. |
|---|---|---|---|---|
|  |  |  |  |  |
|  |  |  |  |  |
|  |  |  |  |  |
|  |  |  |  |  |
|  |  |  |  |  |

### DISCHARGE/TEACHING INSTRUCTIONS

### PATIENT BEHAVIORS/OBSERVATIONS/EVALUATION/INTERVENTIONS (NURSES' NOTES)

24-06 PATIENT RESTING c̄ EYES CLOSED HOB ↑ VSS PULSE
130-150 TELE # 21 AFIB c̄ FREQ PVC HEPLOCK PATENT
+ FLUSHED O₂ ON CONT. PT HAS LOOSE NO PRODUCTIVE
COUGH JEVITY FS THROUGH KANGAROO PUMP @ 100°
PT RECEIVED ALL MEDS THROUGH FT - TOLERATED well.
FOLEY IRRIGATED c̄ NS 50cc ↑ 50cc RETURN c̄ SOME
BLD CLOTS. FOLEY DRAINED 325cc OF DRK AMBER URINE
c̄ CLOTS  RECOGNIZES RELATIVES - NEURO VS
INTACT  UP IN CHAIR c̄ ASSIST  EMESIS - 50cc
0614 patient bathed - turned freq - up in chair
D̄ mist - alert @ times ↓ lg on stool -
foley patent. Jevity FS through K pump @ 100/HR
tol well. occasional prod. cough pt.
resting @ intervals. VSS - pulse reg
135-160 tele # 21 Afib c̄ freq PVC
Heplock patent + flushed  O₂ on cont.
Good day. Urine output - 40cc
15-23 PT CONFUSED AT TIMES - UP IN CHAIR X1
FAMILY VISITED SHARED CONCERN OF PTS
CONFUSION. O₂ ON CONT. STOOL X1 FOLEY
PATENT JEVITY FS THRU K PUMP TOL WELL
HEPLOCK PATENT - FLUSHED  TELE # 21 AFIB OCC
PVC  IV INFUSING  PATIENT RESTING COMFORTABLY
NO COMPLAINTS OF PAIN OR NAUSEA URINE
OUTPUT - 450cc

**PATIENT RECORD - 4**

F I G U R E   8-14 • *Continued*

SAINT, JOSEPH          MR 426-743
10/31/1939  M  57       963997
08/05/96  HOPES, HY

Admission Date _6/10/ XX_ Time _1200_ Room _T7_

Patient prefers to be called _Joe_

Primary Language Spoken _English_

**MODE OF ADMISSION**

☒ Ambulatory          Admitted from _home_          Patient oriented to room:  ☒ Yes  ☐ No

☐ Wheelchair          Valuables in safe:  ☐ Yes  ☐ No

☐ Stretcher          Identiband checked:  ☐ Yes  ☐ No

☐ _____

**Vital signs:**  Temp _98.6_  Pulse _80_  Respirations _20_

Blood Pressure:  Right _138/90_  Left _140/90_

Does patient smoke:  ☒ Yes  ☐ No  Packs / day _one_

Does patient drink alcoholic beverages:  ☒ Yes  ☐ No  Amount _1 drink/day_

Height _6'11'_ actual / stated  Weight _210_ actual / stated  Special diet / restriction _none_

Has patient experienced a change in weight in the last 6 months:  ☐ Yes  ☒ No  Amount _____  ☐ Gained  ☐ Lost

Signature _Barbara Smythe_  ⊛ R.N., L.P.N., N.A.  Date _6/10/XX_  Time _1250_

**MEDICATION PROFILE:**  (PRESCRIPTION AND NON-PRESCRIPTION)  Include eye drops, insulin, ointment, bowel care, etc.

| DRUG NAME AND DOSE | HOW OFTEN | DATE / TIME OF LAST DOSE | SENT TO PHARMACY | LEFT AT BEDSIDE | AT HOME | SENT HOME |
|---|---|---|---|---|---|---|
| Dicumerol  100mg | Tid | 0900 | | | ✓ | |
| Tagamet | Tid & hs | 0900 | | | ✓ | |
| | | | | | | |
| | | | | | | |
| | | | | | | |
| | | | | | | |

Cortisone therapy:  ☐ Yes  ☒ No  When _____  Therapy length _____

Injections _____  Oral _____

**ALLERGIES**

☐ None known          **Substance**                              **Reaction**

_Morphine_                                      _nausea_

_Aspirin_                                        _rash_

_Tomatoes_                                       _rash_

_____

Patient's stated reason for admission and physical complaints: _Severe chest pain,_
_shortness of breath coughing_

Physician notified at admission: _____ ✓

Attending _Dr Hy Hopes_  Date _6/10/XX_ Time _1220_

Resident _Dr Cynthia Spence_  Date _6/10/XX_ Time _1225_

Emergency Contact _Jennie Saynt_  Phone Number _861 1902_

Signature _Barbara Smythe_ R.N., L.P.N.  Date _6/10_ Time _1300_

MR-509-98 (9/91)

**PATIENT ADMISSION**

FIGURE 8–15 • Nurses' admission record. *Illustration continued on following page*

**DIABETIC INFORMATION**

Do you have diabetes?  ☐ Yes  ☒ No     If yes, please complete the following questions:

Do you take insulin at home?                       ☐ Yes  ☐ No

Do you check blood sugars at home?            ☐ Yes  ☐ No

Diabetes Educator notified?                         ☐ Yes  ☐ No

Diet Office notified?                                       ☐ Yes  ☐ No

**MEDICAL HISTORY**  (Pertinent / Current)

Illnesses (acute / chronic) _____

Recent hospitalizations _____

Recent surgeries ___ *Laparoscopic cholecystectomy* _____

Injuries / accidents ___ *fractured left radius* _____

Recent exposure to infections ___ *pneumonia approx 6 months ago* ___

Current infections ___ *none.* _____

Pacemaker _____ *no* _____

Do you have an Advanced Directive / Living Will?     ☐ Yes  ☒ No     If yes, please submit copy.

Durable Power of Attorney for Health Care?     ☐ Yes  ☒ No     If yes, please submit copy.

Are you a designated organ donor?     ☐ Yes  ☒ No

Name and relationship of person providing information if other than patient: _____

**PROSTHESIS / APPLIANCES / VALUABLES**

| ITEM | | | YES | NO | TAKEN HOME | LOCKED IN SAFE | LEFT AT BEDSIDE |
|---|---|---|---|---|---|---|---|
| GLASSES | | | | | | | |
| CONTACT LENSES | ☒ L | ☒ R | ✓ | | | | |
| HEARING AID | ☐ L | ☐ R | | | | | |
| DENTURES: FULL | ☐ U | ☐ L | | | | | |
| DENTURES: PARTIAL | ☐ U | ☐ L | | | | | |
| MOBILITY APPLIANCE | | | | | | | |
| OTHER (Identify): | | | | | | | |
| VALUABLES | | | | | | | |

Signature ___ *Barbara Smythe* ___ (R.N.), L.P.N.   Date _6/10/XX_   Time _1230_

**PATIENT ADMISSION 2**

FIGURE 8–15 • *Continued*

## 8. Graphic or Clinical Record

The **clinical record** (Fig. 8–16) is a graphic representation of the patient's vital signs (temperature, pulse, respiration, and blood pressure) for a given number of days. Vital signs are ordered by the doctor, or taken according to the hospital routine.

It is the task of the health unit coordinator or nursing personnel to graph the vital signs on the clinical record. (Temperature may be calibrated in degrees Fahrenheit or degrees Celsius.)

## 9. Medication Administration Record

All medications given by nursing personnel are recorded on the **medication administration record (MAR)** (Fig. 8–17). As new medications are ordered by the doctor, the date, drug, dosage, administration route, and time frequency for administration of the medication are written on this form. This task is part of the transcription procedure and, therefore, is the responsibility of the health unit coordinator in many health care facilities.

## 10. Nurses' Discharge-Planning Form

The **nurses' discharge-planning form** (Fig. 8–18) is used to prepare the client for discharge from the health care facility. The nurse usually records information about the patient's health status at the time of discharge and provides instructions for the patient to follow after discharge from the health care facility.

## 11. Physicians' Discharge Summary

The physicians' discharge summary (Fig. 8–19), which is used by the physician to summarize the treatment and diagnosis the patient received while hospitalized, includes discharge information. The physician also lists the diagnosis and procedures that will be DRG-coded for reimbursement purposes.

## PREPARING THE CHART

Each health care facility has specific standard forms that are placed on all patients' charts. These forms are assembled by the health unit coordinator, clipped together, and set aside to be used once the patient has been admitted. These assembled forms are often referred to as the **admission packet**.

Upon admission, the forms in the admission packet are identified either with the patient's ID labels or imprinted with the patient's imprinter card. The forms that need dates and days of the week are filled in (Fig. 8–20) and are then placed behind the proper chart divider.

TO THE STUDENT

To practice preparing a patient's chart, complete **Activity 8–2** in the Skills Practice Manual.

## SUPPLEMENTAL CHART FORMS

Supplemental chart forms are additional to the standard forms and are added to the client's charts according to their specific care and treatment. For example, if the client is a diabetic and is receiving medication and being monitored, the supplemental form (diabetic record) will be added to the chart. This allows for information to be recorded separately from other data, making it easier for interpretation.

It is the responsibility of the health unit coordinator to obtain the needed forms, identify the form by using an ID label or imprinter, and place the form behind the proper chart divider in the chart holder.

## 1. Anticoagulant Therapy Record

The **anticoagulant record** (Fig. 8–21) is used to maintain a record of blood test results and the anticoagulant medication received by the client who is undergoing anticoagulant therapy. A flowsheet allows the doctor to make a comparison of the patient's blood test results and the medications prescribed over time.

## 2. Diabetic Record

The **diabetic record** (Fig. 8–22) is placed in the charts of patients who are receiving medication for diabetes. The results of the blood tests and urine studies performed to

967 896
MART TED
DR Y STOCKS
M 4C MEC INS

## GRAPHIC CHART (Fahrenheit)

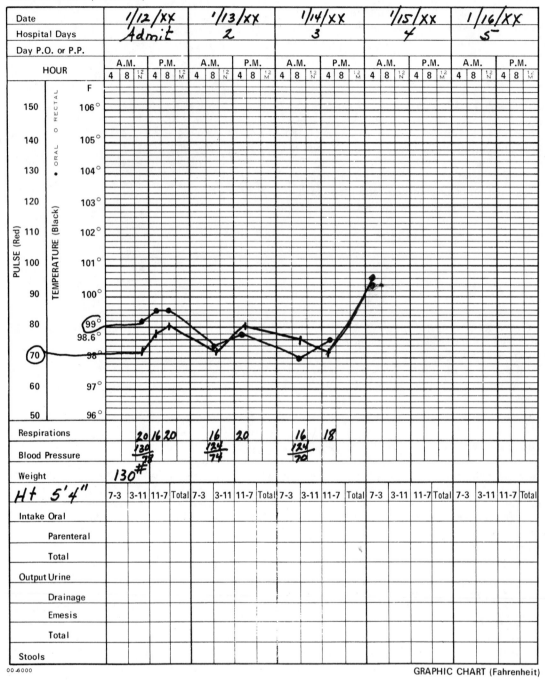

A

**F I G U R E  8–16** • Graphic or clinical record. (*A*) Fahrenheit. (*B*) Celsius (centigrade) with military time. *Illustration continued on opposite page*

967 896
MART TED
DR Y STOCKS
M 40 MED INS

## GRAPHIC CHART (Centigrade)

| Date | 1/12/XX | 1/13/XX | 1/14/XX | 1/15/XX | 1/16/XX |
|---|---|---|---|---|---|
| Hospital Days | Admit | 2 | 3 | 4 | 5 |
| Day P.O. or P.P. | | Surgery | 1 | 2 | 3 |

Temperature/Pulse graphic chart with hourly columns (0400, 0800, 1200, 1600, 2000, 2400) for each date.

| Respirations | | 20 | 18 | 18 20 18 | 22 20 20 22 22 22 | | |
| Blood Pressure | | 140/84 | 150/88 | 146/86 | | |
| Weight | | 146# | | | | |

Ht. 5'5"

| | 0700-1500 | 1500-2300 | 2300-0700 | Total | 0700-1500 | 1500-2300 | 2300-0700 | Total | 0700-1500 | 1500-2300 | 2300-0700 | Total | 0700-1500 | 1500-2300 | 2300-0700 | Total | 0700-1500 | 1500-2300 | 2300-0700 | Total |
|---|---|---|---|---|---|---|---|---|---|---|---|---|---|---|---|---|---|---|---|---|
| Intake Oral | | | | | | 100 | 100 | 200 | 500 | 300 | 1000 | | | | | | | | | |
| Parenteral | | | | | 500 | 500 | 1000 | | | | | | | | | | | | | |
| Total | | | | | 500 | 600 | 1100 | | | | | | | | | | | | | |
| Output Urine | | | | | 200 | 400 | 600 | 200 | 400 | 200 | 800 | | | | | | | | | |
| Drainage | | | | | | | | | | | | | | | | | | | | |
| Emesis | | | | | | 60 | 60 | | | | | | | | | | | | | |
| Total | | | | | 200 | 460 | 660 | 200 | 400 | 200 | 800 | | | | | | | | | |
| Stools | | | | | | | | | | | | | | | | | | | | |

00-6001

GRAPHIC CHART (Centigrade)

B

F I G U R E  8–16 • Continued

**MEDICATION RECORD**

SAINT, JOSEPH   MR 426-743
10/31/1939  M  57   963997
08/05/96  HOPES, HY

| | ROOM NO. 224-2 | | | ROOM NO. 224-2 | | | ROOM NO. 224-2 | | |
|---|---|---|---|---|---|---|---|---|---|
| | LAST NAME *Smyth* | | | LAST NAME *Smith* | | | LAST NAME *Smyth* | | |
| | P.O. DAY | | | P.O. DAY | | | P.O. DAY | | |

| # | DATE | DRUG / DOSE / ROUTE | DATE DC | SCHEDULE | DATE 11-7 | 7-3 | 3-11 | DATE 11-7 | 7-3 | 3-11 | DATE 11-7 | 7-3 | 3-11 |
|---|---|---|---|---|---|---|---|---|---|---|---|---|---|
| 1 | 8/11 | Dilantin 100mg  I.V. ⓞ R. I.M. | | tid | | 10  2 | 10 | | | | | | |
| 2 | 8/11 | Indocin 25mg  I.V. ⓞ R. I.M. | | bid | | 10 | 10 | | | | | | |
| 3 | 8/11 | Premarin 1.25mg  I.V. ⓞ R. I.M. | | qd | | 10 | | | | | | | |
| 4 | | I.V. P.O. R. I.M. | | | | | | | | | | | |
| 5 | | I.V. P.O. R. I.M. | | | | | | | | | | | |
| 6 | | I.V. P.O. R. I.M. | | | | | | | | | | | |
| 7 | | I.V. P.O. R. I.M. | | | | | | | | | | | |
| 8 | | I.V. P.O. R. I.M. | | | | | | | | | | | |
| 9 | | I.V. P.O. R. I.M. | | | | | | | | | | | |
| 10 | | I.V. P.O. R. I.M. | | | | | | | | | | | |
| 11 | | I.V. P.O. R. I.M. | | | | | | | | | | | |
| 12 | | I.V. P.O. R. I.M. | | | | | | | | | | | |
| 13 | | I.V. P.O. R. I.M. | | | | | | | | | | | |
| 14 | | I.V. P.O. R. I.M. | | | | | | | | | | | |
| 15 | | I.V. P.O. R. I.M. | | | | | | | | | | | |
| 16 | | I.V. P.O. R. I.M. | | | | | | | | | | | |
| 17 | | I.V. P.O. R. I.M. | | | | | | | | | | | |
| 18 | | I.V. P.O. R. I.M. | | | | | | | | | | | |
| 19 | | I.V. P.O. R. I.M. | | | | | | | | | | | |
| 20 | | I.V. P.O. R. I.M. | | | | | | | | | | | |
| 21 | | I.V. P.O. R. I.M. | | | | | | | | | | | |
| 22 | | I.V. P.O. R. I.M. | | | | | | | | | | | |
| 23 | | I.V. P.O. R. I.M. | | | | | | | | | | | |
| 24 | | I.V. P.O. R. I.M. | | | | | | | | | | | |
| 25 | | I.V. P.O. R. I.M. | | | | | | | | | | | |
| 26 | | I.V. P.O. R. I.M. | | | | | | | | | | | |
| 27 | | I.V. P.O. R. I.M. | | | | | | | | | | | |
| 28 | 8/13 | Compazine 100mg  I.V. P.O. R. ⓞ | 8/16 | q4h prn IV | 2³⁰ RT | | | | | | | | |
| 29 | 8/13 | Ambien 5mg  I.V. P.O. R. I.M. | 8/16 | hs prn | | | 10 | | | | | | |
| 30 | 8/13 | Demerol 50mg  R. ⓘⓜ | 8/16 | q4h prn | | 8³⁰ LT | | | | | | | |
| | | | | | MN | MN | MN | MN | MN | MN | MN | MN | MN |

**CODES**

| | | |
|---|---|---|
| | O - NOT GIVEN | ABD - ABDOMEN |
| LU - LUQ | LT - LT. THIGH | LA - LT. ARM |
| RU - RUQ | RT - RT. THIGH | RA - RT. ARM |
| OD - RT. EYE | OS - LT. EYE | OU - BOTH EYES |
| IVPB - IV PIGGYBACK | SQ - SUBCUTANEOUS | |

IDIOSYNCRACIES
*Morphine*

DIAGNOSIS
*Chole cystitis*

**MEDICATION RECORD**

MR - 1012 REV. 12/84

FIGURE 8-17 • Medication administration record. Front.

*discharge*

**Home Instructions**

SAINT, JOSEPH          MR 426-743
10/31/1939  M  57          963997
08/05/96  HOPES, HY

Name ___Joseph Saint___

Attending Physician ___Dr. Hy Hopes___

Activity Guidelines (None indicated ☐ )          **Room Checked For Patient Belongings** ☐

___as tolerated___

Diet/Nutrition (None indicated ☐ ) .

___low fat diet___
___small meals___

Treatments/Procedures/Dressings (None indicated ☐ )

___may shower.___

Home Medications (None indicated ☐ )          **Patients Own Medications Returned** ☐ Yes   ☐ No

| Name | Dose | Times | Special Considerations |
|------|------|-------|------------------------|
| Percodan | ҉ | every 4 hours | for pain |
| Compazine | ҉ | every 4 hours | for nausea |
|  |  |  |  |
|  |  |  |  |
|  |  |  |  |
|  |  |  |  |
|  |  |  |  |
|  |  |  |  |

See General Information on Medication Use printed on the back of this form.

Food/Medication Instruction Sheet Provided   ☒ Yes   ☐ None Indicated

Additional Information Provided (Handouts, (Brochures))  ☐ None Indicated

___post op laparoscopic cholecystectomy instructions___

Physician or Agency Referrals          Contact Person          Phone Number

I understand the guidelines for my care at home.

___Joe Saint___                ___Mary Smith___                6/8
Responsible Person          LPN/RN/MD                Date

WHITE - Chart Copy; CANARY - Patient Copy; PINK - Physician Copy

09-9268 6/82 Rev. 9/94

FIGURE 8–18 • Nurses' discharge planning form.

Patient Label

## CODING SUMMARY

Attending Physician *Marietta Harris MD*    Other Attending *Pat Anderson MD*

Anesthesia *Philip Ellis MD*    Assistant Surgeon *Casey Hershfield MD*

Intern/Resident *Connie Estralla MD*

Consultant(s) *Richard Weber M.D.*    Date of Admission *11-6-XX*

Date of Discharge *11-21-XX*

| Principal Diagnosis (Condition after study that occasioned the admission) | H.I.M.S. Codes |
|---|---|
| End Stage Renal Disease | 403.9 |

| Secondary Diagnosis (Including complications and co-morbidities if applicable) | H.I.M.S. Codes |
|---|---|
| Diabetes Mellitus | 250.41 |
| Blindness Secondary to Diabetic Retinopathy | 250.51 |
| Hypertension | 369.00 |

| Procedure(s) and Date(s) (List Principal Procedure first. Principal Procedure should be for definitive treatment.) | H.I.M.S. Codes |
|---|---|
| Kidney Transplant                11-8-XX | 55.69 |
| Excision of Tenckhoff catheter 11-8-XX | 54.99 |

**DISCHARGE STATUS:**

☑ 1. Home          ☐ 5. Other Type Institute      ☐ 20. Expired
☐ 2. Other Acute Care   ☐ 6. Home Health Care        ☐ Autopsy
☐ 3. Skilled Nursing Facility  ☐ 7. Against Medical Advice   ☐ No Autopsy
☐ 4. Intermediate Care Facility  ☐ 8. Home with I.V. Therapy  ☐ Coroner's Case

ATTENDING PHYSICIAN
OR CHIEF _____ *Marietta Harris MD* _____ Date *11-21-XX*
(Signature Optional)

THIS SECTION TO BE UTILIZED BY HEALTH INFORMATION MANAGEMENT SERVICES

Hospital Service *Vascular Surgery* By *WK*

Coding *E MIC*

Analysis *WK*

00-0627 11/83 Rev. 10/95

Patient Label

**F I G U R E   8–19 •** Physicians' discharge summary sheet.

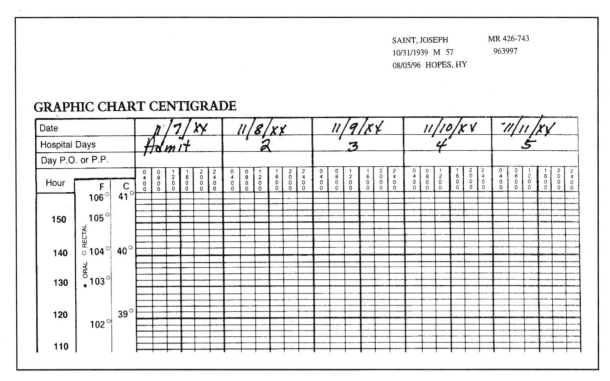

SAINT, JOSEPH            MR 426-743
10/31/1939 M 57         963997
08/05/96 HOPES, HY

### GRAPHIC CHART CENTIGRADE

F I G U R E   8–20 • Chart with headings filled in.

monitor the effect of the diabetic medications are also recorded on the diabetic record.

### 3. Consultation Form

The patient's attending physician may wish to obtain the opinion of another doctor. In this event, he or she requests a consultation by writing it on the doctors' order sheet. A **consultation form** (see Fig. 18–1), on which the consultant may write his or her findings, is placed on the front of the chart by the health unit coordinator. A consultation may also be dictated and appears on the patient's record as a typewritten report. Additional information regarding consultations are found in Chapter 18.

### 4. Operating Room Records

The number of forms required to maintain a record of a patient's operation varies. The records are utilized by operating room personnel, the anesthesiologist, and recovery room personnel (see Figs. 19–16A and B). Additional responsibilities regarding the surgery chart are found in Chapter 19.

### 5. Therapy Records

Health care facilities use individual record sheets for recording treatments. It is possible to have record sheets for physical medicine, respiratory care, diet therapy, radiation therapy, occupational therapy, and others. These departments are discussed elsewhere in Section III (Fig. 8–23).

### 6. Parenteral Fluid or Infusion Record

A patient who receives an intravenous infusion may have a **parenteral fluid record** (Fig. 8–24) placed in his or her chart. This form, when completed, is a written record of types and amounts of intravenous fluids administered to the patient. If computing bedside charting is in use, the parenteral fluid record or vital signs record may be initiated when the information is entered into the computer.

### 7. Vital Signs Record

The **vital signs record** (Fig. 8–25) is used when vital signs are taken more often than every 4 hours.

### 8. Pathway Worksheets

A recent trend in many hospitals is to use clinical pathways, a tool for tracking patient progress in a managed care system. Clinical pathways are preestablished based on the medical diagnosis (Fig. 8–26).

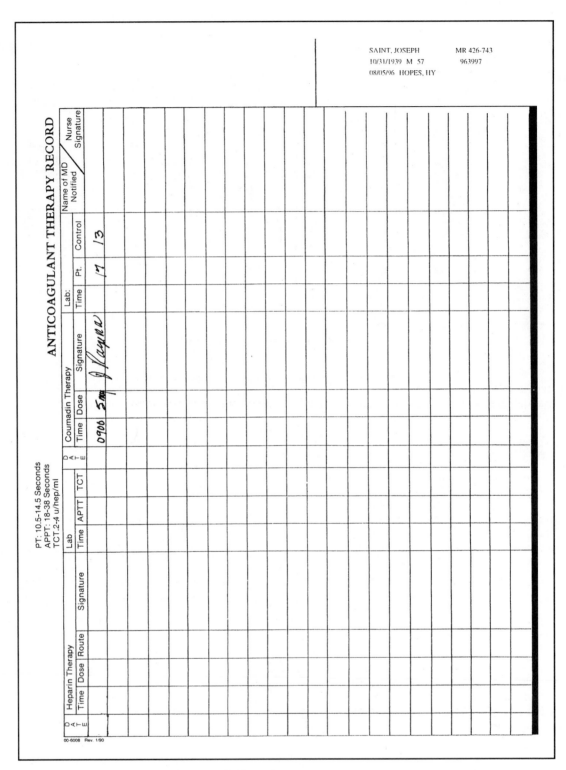

F I G U R E  8–21 • Anticoagulant therapy record.

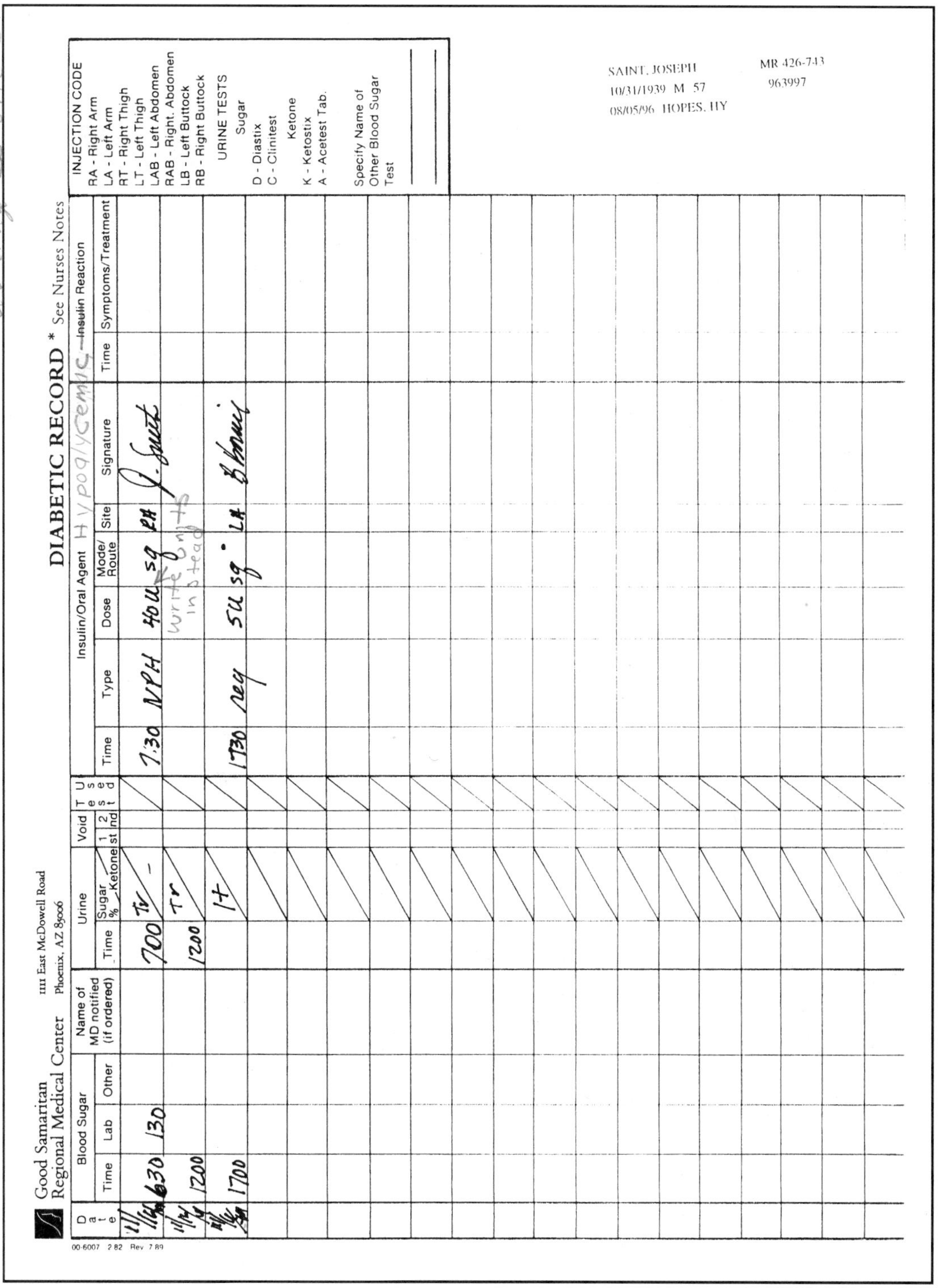

*Handwritten margin notes:*

might be on this flow sheet

Hg A1C average BS over 3 month period

**Good Samaritan Regional Medical Center**
1111 East McDowell Road
Phoenix, AZ 85006

00-6007  2 82  Rev 7 89

## DIABETIC RECORD * See Nurses Notes

SAINT. JOSEPH
10/31/1939  M  57
08/05/96  HOPES. HY

MR 426-743
963997

**INJECTION CODE**
RA - Right Arm
LA - Left Arm
RT - Right Thigh
LT - Left Thigh
LAB - Left Abdomen
RAB - Right. Abdomen
LB - Left Buttock
RB - Right Buttock

**URINE TESTS**
Sugar
D - Diastix
C - Clinitest
Ketone
K - Ketostix
A - Acetest Tab.

Specify Name of Other Blood Sugar Test

*Handwritten:* Hypoglycemic

*Handwritten note near Mode/Route:* write units instead

| Date | Blood Sugar Time | Lab | Other | Name of MD notified (if ordered) | Urine Time | Sugar % | Ketone | Void 1st | 2nd | T.U. | Time | Type | Dose | Mode/Route | Site | Signature | Insulin Reaction Time | Symptoms/Treatment |
|---|---|---|---|---|---|---|---|---|---|---|---|---|---|---|---|---|---|---|
| 11/26 | 0630 | 130 | | | 700 | Tr | − | | | | 1:30 | NPH | 40u sq | eh | J. Sutt | | |
| 11/26 | 1200 | | | | 1200 | Tr | | | | | | | | | | | |
| 11/26 | 1700 | | | | | | 1+ | | | | 1730 | reg | 5u sq | LA | B. mui | | |

F I G U R E  8-22 • Diabetic record.

INSTITUTE OF REHABILITATION MEDICINE
**PROGRESS NOTES**
Home Care, Orientation & Mobility, Occupational
Therapy, Physical Therapy, Speech Pathology
& Orthotics

967 896
MART TED
DR Y STOCKS
M 40 MED INS

| DATE & SERVICE | P.T. |
|---|---|
| 11/12/xx | Patient seen bid in a.m. for exercise in supine position. Ambulated 25' c̄ arm support + minimal assistance for balance. In p.m. pt seen for ambulation 25' C/o light headache so returned to bed.
R. Wentcomb, RPT |
| 11/13/xx | In a.m arm ROM 5-10 reps in all planes. Pt. cooperated c̄ program. Transferred to chair for 10 min.
R. Wentcomb, RPT |

FIGURE 8–23 • Therapy records. (A) Physical therapy progress notes. (B) Respiratory treatment record. (C) Dietetic therapy progress notes. *Illustration continued on opposite page*

## CONSENT FORMS

### Surgery or Procedure Consent Form

There are a number of conditions that require the client or a responsible party to sign a special form granting permission to perform surgery or other invasive procedures upon the patient (Fig. 8–27).

The client who is hospitalized for surgery is required to sign a form permitting his or her doctor to perform the surgery named on the consent form. The form should not be signed until the physician has explained the surgery or procedure and its risks, alternatives, and likely outcomes (informed consent). After receiving an explanation, a competent patient can give informed consent.

Other procedures requiring consent forms to be signed by the patient or a responsible party are covered in chapters related to the specific procedures.

The health unit coordinator may prepare the consent form for the physician or nurse to take to the patient for the patient's signature.

If the surgery should be cancelled, the surgery permit is still valid unless the doctor or the surgical procedure has been changed.

Consent forms for surgery and certain other procedures are legal agreements between the patient and the physician. In some health care facilities it may be the physician's responsibility to write the name of the doctor who is to perform the surgery or procedure, as well as writing the name of the procedure to be done.

### Procedure for Preparing Consent Forms

In facilities in which the health unit coordinator may still fill in some portions of the consent form, the following procedure may be used.

1. Stamp the consent form with the patient's imprinter card or affix the patient's ID label to the form. Some physicians who are incorporated may have preprinted consent forms with their legal business name, which should be used.

2. Write in ink the first and last names of the doctor who is to perform the surgery or procedure. The name of

DEPARTMENT OF RESPIRATORY CARE

### TREATMENT RECORD

967 901
SAAKE PETE
DR B GOOD
M 46 MED INS

| DATE | |
|------|--|
| 11/19/xx | SVN Rx given c̄ 0.2 cc Alupent +2cc N.S via N/P c̄ C/A at 5 L/M X 10 min. Pulse 104 and stable. Breath sounds essentially clear. Pt. tolerated Rx well. Productive cough c̄ sm. amt. thin white sputum |
| | Bonnie Flowers RT. |

B

### DIETETIC PROGRESS NOTES

967 900
CIDER IDA
DR C BARRELL
F 58 SURG INS

| DATE | |
|------|--|
| 2/1/xx | Appetite poor X 4 mo. 150# → 124# States Dr. told her to avoid all fruits and juices and also no red meat. Pt does not tolerate milk products except cheese. Does not tolerate Ensure and Sustacal (diarrhea) Takes Vit. C + E. at home. Pt is 58 yr. old female c̄ lung cancer and mass in abdomen. Also dehydrated. Has med. visceral protein loss. Diet: Soft c̄ Sustacal supplement. |
| | Doris Kay, R.D. |

C

FIGURE 8–23 • *Continued*

967 896
MART TED
DR Y STOCKS
M 40 MED INS

## PARENTERAL FLUID SHEET

| DATE | TIME STARTED | TYPE OF SOLUTION, RATE, SITE MODE OF ADMINISTRATION SIZE & KIND-NEEDLE/CANNULA | STARTED BY | MEDICATION ADDED BY | AMT. INF. | TIME DISC. BY | REMARKS |
|---|---|---|---|---|---|---|---|
| 9/26/XX | 1100 | 1000 cc D₅W @125 cc/h Lt hand c̄ #21 Butterfly | H. Jones | | 1000 cc | 1900 | No redness or edema at site |
| | | | | | | | |
| | | | | | | | |
| | | | | | | | |
| | | | | | | | |

F I G U R E  8–24 • Parenteral fluid or infusion record.

the surgeon may be found on the doctors' order sheet or on the surgery schedule. For procedures performed by other departments that require consent forms, the health unit coordinator must contact the individual department for the name of the doctor who is to perform the procedure.

3. Write out in full in ink the surgery or procedure to be performed. (The physician writes the surgical or diagnostic procedure on the physicians' order sheet.) Do not use abbreviations; for instance, if the procedure is the "amputation rt index finger," the consent form should read "amputation of the right index finger."

967 896
MART TED
DR Y STOCKS
M 40 MED INS

## VITAL SIGNS RECORD

DATE  11/6/XX

| Time | BP | T | P | R | Oral | N/G | IV | Blood | Misc. | Urine | N/G | Stool | Emesis | Misc. | Spec. Grav. | CVP |
|---|---|---|---|---|---|---|---|---|---|---|---|---|---|---|---|---|
| | | | | | | INTAKE | | | | | OUTPUT | | | | | |
| 0900 | 110/50 | 98 | 60 | 16 | | | 100cc | | | | | | 50cc | | | |
| 1000 | 112/54 | 98⁴ | 64 | 16 | 60cc | | 100cc | | | 100 cc | | | | | | |
| 1100 | 112/57 | 98⁴ | 60 | 18 | 60cc | | 100cc | | | | | Ṫ | | | | |
| 1200 | 110/56 | 98⁸ | 68 | 18 | 60cc | | 100cc | | | 150cc | | | 100cc | | | |
| | | | | | | | | | | | | | | | | |

F I G U R E  8–25 • Vital signs record.

History: _____
IV: _____

Procedures: _____

A = achieved - N = not achieved

| | Pre-hospital | Day of Surgery | Post-op day 1 | PO day 2 | PO day 3 | PO day 4 Discharge |
|---|---|---|---|---|---|---|
| | | Date | Date | Date | | |
| Consult | Medical Clearance if necessary | PT consult in PM | PT therapy BID | PT BID Home Care and SS as appr | PT BID | PT |
| Tests | CXR, CBC, UA, PT, SMA20, EKG, Labs appropriate for age & health 72 hrs before | T & C 2 units (pre-op) (autologous when able) X-ray (in PACU) | H & H ☐ PT (If on coumadin) ☐ | H & H ☐ PT ☐ | H & H ☐ PT ☐ | PT ☐ |
| Mobility | | dangle - stand prn | Knee exercises Chair BID (30 min) - up for dinner Stand/Amb | Cont exercises - Amb BID Chair BID (45 min) - up for lunch and dinner BRP | Continue mobility Chair (60 min) - up for all meals | Continue mobility Chair (60 min) - up for all meals |
| Treatments | | Trapeze Drain IV therapy, incentive spir q2° DVT prophylaxes : (TED, foot compression device, coumadin , Lovenox) CPM 0 - 40° in PACU | Trapeze Drain Cap IV, incentive spir q2° DVT prophylaxes CPM 0 - 50° | Trapeze DC drain Cap IV, incentive spir q2° DVT proph Dressing change by physician CPM 0 - 60° | Trapeze Incentive spirometer DC IV DVT proph CPM 0 - 70° | CPM 0 - 80° |
| Meds | | Pain Med (IV, IM) Pt states pain relief: A N Antibiotics | Pain Med (IV, IM) Pt states pain relief: A N DC Antibiotics | PO pain meds Pt states pain relief: A N | PO pain meds prn Pt states pain relief: A N | PO pain meds prn Pt states pain relief: A N |
| Nutrition Metabolic | | DAT ____ | DAT ____ | DAT ____ | DAT ____ | DAT ____ |
| Elimination | | Cateter of choice prn st cath foley after 3rd time | DC foley | Eval. bowel function (BCOC) | Bowel movement: A N | Bowel movement: A N |
| Health /Home Management | | | Screen for Home Care & Social Service needs | Prescription for home equipment identified by PT Order equipment | Complete transfer form | ☐ Home ☐ ECF |
| Health Perception | TKA pre-op teaching by Interdisciplinary Team | Review: ☐ TCDB, ☐ incentive spirometry, ☐ ankle pumps, ☐ ROM to arms, ☐ CPM, ☐ pain management | Instruct on: ☐ knee precautions | Instruct on: ☐ incisional care ☐ pain management | Discharge teaching: ☐ Medication ☐ review knee book | ☐ Written discharge instructions to patient and family |
| Signature | | | | | | |
| Signature | | | | | | |
| Signature | | | | | | |

| Outcomes | | | Date met/initials |
|---|---|---|---|
| 1. In-out of bed | ☐ indep or with min assist | ☐ mod - max assist | |
| 2. On-off commode or chair | ☐ indep or with min assist | ☐ mod - max assist | |
| 3. Ambulates with assistive devices. | ☐ 75 feet indep or with min asst | ☐ 50 feet | |
| 4. AROM | ☐ 0 - 70 - 90° | ☐ 0 - 60° | |

| Outcomes | | Date met/initials |
|---|---|---|
| 5. Evidence of wound healing, no drainage | | |
| 6. Performs total knee exercises without assistance | | |
| 7. Re-establish elimination pattern. | | |
| 8. Utilizes oral analgesics for pain control. | | |

F I G U R E  8–26 • Clinical pathway for total knee arthroscopy.

## CONSENT FORM

1. I authorize and direct ___Roderick Curitan___, ("Physician"), and/or such associates and assistants as the Physician chooses, to perform upon ___Darina Parker___ ("Patient"), the following procedure(s): ___bilateral salpingo-oophorectomy___ ___write out in full no Abr.___

2. I also authorize the Physician to perform any other procedures that, in the Physician's judgment, are reasonable and necessary for the Patient's well-being, including, but not limited to, the administration of anesthesia and the performance of pathology and radiology services.

3. For purposes of medical education, I authorize the Physician to admit observers to the operating room.

4. The Physician has explained to me the nature, purpose, and possible consequences, risks, and complications of the procedure, as well as alternative methods of treatment. I understand that the explanation I have received is not exhaustive and that other, more remote risks and consequences may occur. I understand that a more detailed and complete explanation of any of the foregoing matters will be given to me if I so desire. No warranty or guarantee has been made to me regarding the results or cure that may be obtained.

5. I understand that my private attending Physician and any anesthesiologists, radiologists, pathologists, or other private physicians who may be involved in the Patient's care are not employees or agents of this hospital, nor are they controlled by this hospital. Rather, they are independent contractors who act on the Patient's behalf using independent medical judgment. The only exceptions are employees of the hospital who provide these services.

6. I authorize the hospital pathologist to dispose of any severed tissue, body part, or explant as the pathologist best sees fit, <u>except</u> (specify desired disposal):

_____

_____

**BY SIGNING THIS FORM, I HEREBY CERTIFY THAT I HAVE READ AND UNDERSTAND THIS CONSENT FORM IN ITS ENTIRETY, THAT ALL STATEMENTS MADE HEREIN ARE TRUE, AND THAT I CONSENT TO ALL TERMS STATED HEREIN.**

___Darina Parker___      ___8/10/xx___
Signature of Patient or Authorized Decision-Maker* (Specify Relationship)    Date & Time

___Bertha Callahan___      ___8/10/xy___
Signature of Witness/Two Witnesses Required for Telephone Consent    Date & Time

*If not signed by Patient, specify reason:
_____ Patient is a minor;
_____ Patient is unable to sign because:_____

## CONSENT FORM

MR-10-303 (2/94)

F I G U R E  8–27 • Surgery consent form.

4. All written information must be spelled correctly and written legibly.
5. Do not record the date and time. This will be completed by the person obtaining the client's signature.

The patient may be required to sign other permit or release forms during her or his hospitalization. The following are examples of situations that usually require a signature by the patient or the patient's representative.

1. Release of side rails (Fig. 8–28)
2. Refusal to permit blood transfusion (Fig. 8–29)
3. Consent form for human immunodeficiency virus (HIV) testing (Fig. 8–30)

---

**RELEASE OF SIDE RAILS**

Having been informed by Good Samaritan Hospital that protective side rails should be placed on my bed and raised for my personal protection, I hereby instruct the hospital and its employees not to place or raise protective side rails on my bed and hereby assume all risks in connection therewith and fully release the said hospital, its employees and my physician from any and all liability for any injury or damage to me by reason of its failure to place or raise protective side rails on my bed.

Signature_____

Room No._____

Witness_____

Witness_____

Date_____Hour_____ .M.

51-98                                                                                Release of Side Rails

---

F I G U R E  8–28 • Release of side rails forms.

PATIENT LABEL

### Refusal To Permit Blood Transfusion

1.  I request that no blood derivatives be administered to _Richard Kramer_
    during this hospitalization.                                       (patient name)

2.  I hereby release the hospital, its personnel and the attending physician from any responsibility whatever for
    unfavorable reactions or any untoward results due to my refusal to permit the use of blood or its derivatives.

3.  I fully understand the possible consequences of such refusal on my part.

_____    _9/10/xx_    _1200_
Patient's Signature                    Date          Time

_____
Signature of parent, legally appointed guardian or responsible person
(for patients who cannot sign)

_Alan Carlo_          _9/10/xx_    _1200_
Witness                Date           Time

_Donna Small_         _9/10/xx_    _1200_
Witness                Date           Time

00-0038 6/90                                    **REFUSAL TO PERMIT BLOOD TRANSFUSION**

F I G U R E  8–29 • Form for refusal to permit blood transfusion.

**CONSENT FOR HIV TESTING**

1. My physician, _____, has recommended that I (my child) receive a blood test to detect the presence of antibodies to Human Immunodeficiency Virus (HIV), the virus that causes Acquired Immune Deficiency Syndrome (AIDS). I consent to this testing.

   It has been explained to me that in some cases the tests may be positive when I have (my child has) not been infected with HIV. This is a false positive.

   If the screening is positive, a second confirming test is done.

   I understand that a negative result usually means that I have (my child has) not been exposed to HIV. However, there is a possibility of a false-negative result, especially in the time period immediately after exposure to the virus.

2. I have been advised by my physician and I understand the following:

   - Positive test results could mean that I have (my child has) been exposed to the HIV; this would not necesarily mean that I have (my child has) AIDS, or will develop AIDS.

   - That if I am (my child is) HIV positive, I (my child) can transmit the virus to other individuals by sexual contact, by sharing needles, or by the donation of organs, blood, and blood products.

   - That if I am (my child is) HIV positive, I (my child) should not donate blood or blood products, or body organs because the virus can be transmitted to the recipient.

3. I understand that Arizona State Law and Regulations require the reporting of HIV cases to the Department of Health Services and that if my (my child's) test results are positive, they will be submitted to the Arizona Department of Health Services, and others whose authority is established by law, regulation, or court order.

4. I also understand that my request for the test and the test results will be part of my (my child's) Hospital medical record and may therefore be requested by others, including insurers, third party payors or other individuals as outlined in the Conditions of Admission.

I have been given the opportunity to ask quesitons, I understand what is involved in HIV testing, and I freely consent to it.

_____          _____
DATE                                                              SIGNATURE

_____          _____
LEGAL GUARDIAN                                             WITNESS SIGNATURE
(If patient cannot sign or under age)

**F I G U R E   8–30** • Consent form for human immunodeficiency virus (HIV) testing.

4. Consent to receive blood transfusion (Fig. 8–31)

> **TO THE STUDENT**
>
> To practice preparing a consent form for surgery, complete **Activity 8–3** in the Skills Practice Manual.

Some health care facilities may allow the health unit coordinator to witness the signing of consent forms. The health unit coordinator signs as a witness to the patient's signature and not as a witness to the content of the consent. There are several general rules for the health unit coordinator to remember when serving in this capacity.

1. The patient must not be under the influence of any "mind-clouding" medications.
2. The client must be of legal age (18 in most states).
3. The client must be mentally competent.

Check with your instructor or the hospital policy manual for other rules that may apply.

## METHODS OF ERROR CORRECTION

Since the chart is considered a legal document, information recorded on a chart form must not be erased or oblit-

**CONSENT FOR TRANSFUSION**

**OF BLOOD OR BLOOD PRODUCTS**

1. My physician has informed me that I need, or may need during treatment, a transfusion of blood and/or one of its products in the interest of my health and proper medical care.

2. My physician has explained to me the nature, purpose and possible consequences of the procedures relating to transfusion, as well as significant risks involved, possible complications of and alternatives to transfusion and possible options of obtaining blood and blood products. I understand that transfusion involves some risks to the patient even though precautions are taken. I also understand that despite the exercise of due care, the transfusion of blood and blood products may transmit infectious diseases such as hepatitis or HIV (AIDS) or may result in an allergic reaction of the patient.

3. The alternatives to transfusion, including the risks and consequences of not receiving this therapy, have been explained to me.

4. I have had the opportunity to ask questions.

5. I consent to transfusion(s) as ordered by my physician(s) during my hospitalization.

_____     _____     _____
Signature of Patient                               Date                  Time

_____     _____     _____
Signature of Parent/Guardian or                 Date                  Time
Responsible Person (for minors or
patients who are unable to sign)

_____     _____     _____
Witness                                             Date                  Time

MR-2320 (8/91)

F I G U R E  8–31 • Consent form for receiving blood transfusion.

erated by pen, by pasting over, or by liquid correction fluid. Only certain methods of correcting errors recorded on the chart are permitted.

Chart forms that are imprinted with an incorrect imprinter card or with the wrong imprinter card or affixed with the wrong or incorrect ID label may be destroyed if no notations have been made on them. If the chart form has notations on it, the chart form cannot be destroyed. The correct information may be imprinted with the patient's imprinter card next to or below the error. It is also

*11/7/XX mistaken entry W. Andrew CHUC*

967-811 MR 243-687          967-801    MR-243-687
Kay, JoAnn                  Kay, JoAnn
A. Heart                    A. Hart
F 39 Ortho CHAMPUS          F 39 Ortho CHAMPUS

NURSES NOTES

F I G U R E  8–32 • Method for correcting imprinting error.

permissible to print the information in ink by hand. After the correct information has been placed on the chart form, an **X** should be made across the incorrect information and "mistaken entry" written above the first line. The date, your first initial, your last name, and your status should appear next to the words *mistaken entry* (Fig. 8–32).

To correct an error of a written entry made on a chart form, draw (in ink) one single line through the error. Record "mistaken entry" with the date, your first initial, your last name, and your status in a blank area near (directly above or next to) the error (Fig. 8–33). Follow your facility policy for correction of erroneous computer entries.

The procedure for correcting an error on the graphic sheet is covered in Chapter 21.

```
T O  T H E  S T U D E N T
```

To practice correcting imprinter errors and written errors on a chart form, complete **Activities 8–4** and **8–5** in the Skills Practice Manual.

## MAINTAINING AND MANAGING THE CLIENT'S CHART

As the person in charge of the clerical duties on the nursing unit, you are responsible for maintaining the patient's chart.

Duties in the maintenance of the client's chart are:

1. Place all charts in proper sequence (usually according to room number) in the chart rack when they are not in use.
2. Keep a record of the location of the patient's chart when it is removed from the unit.
3. Make sure you know the identity of the persons who have access to the charts.
4. Place new chart forms in the chart before the immediate need arises. In many health care facilities, this is referred to as "stuffing the chart." Imprint or label the forms with proper identification before placing them in the chart. Depending on hospital policy, new forms placed in the progress notes section may be placed at the end so the notes read like a book. New forms for doctors' orders are placed on top of old orders for the doctor's convenience. The new form may be folded in half to show the old form has not been completely used.
5. Place diagnostic reports in the correct patient's chart behind the correct divider. (It is the practice in many hospitals for a nurse to check all diagnostic reports before the health unit coordinator places them in the chart.)
6. Review the client's charts frequently for new orders.
7. Properly identify the patient's chart so that it can easily be located at all times.

## MEDICATION RECORD

*Routine Medications*

◯ - CIRCLE ALL DOSES NOT GIVEN - STATE REASON IN NURSES NOTES

| DATE | | | | 11/6/XX | 11/7/XX | 11/8/XX | 11/9/XX | 11/10/XX |
|---|---|---|---|---|---|---|---|---|
| DAY OF WEEK | | | | Sun. | Mon. | Tues. | Wed. | Thurs. |
| MEDICATION      ~~prednisolone~~  11/6/84 mistaken entry  A. Hay. Chuc | | | 11-7 | | | | | |
| | | | 7-3 | | | | | |
| DOSE   5 mg | ROUTE | FREQUENCY | 3-11 | | | | | |
| MEDICATION    *Prednisone* | | | 11-7 | | | | | |
| | | | 7-3 | | | | | |
| DOSE   5 mg | ROUTE   p.o. | FREQUENCY   Bid. | 3-11 | | | | | |
| MEDICATION | | | 11-7 | | | | | |
| | | | 7-3 | | | | | |
| DOSE | ROUTE | FREQUENCY | 3-11 | | | | | |
| MEDICATION | | | 11-7 | | | | | |
| | | | 7-3 | | | | | |
| DOSE | ROUTE | FREQUENCY | 3-11 | | | | | |
| MEDICATION | | | 11-7 | | | | | |
| | | | 7-3 | | | | | |
| DOSE | ROUTE | FREQUENCY | 3-11 | | | | | |
| ~~MEDI~~CATION | | | 11-7 | | | | | |
| | ROUTE | FREQUENCY | | | | | | |

F I G U R E  8–33 • Method for correcting a written error on the chart.

8. Check the charts for reports of routine admission studies.
9. Check the charts to be sure all the forms are imprinted or labeled with the correct patient's name. Chart forms should be in the proper sequence.
10. Check the chart frequently for the information form. Physicians may remove the copy for billing purposes. If the form is missing, obtain another copy from the admitting department.
11. Assist physician's or other professionals in locating the client's chart.

## SPLITTING OR THINNING THE CHART

The chart of a patient who remains in the health care facility for a long time becomes very full and eventually does not fit within the chart holder. When this occurs, the health unit coordinator is requested to "thin" or "split" the chart. To thin the chart, certain categories of chart forms may be removed and placed in an envelope for safekeeping on the unit.

To thin the chart:

■ Remove early graphic records, nurses' notes, medication forms and often other forms that are no longer needed in the chart folder.
■ Place the forms in an envelope.
■ Place the chart's ID on the envelope.

■ Record the date, the time, and your initials on the envelope.
■ If the client is transferred to another unit, transfer the envelope with the client's chart.
■ If the patient is discharged, return all the forms to the chart in the proper sequence.

## REPRODUCTION OF CHART FORMS WITH INFORMATION

There are occasions that necessitate the use of a copier to reproduce portions of a patient's chart. For example, when a patient is discharged to another health care facility, to ensure the continuity of care the attending physician requests that specific information on the patient's chart be reproduced. The entire chart or the specified forms are taken to the health records department for reproduction. After the forms are reproduced on the copier, the original forms are replaced in the chart and the copied records are sent to the receiving facility. In some health care facilities, copying the client chart forms is the responsibility of the health unit coordinator.

## SUMMARY

The chart is a record of care rendered and the client's response to care during hospitalization. The nursing unit to which the client is assigned adds forms to the chart. The record is a legal document and should be maintained as such. Standard forms are placed on all client's charts; supplemental forms may be added according to the need dictated by the patient's treatment and care. The purpose of the forms is the same for each hospital; but the sequence of forms in the chart, color of ink used, and the placement of blank forms that are added may differ from hospital to hospital. The information contained in the client's chart must always be regarded as confidential.

## REVIEW QUESTIONS

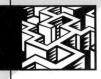

1. A client who has been admitted to the health care facility at least overnight for treatment and care is called an

   _out patient_ .

2. A plastic card containing individual patient information is a(n)

   _Imprinting Card_ .

3. To properly maintain a client's chart, the health unit coordinator should do the following:

   a. _place in proper sequence when not in use_

   b. _Keep a record of Location of chart when removed from unit_

   c. _Know Identities of those who have access to chart_

   d. _place new forms in chart before needed_

   e. _place diagnostic reports behind correct dividers_

   f. _Review frequently for New Orders_

   g. _check all forms for correct patient Name_

   h. _check chart frequently for Information form_

   i. _assist physicians & other professionals in Locating chart_

4. State the purpose of the following:

   a. physicians' order form: _request for care & treatment for the patient_

   b. graphic record: _graphic representation of patients vital signs over a set period of days_

   c. progress record: _physicians record of patients progress during their hospitalization_

   d. history and physical form: _provides medical history medical problem and Review of body systems_

   e. nurses' notes and activity flowsheet: _used to record patient observations by the nurse_

   f. medication and administration record: _to record all medications administered to the patient_

   g. face sheet or information form: _to summarize the patients hospital stay_

5. A supplemental chart form is (define): _additional forms used for specific conditions of patients_

Two examples of a supplemental chart form are _operating room records_ and _Therapy records_ .

6. List six reasons for keeping a chart on each client.

a. _means of communication_

b. _planning patient care_

c. _research_

d. _educational purposes_

e. _Legal document for protection for everyone_

f. _written record of Illness treatment care outcome_

7. A patient receiving care by a health care facility but not admitted overnight is referred to as an _out patient_ .

8. A group of chart forms prepared by the health unit coordinator to be used for new patients is usually called a(n) _admission packet_ .

9. A device used to place identifying information on chart forms or requisitions is called a(n) _Imprinter device_ .

10. Explain how the health unit coordinator may maintain the confidentiality of the patient's chart. _request Identification from anyone wanting to see chart do not discuss information_

11. Describe how to correct the following errors on a chart form:

a. an imprinter error

_no notations may be destroyed If notations place correct Information next or below error and cross out Incorrect information, Write date mistaken entry and first Initial Last name + title_

b. a written entry error

_draw a single line of Ink through the error write date mistaken entry First Initial, last name + status_

12. Three-thirty PM in military time is _1530_ .

13. Twenty-three forty-five military time in standard time is _11:45_ .

14. Define:

a. stuffing charts _putting in extra forms in all the patients c_

b. "split" or thinned chart _portions removed temporarily when chart becomes to Large_

c. identification labels _Preprinted labels containing patient ↑ Last_ _for identification of records ↑ information_

d. name alert _When two or more patients have same name_ _method of alerting staff_ _on unit_

## References

Arizona Hospital Association: *Consent Manual*, revised ed. Phoenix, 1977.

DuGas, Beverly Witter: *Introduction to Patient Care*, 3rd ed. Philadelphia, W. B. Saunders Co., 1977.

Ellis, Janice Rider, Nowlin, Elizabeth Ann, and Patricia M.: *Modules for Basic Nursing Skills*. Boston, Houghton Mifflin, 1977.

Ignatavicius, Donna D, Workman, M. Linda, and Mishler, Mary A: *Medical-Surgical Nursing—A Nursing Process Approach*, 2nd ed. Philadelphia, W. B. Saunders Co., 1995.

Iyer, Patricia W.: New trends in charting. *Nursing 91* January 1991, p. 48.

Iyer, Patricia W.: Thirteen charting rules. *Nursing 91* June 1991, p. 40.

Readey, Helen, Teague, Mary, and Readey, William, III: *Introduction to Nursing Essentials—A Handbook*. St. Louis, The C. V. Mosby Co., 1977.

Wood, Lucille A. and Rambo, Beverly J. (eds.): *Nursing Skills for Allied Health Services*, vol. 1, 2nd ed. Philadelphia, W. B. Saunders Co., 1977.

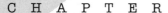

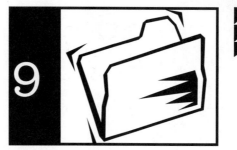

# 9

# TRANSCRIPTION OF DOCTORS' ORDERS INCLUDING THE RECORDING OF TELEPHONED PHYSICIANS' ORDERS

## C H A P T E R    O B J E C T I V E S

*Upon completion of this chapter, you will be able to:*

1. Define the terms in the vocabulary list.
2. Describe the health unit coordinator's role in executing doctors' orders.
3. Name two criteria the health unit coordinator can use to recognize a new set of doctors' orders that need transcription.
4. List the four categories of doctors' orders and explain the characteristics of each.
5. Describe the purpose of and process for kardexing.
6. List five areas commonly found on the Kardex form.
7. Describe the purpose of and process for ordering doctors' orders.
8. Name the symbols used in transcribing doctors' orders, and describe the purpose of and process for using each.
9. Describe the purpose of and process for signing-off doctors' orders.
10. Explain why all entries on the doctors' order sheet are recorded in ink.

11. List in order the 10 steps of transcription.
12. Discuss why accuracy is important in the transcription procedure.
13. Discuss the types of errors that may occur during the transcription procedure and the methods of avoidance that may be used.
14. List seven guidelines for recording telephoned physicians' orders

## V O C A B U L A R Y

**Flagging** • A method used by the doctor to notify the nursing staff that she or he has written a new set of orders   *red or yellow*

**Kardex** • A portable file   *not a legal document*

**Kardex Form** • A form used by the nursing staff to maintain a current patient profile; the Kardex form is filed in the Kardex file

**Kardexing** • The process of recording doctors' orders on the Kardex form

**One-Time** or **Short-Series Order** • A doctor's order that is executed according to the qualifying phrase, and then is automatically discontinued

**Ordering** • The process of ordering diagnostic procedures, treatments, or supplies from hospital departments other than nursing

**Requisition** • The form used to order diagnostic procedures, treatments, or supplies from hospital departments other than nursing

**Set of Doctors' Orders** • An entry of doctors' orders made at one time on the doctors' order sheet, dated, and signed by the doctor; may include one or more orders

**Signing-Off** • A process of recording data on the doctors' order sheet to indicate the completion of transcription of a set of doctors' orders

**Standing Order** • A doctor's order that remains in effect and is executed as ordered until the doctor discontinues or changes it *postop orders*

*admit telemetry*

**Standing PRN Order** • Same as a standing order, except that it is executed according to the patient's needs

**Stat Order** • A doctor's order that is to be executed immediately, then automatically discontinued

**Symbols** • Notations written in ink on the doctors' order sheet to indicate completion of a step of the transcription procedure

**Telephoned Orders** • Orders for a client telephoned to a health care facility by the doctor

# DOCTORS' ORDERS

During the client's stay in a health care facility, the doctors' orders for a patient's care are expressed in handwriting or typewriting on the doctors' order sheet. These orders include such things as diagnostic procedures, medications, surgical treatment, diet, patient activities, discharge, and so forth. As you will recall from Chapter 8 written doctors' orders are a legal document and become a permanent record of the care prescribed during a client's hospital stay.

The doctor writes all of the orders in black or blue ink, dates them, and signs each entry. He or she also records the time that the orders are written. An entry may be *one or more orders*; this is referred to as a **set of doctor's orders**. The doctor indicates to the nursing staff that he or she has written a new set of orders by **flagging** the chart. Flagging techniques vary among health care facilities. New orders can also be identified by date, absence of symbols, and absence of sign-off information. See Figure 9–1 for an example of written doctors' orders. Sometimes the doctor may write new orders and forget to flag the chart. Always check for new orders before returning a chart from the counter into the chart rack.

If the new orders are recorded at the top of the doctors' order sheet, check the previous sheet to see if the orders are continued from it. Also if orders are recorded near the bottom of the doctors' order sheet, make diagonal lines across the sheet so new orders will not be recorded there

**PHYSICIAN'S ORDER SHEET**   4052-3987
3W   Joint, Jane L.   F-25
318-2 Dr. T. Arthro

| Date Ordered | Physician's Orders |
|---|---|
| 6-4-00 | CBR (Complete bed rest*) |
| 10:45AM | CBC (Complete blood count, laboratory tests*) |
| | consultation with Dr. F. L. Payne |
| | please call |
| | Dr. T. Arthro |
| | |
| | |
| | |
| | |
| | |
| | |

F I G U R E 9–1 • An example of a set of written doctors' orders. *Note: The typed interpretations of the abbreviations shown with an asterisk here and in Figures 9–7, 9–8, 9–9B, 9–10C, 9–11, and 9–12 are included for your information and would not be seen on a typical set of orders. These abbreviations will be covered in succeeding chapters.

7-10-00 ord 143 k lytes STAT
0900 pesent Persantin 50 mg p o @ 1700, 1900, 2100
  day of admit only
  k Dalmane 30 mg po 1t5 prn sleep
  k Consent on chart & signed: Retrograde
  L heart cath L Ventriculography,
  selective coronary arteriography
  k Upad bil
                              Dr. I. M. Hart
7-10-00 1000  Jane Dalmin, CHUC

MR-20B-306 (Rev. 7/89)                    **PHYSICIAN'S ORDERS**

F I G U R E  9–2 • Diagonal lines drawn at the bottom of a nearly filled doctors' order sheet.

**PHYSICIAN'S ORDER SHEET** 3W  4052-3987
                                   Joint, Jane L.  F-25
                            318-2 Dr. T. Arthro

| Date Ordered | Physician's Orders |
| --- | --- |
| 6-4-00 10:30 AM | May have regular diet T.O. Dr T Arthro / Ray Nee CHUC |

F I G U R E  9–3 • An example of a telephoned doctors' order recorded by a certified health unit coordinator.

then continued on the following page. When this happens it is easy to miss the orders at the bottom of the first page (Fig. 9–2).

## RECORDING TELEPHONED PHYSICIANS' ORDERS

With the restructuring programs that are taking place in health care facilities today, many duties are added to positions while others are expanded. Recording of physicians' orders by the health unit coordinator fits under this heading. In the past, recording physicians' orders by the health unit coordinator has varied much among facilities; some did not allow it, some allowed it with restrictions, such as recording all orders except medication, and some allowed the full recording of orders.

Now it appears that facilities are expanding this duty for health unit coordinators; therefore, we are giving it more emphasis in this text. We are including it in this chapter so you have an opportunity to practice recording orders as you learn each category of doctors' orders in the following chapters.

Recording of physicians' orders is a serious matter, since error could cause harm to the patient. Accuracy is an absolute must. Follow the guidelines listed below to ensure accuracy in recording the orders.

### Guidelines for Recording Physicians' Orders

1. Make sure you have the correct chart. Check both the chart spine and the identifying information on the doctor's order sheet.
2. Begin recording the orders directly below the last entry on the doctor's order sheet. In other words, do not leave a space between your entry and the last entry.
3. Record the orders in ink.
4. Record the date and time.
5. Record each order as the doctor states it. Do not hesitate to ask questions if you do not understand what is being said.
6. Read the entire set of orders back to the physician. *DO NOT SKIP ANY PART OF THIS STEP*.
7. Sign the orders as shown in Figure 9–3.

The physician is expected to cosign the orders within 24 hours.

### TO THE STUDENT

To prepare for recording telephoned doctor's orders, complete **Activity 9–1** in the Skills Practice Manual.

## CATEGORIES OF DOCTORS' ORDERS

Doctors' orders may be categorized according to when they are carried out and the length of time they are in effect. The transcription procedure varies according to the category of the order; therefore, it is necessary for you to be able to recognize each category. The four categories are (1) standing, or continuing, orders; (2) standing, or continuing, PRN orders; (3) one-time, or short-series orders; and (4) stat orders.

### Standing, or Continuing, Orders

The majority of doctors' orders fall into this group. Standing orders are in effect and executed routinely as ordered until they are discontinued or changed by a written doctor's order. For example, in the order

#### BP tid

the doctor has ordered the patient's blood pressure (BP) to be taken and recorded three times a day (tid). A time sequence such as 10:00 AM, 2:00 PM, and 6:00 PM is set up for the blood pressure to be taken daily. This routine continues until changed or discontinued by the doctor. Another example of a standing order—

#### Regular Diet

—means that the patient receives a regular diet each day of his or her hospital stay unless the order is changed or discontinued by the doctor.

### Standing, or Continuing, PRN Orders

The Latin words *pro re nata*, meaning "as circumstances may require," are abbreviated as **prn** and are used by the doctor in a written order to indicate that the order is to be executed as needed. Standing prn orders, like standing orders, are in effect until changed or discontinued by the doctor. They differ from standing orders in that they are executed according to the clients' needs. For example, in the order

#### Aspirin 650 mg q4h *prn headache*

the nurse may give 650 mg of aspirin as often as every 4 hours (q4h) as needed by the client to relieve a headache. This does *not* mean the patient necessarily receives the medication every 4 hours, as he or she may not have a headache at those times; therefore, it is impossible to set up a time sequence as we discussed with the standing order.

In the order

#### Compazine 10 mg IM q6h *nausea or vomiting*

the doctor uses a *qualifying phrase, **nausea or vomiting**,* to indicate it is a *prn* order.

*Remember:* A prn order may be recognized either by the abbreviation prn or by the content of a qualifying phrase and is in effect until changed or discontinued by the doctor.

## One-Time or Short-Series Order

The doctor may want a treatment or medication carried out once only or for a short series. This is indicated by a qualifying phrase, such as *give at 2:00 PM* or *give tonight and in AM*. Upon completion of the one time or short series, the order is automatically discontinued. For example, in the order

### give patient TW enema this PM

*this* PM makes it a one-time order—thus, the order is discontinued after the enema is given.

Another example; in the order

### Blood pressure q2h till awake

*till awake* makes it a short-series order.

*Remember:* A one-time or short-series order may be recognized by the content of the qualifying phrase and is automatically discontinued after completion.

## Stat Orders

*Stat* is the abbreviation for the Latin word *statim*, which means "at once." When included in a doctor's order it indicates that the order is to be carried out immediately. Stat orders are usually written during an emergency or for patients who are critically ill. Because of the urgency of stat orders, they are communicated to the nurse immediately and are transcribed first when included in a set of orders. Stat orders are recognized by the word *stat* included in the order, for example,

### CBC (complete blood count) stat

In the orders:

### CBC now

or

### CBC immediately

the words *now* and *immediately* are *usually* categorized under stat orders and should receive urgent attention.

---

**H I G H L I G H T**

Categories of Doctors' Orders

- **Standing:** In effect and given routinely until discontinued or changed by the doctor
- **Standing PRN:** In effect and given as needed by the patient until automatically discontinued or changed by the doctor
- **One-time or short-series:** In effect for one time or a short period, automatically discontinued when the order has been completed
- **Stat:** Given immediately, then automatically discontinued

---

## THE KARDEX FILE AND KARDEX FORM

A portable file, often referred to as the Kardex, is maintained by each nursing unit. The Kardex is made up of Kardex forms, one for each patient on the unit. Approximately 15 to 20 individual patient Kardex forms are filed in one Kardex file; large nursing units of 30 or more patients may maintain two Kardex files. Patient information such as room number, name, doctor's name, and diagnosis is recorded at the bottom of the Kardex form, so that, when filed in the Kardex file, this information remains visible for each location of each client's Kardex form (Fig. 9–4).

Five main areas common to most Kardex forms are:

1. Activity
2. Medication
3. Diet
4. Treatment
5. Diagnostic studies

Other areas, such as vital signs or weight, may also be included on the form.

The Kardex form may also include an area for a patient care plan. This area is completed by the nursing staff. The purpose of the Kardex is to maintain a current profile of patient information, doctors' orders, and the patient's nursing needs. It provides a quick reference for the nursing staff, and it is also used for planning and designating patient care and for reporting patient information to the oncoming shift. The design of the Kardex form varies according to hospital and nursing unit needs. However, the basic concept remains constant. See Figure 9–5 for a typical Kardex form. Some hospitals are using a computerized kardexing system, eliminating the need for the Kardex form and the Kardex holder.

## Kardexing

*Pencil        Allergies in Red*

**Kardexing** is the process of recording all new doctors' orders onto the patient's Kardex form. The purpose of kardexing all the doctors' orders is to communicate new orders to the nursing staff and to update the client's profile on the Kardex form. Kardexing is usually done in pencil, since new doctors' orders may involve changing or discontinuing an existing order. However, information not subject to change, such as the patient's name, is usually recorded in ink.

Accuracy in kardexing is absolutely essential. An error could result in the client's receiving the wrong and perhaps harmful treatment. The patient's Kardex form is not considered a legal document and in the past it was usually discarded when the patient was discharged from the hospital. However, the present trend is toward filing the nursing care plan portion of the Kardex form with the patient's chart in the health records department.

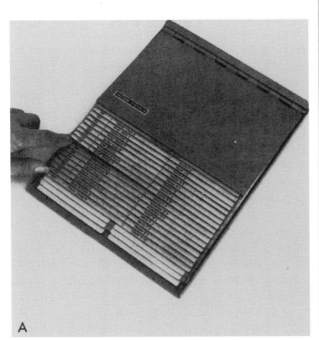

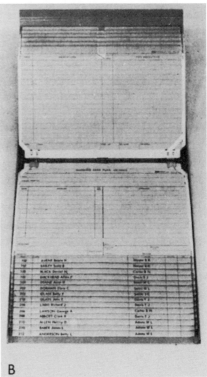

F I G U R E   9–4 • A portable file (often referred to as a Kardex) shown as it appears closed (*A*) and open (*B*). (Courtesy of Acme Visible Records, Inc.)

## Ordering

**Ordering** is the process of inputting the doctors' orders into the computer or of copying the doctors' order onto a requisition (Fig. 9–6). Whichever method is used, the purpose of ordering is to forward the doctors' orders to the various hospital departments that will execute the order.

Doctors' orders that involve diagnostic procedures, treatment, or supplies other than nursing usually require the ordering step. Ordering by requisition requires the health unit coordinator first to imprint the requisition with patient information and, second, to copy or fill in the pertinent data from the doctors' orders. Ordering by computer requires the health unit coordinator to select the clients' name from a computer screen, then to input the information into the computer.

### SYMBOLS

As the health unit coordinator completes a part of the transcription procedure, he or she places a **symbol** on the doctors' order sheet to indicate completion of the task. The symbol is written in ink (since the doctors' order sheet is a legal document) in front of the doctors' order (Fig. 9–7). Some hospitals prefer the health unit coordinator to record the symbol in red ink to contrast with the doctors' written orders.

By using symbols, the health unit coordinator has a written record of the steps completed and reduces the possibility of forgetting to complete a part of the transcription procedure. Omission can cause delay in treatment, which may slow down or be harmful to the patient's recovery.

Below are listed the symbols we will use in this textbook; however, symbols vary among hospitals. Your instructor, therefore, may wish you to become familiar with a different set of symbols commonly used in hospitals in your area.

**K**  Indicates the order has been transcribed on the patient's Kardex form. It is also used to indicate that a discontinued order has been erased from the Kardex.

**Ord**  Indicates diagnostic tests, treatments, or supplies have been ordered by either computer or requisition. If using the computer method, record the computer order number by the symbol "ord."

**M**  Indicates transcription of a medication order on the medication administration record form.

**Called and Time**  Indicates completion of a telephone call necessary to complete the doctor's order. Record the name of the person who received the call.

**PC sent**  Indicates that the pharmacy copy of the physicians' order sheet was forwarded to the pharmacy. Record the time the copy was sent.

### SIGNING-OFF DOCTORS' ORDERS

**Signing-off** is the process used to indicate completion of the transcription procedure of a set of doctors' orders. To

**KARDEX FORM A**

| DATE ORD | STANDING MEDICATIONS | STOP DATE | DATE ORD | STANDING PRN MEDICATIONS | STOP DATE |
|---|---|---|---|---|---|
| | | | | | |
| | | | | | |
| | | | | | |
| | | | | | |
| | | | | | |
| | | | | | |
| | | | | | |
| | | | | | |
| | | | | | |
| | | | | | |
| | | | | | |
| | | | | | |
| | | | | | |
| | | | | | |
| | ONE TIME MEDICATIONS | | | | |
| | | | | ALLERGIES | |
| | | | | | |
| | | | | | |
| | NAME | | | | |

A

FIGURE 9–5 • Typical Kardex form. (A) Upper Kardex form. *Illustration continued on opposite page*

sign off, the health unit coordinator records the date, time, and his or her name and status (may use abbreviation HUC or CHUC if certified) on the line directly below the doctor's signature, as shown in Figure 9–8. Once again, this is done in ink, because the doctors' order sheet is a legal document. In the past it was common practice to have a registered nurse cosign the transcribed orders. However, with the recognition of health unit coordinator competency by national certification and upgraded educational standards, this procedure is no longer practiced in many hospitals.

The sign-off procedure varies among health care facilities. For example, some health care facilities use a different color ink for the sign-off procedure, to distinguish it from the written doctors' orders, and some require the health unit coordinator to draw a line below the sign-off data.

## TRANSCRIPTION OF DOCTORS' ORDERS

**Transcription of doctors' orders** is a written process used to communicate doctors' orders to the nursing staff and other hospital departments. The transcription procedure includes kardexing, ordering, using symbols, the signing-off process, and sometimes other steps. How the health unit coordinator goes about performing this procedure varies among health care facilities and from individual to individual.

For learning purposes we have outlined ten steps that make up the transcription procedure. it is important to note that each type of doctors' orders may require *some or all* of the steps to complete the transcription procedure. Always *compare each order with the ten steps of transcription* when choosing the steps that are required for complete

**KARDEX FORM B**

| ACTIVITY | DATE ORD | TREATMENTS | DATE ORD | LABORATORY | DATE ORD | DIAGNOSTIC IMAGING | DATE TO BE DONE |
|---|---|---|---|---|---|---|---|
|  |  |  |  |  |  |  |  |
|  |  |  |  |  |  |  |  |
|  |  |  |  |  |  |  |  |
|  |  |  |  |  |  |  |  |
| DIET |  |  |  |  |  |  |  |
|  |  |  |  |  |  |  |  |
| VITAL SIGNS |  |  |  |  |  |  |  |
|  |  |  |  |  |  |  |  |
|  |  |  |  |  |  |  |  |
|  |  |  |  |  |  |  |  |
| WEIGHT |  |  |  |  |  |  |  |
| IV |  | PULMONARY FUNCTION |  | PRE OP ORDERS |  | DIAGNOSTIC STUDIES |  |
|  |  | RESPIRATORY CARE |  | DAILY LAB |  |  |  |
| I & O |  |  |  |  |  |  |  |
| RETENTION CATH (FOLEY) □ HEALTH RECORDS _____ |  | PHYSICAL MEDICINE |  |  |  |  |  |
| ADM. DATE |  | CONSULTATIONS: |  | SURGERY: DATE: |  |  |  |

NAME                           DOCTOR                       AGE            DIAGNOSIS

B

F I G U R E  9–5 *Continued* • (*B*) Lower Kardex form.

transcription of each order. Using this procedure allows for the simplest yet most efficient method for transcribing doctors' orders.

The 10 steps of transcription are listed, followed by a more detailed explanation of how to perform each step.

## Ten Steps for Transcription of Doctors' Orders

1. Read the complete set of doctors' orders.
2. Send the pharmacy copy of the doctors' order sheet to the pharmacy department.
3. Complete stat orders.
4. Select the patient's name from the census on the computer screen or collect all necessary forms.
5. Order diagnostic tests, treatments, and supplies.
6. Kardex all doctors' orders.
7. Complete medication orders.
8. Place telephone calls as necessary to complete doctors' orders.
9. Recheck your performance of each step for accuracy and thoroughness.
10. Sign-off the completed set of doctors' orders.

Below is a procedure for carrying out the 10 steps of transcription. Refer to this often as you practice the transcription exercises in the Skills Practice Manual. Adapt it to the procedure of your health care facility.

TO THE STUDENT

To prepare for transcribing doctors' orders complete **Activity 9–2** in the Skills Practice Manual.

DR. ORDERING _____

DIAGNOSIS _____

REASON FOR TEST _____

DRAW AT _____ TIME _____ DATE _____

REQUEST BY _____

DATE _____

SURGERY
DATE _____
TIME _____

☐ STAT

☐ ROUTINE

## CHEMISTRY

☐ Acetone
☐ Acid Phos
☐ Albumin
☐ Alk. Phos
☐ Bilirubin, Total
  ☐ Direct
  ☐ Indirect
☐ BUN
☐ Calcium
☐ Cardiac Enzymes
  ☐ CPK (CK)
  ☐ LDH
  ☐ SGOT (AST)

☐ Cholesterol
☐ Creatinine, Serum
☐ Creatinine, Clearance
☐ Drug Screen
☐ Electrolytes
  ☐ Sodium
  ☐ Potassium
  ☐ Chloride
  ☐ Carbon Dioxide
☐ Glucose, Random
☐ Glucose, Fasting
☐ Glucose, _____ hr PP
☐ Glucose Tolerance _____ hr

☐ Iron
☐ TIBC
☐ Lactic Acid
☐ Lipase
☐ Magnesium
☐ Osmolality, Serum
☐ Phosphorus
☐ Protein, Total
☐ SGPT (ALT)
☐ SMA 6
☐ SMA 12
☐ SMA 20 (SMAC)
☐ TRIGLYCERIDES
☐ URIC ACID

| NUCLEAR CHEMISTRY | SEROLOGY | OTHER |
|---|---|---|
| ☐ ACTH<br>☐ Cortisol<br>☐ Folate<br>☐ FSH<br>☐ LH<br>☐ TBG<br>☐ TSH<br>☐ $T_3$<br>☐ $T_4$ | ☐ ANA<br>☐ ASO Titer<br>☐ Cocci Screen<br>☐ HAA<br>☐ CEA<br>☐ Histoplasma<br>☐ Monospot<br>☐ R Factor<br>☐ RPR<br>☐ Rubella Screen<br>☐ Streptozyme<br>☐ VDRL | |

| HEMATOLOGY | COAGULATION | Special Instructions |
|---|---|---|
| ☐ CBC<br>☐ HGB<br>☐ HCT<br>☐ WBC<br>☐ DIFF<br>☐ RBC<br>☐ RBC Indices<br>☐ Reticulocyte Count<br>☐ ESR<br>☐ Sickle Cell Prep. | ☐ Platelet Count<br>☐ APTT (PTT)<br>☐ PT<br>☐ Fibrinogen<br>☐ Bleeding Time<br>☐ Lee White<br>☐ Factor VIII | Drawn by _____<br><br>Date _____<br><br>Time _____<br><br>Spec. # _____ |

## GENERAL LABORATORY REQUISITION

FIGURE 9–6 • A general laboratory requisition.

**PHYSICIAN'S ORDER SHEET**   3W   Joint, Jane L.   F-25

4052-3987

318-2 Dr. T. Arthro

| Date Ordered | Physician's Orders |
|---|---|
| 6-4-00 10:AM K | C B R (Complete bed rest*) |
| # 254 ord K | C B C (Complete blood count, laboratory test*) |
| K | Consultation with Dr. F. L. Payne |
| Called 10:30ª | please call |
| Mary Smith | Dr. T. Arthro |

F I G U R E  9–7 • An example of a doctors' order sheet with the transcription symbols recorded.

**PHYSICIAN'S ORDER SHEET**   3W   Joint, Jane L.   F-25

4052-3987

318-2 Dr. T. Arthro

| Date Ordered | Physician's Orders |
|---|---|
| 6-4-00 10AM K | C B R (Complete bed rest*) |
| # 254 ord K | C B C (Complete blood count, laboratory test*) |
| K | Consultation with Dr. F. L. Payne |
| Called 10:30ª | please call. |
| Mary Smith | Dr. T. Arthro |
| 6-4-00 | 10:45 AM Ella Bowr /C HUC |

F I G U R E  9–8 • An example of a transcribed set of doctors' orders, showing the health unit coordinator's sign-off data.

| Step | Task | Notes |
|---|---|---|
| 1. | Read the complete set of doctors' orders. | Reading the complete set of orders gives an overview of the task at hand. Accurate reading and interpretation of each word of the doctors' orders are vital, since each word or abbreviation carries a specific meaning. |
| 2. | Ordering Medications<br>a. Remove the pharmacy copy of the doctors' order sheet and send it to the pharmacy.<br>b. Write *PC sent* and time on the doctors' order sheet. | Sending a copy of the original doctors' orders to the pharmacy helps avoid medication errors because no rewriting is involved. Completing this step first allows for the patient to receive the medication as soon as possible. |
| 3. | Complete all stat orders. | Stat orders are always transcribed first. |
| 4. | Select the patient's name from the census on the computer screen or collect all necessary forms. | This varies according to the type of doctors' orders included in the set. Collecting all forms at once saves time. |
| 5. | Order all diagnostic tests, treatments, and supplies. | This step includes ordering medications, diagnostic procedures, and treatments and ordering supplies from hospital departments other than the nursing department. |
| | *Computer Method* (see Figs. 4–6 through 4–8, pp. 46 and 47)<br>a. Select clients' name from the census on the viewing screen. | Check both the patient's name and hospital number with the same information on the chart back label. |
| | b. Select the department from the department menu on the viewing screen.<br>c. Select the test, treatment, or supply from the menu on the viewing screen.<br>d. Fill in required information.<br>e. Order tests, treatments, or supplies.<br>f. Write the symbol *ord* and computer number in ink in front of the doctor's order on the doctors' order sheet. | |
| | *Requisition Method* (Fig. 9–9)<br>a. Imprint the requisition form with the patient's imprinter card, or affix the patient's ID label to the requisition. | Selection of the right patient's label or imprinter card is absolutely essential. The wrong selection could easily cause a patient to receive a diagnostic test or treatment intended for another patient. Always compare the name and patient's hospital number you have imprinted or labeled on the requisition form with the same information on the chart back label. *Remember*: There may be more than one patient on the unit with the same last name. Imprint all requisitions at the same time. |
| | b. Place a check mark on the requisition to indicate the test, treatment, or supply being requisitioned.<br>c. Fill in today's date and the date the test or treatment is to be done in the appropriate spaces.<br>d. Write in pertinent data, such as, "patient blind" or "isolation."<br>e. Sign your name and status in the appropriate space on the requisition form.<br>f. Write the symbol *ord* in ink in front of the doctors' order on the doctors' order sheet. | |

*Continued*

**PROCEDURE FOR TRANSCRIPTION OF DOCTORS' ORDERS (Continued)**

6. Kardex all the doctors' orders. Begin with the first order, then proceed to the next until all the orders are completed (Fig. 9–10).
   Complete kardexing by:
   a. Writing the date followed by the order in pencil under the correct column of the Kardex form. Carefully read what is already written in the column to evaluate whether the new order cancels an existing order. If this occurs, erase the existing order. If an order is discontinued, erase it from the Kardex.

   b. Writing the symbol *K* in ink in front of the doctor's order on the doctors' order sheet.
7. Complete medication orders by:
   a. Writing the medication order on the medication administration record.
   b. Placing the symbol *M* in ink in front of the doctor's order on the doctors' order sheet.
8. Place telephone calls as necessary to complete the doctors' orders (Fig. 9–11).
   Upon completing this task, write the symbol *called* and the time called (be sure to include AM or PM or use military time) and the name of the person receiving the call in ink in front of the doctor's order on the doctors' order sheet.
9. Recheck your performance of each task for accuracy and thoroughness.
10. Sign-off the completed set of orders by writing the following in ink on the line directly below the doctor's signature:
    a. date
    b. time
    c. full signature
    d. status
    Figure 9–12 is an example of this step.

Nursing orders that need to be implemented during the shift are often recorded on a chalk board or clipboard in order to bring them to the immediate attention of the nurse.
*Remember*: All doctors' orders are kardexed. Make sure you have selected the right patient's Kardex forms; many patients' Kardex forms are filed in one Kardex. To ensure accurate selection, check the names of the patient and doctor on the Kardex with the imprinted or computer-labeled information on the chart back label.
*Remember*: There may be more than one patient on the unit with the same last name.

This procedure is covered in more detail in Chapter 13.

Doctors' orders may require you to place a telephone call to another department or health agency to schedule appointments, procedures, etc. Recording the persons name receiving the call is helpful if a follow-up is necessary.

It is **important** that you have completed all the tasks of transcription before signing-off.

## Avoiding Transcription Errors

Throughout this chapter we have mentioned the importance of accuracy during the transcription procedure, so errors that may cause serious harm to the patient can be avoided. Consider, for example, the consequences of the health unit coordinator's overlooking a doctor's order during the transcription procedure for the patient to have a stat administration of IV fluid, or the consequences of a health unit coordinator's ordering a diet for a patient who has been ordered by the doctor to have nothing by mouth.

Below we have outlined for you the types of errors that may occur during the transcription procedure and methods you may use to avoid making these errors. *Remember: prevention* is *easier* than cure.

DR. ORDERING _T. Arthro_

DIAGNOSIS _Arthritis_

REASON FOR TEST _fatigue_

DRAW AT ____ TIME ____ DATE ____

REQUEST BY _Ella Bow_

DATE _6-4-00_

SURGERY

DATE ____

TIME ____

☐ STAT

☒ ROUTINE

4052 3987
3W Joint, Jane F-25
318-2 Dr. T. Arthro

## CHEMISTRY

| | | |
|---|---|---|
| ☐ Acetone | ☐ Cholesterol | ☐ Iron |
| ☐ Acid Phos | ☐ Creatinine, Serum | ☐ TIBC |
| ☐ Albumin | ☐ Creatinine, Clearance | ☐ Lactic Acid |
| ☐ Alk. Phos | ☐ Drug Screen | ☐ Lipase |
| ☐ Bilirubin, Total | ☐ Electrolytes | ☐ Magnesium |
|   ☐ Direct |   ☐ Sodium | ☐ Osmolality, Serum |
|   ☐ Indirect |   ☐ Potassium | ☐ Phosphorus |
| ☐ BUN |   ☐ Chloride | ☐ Protein, Total |
| ☐ Calcium |   ☐ Carbon Dioxide | ☐ SGPT (ALT) |
| ☐ Cardiac Enzymes | ☐ Glucose, Random | ☐ SMA 6 |
|   ☐ CPK (CK) | ☐ Glucose, Fasting | ☐ SMA 12 |
|   ☐ LDH | ☐ Glucose, ____ hr PP | ☐ SMA 20 (SMAC) |
|   ☐ SGOT (AST) | ☐ Glucose Tolerance ____ hr | ☐ TRIGLYCERIDES |
| | | ☐ URIC ACID |

| NUCLEAR CHEMISTRY | SEROLOGY | OTHER |
|---|---|---|
| ☐ ACTH | ☐ ANA | |
| ☐ Cortisol | ☐ ASO Titer | |
| ☐ Folate | ☐ Cocci Screen | |
| ☐ FSH | ☐ HAA | |
| ☐ LH | ☐ CEA | |
| ☐ TBG | ☐ Histoplasma | |
| ☐ TSH | ☐ Monospot | |
| ☐ $T_3$ | ☐ R Factor | |
| ☐ $T_4$ | ☐ Rubella Screen | |
| | ☐ Streptozyme | |

| HEMATOLOGY | COAGULATION | Special Instructions |
|---|---|---|
| ☒ CBC | ☐ Platelet Count | |
| ☐ HGB | ☐ APTT (PTT) | |
| ☐ HCT | ☐ PT | |
| ☐ WBC | ☐ Fibrinogen | |
| ☐ DIFF | ☐ Bleeding Time | |
| ☐ RBC | ☐ Lee White | Drawn by _____ |
| ☐ RBC Indices | ☐ Factor VIII | Date _____ |
| ☐ Reticulocyte Count | | Time _____ |
| ☐ ESR | | Spec. # _____ |
| ☐ Sickle Cell Prep. | | |

A        GENERAL LABORATORY REQUISITION I

**F I G U R E  9–9** • An example of a requisitioning step 2 of the transcription procedure. (*A*) A completed requisition. *Illustration continued on opposite page*

| Date Ordered | Physician's Orders |
|---|---|
| | **PHYSICIAN'S ORDER SHEET**   4052-3987<br>3W   Joint, Jane L.   F-25<br>318-2 Dr. T. Arthro |
| 6-4-00 2 PM | C B R  (Complete bed rest*) |
| 🌡 254 ord | C B C  (Complete blood count, laboratory test*) |
| | consultation with Dr. FL Payne, please call |
| | Fowler's position |
| | wt daily  (wt: weight*) |
| | rectal temp. q4h   (q4h: every 4 hours*) |
| | intake and output |
| PC sent | Compazine 10 mg I.M. q4h nausea or vomiting |
| | Dr. T. Arthro |

B

F I G U R E  9–9 Continued • (B) The symbols recorded on the doctors' order sheet to show completion of step 2.

KARDEX FORM A

| DATE ORD | STANDING MEDICATIONS | STOP DATE | DATE ORD | STANDING PRN MEDICATIONS | STOP DATE |
|---|---|---|---|---|---|
| | | | 6/4/00 | Compazine 10mg q4h nausea or vomiting | |
| | | | | | |
| | | | | | |
| | | | | | |
| | | | | | |
| | | | | | |
| | | | | | |
| | | | | | |
| | | | | | |
| | | | | | |
| | | | | | |
| | | | | | |
| | | | | | |
| | | | | | |
| | | | | | |
| | ONE-TIME MEDICATIONS | | | ALLERGIES | |
| | | | | | |
| | | | | | |
| | | | | | |
| | | | | | |

A   NAME   *Joint, Jane L.*

F I G U R E  9–10 • An example of kardexing, step 6 of the transcription procedure. (*A*) and (*B*) The doctors' orders are recorded in pencil on the Kardex forms. (*C*) The symbols recorded on the doctors' order sheet to show completion of step 6. *Illustration continued on opposite page*

| ACTIVITY 6-4-00 | DATE ORD | TREATMENTS | DATE ORD | LABORATORY | DATE ORD | DIAGNOSTIC IMAGING | DATE TO BE DONE |
|---|---|---|---|---|---|---|---|
| *CBR* *Fowler's position* | | | 6-4 | *CBC* | | | |
| **DIET** | | | | | | | |
| **VITAL SIGNS** *6-4-00* *rectal temp q4h* | | | | | | | |
| **WEIGHT** *6-4-00 daily* | | | | | | | |
| **IV** | | PULMONARY FUNCTION | | PRE OP ORDERS | | DIAGNOSTIC STUDIES | |
| **I & O** *6-4-00* | | RESPIRATORY CARE | | DAILY LAB | | | |
| **RETENTION CATH (FOLEY)** ☐ HEALTH RECORDS___ | | PHYSICAL MEDICINE | | | | | |
| **ADM. DATE** *6-4-00* | | CONSULTATIONS: *6-4-00* *Dr. F. L. Payne* | | SURGERY: DATE: | | | |

NAME *Joint, Jane L.*   DOCTOR *T. Arthro*   AGE **25**   DIAGNOSIS *Arthritis*

B

---

**PHYSICIAN'S ORDER SHEET**

4052-3987
3W    Joint, Jane L.    F-25
318-2 Dr. T. Arthro

| Date Ordered | | Physician's Orders |
|---|---|---|
| *6-4-00 2 PM K* | | *CBR*  (Complete bed rest*) |
| *#25 1 ord K* | | *CBC*  (Complete blood count, laboratory test*) |
| *K* | | *consultation with Dr. F. L. Payne, please call* |
| *K* | | *Fowler's position* |
| *K* | | *wt daily*  (wt: weight*) |
| *K* | | *rectal temp q4h*   (q4h: every 4 hours*) |
| *K* | | *intake and output* |
| *PC sent K* | | *Compazine 10 mg. I.M. q4h nausea or vomiting* |
| | | *Dr. T. Arthro* |

C

**F I G U R E   9–10** • *Continued*

## PHYSICIAN'S ORDER SHEET

4052-3987
3W    Joint, Jane L.    F-25
318-2 Dr. T. Arthro

| Date Ordered | Physician's Orders |
|---|---|
| 6-4-00 2PM K | C B R (Complete bed rest*) |
| # 25′ ord K | C B C (Complete blood count, laboratory test*) |
| called 2:30 PM K | consultation with Dr. F. L. Payne. please call |
| Mary Smith    K | Fowler's position |
| K | wt daily (wt: weight*) |
| K | rectal temp q4h (q4h: every 4 hours*) |
| K | intake and output |
| PC sent K | Compazine 10 mg. I.M. q4h nausea or vomiting |
| | Dr. T. Arthro |

F I G U R E  9–11 • An example of using the symbol for placing a telephone call, step 8 of the transcription procedure. *Note:* the figure also shows completion of steps 4 and 5 of the transcription procedures.

## PHYSICIAN'S ORDER SHEET

4052-3987
3W    Joint, Jane L.    F-25
310-2 Dr. T. Arthro

| Date Ordered | Physician's Orders |
|---|---|
| 6-4-00 2PM K | C B R (Complete bed rest*) |
| # 257 ord K | C B C (Complete blood count, laboratory test*) |
| called 2:30 PM K | consultation with Dr. F. L. Payne. please call |
| Mary Smith    K | Fowler's position |
| K | wt daily (wt: weight*) |
| K | rectal temp q4h (q4h: every 4 hours*) |
| K | intake and output |
| PC sent K | Compazine 10 mg. I.M. q4h nausea or vomiting |
| | Dr. T. Arthro |
| 6-4-00 | 3:10 PM    Ella Bow    CHUC |

F I G U R E  9–12 • An example of a transcribed set of doctors' orders, showing step 10 of the transcription procedure, the signing-off of doctors' orders.

| Type of Error | Method of Avoidance |
|---|---|
| ■ *Errors of Omission* | 1. *Always* read and understand each word of doctors' orders. If in doubt, check with a registered nurse or the doctor. |
| | 2. *Always* use symbols. It is especially important for you to write the symbol after you have completed each step of transcription. |
| | 3. When new orders are recorded at the top of the doctors' order sheet, check the previous order sheet to see if these orders are continued from the previous page. |
| | 4. If the set of orders finishs near the bottom of the doctors' order sheet, cross through the remaining space with diagonal lines. |
| | 5. *Always* record the signing off information on the line directly below the doctor's signature to avoid leaving space in which future orders could be written. |
| | 6. *Always* check for new orders before returning a chart from the counter or elsewhere to the chart rack. |
| ■ *Errors of Interpretation* | 1. When in doubt about the correct interpretation of doctors' order, *always* check with the registered nurse or the doctor. |
| ■ *Errors in the Selection of the Patient's Imprinter Card or Errors in Selection of the Patient's name on the Computer Screen* | 1. *Always* compare the patient's name and the hospital number you have imprinted on the requisition form or selected on the computer screen with the same information on the patient's chart cover. *Never* select the imprinter card or computer labels by the patient's room number only. |
| ■ *Errors in the Selection of the Patient's Kardex Form* | 1. *Always* compare the patient's name and the doctor's name on the Kardex form with the same information on the label on the patient's chart cover. Do not use the information on the doctors' order sheet. It may have the wrong information on it. *Never* select by using room number alone. If the patient has been transferred the room number imprinted on chart forms may no longer be correct. |
| | *Note:* Many people on the nursing staff use the Kardex for a quick reference and may flip to another patient's Kardex form while you are transcribing orders. If this should occur, check to see that the Kardex file is returned to the patient's Kardex form that you are working on. |
| ■ *Errors in Reading the Doctor's Poor Handwriting* | 1. When you cannot read an order because of the doctor's handwriting, refer to the progress record form on the chart. The orders are often recorded on this form also, and using this information may assist you in reading the orders on the physicians' order form. If the order remains unclear, ask the doctor who wrote it for clarification. Don't waste time asking others. They will be guessing also. If a doctor has a reputation for poor handwriting, ask him or her to read the orders to you before leaving the unit. |

**HIGHLIGHT**

How to Avoid Errors of Transcription

- Ask the doctor or nurse for assistance if you cannot read or understand a doctors' order.
- Always use patient information from the chart cover to select the computer screen or the imprinter card.
- Always record the sign-off information on the line directly below the doctor's signature.
- Always check the previous page for orders when the orders begin at the top of the page.
- Always void space if three or more lines are left at the bottom of the doctors' order sheet.

## SUMMARY

Transcription of doctors' orders is the single most responsible task you perform as a health unit coordinator. An error may result in a patient being harmed or his or her recovery time being extended. You owe it both to the patient and the health care facility to complete the transcription procedure promptly, accurately, and thoroughly.

**REVIEW QUESTIONS**

1. Why are symbols used as a part of the transcription procedure? _to note that each task has been done_

2. List the information used by the health unit coordinator to completely sign-off a set of doctors' orders.
   _date, time full signature and title_

3. List in order the 10 steps of transcription.
   a. _read the complete set of Doctors orders._
   b. _send the pharmacy copy of pharmacy orders_
   c. _complete stat orders._
   d. _collect necessary forms or select patient name on computer_
   e. _ordering_
   f. _kardexing_
   g. _complete medication orders_
   h. _complete telephone calls_
   i. _Recheck_
   j. _sign off procedures_

4. Explain why doctors' orders, symbols, and sign-offs are recorded in ink on the doctors' order sheet.
   _doctors order sheet is a legal document and therefore ink must be used_

5. Symbols are recorded on the doctors' order sheet (circle one):
   a. after the step is completed
   b. before the step is completed
   c. at any time, as long as they are recorded accurately

6. Orders that need transcription are recognized by (circle one):
   a. the date
   b. the absence of symbols and sign-off

7. Why are the doctors' orders written on the Kardex in pencil? _in case you need to erase to update it or discontinue orders_

8. Why are all doctors' orders recorded on the Kardex? _to communicate new orders to the nursing staff and to update patient information_

9. Define the following terms:
   a. ordering: _the process of ordering medication, dietary, diagnostic tests, treatments, and equipment from other hospital departments_

b. kardexing: _the process of writing all doctors orders on the kardex form & erasing discontinued & changed orders_

c. requisition: _form used to order supplies & diagnostic procedures & equipment_

d. flagging: _method of indicating new doctors orders to the nursing staff._

10. Regarding the doctors' order sheet:

a. which line of the doctors' order sheet is used for the signing-off procedure?
   _the line directly below the doctors signature._

b. why? _to indicate that the doctors order has been transcribed_

11. Why is accuracy necessary in the transcription procedure? _to avoid errors that may cause harm to patients_

12. What symbol is used to indicate completion of:

a.  ordering                          _Ord computer #_

b.  transcription of a medication order    _M_

c.  kardexing                         _K_

d.  telephone call                    _called & time_

e.  pharmacy copy sent                _pc sent_

13. a. You are transcribing a set of doctors' orders. There are three lines remaining at the bottom of the page. You should _draw diagonal lines through left over spaces so new orders cannot be written there_
   Why? _to avoid error of omission_

b. A doctor has just written a set of doctors' orders. She is still on the nursing unit. You cannot tell whether the order reads CBC or CBR. You should _ask the doctor to clarify_
   Why? _to avoid making an error in transcription_

c. When selecting a patient's computer screen, you should obtain the patient information from the _patient chart rack_
   Why? _more apt to be correct them on the imprinted information on the patients chart form._

d. You see three charts lying on the counter. Before returning them to the chart rack you should _check each chart for new orders before returning to rack_
   Why? _doctor might have forgotten to flag his new orders._

14. True or False? All 10 steps of transcription are used to transcribe each category of the doctors' orders. _F_

15. What type of doctors' orders require requisition forms or use of the computer? _for_ _ordering diets, supplies, diagnostic procedures, treatment from other dept in "hospital"_

16. List five areas commonly found on a Kardex form.

    a. _activity_
    b. _medication_
    c. _diet_
    d. _treatment_
    e. _~~allergies~~ diagnostic studies_

17. List the four categories of doctors' orders in the order they are presented in this text and write a brief description of each.

    a. _Standing or continuing - executed as ordered until discontinued_
    b. _Standing or continuing PRN - same as standeded only preformed as needed discontinued when finished_
    c. _One-time or short series - performed once or in short series_
    d. _Stat - carried out immediatly then discontinued_

18. Identify each type of order written below.

    a. blood pressure q3h til alert _~~PRN~~ short series_
    b. morphine 8–12 mg IM q3–4 hr prn pain _PRN standing_
    c. Valium 10 mg PO now _Stat_
    d. Premarin 1.25 mg PO daily _Standing or continuing_

19. How do you recognize a stat order? _Order contains stat, now or immediatly_

20. How do you recognize a standing prn order? _by prn in the order or a qualifying phrase_

21. List the seven guidelines for recording physicians' orders.

    a. _record on correct chart_
    b. _directly below prenoslprders_
    c. _use ink_
    d. _record date + time_
    e. _record Completely_
    f. _read back entire order to doctors_
    g. _sign the order_

## References

Miller, Benjamin F. and Keane, Claire Brackman: *Encyclopedia and Dictionary of Medicine, Nursing and Allied Health*, 3rd ed. Philadelphia, W. B. Saunders Co., 1983.

Stryker, Ruth Perin: *The Hospital Ward Clerk*. St. Louis, The C. V. Mosby Co., 1970.

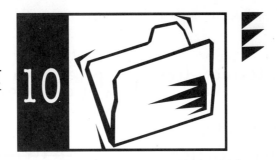

CHAPTER **10**

# PATIENT ACTIVITY, PATIENT POSITIONING, AND NURSING OBSERVATION ORDERS

## CHAPTER OBJECTIVES

*Upon completion of this chapter, you will be able to:*

1. Define the terms in the vocabulary list.
2. Write the meaning of each abbreviation and write the abbreviation for each term in the abbreviation list.
3. Interpret patient activity, patient positioning, and nursing observation orders.

## VOCABULARY

**Activity Order** • A doctors' order that defines the type and amount of activity a hospitalized patient may have

**Afebrile** • Without fever

**Apical Rate** • Heart rate obtained from the apex of the heart

**Axillary Temperature** • The temperature reading obtained by placing the thermometer in the patient's axilla (armpit)

**Blood Pressure** • The measure of the pressure of blood against the walls of the blood vessels

**Commode** • A chair or wheelchair with an open seat, used at the bedside by the patient for the passage of urine and stool

**Febrile** • Elevated body temperature (fever)

**Fowler's Position** • A semisitting position

**Intake and Output** • The measurement of the patient's fluid intake and output

**Neurologic Vital Signs** • The measurement of the function of the body's neurologic system; includes checking pupils of the eyes, verbal response, and so forth

**Nursing Observation Order** • A doctors' order that requests the nursing staff to observe and record certain patient signs and symptoms

**Oral Temperature** • The temperature reading obtained by placing the thermometer in the patient's mouth under the tongue

**Pedal Pulse** • The pulse rate obtained on the top of the foot

**Positioning Order** • A doctors' order that requests that the patient be placed in a specified body position

**Pulse Oximetry** • A noninvasive method to measure the oxygen saturation of arterial blood

**Pulse Rate** • The number of times per minute the heartbeat is felt through the walls of the artery

**Radial Pulse** • Pulse rate obtained on the wrist

**Rectal Temperature** • The temperature reading obtained by placing the thermometer in the patient's rectum

**Respiration Rate** • The number of times a patient breathes per minute

**Temperature** • The quantity of body heat, measured in degrees—either Fahrenheit or Celsius

**Tympanic Membrane Temperature** • The temperature reading obtained by placing an aural (ear) thermometer in the patient's ear

**Vital Signs** • Measurements of body functions, including temperature, pulse, respiration, and blood pressure

## ABBREVIATIONS

| Abbreviation | Meaning | Example of Usage on a Doctors' Order Sheet |
|---|---|---|
| A & O | alert and oriented | BRP when A & O |
| ABR | absolute bedrest | ABR tonight |
| ad lib | as desired | Up ad lib |
| amb | ambulatory, ambulate | Amb today |
| as tol | as tolerated | Up as tol |
| ax | axillary or axilla | Ax temp |
| bid | two times a day | amb bid |
| BP | blood pressure | BP q 15 min ×4 |
| BR | bedrest | BR c̄ BRP |
| BRP | bathroom privileges | BRP starting tomorrow |
| BSC | bedside commode | May use BSC |
| c̄ | with | Up c̄ help |
| CBR | complete bed rest | CBR today |
| CMS | circulation, motion, and sensation | Check CMS fingers rt hand |
| CVP | central venous pressure | Measure CVP q4h |
| DC | discontinue | DC BSC |
| HOB | head of bed | ↑ HOB |
| h, hr, hrs | hour, hours | Flat in bed for 8 h |
| I & O | intake and output | Strict I & O |
| lt | left | ↑ lt arm on pillow |
| min | minutes | Up in chair for 5 min today |
| NVS | neurologic vital signs | NVS q4h & record |
| ° | degree or hour | Elevate head of bed 30° |
| OOB | out of bed | OOB ad lib |
| P | pulse | BP & P q4h |
| prn | as necessary | Up prn |
| q | every | wt q day |
| qd | every day or daily | wt qd |
| qid | four times a day | VS qid |
| qod | every other day | wt qod |
| q-h | every (fill in number) hour | Check VS q2h |
| R | rectal | R temp |
| RR | respiratory rate | Monitor RR q1h |
| rt | right | ↑ rt arm on pillow |
| Rt | routine | Rt VS |
| SOB | shortness of breath | Evaluate for SOB & notify physician |
| temp | temperature | rectal temp |
| tid | three times a day | up in chair tid |
| TPR | temperature, pulse, respiration | TRP & BP q4h |
| VS | vital signs | VS q4h |
| wt | weight | wt daily |
| ↑ | increase, above, or elevate | ↑ arm on 2 pillows |
| ↓ | decrease, below, or lower | if BP ↓ 100/60 call me |

## EXERCISE 1

Write the abbreviation for each term listed below.

1. complete bed rest    _CBR_
2. with    _c̄_
3. alert and oriented    _A & O_
4. four times a day    _qid_
5. degree or hour    ____
6. blood pressure    _BP_
7. every    _q_
8. ambulatory    _amb_
9. absolute bedrest    _ABR_
10. increase or elevate    _↑_
11. bathroom privileges    _BRP_
12. respiratory rate    _RR_
13. as desired    _ad lib_
14. every other day    _qod_
15. two times a day    _bid_
16. every day    _qd_
17. three times a day    _tid_
18. every hour    _q-h_
19. temperature    _temp_
20. as tolerated    _as tol_
21. right    _rt_
22. left    _Lt_
23. discontinue    _DC_
24. vital signs    _VS_
25. intake and output    _I & O_
26. out of bed    _OOB_
27. minutes    _min_

28. weight _____ wt
29. bed rest _____ BR
30. rectal _____ Ⓡ
31. axilla or axillary _____ ax
32. temperature, pulse, respiration _____ TPR
33. pulse _____ P
34. hour _____ h, hr, hrs
35. as necessary _____ prn
36. neurologic vital signs _____ NVS
37. below _____ ↓
38. head of bed _____ HOB
39. bedside commode _____ BSC
40. every 4 hours _____ q4h
41. circulation, motion and sensation _____ CMS
42. shortness of breath _____ SOB
43. central venous pressure _____ CVP

18. amb _____ ambulate
19. qod _____ every other day
20. qd _____ every day
21. bid _____ twice a day
22. qid _____ 4 times a day
23. qh _____ every hour
24. ABR _____ absolute bedrest
25. temp _____ temperature
26. as tol _____ as tolerated
27. I & O _____ Intake & Output
28. q _____ every
29. P _____ Pulse
30. ax _____ axilla or axillary
31. R _____ Rectal
32. prn _____ as necessary
33. RR _____ respiration rate
34. q4h _____ every 4 hours
35. hrs _____ hours
36. NVS _____ neurological vital signs
37. ↓ _____ decrease, lower, below
38. Rt _____ routine
39. SOB _____ shortness of breath
40. HOB _____ head of bed
41. BSC _____ bedside commode
42. CMS _____ circulation motion & sensation
43. CVP _____ Central venous pressure

# EXERCISE 2

Write the meaning of each abbreviation listed below.

1. lt _____ left
2. rt _____ right
3. DC _____ discontinue
4. VS _____ Vital Signs
5. BP _____ Blood Pressure
6. tid _____ three times a day
7. CBR _____ Complete bed rest
8. c̄ _____ with
9. TPR _____ Temperature, Pulse, Respiration
10. BR _____ Bedrest
11. min _____ minute
12. BRP _____ Bathroom Privileges
13. ad lib _____ as desired
14. ↑ _____ Increase above elevate
15. OOB _____ out of bed
16. A & O _____ alert & orientated
17. wt _____ weight

## PATIENT ACTIVITY ORDERS

## Background Information

Patient activity refers to the amount of walking, sitting, and so forth that the patient may do in a given period during his or her hospital stay. The prescribed activity changes to coincide with the client's stage of recovery. For example, following major surgery the doctor will want the patient to remain in bed; as the patient recovers, the doctor increases the activity accordingly. The doctor indicates the degree of activity the patient should have by writing an activity order on the doctors' order sheet. Common activity orders are listed below with an interpretation.

**COMMUNICATION AND IMPLEMENTATION OF PATIENT ACTIVITY, PATIENT POSITIONING, AND NURSING OBSERVATION ORDERS**

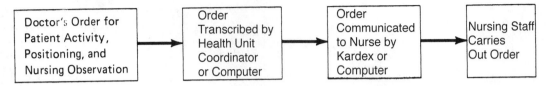

These orders are written in abbreviated form as the doctor would write them on the doctors' order sheet, *with one exception*: they are not written in a doctor's handwriting. Reading doctors' handwriting can be a difficult task. However, the repetitive reading of doctors' handwritten orders soon prepares you to become an expert in this area. For assistance with abbreviations, refer to the abbreviation list at the beginning of the chapter.

## Doctors' Orders for Patient Activities

### CBR
The patient is to remain in bed at all times.

### BR c̄ BRP
The client may use the bathroom for the elimination of urine and stool, but otherwise must remain in bed.

### Dangle tonight
The patient may sit and dangle his feet over the edge of the bed. The doctor may specify the number of times per day the patient should dangle, such as *Dangle bid*; or he or she may specify a period of time, such as *Dangle 5 min tid*.

### Use bedside commode or use BSC
The patient may use a portable commode at the bedside.

### Up c̄ help
The client may be out of bed when assisted by a member of the nursing staff.

### Up in chair
The patient may sit in a chair. The doctor may specify the length of time and/or number of times per day, especially if he or she orders this activity following CBR. Example: *Up in chair 5 min tid*.

### BRP when A & O
The patient may use the bathroom as desired when alert and oriented.

### Up in hall
Patient may walk in the hall.

### Up as tol
The patient may be out of bed as much as he or she can physically tolerate.

### Up ad lib
The patient has no restriction on activity.

### OOB
The patient may be out of bed. The doctor may qualify this order with another statement, such as *OOB bid*.

### Amb
This is another way of saying the patient may be up as desired.

### May shower
The patient may have a shower. A doctors' order is necessary for a hospitalized patient to have a shower or tub bath.

---
**TO THE STUDENT**

To practice transcribing an activity order, complete **Activity 10–1** in the Skills Practice Manual.
---

## PATIENT POSITIONING ORDERS

## Background Information

Patient positioning is often determined by the nursing staff; however, the doctor may want the patient to remain in a special body position to maintain body alignment, promote comfort, and facilitate body functions. For example, the doctor may order the head of the bed to be elevated to ease the patient's breathing, or he or she may want the nurse to turn the patient to the unaffected side to promote healing. The doctor indicates a special position by writing the order on the doctors' orders sheet. Since it would be impossible to discuss all patient positioning orders, only those that are most typical are described here. The following positioning orders are written in the same terms as you will find them on a doctors' orders sheet. Refer to the abbreviation list at the beginning of the chapter for assistance.

## Doctors' Orders for Patient Positioning

### Elevate head of bed 30° or ↑ HOB 30°
The head of the bed is to be elevated 30 degrees. (The degree of elevation may vary according to the purpose of

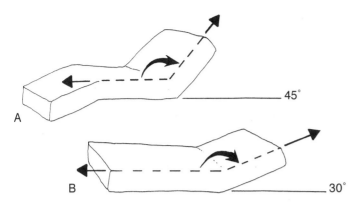

F I G U R E   10–1 • (*A*) Fowler's position. (*B*) Semi-Fowler's position.

the order; for example, the doctor may write ↑ *head of bed 20°*.)

### Elevate lt arm on two pillows

The left arm is to be elevated on two pillows. Variations of this order include the degree of elevation and also include other limbs; for example, *Elevate rt foot on pillow*.

### Fowler's position

The client is placed in a semisitting position by elevating the head of the bed approximately 18–20 inches or 45 degrees with a slight elevation of the knees. The semi-Fowler's position is the same as Fowler's but with the head of the bed elevated 30° (Fig. 10–1).

### Log roll

The patient is turned from side to side or side to back while keeping the back straight like a log with a pillow between the knees.

### Turn to unaffected side

The doctor wishes the patient to lie on the side that is free of injury.

### Flat in bed for 8 h no pillow

The client is to remain flat in bed for 8 hours, after which the standing activity order is resumed.

### Turn q2h

The client's position is changed every 2 hours to prevent skin breakdown (bedsores).

---

**TO THE STUDENT**

To practice transcribing a patient positioning order, complete **Activity 10–2** in the Skills Practice Manual.

---

## NURSING OBSERVATION ORDERS

## Background Information

The doctor may wish to have the nursing staff make periodic observations of the patient's condition; these obser-

vations are referred to as *signs and symptoms*. Some doctors may write "call orders" indicating she or he is to be called in the event of certain circumstances. For example, call if P ↑ 110, R ↓ 10, T ↑ 101°, B/P systolic ↑ 160, diastolic ↑ 90. The doctor may need this information to assist in diagnosing the patient's illness or interpreting the patient's progress. The doctor writes an order to request the information wanted. It is difficult to record all doctors' orders that you will encounter in this area; however, we have outlined some of the more common ones for you below, written as you may find them on the doctors' orders sheet. For assistance with the interpretation of the abbreviations, refer to the abbreviation list at the beginning of the chapter.

## Doctors' Orders for Nursing Observation

### VS q4h

The client's vital signs are to be taken and recorded every 4 hours. Vital signs include *temperature* (Fig. 10–2), *pulse rate, respiration rate,* and *blood pressure reading*. The temperature may be taken using an aural thermometer, an oral thermometer or rectal thermometer. Oral and rectal thermometers may be glass or electric (Fig. 10–2). The results of the temperature will indicate whether the patient is febrile or afebrile. The pulse is obtained from the radial artery in the wrist, unless otherwise indicated. Variations of this type of order may include other time sequences and can read, for example, *VS q1h, VS q2h,* or may include a qualifying phrase, such as *VS q1h until stable then q4h*.

### BP qh × 4

The blood pressure is to be taken and recorded every hour for 4 hours. Variations to this order may involve other time sequences, such as *BP q4h, BP tid,* and so forth, or a qualifying phrase, such as *BP q3h while awake* or *BP q4h if ↓ 100/60 call me*.

### Observe for SOB and notify physician

The patient will be observed for shortness of breath and, if severe, the nurse will notify the physician of the patient's condition.

### Apical rate

The patient's heart rate is to be taken at the apex of the heart with a stethoscope.

### Check pedal pulse R foot q2h

The pulses are obtained from an artery (dorsalis pedis) on top of the foot.

### NVS q2h

The patient's neurologic vital signs are taken and recorded every 2 hours.

### I & O

The client's fluid intake and output is measured and recorded at the completion of each shift. It is then calculated for 24-hour periods. See Figure 10–3, a typical intake and output form used by the nursing staff to calculate the patient's intake and output for an 8-hour shift.

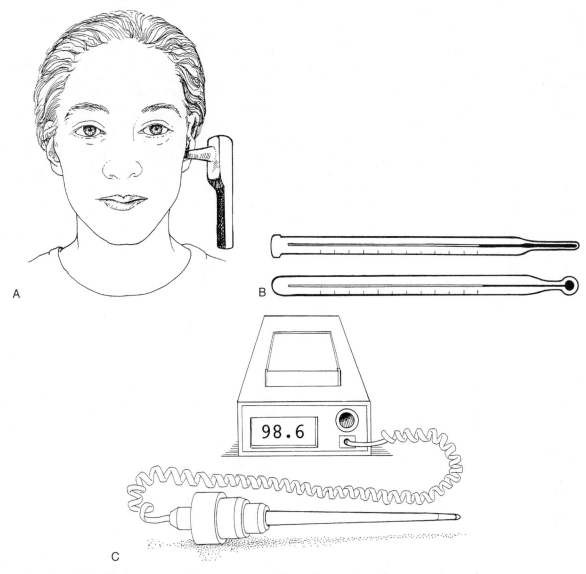

**F I G U R E   10–2 •** Types of thermometers. (*A*) Aural—used to take tympanic membrane tempera-ture in the ear. (*B*) Glass—used to take oral, rectal, and axillary temperatures. (*C*) Electric—used to take oral and rectal temperatures.

### wt daily

The patient is to be weighed daily and the weight re-corded. A variation of this order may be *wt qod*.

### Tympanic membrane temp q4h

The temperature is to be measured every 4 hours, using the aural thermometer (see Fig. 10–2) as opposed to the oral method. A third method of measuring the body tem-perature is the axilla method. The doctor's order for this method may read, *axillary temp q4h*. A fourth is the rectal method. The doctors' order will read, *rectal temp q4h*.

### CVP q2h

A catheter is inserted, usually through the right or left subclavian vein, and threaded through the vein until the tip reaches the right atrium of the heart (see Fig. 11–11). The catheter is inserted by the doctor; the pressure read-ings are done by the nurse.

### Pulse oximetry q4h

The oxygen saturation of arterial blood is to be measured every 4 hours. A portable pulse oximeter with a special sensor is used. Pulse oximetry may be performed by the nursing staff or respiratory therapist. The sensor may be left in place for continuous monitoring.

### Check CMS fingers rt hand

The circulation, motion, and sensation of the patient's right-hand fingers are to be checked as often as the nurse determines it to be necessary. This type of order specifies observation of the patient's signs and symptoms relative to the patient's diagnosis and treatment. For example, this order was written following the application of a cast to the patient's right arm and hand. *Check for rectal bleeding and observe for headaches and dizziness* are two other exam-ples of this type of order.

## 24 HOUR INTAKE AND OUTPUT

Name _Mary Ryan_
Room _403A_
Date _9 / 10 / 98_

| Shift | Fluid Intake | | | Fluid Output | | Other | Stools |
|---|---|---|---|---|---|---|---|
| | Oral | I.V. | Piggy Back | Urine | Emesis | Suction ☐ | |
| 0700-1500 | 0830  100cc / 30cc<br>1000  320cc<br>1200  500cc<br>1500  210 | Credit _300_<br>Add _1000_<br>Add _____ | 50 | 0730  200cc<br>1100  300cc<br>1300  175cc | 200cc | | x 1 lg amt |
| 8 hr. | 1160 | | 50 | 675 | | | |
| 1500-2300 | | Credit _500_<br>Add _____<br>Add _____ | | | | | |
| 8 hr. | | | | | | | |
| 2300-0700 | | Credit _____<br>Add _____<br>Add _____ | | | | | |
| 8 hr. | | | | | | | |
| 24 hr. | | | | | | | |

Iced Tea - 6 oz. (180 cc)
Water Glass - 6 oz. (180 cc)
Milk (carton) - 8 oz. (240 cc)
Fruit Juice - 4 oz. (120 cc)
Soup - 4 oz. (120 cc)
Ice Cream - 3 oz.(90 cc)
Jello - 3.5 oz. (105 cc)

Cup of Coffee or Tea - 7 oz. (210 cc)
Styrofoam Cup - 150 cc
Paper Cup - 150 cc
Coffee Creamer - .5 oz. (15 cc)
Cereal Creamer - 2 oz. (60 cc)
Coca Cola and Sprite - 12 oz. (360 cc)
$H_2O$ Pitcher - 30 oz. (900 cc)

FIGURE  10–3 • An intake and output form.

**HIGHLIGHT**

Vital signs are measured to detect changes in the patient's condition, assess response to treatment, and recognize life-threatening situations. Accurate recording of vital signs is essential. Vital signs consist of:

Blood pressure
Pulse
    Apical
    Radial
    Pedal
    Femoral
    Carotid
    Popliteal
Temperature
    Oral
Tympanic membrane
    Axillary
    Rectal
Respirations

TO THE STUDENT

To practice transcribing a nursing observation order, complete **Activity 10–3** in the Skills Practice Manual.

   To practice transcribing, automatically cancelling, and discontinuing doctors' orders, complete **Activity 10–4** in the Skills Practice Manual.

   To practice transcribing a review set of doctors' orders, complete **Activity 10–5** in the Skills Practice Manual.

TO THE STUDENT

To practice recording telephoned doctors' orders and to practice recording telephoned messages, complete **Activities 10–6** and **10–7** in the Skills Practice Manual.

## SUMMARY

Transcription of doctors' orders is a major responsibility in health unit coordinating. This chapter introduced you to doctors' orders for patient activity, patient positioning, and nursing observation. Refer back to this chapter as needed.

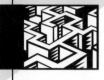

**REVIEW QUESTIONS**

1. Define the following terms:

   a. nursing observation orders: _a doctors order that requests the nursing staff to observe record certain patient signs + symptoms_

   b. activity order: _a doctors order defining the type and amount of activity the patient can have_

   c. positioning order: _a doctors order that specifies the the position of that patients body is to be placed in_

   d. vital signs: _the measuring of body functions which include temp, pulse, respiration, and blood pressure_

   e. temperature:

      i. oral: _glass or electric temperature taken from mouth_

      ii. rectal: _temperature taken from rectum using electric or glass thermometer_

      iii. axillary: _temperature reading taken from under the arm, with glass thermometer_

      iv. tympanic membrane: _temperature reading taken from the tympanic membrane in the ear_

   f. pulse oximetry: _method of measuring oxygen saturation of arterial blood._

   g. febrile: _elevated body temperature_

   h. afebrile: _without fever_

2. Write out each doctors' order in the space provided.

   a. CBR _Complete bed rest_

   b. BR c̄ BRP when A & O _bed rest with bathroom privileges when + oriented alert_

   c. wt qod _weight every other day_

   d. VS qid _Vital Signs 4 times a day_

   e. TPR & BP tid _Temp, Pulse, respiration and Blood pressure three times a day_

   f. ↑ head of bed 20° _elevate head of bed to 20 degrees_

g. check dressing prn _____ check dressing as necessary _____

h. temp R or ax only _____ temperature rectal or axillary only _____

i. NVS q2h _____ neurological vital signs every 2 hours _____

j. I & O q shift _____ Intake and Output every shift _____

k. OOB ad lib _____ Out of bed as desired _____

l. up as tol _____ up as tolerated _____

m. TPR & BP q4h _____ vital signs every 4 hours _____

n. amb today _____ ambulate today _____

o. DC VS _____ discontinue vital signs _____

p. ↑ HOB 30° _____ elevate head of bed 30° degrees _____

q. may use BSC _____ may use bedside commode _____

r. log roll q2h _____ log roll every 2 hours _____

s. check CMS toes lt foot _____ check circulation motion sensation of the toes of the left foot _____

t. CVP q3h _____ Check Central Venous Pressure every three hours _____

u. call me if pt SOB _____ call me if patient has shortness of breath _____

## References

Blackburn, Elsa: *Health Unit Coordinator*, 1st ed. Englewood Cliffs, NJ, Prentice-Hall Inc., 1991.

Brunner, Lillian Sholts and Suddarth, Doris Smith: *Textbook of Medical-Surgical Nursing*, 5th ed. Philadelphia, J. B. Lippincott Co., 1984.

Hegner, Barbara and Caldwell, Esther: *Nursing Assistant: A Nursing Process Approach*, 7th ed. New York, Delmar Publishers Inc., 1995.

Lammon, Carol, Foote, Anne, Leli, Patricia, Ingle, Janice, and Adams, Marsha: *Clinical Nursing Skills*. Philadelphia, W. B. Saunders Co., 1995.

Readey, Helen et al.: *Introduction to Nursing Essentials: A Handbook*. St. Louis, The C. V. Mosby Co., 1977.

Wood, Lucille A. and Rambo, Beverly J.: *Nursing Skills for Allied Health Services*, vol. 1, 2nd ed. Philadelphia, W. B. Saunders Co., 1977.

CHAPTER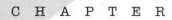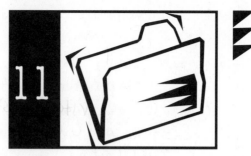

# NURSING TREATMENT ORDERS

## CHAPTER OBJECTIVES

*Upon completion of this chapter, you will be able to:*

1. Define the terms in the vocabulary list.
2. Write the meanings of the abbreviations and the abbreviations for the terms on the abbreviations list.
3. Describe the function of the central service department with regard to nursing treatment orders.
4. Explain why reusable equipment should be returned to the central service department as quickly as possible.
5. List and describe the types of items stored on the central service department stock supply cart on the nursing units.
6. List and describe the types of items stored in the central service department.
7. Demonstrate the procedure to order supplies/equipment from the central service department using the requisition and/or computer method.
8. Describe four types of enemas.
9. Compare the purposes of the two types of urinary catheterization procedures.
10. List four reasons for administering intravenous therapy.
11. Explain the various methods of administering intravenous therapy.
12. List three parts of an intravenous therapy order and give an example of each.
13. Describe the various types of blood transfusions.
14. Explain the health unit coordinator's role in obtaining blood from the blood bank and the correct storage of blood.
15. Describe the various suction devices and explain their uses.
16. Explain the uses for heat and cold applications and list the devices used for heat and cold therapy.
17. List and explain the various types of doctors' orders for patient comfort, safety, and healing.
18. Explain the reasons for obtaining blood glucose levels.

## VOCABULARY

**Autologous Blood** • The patient's own blood donated previously for transfusion as needed by the patient; also called autotransfusion

**Binder** • A cloth or elastic bandage usually used for abdominal or chest support

**Urinary Catheter** • A tube used for removing urine or injecting fluids into the bladder

**Retention Catheter** • A catheter that remains in the bladder

**Nonretention Catheter** • A catheter that is removed from the bladder upon completion of the catheterization procedure

**Central Venous Line** or **Central Venous Catheter** • A catheter is threaded through to the superior vena cava or right atrium used for the administration of intravenous therapy

**Donor-Specific** or **Donor-Directed Blood** • Blood donated by relatives or friends of the patient to be used for transfusion as needed

**Egg-Crate Mattress** • A foam rubber mattress

**Enema** • The introduction of fluid into the rectum

**Foley Catheter** • A type of retention catheter

**Gastric Suction Machine** • An electronic machine used to remove gastric contents

**Harris Flush** • A return flow enema

**Hemovac** • A disposable suction device

**Heparin Lock; Buffalo Cap** • A venous access device (also called intermittent infusion device) placed on a peripheral intravenous catheter when used intermittently

**In AM** • To be done the following morning

**Incontinence** • Inability of the body to control the elimination of urine and/or feces

**Infusion Pump** • A device used to regulate flow or rate of intravenous fluid. It is commonly called an I-med pump

**Intermittent** • Having periods of cessation of activity

**Intermittent IV Line** • An access into a vein by means of a venous access device; used to give medication at intervals

**Intravenous Infusion** • The administration of a large amount of fluid through a vein

**Irrigation** • Washing out of a body cavity or wound

**K-Pad** • An electric device used for heat application (also called a K-thermia pad, aquathermia pad, or aquamatic pad)

**Nasogastric Tube** • A tube that is inserted through the nose into the stomach

**Nursing Treatment Orders** • Doctors' orders for treatments performed by the nursing staff

**Peripheral Intravenous Catheter** • A catheter that begins and ends in the extremities of the body; used for the administration of intravenous therapy

**Rectal Tube** • A plastic or rubber tube designed for insertion into the rectum; when written as a doctor's order, *rectal tube* means the insertion of a rectal tube into the rectum to remove gas and relieve distention

**Restraints** • Devices used to control patients exhibiting dangerous behavior or to protect the patient

**Sheepskin** • A pad made out of lamb's wool or synthetic material; used to prevent pressure sores

**Sitz Bath** • Application of warm water to the pelvic area

**This AM** • To be done this morning

**Throat Suction Machine** • An electric machine or wall mount used to remove secretions that may block the airway

**Transfusion** • Transfer of blood, or one of its components, from one person to another

**Urinary Catheterization** • Insertion of a catheter through the urethra into the bladder

**Urine Residual** • The amount of urine left in the bladder after voiding

**Venipuncture** • Needle puncture of a vein

**Void** • To empty, especially the urinary bladder

## ABBREVIATIONS

| Abbreviation | Meaning | Example of Usage on a Doctors' Order Sheet |
| --- | --- | --- |
| @ | at | Run IV @ 100 cc/hr |
| abd | abdominal | Up c̄ abd binder |
| ac | before meals | Accu-Chek ac and hs |
| A-E | antiembolism | A-E hose on when up |
| ASAP | as soon as possible | Start IV ASAP |
| cath | catheterize | Cath q8h prn |
| CBI | continuous bladder irrigation | CBI c̄ NS 50 cc/hr |
| cc | cubic centimeter (equivalent to milliliter [mL]) | IV 1000 cc 5% D/W 125 cc/hr |
| cm | centimeter | Chest tube 20 cm neg pressure |
| con't | continue, continuous | Foley cath to con't drainage |
| CVC | Central venous catheter | Blood draws through CVC |
| D/RL | dextrose in Ringer's lactate | IV 1000 cc 5% D/RL at 125 cc/hr |
| D5W (5% D/W) | 5% dextrose in water | 1000 mL D5W @ 125 mL/hr |
| D/W | dextrose in water | 1000 mL 5% D/W at 125 mL/hr |
| DW | distilled water | Irrig cath prn c̄ DW |
| ETS | elevated toilet seat | Order elevated toilet seat for home use |
| gtt(s) | drop(s) | IV @ 60 gtts/min |
| H₂O₂ | hydrogen peroxide | Irrigate wound c̄ H₂O₂ & NS equal strength |
| hs | bedtime, hour of sleep | Give TWE hs |
| irrig | irrigate | Irrig cath c̄ NS prn |
| IV | intravenous | Con't IVs as ordered |
| IVF | intravenous fluids | DC IVF at 1000 today |
| KO | keep open | KO IV c̄ 1000 cc 5% D/W |
| min, m | minute | Run @ 30 gtts/min |
| mL | milliliter | IV 1000 mL 5% D/W |
| MR | may repeat | SSE now MR × 1 |
| nec | necessary | SSE now MR if nec |
| NG | nasogastric | Insert NG tube |
| NS | normal saline | Give NS enema now |
| ORE | oil retention enema | ORE today |
| p̄ | after | Up p̄ breakfast |
| PAS | pulsatile antiembolism stockings | PAS to both legs |

*for test*

| PICC | peripherally inserted central catheter | Insert PICC, follow protocol |
|------|------|------|
| RL, LR | Ringer's lactate, lactated Ringer's | 1000 mL RL 125 mL/h |
| sol'n | solution | Irrig cath c̄ NS sol'n |
| SSE | soap suds enema | SSE now |
| st | straight | Retention cath to st drain |
| TCDB | turn, cough, and deep breathe | TCDB q2h |
| TEDs | antiembolism stockings | Apply TEDs |
| TKO | to keep open | IV TKO c̄ 5% D/W |
| TWE | tap water enema | Give TWE |
| VAD | venous access device | Use VAD for blood draws |
| Δ | change | Δ catheter daily |
| / | per, by | Run IV @ 150 cc/hr |

## E X E R C I S E  1

Write the abbreviation for each term listed below.

1. soap suds enema — SSE
2. keep open — KO
3. may repeat — MR
4. solution — sol'n
5. necessary — prn
6. centimeter — cm
7. tap water enema — TWE
8. nasogastric — NG
9. normal saline — NS
10. dextrose in Ringer's lactate — D/RL
11. bedtime — ~~prn~~ hs
12. distilled water — DW
13. at — @
14. oil retention enema — ORE
15. dextrose in water — D/W
16. irrigate — Irrig
17. intravenous — IV
18. catheterize — cath
19. Ringer's lactate — RL ∩ LR
20. straight — st
21. cubic centimeter — cc
22. after — p̄

23. abdominal — ~~ABD~~ abd
24. turn, cough, and deep breathe — TCDB
25. minute — min
26. drops — gtt
27. change — Δ
28. as soon as possible — ASAP
29. per — /
30. hydrogen peroxide — $H_2O_2$
31. before meals — ac
32. antiembolism — A-E
33. continue — con't
34. continuous bladder irrigation — CBI
35. to keep open — TKO
36. antiembolism stockings — AS
37. milliliter — ml
38. pulsatile antiembolism stockings — PAS
39. intravenous fluids — IVF
40. elevated toilet seat — ETS
41. peripherally inserted central catheter — PICC
42. venous access device — VAD
43. central venous catheter — CVC

## E X E R C I S E  2

Write out each doctors' order in the space provided

1. *1000 mL 5% D/RL, 125 mL/hr then DC* on at then Discard for 125 milliliters per hour
   1000 milliliters of 5 percent Dextrose in Ringers Lactate

2. *SSE hs MR × 1*
   Soap suds Enema at bedtime may repeat one tim

3. *Give ORE follow c̄ TWE if nec*
   Give oil retention enema and follow with tap water enema if necessary

4. *Irrig cath tid c̄ NS sol'n*
   Irrigate catheter 3 times a day with normal saline solution

5. *IV KO c̄ 1000 cc 5% D/W*
   Intravenous keep open with 1000 cubic centimeters of 5% Dextrose in water

6. *Insert NG tube*
   Insert Nasogastric tube

7. *TCDB q2h*

 *turn cough and deep breath every 2 hours*

8. *Δ IV tubing ASAP*

 *change Intravenous tubing as soon as possible*

## COMMUNICATION WITH THE CENTRAL SERVICE DEPARTMENT

The **central service department (CSD)** distributes the supplies used for nursing procedures. **Central processing department (CPD)**, **products and materials (PAM)**, and **supplies, processing, and distribution (SPD)** are other names used for the central service department. Although CSD supplies are frequently used without being a part of the doctors' orders, obtaining these supplies for the nursing staff may be a step of the transcription procedure for nursing treatment orders. For example, in the order *foot board to bed*, the health unit coordinator orders the foot board from the central service department. It is therefore necessary for you to be familiar with frequently used central service department items and to learn your hospital's system for obtaining them.

The system for obtaining central service supplies varies among hospitals; thus it is impossible to outline one procedure to cover all hospital systems. However, one common practice is to store disposable or frequently used items on the nursing unit. This is often referred to as the **CSD stock supply**. Many hospitals have an exchange cart system. The carts are supplied with frequently used items and exchanged every 24 hours. The unit receives another completely supplied cart while CSD replenishes the used cart. See the following for a list of items commonly stored in the stock supply. Reusable or infrequently used items are stored in the central service department. See the following for items commonly obtained from the central service area.

### A LIST OF ITEMS THAT MAY BE STORED IN THE CENTRAL SERVICE DEPARTMENT

Alternating pressure pad
Egg-crate mattress
Antiembolism stockings
Pulsatile antiembolism stockings and pump
Colostomy irrigation bag
Stomal bag
Elastic abdominal binder
Foot board
Foot cradle
Gastric suction machine
Nasogastric tube
Feeding tube
Feeding infusion pump and tubing
Throat suction machine
Throat suction catheter
IV infusion pump with tubing
Hypothermia machine
Ice bag
K-pad with motor
Restraints
Sheepskin
Sitz bath, disposable
Vaginal irrigation kit
Sterile trays
 Tracheostomy
 Paracentesis
 Bone marrow
 Spinal tap
 Thoracentesis
 Central line

### A LIST OF ITEMS THAT MAY BE STORED IN THE CSD STOCK SUPPLY ON THE UNIT

Enema bag
Fleet enema
Rectal tube
Retention catheter tray (Foley, indwelling)
Nonretention catheter tray
Irrigation tray
Continuous bladder irrigation solution and tubing
IV solutions
IV catheters and IV needles
IV tubing
Blood tubing
Intermittent injection caps
Tissue
Lotion
Oral care supplies
Powder
Sterile gloves
Exam gloves
Masks
Syringes
Disposable suture removal kits
Dressings
 Abdominal pads
 4 × 4 gauze
 2 × 2 gauze
 Kling
 Vasoline gauze
 Telfa
Irrigating solutions
 500 cc sterile water
 1000 cc sterile water
 500 cc normal saline
 1000 cc normal saline

The health unit coordinator, when transcribing a treatment order, orders only those items stored in the central service department, since the nursing staff can quickly obtain the items needed from the CSD stock supply. Items from CSD are ordered by computer or by completing a requisition. It is important to remember that supplies used from the CSD stock supply are also charged to the patient. This is done by completing a requisition or removing a label from the supply package and placing it in a CSD charge book on the patient's charge card (Fig. 11–1). The person removing the needed supplies is responsible for the charging process. Figure 11–2 is an example of central service requisition or computer screen.

Many items, such as enema bags or urinary catheterization trays, used for nursing treatments are *disposable*. This means that once the item has been used by the patient, it is either discarded or given to the patient for future use. The patient is charged for the disposable equipment.

Other items are *reusable*. They are cleaned or sterilized, if necessary, after use by a patient. The item is then available for another patient. The patient usually pays a fee for the use of these items. When the doctor writes an order to discontinue a reusable item, such as a gastric suction machine, it is important for the health unit coordinator to notify the nursing staff to discontinue the equipment as soon as possible so the equipment can be returned to the central service department. Once there, if there is a rental charge, it can be terminated and the equipment readied for use by other patients.

Equipment is discussed and illustrated throughout this chapter as it relates to nursing treatment orders. Although you will not use the equipment yourself, being able to recognize frequently used items helps you in the ordering step of the transcription procedure.

FIGURE 11–1 • CSD patient charge card.

## HIGHLIGHT

The health unit coordinator can best assist the nursing staff when transcribing nursing treatment orders by learning about the equipment and supplies on the unit where you work so you can have the items needed by the staff to carry out the treatments.

- Learn which items are stored on the unit, and do not order them from CSD.
- Learn the items stored in CSD and order those. If patient information, such as weight, is needed record this information when ordering the item.
- Know which items are disposable and which are reusable and return reusable items to CSD immediately after the patient is finished using them.

When you begin your clinical experience or employment, begin a list of supplies and equipment and where they are stored and particulars about obtaining them. This will be a handy reference until you commit this knowledge to memory.

## INTESTINAL ELIMINATION ORDERS

### Background Information

Enemas, rectal tubes, and colostomy irrigations are treatments used to remove stool and/or flatus (gas) from the large intestine.

An enema is the introduction of fluid into the rectum for the purpose of relieving distention (trapped gas) or constipation, or to prepare the patient for surgery or diagnostic tests. Common types of enemas are:

1. Oil retention
2. Soap suds
3. Tap water
4. Normal saline

Figure 11–3 is an example of a disposable enema bag used to administer these types of enemas.

| | | |
|---|---|---|
| ALTERNATING PRESSURE PAD | | |
| EGG-CRATE MATTRESS | | |
| ANTIEMBOLISM STOCKINGS | SIZE | |
| PULSATILE ANTIEMBOLISM STOCKINGS | | |
| COLOSTOMY IRRIGATING BAG | | |
| STOMAL BAGS | SIZE | |
| ELASTIC ABDOMINAL BINDER | SIZE | |
| FOOT BOARD | | |
| FOOT CRADLE | | |
| GASTRIC SUCTION MACHINE | | |
| NASOGASTRIC TUBE<br>    TYPE | SIZE | |
| FEEDING TUBE<br>    TYPE | SIZE | |
| FEEDING INFUSION PUMP AND TUBING | | |
| THROAT SUCTION MACHINE | | |
| THROAT SUCTION CATHETERS | SIZE | |
| IV INFUSION PUMP WITH TUBING | | |
| HYPOTHERMIA MACHINE | | |
| ICE BAG | | |
| K-PAD WITH MOTOR | SIZE | |
| RESTRAINTS<br>    TYPE | | |
| SHEEPSKIN | | |
| SITZ BATH, DISPOSABLE | | |
| VAGINAL IRRIGATION KIT | | |
| OTHER | | |

REQUESTED BY _____
DATE _____

STERILE TRAYS

| |
|---|
| TRACHEOSTOMY |
| PARACENTESIS |
| BONE MARROW |
| SPINAL TAP |
| THORACENTESIS |
| CENTRAL LINE |
| OTHER |

F I G U R E  11–2 • An example of CSD requisition.

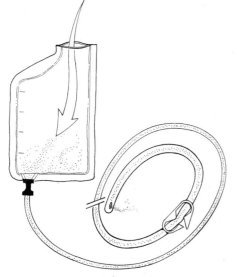

F I G U R E  11–3 • A disposable enema bag.

*Fleet enema* is a disposable commercially prepackaged sodium phosphate enema that is frequently used (Fig. 11–4).

The order for a **rectal tube** means the insertion of a disposable plastic or rubber tube into the rectum for the purpose of relieving distention. The rectal tube may be attached to a flatus bag that captures the flatus (Fig. 11–5).

**Harris flush** is a return-flow enema and is used to relieve distention. A disposable enema bag is used to inject fluid into the rectum. The fluid is allowed to return into the bag. The process is repeated several times.

**Colostomy** (an artificial opening in the colon for passage of stool) **irrigation** (the flushing of fluid) resembles an enema and is used to regulate the discharge of stool. Figure 11–6 shows a disposable colostomy irrigation bag used for this treatment.

A doctors' order is required for the administration of enemas, rectal tubes, and colostomy irrigations. The order contains the name of the treatment, the type (when pertinent), and the frequency. If the frequency is not indicated

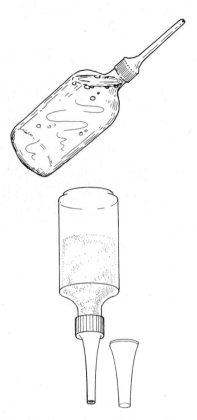

F I G U R E   11–4 • Commercially prepackaged enema.

(such as in the order *tap water enema*), it is considered a one-time order.

Examples of intestinal elimination orders are listed below as they are usually written on the doctors' order sheet. Refer to the abbreviations list at the beginning of the chapter for interpretation of the abbreviations.

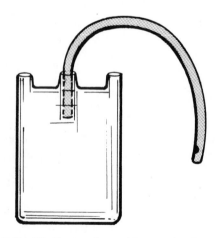

F I G U R E   11–5 • A disposable rectal tube in a flatus bag.

## Doctors' Orders for Intestinal Elimination

1. *TWE now MR × 1 prn*
2. *Give ORE followed by NS enemas this AM*
3. *Harris flush for abdominal distention*
4. *NS enemas until clear*
5. *Give Fleet enema qd prn constipation*
6. *Colostomy irrig daily c̄ tap water*
7. *Rectal tube prn for distention*

## URINARY CATHETERIZATION ORDERS

### Background Information

Urinary catheterization is the insertion of a tube called a **catheter** through the urethra into the bladder for the purpose of removing urine. The tube is usually made of plastic, and it varies in size. The doctor may order two types of catheterization procedures: retention and nonretention. Disposable sterile catheterization trays are used. Because different equipment is needed for each procedure, two types of catheter trays are available. One is used for the insertion of the retention catheter and the other is used for the insertion of the nonretention catheter. Each tray is marked with the size and type of catheter it contains.

A **nonretention catheter**, sometimes referred to as a **straight catheter**, is used to empty the bladder, to collect a sterile urine specimen, or to check residual. **Residual** is the amount of urine remaining in the bladder after voiding. The nonretention catheter is removed from the bladder after completion of the procedure (Fig. 11–7).

A **retention catheter** (also called an **indwelling** or **Foley catheter**) remains in the bladder and is usually connected to a drainage system that allows for continuous flow of urine from the bladder to the container. Doctors refer to this type of drainage system as a **straight drain** (Fig. 11–8).

The doctor may order the retention catheter to be irrigated on an intermittent or continuous basis to maintain patency (to keep the catheter open). This is referred to as a closed system (Fig. 11–9) and is usually used for those who have had surgery involving the urinary or reproductive system. The open irrigation system is used for irrigating the catheter at specific intervals. The open system requires the nurse to open a closed drainage system and insert an irrigation solution. A disposable irrigation tray is used for this procedure. The doctor indicates the solution to be used (normal saline, acetic acid, distilled water). For continuous and intermittent irrigation, special set-ups are used (Fig. 11–9).

Several types of typical doctors' orders related to urinary catheterizations are listed below, recorded in abbreviated form as they would appear on the doctors' order

## COMMUNICATION AND IMPLEMENTATION OF NURSING TREATMENT ORDERS

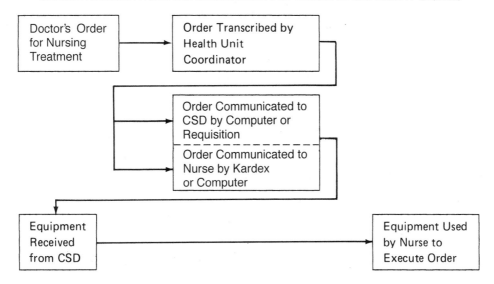

sheet. Refer to the abbreviations list at the beginning of the chapter for assistance with abbreviations.

## Doctors' Orders for Catheterization

### Nonretention Catheter

- *May cath q8h prn*
- *Catheterize now*
- *Cath prn*
- *Cath in 8 hr if unable to avoid*
- *Cath for residual*
- *Stand to avoid p̄ 4 PM—cath if nec*

### Retention Catheter

- *Insert Foley*
- *Retention cath to st drain*

- *Insert Foley cath for residual; if over 200 mL, leave in*
- *DC cath in AM if unable to void in 6 h reinsert*
- *DC cath this AM*
- *Clamp cath 4 hr then drain*

### Retention Catheter Irrigation

- *CBI; use NS @ 50 mL/hr*
- *Irrig Foley c̄ NS bid*
- *Irrig cath prn patency*
- *Intermittent CBI q4h × 6*

> ### TO THE STUDENT
>
> To practice transcribing intestinal elimination and urinary catheterization orders, complete **Activity 11–1** in the Skills Practice Manual.

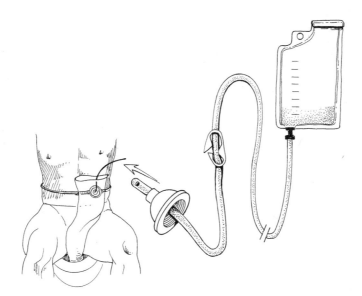

F I G U R E  11–6 • A disposable colostomy irrigation apparatus.

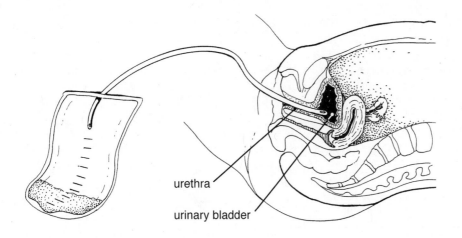

F I G U R E  11–7 • A nonretention catheter in place.

urethra

urinary bladder

## INTRAVENOUS THERAPY ORDERS

### Background Information

Until 1949 intravenous therapy consisted of the administration of simple solutions, such as water and normal saline, through peripheral veins. Equipment was a glass bottle, rubber tube, and a needle. Today, intravenous therapy is the parenteral administration of fluids, medications, nutritional substances, and blood transfusion through peripheral veins and through central venous lines. The availability of sophisticated equipment allows intravenous therapy to be administered to the patient at home as well as in the hospital. Fluids can be administered continuously or intermittently and intravenous administration is done by the nurse, by the patient, or by the patient's family. The purpose of the intravenous therapy is to:

- Administer nutritional support such as TPN (covered in Chapters 12 and 13)
- Provide for intermittent or continuous administration of medication
- Transfuse blood or blood products
- Maintain or replace fluids and electrolytes

### Intravenous Therapy Catheters and Devices

#### Peripheral Intravenous Therapy

In peripheral intravenous therapy, peripheral refers to the blood flow in the extremities of the body. To administer therapy, the needle or cannula is inserted into a vein in the arm, leg, head, hand, or foot. The needle or cannula is short, less than 2 inches, so that it ends in the extremity. It is not threaded to the larger veins or the heart as in

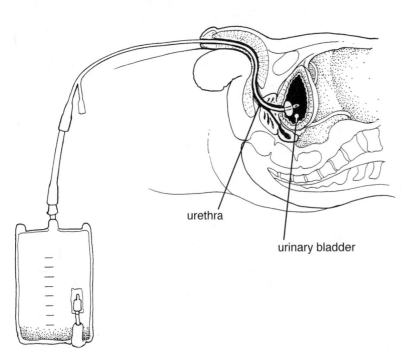

F I G U R E  11–8 • A retention catheter in place and connected to a drainage bag.

urethra

urinary bladder

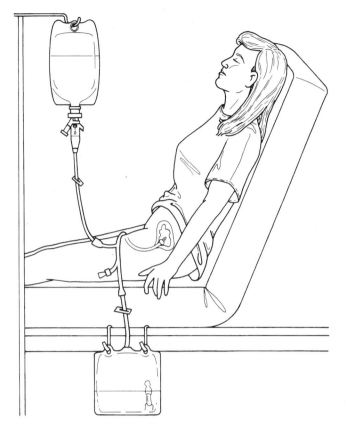

**FIGURE 11–9 •** A set-up used for intermittent or continuous bladder irrigation.

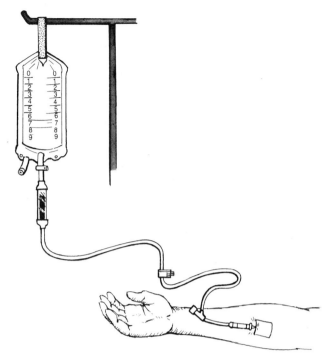

**FIGURE 11–10 •** Peripheral intravenous therapy (venipuncture).

central venous therapy (Fig. 11–10). Peripheral intravenous therapy is:

- Initiated by the nurse at the bedside
- Usually started in a vein in the arm by a venipuncture
- Used for short-term IV therapy, a week or less
- Basic and easiest to initiate
- Commonly used in hospitals

### Central Intravenous Therapy

In central intravenous therapy, central refers to the blood flow in the center of the body. To administer therapy the catheter is inerted into the jugular or subclavian vein or arm and threaded to the superior vena cava or right atrium of the heart. A central venous catheter (CVC) is used. It is commonly referred to as a central venous line, subclavian line, or venous access device (VAD) (Fig. 11–11).

#### Types of Central Venous Catheter

A peripherally inserted central catheter (PICC or PIC) is:

- Initiated by the doctor or by a nurse certified in the procedure at the bedside, and requires a consent form
- Inserted in the arm and advanced until the tip lies in the superior vena cava

- X-rayed to verify placement
- Used when therapy is needed longer than 7 days
- Used for antibiotic therapy, TPN, chemotherapy, or continuous antibiotic therapy
- Can by used for blood draws

A percutaneous central venous catheter is:

- Sometimes referred to as a subclavian line
- Initiated by the doctor at the bedside and requires a consent form
- Inserted through the skin directly into the subclavian (most common) or jugular vein and advanced until the tip lies in the superior vena cava or right atrium of the heart
- X-rayed to verify placement
- Used for short-term therapy, 7 days to several weeks
- Used for antibiotic therapy, TPN, chemotherapy, or continuous antibiotic therapy
- Can be used for blood draws

A tunneled catheter is:

- Initiated by the doctor, is considered a surgical procedure, and requires a consent form
- Inserted through a small incision made near the subclavian vein
  - A catheter is inserted here and advanced to the superior vena cava
  - A device called a tunneler is used to exit the catheter low in the patient's chest

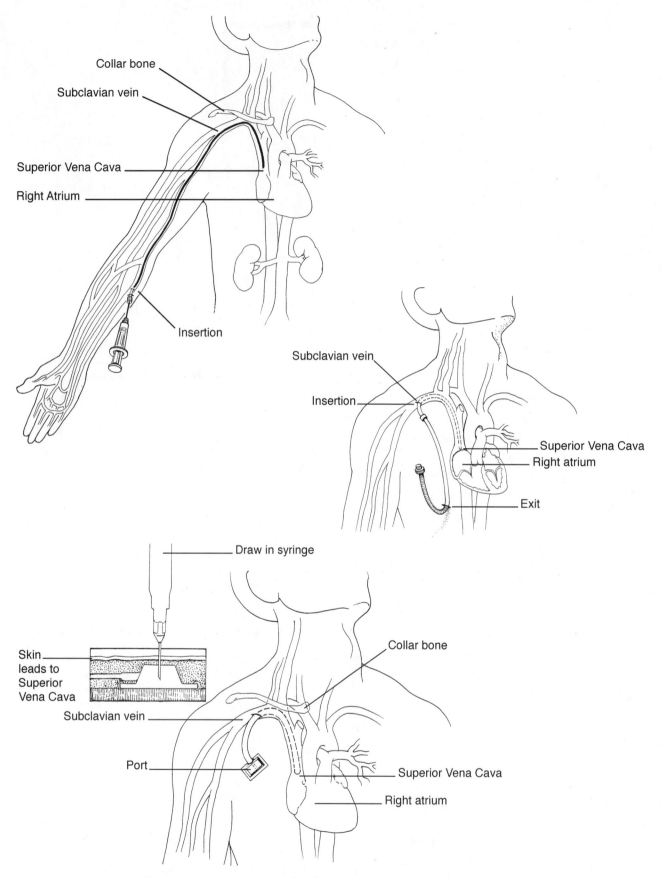

F I G U R E   11–11 • Types of central venous catheters.

- This allows for the patient to administer their own therapy and the tips can be placed under clothing
- Hickman, Raaf, Groshong, and Boviac are types of tunneling catheters
- Inserted for long-term IV therapy, longer than a month
- Is used for home care, in long-term care facilities, and for self-administration
- Can be used for blood draws

An implanted port is:

- A surgical procedure, performed by the doctor in a surgical setting
- Inserted into the subclavian or jugular vein
  - A port (container) is implanted under the skin in the chest wall
  - The incision is closed and the device cannot be seen but can be identified by a bulge
  - Implanted ports differ from other long-term catheters in that there are no external parts, they are located under the skin, and do not require daily care
  - A special needle is inserted into the port to administer the therapy
  - Port-A-Cath and Med-I-Port and Infus-A-Port are types of implanted ports
- Used for long-term and or intermittent use, often used for chemotherapy administration

### Intermittent Infusion Devices

The intermittent infusion device, also referred to as a venous access device (VAD), is used to establish an intermittent line when IV fluids are no longer needed but IV entry is still required. It is commonly used for the administration of medication. It consists of a plastic needle with an attached injection cap. The device is kept patent by heparin or saline flushes administered at specific intervals. It is commonly referred to as heparin lock, hep lock, or buffalo cap (Fig. 11–12).

An **infusion pump** is an electrical device used in the administration of intravenous fluid. It is used to measure a precise amount of fluid to be infused for a stated amount

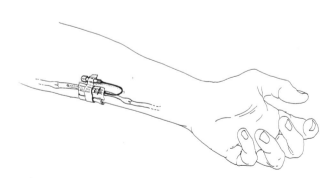

F I G U R E 11–12 • Intermittent infusion device (heparin lock).

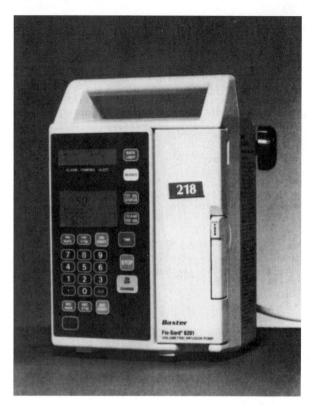

F I G U R E 11–13 • Infusion pump. (From Ignatavicius, Donna D., Workman, Linda M., and Mishler, Mary A.: *Medical-Surgical Nursing*: *A Nursing Process Approach*, 2nd ed. Philadelphia, W. B. Saunders Co., 1995, with permission.)

of time. The pump is ordered from CSD and is manufactured under several brand names (Fig. 11–13).

## FLUIDS AND ELECTROLYTES

The doctors orders the type, the amount, and the flow rate of the solutions to be given. For example, in the IV order

*1000 mL 5% D/W @ 125 mL/hr*

5% D/W is the type of solution. There is a large variety of solutions on the market, and the doctor must select the one that best meets the patient's needs.

Continuing this example, 1000 mL is the amount of solution the doctor wants the patient to have. Solutions are most commonly packaged in amounts of 1000 mL; however, 250 mL or 500 mL may also be ordered.

The notation 125 mL/hr indicates the rate of flow per hour of the solution into the vein. Other examples of phrases used in stating the rate of flow are *60 gtts per min, to run for 8 hr*; or *to keep open* (usually 50 to 60 mL/hr).

Frequently, the health unit coordinator is required to order IV solutions at specific intervals; therefore, it is necessary to know the length of time it takes the IV to infuse. An IV of 1000 mL running at 125 mL/h runs for 8 hours

(1000 mL ÷ 125 mL = 8 hours). How many hours will an IV running at 100 mL/h take to infuse?*

Below are listed several one-time, continuous, and discontinuation IV orders, written in abbreviated form as commonly seen on the doctors' order sheet. Use the abbreviations list at the beginning of the chapter for assistance in interpreting these, if necessary.

## Doctors' Orders for Intravenous Therapy

- *1000 mL LR 125 mL/h then DC*
- *Con't IVs alternate 1000 cc/RL c̄ 1000 cc 5% D/W each to run for 8 h via CVC*
- *KO IV rate 30 cc/h c̄ 5% D/W*
- *DC IV when present bottle is finished*
- *5% D/RL 100 cc/h follow c̄ 1000 cc 5% Isolyte M at same rate*
- *IVs*
  - a. *1000 mL 5% D/LR via Groshong cath*
  - b. *1000 cc 5% D/W plus 20 mEq KCl to run at 125 cc/h*
- *IV 1000 cc D 5%/½NS @ 100 cc/h if pt not tol fluids*
- *DC IV fluids, convert to hep lock IV*
- *Have IV team insert PICC*
- *Use Port-A-Cath for blood draws*

### HIGHLIGHT

To determine the amount of time it will take for IV infusion, divide the number of milliliters in the IV bag by the rate of flow. In the doctors' order *1000 mL 5% D/W @ 125 mL/h*, divide 1000 by 125. The answer is 8. The IV will run for 8 hours. Use this information to order the number of 1000-mL IV bags needed for a given amount of time.

## TRANSFUSION OF BLOOD, BLOOD COMPONENTS, AND PLASMA SUBSTITUTES

### Background Information

An intravenous infusion of blood is called a **transfusion**. It is usually ordered for patients who have lost blood because of hemorrhage from trauma or surgery. A consent form must be signed by the patient prior to the administration of blood and blood products (see Fig. 8–31).

The use of the whole blood for transfusion is gradually lessening, and only parts or components of blood are being used. You will find the following in transfusion orders:

---

*The answer is 10 hours.

### COMMON COMMERCIALLY PEPARED IV SOLUTIONS*

- Sodium chloride 0.45% (NaCl 0.45%, or half-strength NaCl)
- Sodium chloride 0.9% (NaCl 0.9%, or normal saline)
- 5% dextrose in water (5% D/W, or D5W)
- 10% dextrose in water (10% D/W, or D10W)
- 5% dextrose in 0.2% sodium chloride (5% D/0.2% NaCl)
- 5% dextrose in 0.45% sodium chloride (5% D/0.45% NaCl)
- 5% dextrose in 0.9% sodium chloride (5% D/0.9% NaCl)
- Lactated Ringer's solution with 5% dextrose (LR/5%D)
- 5% dextrose in 0.2% normal saline
- 5% dextrose in 0.45% normal saline
- Lactated Ringer's solution

---

*There are other IV solutions containing essential body elements that are sold under trade names. For example, McGaw, a manufacture of parenteral fluids, markets an IV solution with electrolytes as Isolyte M. The same formula is sold by Abbott Laboratories as Ionosol T.

Your instructor will give you the trade names used in your hospital.

- Packed cells (red blood cells) (frequently used)
- Plasma
- Platelet concentrate
- Washed cells
- Fresh frozen plasma (FFP)
- Cryoprecipitates
- Granulocytes
- Albumin
- Gamma globulins
- Factor VIII

**Type and crossmatch**, a laboratory study made to determine the type and compatibility of the blood, is done before the patient receives blood or certain blood components. This test is performed in the blood bank division of the hospital laboratory. The blood bank also obtains and stores blood and blood components (see "Blood Bank" in Chapter 14).

The equipment used for infusion of blood is similar to that used for the infusion of regular intravenous solutions. Blood is packaged in plastic containers and ordered by the unit. The intravenous tubing used for blood contains a filter. Normal saline solution is usually used along with the administration of blood. All equipment items must be disposed of.

The transfusion of blood is a potentially dangerous procedure. Special precautions are taken by the nursing staff to ensure the correct administration of blood. Proper storage of blood is also essential to ensure safe administration. Blood is stored in the blood bank, in a special refrigerator designed to maintain constant temperature for safe storing of the blood. It is often the health unit coordinator's responsibility to pick up the blood from the blood bank and bring it to the nursing unit. *If blood for two different patients is to be obtained from the blood bank at the same time, two different health care personnel should pick up the blood.* It is important for the health unit coordinator to know that if the blood is not used immediately it must be returned to the blood bank for storage. Blood should not be stored in the refrigerator on the nursing unit because a safe even temperature cannot be maintained.

Planning for blood transfusions is becoming common practice because it eliminates the risk of acquiring blood-borne infections such as human immunodeficiency virus (HIV) or hepatitis B. Patients, family, or friends may donate blood for a patient in advance. The patient's own blood transfusion is called **autologous** or **autotransfusion**; blood of relatives or friends is called **donor-directed**, or **donor-specific**. Blood may also be collected from a surgical site, which is then transfused back to the patient. The blood is collected in a device called a **cell-saver**, or **autotransfusion system**.

Plasma extenders or plasma substitutes are ordered by the doctor to increase the level of circulating fluid in the body. They are obtained from the pharmacy. Rheomacrodex or dextran 40 is commonly ordered.

## DOCTORS' ORDERS FOR TRANSFUSION OF BLOOD, BLOOD COMPONENTS, AND PLASMA SUBSTITUTES

The following orders for the administration of blood, blood components, and plasma substitutes are performed by the nurse; however, the transcription procedure requires the ordering step of transcription. Blood bank ordering is described in Chapter 14, "Laboratory Orders." Transcription practice is also included in Chapter 14.

- *Give 2 units of whole blood now*
- *Give 1 unit of packed cells tonight and one in the* AM
- *Give 2 units of plasma stat*
- *Give 500 cc dextran 40 p̄ surgery*
- *Transfuse 1 unit of autologous blood today*
- *Autotransfusion per protocol*

---

### HIGHLIGHT

Obtaining Blood

- When 2 units of blood are ready to be transfused to different patients at the same time, have two individuals pick up 1 unit each to avoid giving the blood to the wrong patient.
- When blood is brought to the unit and for some reason cannot be given immediately, return the blood to the blood bank for storage where the storage temperature will ensure the safety of the blood.

---

**TO THE STUDENT**

To practice transcribing intravenous therapy orders, complete **Activity 11–2** in the Skills Practice Manual.

Doctors' orders or total parenteral nutrition and for intravenous medication are covered in Chapter 13.

## SUCTION ORDERS

### Background Information

Suction apparatus—tubes, suction machines, and so forth—may be ordered by the doctor to remove fluid or air from the body cavities and surgical wounds. Suction may be ordered intermittently or continuously. It may be accomplished manually or by machine. Some types of suction apparatus are set up by the doctor during surgery, and some—a gastric suction, for example—may be initiated by the nursing staff. The doctor may write orders for the establishment, maintenance or removal of suction equipment.

Doctors' orders relating to suctioning are listed below, with a brief interpretation. Refer to the abbreviations list at the beginning of the chapter for assistance, if necessary.

### Doctors' Orders for Suctioning

- *Insert NG tube, connect to intermittent low gastric suction*

The nurse or doctor inserts a nasogastric tube through the nose or mouth into the stomach. The tube is then connected to a gastric suction machine. There are a variety of portable machines and wall-mounted suction units (Fig. 11–14). These machines provide an intermittent removal of gastric contents and are usually set on low. (A high pressure setting is never used without specific orders.) Gastric suction is often ordered following gastrointestinal or other abdominal surgery, to prevent vomiting or for various other reasons. The gastric suction machine is a reusable item; however, the tube is disposable. *Levin* and *Salem sumps* are examples of tubes that may be used (Fig. 11–15).

- *Irrig NG q4h c̄ 30 mL NS*

The nurse irrigates the nasogastric tube every 4 hours with 30 mL of normal saline. An irrigation tray, usually disposable, is used for this procedure. Normal saline is packaged in 500-mL, 1000-mL, or 2000-mL containers. The nurse should be consulted as to the amount needed.

- *Clamp NG tube intermittently q1h*

A clamp is applied to the NG tube or a plug is inserted in the distal end of the tube at 1-hour intervals and then reconnected to the suction machine for 1-hour intervals.

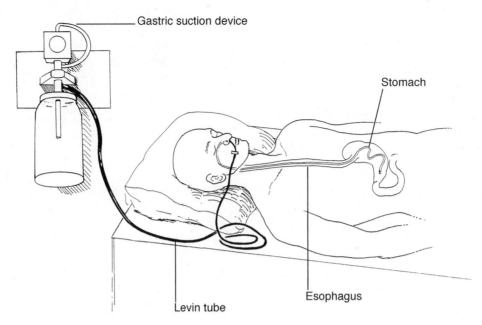

FIGURE 11–14 • Gastric suctioning equipment. Wall unit.

■ *Remove NG tube and gastric suction*
This is a typical example of an order to discontinue the gastric suction.

■ *Suction throat prn to clear airway*
Because of paralysis, coma, and various other conditions, patients may have difficulty swallowing, and secretions may collect in the throat that block the airway. These secretions are removed by a catheter attached to an electric throat suction apparatus. Many hospitals have a throat suctioning machine installed in the wall. However, if this is not available, a portable electric suction machine is obtained from CSD (Fig. 11–16). The suction machine is a reusable item, but the suction catheters are disposable.

■ *Suction tracheostomy prn*
A tracheostomy is an artificial opening into the trachea (windpipe), performed to facilitate breathing. When the patient is unable to cough, suctioning is necessary to remove secretions. Electric wall or portable electric throat suction machines are used (Fig. 11–17).

■ *Chest tube 20 cm neg pressure*
Chest tubes are inserted to reexpand the lungs by removing air or fluids that collect in the pleural cavity. The chest tube is connected to a closed chest-drainage system, such as Pleur-evac, then connected to a vacuum source, such as wall suction. The Pleur-evac and chest tubes are disposable items (Fig. 11–18).

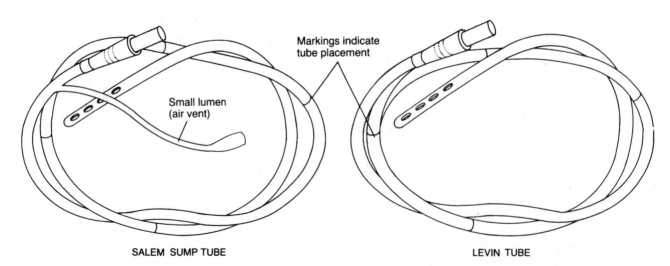

FIGURE 11–15 • Two types of nasogastric tubes. (From Ignatavicius, Donna D., Workman, Linda M., and Mishler, Mary A.: *Medical-Surgical Nursing: A Nursing Process Approach*, 2nd ed. Philadelphia, W. B. Saunders Co., 1995, with permission.)

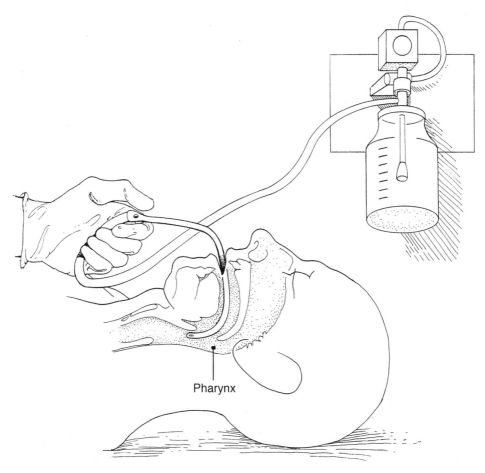

F I G U R E  11–16 • Throat suctioning apparatus.

■ *Keep Hemovac compressed*

A Hemovac is a disposable wound-suction device attached to an incisional drain during surgery. The above order is for maintenance, as the Hemovac only exerts suction when the nurse keeps it compressed. The doctor may also write the order *routine Hemovac care*, considering compression to be part of the nursing procedure (Fig. 11–19A).

■ *Empty the Jackson-Pratt (J-P) q shift and record*

The Jackson-Pratt drain is a disposable wound-suction device that must be compressed to create suction (Fig. 11–19B).

| TO THE STUDENT |
| --- |

To practice transcribing suction orders, complete **Activity 11–3** in the Skills Practice Manual.

## HEAT AND COLD APPLICATION ORDERS

## Background Information

Heat and cold treatments are ordered for the patient by the doctor. Heat treatment is used to promote comfort, relaxation, and healing; to reduce pain and swelling; and to promote circulation. Cold treatment may be used to relieve pain, reduce inflammation, control hemorrhage, and decrease circulation.

Various methods for application of heat and cold are used, and thus there are a variety of doctors' orders to prescribe the methods intended. Typical doctors' orders for the common procedures used for heat and cold applications are listed below with an explanation.

## Doctors' Orders for Heat Applications

■ *K-pad to lower lt arm 20 min qid*

An **aquamatic K-pad** is a device in which the water is electrically heated in a container and circulated through a network of tubes in a pad. K-pads are used for the application of continuous dry heat to various parts of the body. They are manufactured in different sizes and shapes, designed to apply heat to certain body parts; for example, a long narrow pad is used to apply heat to the neck, while a broad, long pad is used to apply heat to the back. When ordering the K-pad from the central service department, it is important to indicate the size and shape needed to suit the doctor's order. The temperature for the water in

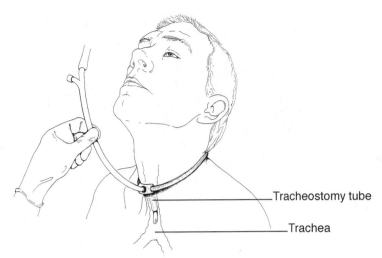

F I G U R E  11–17 • Suctioning of a tracheostomy.

Tracheostomy tube

Trachea

the K-pad is preset in CSD. A doctor's order for a temperature setting higher than one approved by the hospital must be communicated to CSD, since the CSD personnel can make the setting change. The K-pad is a reusable item (Fig. 11–20).

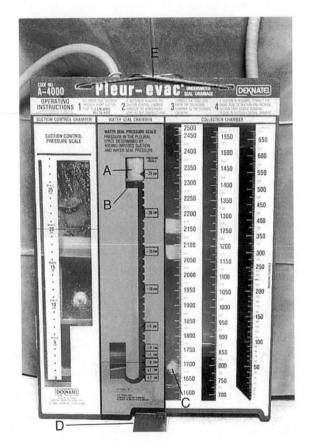

F I G U R E  11–18 • Pleur-evac—one of many available brands of chest draining systems.

■ *Hot compresses to abscess on lt ankle 10 min qh*
Hot compresses are warm, wet gauze applied to a body part. They are used to treat small areas of the body. Usually, disposable items are used for this procedure.

■ *Soak rt hand 20 min in warm NS solution q4h while awake*
A soak is usually ordered to facilitate healing. For this order the right hand is placed in a container of the prescribed solution to soak for 20 minutes every 4 hours while the patient is awake.

■ *Sitz bath 30 min tid*
A sitz bath is used for the application of warm water to the pelvic area. Special tubs and chairs may be used for this procedure, and are usually part of the unit equipment and do not need to be obtained from CSD. Disposable basins are available from CSD (Fig. 11–21).

## Doctors' Orders for Cold Applications

■ *Alcohol sponge for temp over 102°*
Alcohol sponge is the bathing of a patient with a solution of alcohol and water for the purpose of reducing the patient's temperature

■ *Ice bag to scrotum as tolerated for 24 hr*
An ice bag is a rubber or plastic container filled with ice. It is a reusable item obtained from CSD. Commercially prepared disposable ice bags are also available for use.

■ *Hypothermia machine PRN if temp ↑ 104°*
The hypothermia machine circulates fluid through a network of tubing in a mattress-sized pad. It is used for prolonged cooling and to reduce body surface temperature (Fig. 11–22). This is a reusable item and is returned to the CSD when discontinued by the doctor.

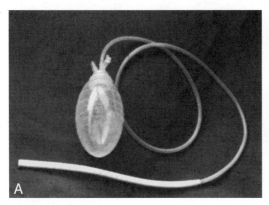 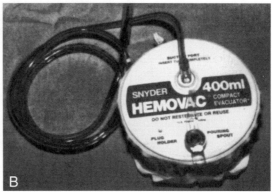

FIGURE 11–19 • (*A*) Jackson-Pratt. (*B*) Hemovac. A disposal wound suction apparatus. (From Ignatavicius, Donna D., Workman, Linda M., and Mishler, Mary A.: *Medical-Surgical Nursing*: *A Nursing Process Approach*, 2nd ed. Philadelphia, W. B. Saunders Co., 1995, with permission.)

## COMFORT, SAFETY, AND HEALING ORDERS

### Background Information

The nursing staff determines and performs many tasks to promote the comfort, safety, and healing of the client. However, you will encounter doctors' orders relating to these areas also. Because such orders are so varied, only typical examples with the interpretation of each are listed below.

### Doctors' Orders for Patient Comfort, Safety, and Healing

■ *Sheepskin on bed*
A sheepskin (may also be referred to as lamb's wool or bed puff) is made either of lamb's wool or of a synthetic material. It measures approximately three quarters of the length and the same width as the bed. The sheepskin is placed directly below the patient and is used to relieve pressure and prevent bedsores (decubitus ulcers). A sheepskin is usually considered a disposable item.

■ *Alternating pressure (A-P) pad*
The alternating pressure pad is a mattress-sized pad that provides alternating distribution of air through channels in the pad and is used to relieve pressure and promote circulation. This is a reusable item. A Lapidus pad, egg-crate mattress, or water bed may also be ordered for comfort, prevention of sores, or healing.

■ *Foot board on bed*
A board is placed at or near the foot of the bed so that the patient's feet, when placed against it, are at a right angle

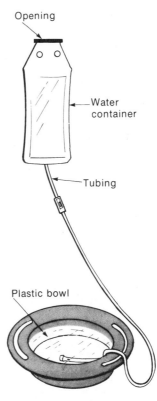

FIGURE 11–21 • A disposable sitz bath apparatus. (Courtesy of Baxter Travenol Laboratories, Inc.)

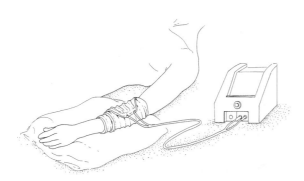

FIGURE 11–20 • Aquamatic K-pad.

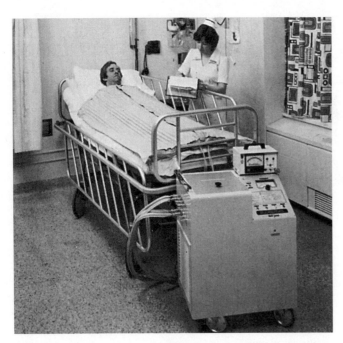

**F I G U R E  11–22** • A hypothermia machine. (Courtesy of Cincinnati Sub-zero Products.)

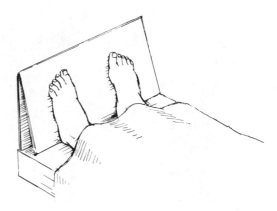

**F I G U R E  11–23** • A foot board.

to the bed. It is used to prevent footdrop of patients who are in bed for long periods (Fig. 11–23). A foot board is a reusable item.

■ *Foot cradle*

A cradle is a metal frame placed on the bed to prevent the top sheet from touching a specified part of the body. A foot cradle is a reusable item.

■ *Immobilizer to lt knee 20° flexion*

**Immobilizers** are used to keep a limb or body part in alignment (Fig. 11–24). Immobilizers are reusable.

■ *OOB with elastic abd binder*

An elastic abdominal binder is often ordered following surgery for patient support (Fig. 11–25). It is a disposable item. It is usually necessary to include the measurement of the patient's waist and hips on the requisition to obtain the correctly sized binder. The doctor may also order an elastic binder for the chest.

■ *Egg-crate mattress*

The egg-crate mattress is a foam rubber pad resembling an egg crate or carton used to distribute body weight more evenly (Fig. 11–26). It is a disposable item.

■ *Air therapy bed*

The **air therapy bed** is a low-air-loss therapy bed. Types include Respair, Flexicare, and Kinair. The health unit coordinator must include the patient's height and weight when ordering the bed.

■ *Sling to rt arm when up*

A **sling** is a disposable bandage used to support an arm (Fig. 11–27).

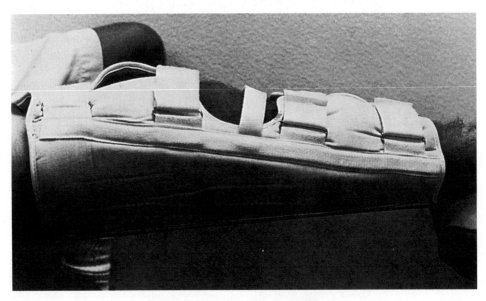

**F I G U R E  11–24** • Immobilizer.

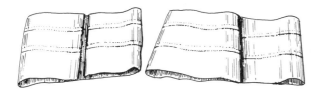

F I G U R E  11–25 • An elastic binder.

■ *Elastic stockings to both legs*

Elastic stockings or antiembolism hose (AE hose) are made in various sizes and lengths and are ordered to promote circulation to the lower extremities and therefore prevent blood clots or emboli. They are disposable. The nurse needs to measure the patient's leg before you can order. The doctor should also indicate thigh length (TL) or knee length (KL) (Fig. 11–28)

■ *Soft restraints prn for agitation and patient safety*

When they are absolutely necessary for patient safety, the doctor orders restraints to be used. There are various methods of restraint, and several types of commercial equipment are available (Fig. 11–29).

■ *May shampoo hair*

A doctor's order is necessary for the hospitalized patient to have a shampoo. The appropriate equipment is usually requisitioned from CSD and is reusable.

■ *Change surgical dressings bid*

A bandage or other application over an external wound is called a dressing. Items used for this treatment are disposable

■ *PAS*

An electrical pump is used with pulsatile antiembolism stockings to provide alternating pressure and thereby pre-vent clots from forming in the legs from inactivity. The stockings are disposable; the pump is reusable.

■ *TCDB q2h*

The nursing staff turn the patient to a different position (right side, left side, back) every 2 hours and encourage him or her to take deep breaths and cough. TCDB is frequently ordered following surgery.

■ *ET nurse referral*

ET is the abbreviation for enterostomal therapist. The term is now outdated but is used to refer to the nurse who specializes in stoma and wound care. The ET nurse is notified and she or he performs the care needed by the patient. Figure 11–30 is a stomal bag used for ostomy care.

■ *Give warm water vaginal irrigation (douche) in AM*

---

**TO THE STUDENT**

To practice transcribing heat and cold applications, comfort, safety, and healing orders, complete **Activity 11–4** in the Skills Practice Manual

---

## BLOOD GLUCOSE MONITORING ORDERS

Blood glucose monitoring is routinely performed by the nursing staff for diabetic patients or patients who are receiving nutritional support (total parenteral nutrition). A special device is used to obtain capillary blood, usually from the patient's finger. A drop of blood is placed on a chemically treated strip. The strip is placed in a blood glu-

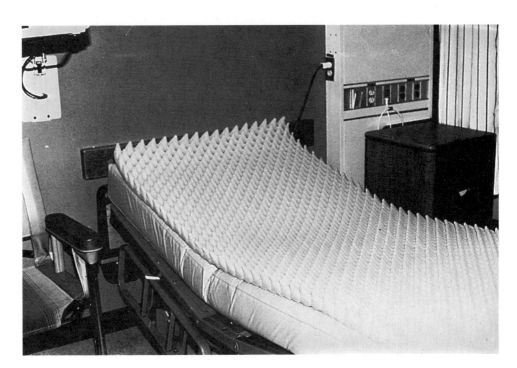

F I G U R E  11–26 • An egg-crate mattress.

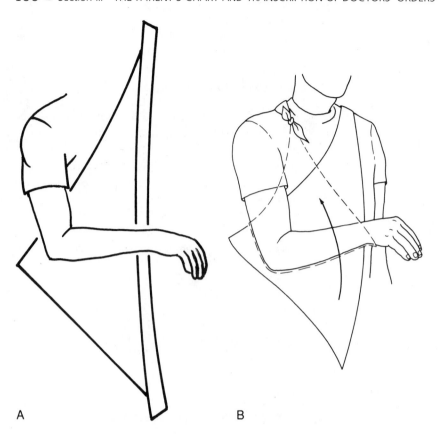

A                                B

FIGURE 11–27 • A sling. (From deWit, Susan C.: *Rambo's Nursing Skills for Clinical Practice*, 4th ed. Philadelphia, W.B. Saunders Co., 1994, with permission.)

cose monitor. The monitor will display the results of the blood glucose in numbers. The nurse uses the results of the blood glucose level to administer or adjust insulin dosage according to the doctors' orders (see Chapter 14). The order is written in the nursing treatment column of the Kardex form during the transcription procedures.

## Doctors' Orders for Blood Testing for Glucose

### ■ *Accu-Chek ac and hs*

Accu-Chek is a type of commercial blood glucose monitor used to check the glucose level of blood. The doctor has ordered the test to be done four times a day.

### ■ *Blood glucose monitoring q6h. Call if ↑ 400*

The doctor has ordered that blood glucose be checked every 6 hours by using a blood glucose monitor; the doctor should be called if the reading is over 400.

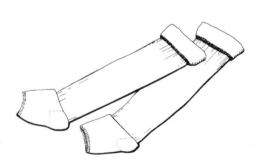

FIGURE 11–28 • Elastic stockings.

**HIGHLIGHT**

Types of Nursing Treatment Orders
- Intestinal elimination orders
- Urinary catheterization orders
- Intravenous therapy orders
- Blood transfusion orders
- Suction orders
- Heat and cold application orders
- Comfort, safety, and healing orders
- Blood glucose monitoring orders

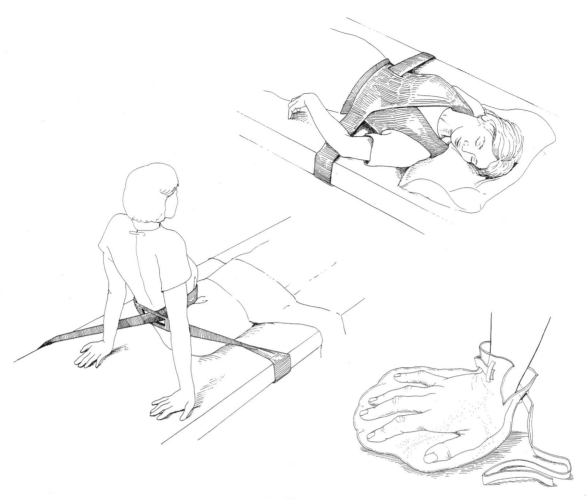

FIGURE  11–29 • Types of restraints.

## SUMMARY

The transcription procedure for nursing treatment orders is fairly simple once you become familiar with the equipment necessary to implement each order. Ordering the wrong equipment only delays the treatment and probably would not harm the patient. However, when in doubt about the equipment needed, check with the nurse in charge or with the central service department. The health unit coordinator who is able to recognize the equipment and its uses and effectively use the central service system plays an invaluable role in helping the nursing staff to practice quality patient care.

TO THE STUDENT

To practice recording telephone physicians' orders, complete **Activity 11–7** in the Skills Practice Manual.

To practice recording telephone messages, complete **Activity 11–8** in the Skills Practice Manual.

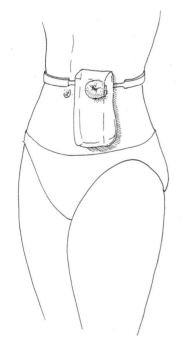

FIGURE  11–30 • Stomal bag covering a colostomy.

**REVIEW QUESTIONS**

1. List seven types of nursing treatment orders.

   a. intestinal elimination   e. suction

   b. urinary catheterization   f. heat + cold application

   c. intravenous therapy   g. blood glucose monitoring

   d. blood transfusion

2. Underline those terms in the list below that may be included in an order relating to urinary catheterization.

   | | | |
   |---|---|---|
   | rectal tube | catheter | Boviac |
   | Foley | Hemovac | |
   | Levin | colostomy | |
   | residual | Port-A-Cath | |

3. List three types of enemas a doctor may order.

   a. oil retension

   b. soap suds

   c. fleets

4. In the order *Give ORE enema in* AM, the doctor wants the order done:
   a. this AM
   b. tomorrow AM

5. Define:

   a. sitz bath   application of warm water to the pelvic area

   b. Hemovac   for drainage of a wound. a disposable suction device.

   c. restraints   devices used to restrain patients to control behavior or for protection

   d. nursing treatment orders   a doctors order for treatment to be preformed by a nurse

6. List two types of electric suction apparatus.

   a. Gastric

   b. throut

7. *IV c̄ 1000 mL 5% D/W*
   The above is an IV order. Is it complete? __NO__ Yes. _____ No. If you checked no, tell what is missing. How much per hour is given o flow rate

8. The central service system in your hospital includes a central service stock supply on the nursing unit. Below are examples of doctors' orders. Place a check in the space provided by those orders that require you to order supplies as a part of the transcription procedures.

Write the supplies you would order. (Use the two lists of items given earlier in the chapter as references to answer this question.)

ORDERS:

a. *SS enema till clear* _____

b. *Insert NG connect to intermittent gastric suction* ✓

gastric tube

c. *Retention cath to st drain* _____

d. *Keep Hemovac compressed* _____

e. *PAS* ✓

pulsatile antiembolism stocking

f. *K-pad to shoulder* ✓

K-pad

g. *Sitz bath 20 min tid* ✓

disposable sitz bath

h. *Ice bag to lt hand* ✓

Ice bag

i. *Irrig cath prn patency* _____

j. *Sheepskin* ✓

sheepskin

k. *1000 mL 5% D/W to run at 125 mL/hr* _____

l. *Foot cradle on bed* ✓

foot cradle

m. *Change dressing prn* _____

9. Rental equipment should be promptly returned to the central service department because:

a. the patient is charged for the equipment and the charge has to be terminated

b. it may be needed for other patients

10. The registered nurse asked you to pick up a unit of packed cells from the blood bank. When you return to the nursing unit with the packed cells, the nurse tells you she is not able to start the transfusion for an hour. Explain what you would do with the packed cells until then.

return to the blood bank

11. Below is a list of CSD equipment. Identify the items as reusable by writing "R" in the space provided, or disposable by writing "D" in the space provided.

a. Fleet enema — D          m. IV tubing — D

b. sheepskin — D            n. blood tubing — D

c. Pleur-evac — D           o. foot board — R

d. catheter irrigation tray — D   p. Hemovac — D

e. foot cradle — R          q. alternating pressure pad — R

f. egg-crate mattress — D   r. PAS pump — R

g. nasogastric tube — D     s. sling — D

h. enema bag — D            t. feeding tube — D

i. immobilizer — R          u. K-pad — R

j. retention catheter tray — D   v. hypothermia machine — R

k. throat suction machine — R   w. gastric suction machine — R

l. elastic abdominal binder — D

12. Briefly describe the function of the CSD as it relates to nursing treatment orders.

_____

_____

_____

13. Compare the function of a retention catheter to the function of a nonretention catheter.

retention catheter remains in the bladder to allow for continuous flow of urine nonretention empties the bladder and is removed.

14. Place a check mark by each of the routes of intravenous administrations that may be initiated by the nurse.

a. ___✓___ venipuncture (peripheral)

b. ___✓___ tunneled venous line

c. _____ implanted port

d. ___✓___ PICC

e. _____ percutaneous venous catheter

15. Define

a. autotransfusion

transfusion using the patient's own blood

_____

b. heparin lock

a venous access device

_____

c. donor-specific blood

_blood donated by a friend or relative_

16. Place a check mark by each of the following that are types of tunneling catheters.

a. _____ Levin                   e. _____ Hemovac

b. _✓_ Hickman                   f. _____ Boviac

c. _____ Port-A-Cath             g. _____ PICC

d. _✓_ Groshong                  h. _✓_ Raaf

17. Which of the following is not a central venous line?

a. tunneling catheter                  _____

b. PICC                                _____

c. percutaneous central venous line    _____

d. peripheral intravenous              _✓_

18. Rewrite the following doctors' orders using abbreviations; or to practice writing doctors' orders, have someone read the order to you while you record them, once again using the abbreviations you have learned.

a. Have the intravenous team insert a peripherally inserted central catheter. _Have IV team insert PICC_

b. Continuous intravenous alternate with one thousand cubic centimeters of Ringer's lactate with one thousand cubic centimeters of dextrose and water to run at one hundred twenty-five cubic centimeters per hour via central venous catheter. _Con't IV alternate c̄ 1000 cc RL c̄ 1000 cc D/W TRA 125 cc/hr via CVC_

c. Irrigate nasogastric tube every four hours with thirty milliliters of normal saline. _Irrig NG tube q4h c̄ 30 mL NS_

## References

Ignatavicius, Donna D, Workman, M. Linda, and Mishler, Mary A.: *Medical-Surgical Nursing: A Nursing Process Approach*, 2nd ed. Philadelphia, W. B. Saunders Co., 1995.

*Nursing Policy and Procedure Manual*. St. Joseph's Hospital and Medical Center, Phoenix, AZ.

Rambo, Beverly J. and Wood, Lucille A.: *Nursing Skills for Clinical Practice*. Philadelphia, W. B. Saunders Co., 1982.

Taylor et al.: *Fundamentals of Nursing, The Art and Science of Nursing Care*. Philadelphia, J. B. Lippincott, 1989.

Terry, Judy, et al (eds): *Intravenous Therapy: Clinical Principles and Practice*. Philadelphia, W. B. Saunders Co., 1995.

Wood, Lucille A. and Rambo, Beverly J.: *Nursing Skills for Allied Health Services*, vol. 2, 2nd ed. Philadelphia, W. B. Saunders Co., 1977.

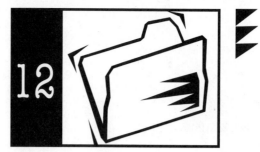

CHAPTER **12**

# DIETARY ORDERS

## CHAPTER OBJECTIVES

*Upon completion of this chapter, you will be able to:*

1. Define the terms listed in the vocabulary list.
2. Write the meaning of the abbreviations in the abbreviations list
3. Describe two methods of sending dietary orders to the dietary department.
4. Interpret the dietary orders included in this chapter.
5. List the diets that provide change in the consistency of food.
6. Identify five special diets.
7. List four diets that may be selected for the patient who is on *diet as tolerated*.
8. Identify types of tube feeding formula and feeding tubes, an infusion pump, and methods of administration of tube feedings.

## VOCABULARY

**Calorie** • A measurement of energy generated in the body by the heat produced after food is eaten

**Dietitian** • A person with a minimum of 4 years of college training in the science of nutrition

**Diet Order** • A doctor's order that states the type and amount of food and liquids the patient may receive

**Enteral Feeding Set** • Includes equipment needed to infuse tube feeding; includes plastic bag for feeding solution and may be ordered with or without pump

**Gastrostomy Feeding** • Feeding by means of a tube inserted into the stomach through an artificial opening in the abdominal wall

**Gavage** • Feeding by means of a tube inserted into the stomach, duodenum, or jejunum, through the nose, also called *tube feeding*

**Ingestion** • The taking in of food by mouth

**Kangaroo Pump** • A brand name of a feeding pump used to administer tube feeding

**Nothing by Mouth** • No food or liquids taken by mouth

**Nutrients** • Substances derived from food, which are utilized by body cells, for example, carbohydrates, fats, proteins, vitamins, minerals, and water

**Percutaneous Endoscopic Gastrostomy** • Insertion of a tube through the abdominal wall into the stomach using endoscopic guidance

**Registered Dietitian** • One meeting qualifications of the Commission on Dietetic Registration of the American Dietetic Association

**Regular Diet** • A diet that consists of all foods, designed to provide good nutrition *general* *whatever patient want*

**Therapeutic Diet** • A regular diet with modifications or restrictions (also called a *special diet*)

**Tube Feeding** • Administration of liquids into the stomach, duodenum, or jejunum, through a tube

*dialysis\
protien restricted*

# A B B R E V I A T I O N S

| Abbreviation | Meaning | Example of Usage on a Doctor's Order Sheet |
|---|---|---|
| ADA | American Diabetic Association | 1000 cal ADA diet |
| cal | calorie | 800 cal diet |
| CHO | carbohydrate | high protein, low CHO diet |
| chol | cholesterol | low chol diet |
| cl | clear | cl liq diet |
| DAT | diet as tolerated | DAT |
| FF | force fluids | soft diet FF |
| FS | full strength | Δ Jevity FS @ 50 mL/h |
| gen | general | gen diet |
| liq | liquid | full liq diet |
| MN | midnight | NPO MN |
| Na | sodium | 400 mg Na diet |
| NAS | no added salt | reg diet, NAS |
| NPO | nothing by mouth | NPO after midnight |
| NSA | no salt added (same as NAS) | |
| PEG | percutaneous endoscopic gastrostomy | PEG in AM |
| RD | registered dietitian | |
| reg | regular | reg diet |
| TRA | to run at | Ensure TRA 1000 cc/h |

## EXERCISE 1

Write the abbreviation for each term listed below.

1. general — gen
2. sodium — NA
3. midnight — MN
4. nothing by mouth — NPO
5. regular — reg
6. clear — cl
7. calorie — cal
8. American Diabetic Association — ADA
9. liquid — liq
10. cholesterol — chol
11. diet as tolerated — DAt
12. force fluids — FF
13. carbohydrate — CHO
14. no salt added — NSA

15. to run at — TRA
16. full strength — FS
17. percutaneous endoscopic gastrostomy — PEG
18. no added salt — NAS
19. registered dietitian — RD

## EXERCISE 2

Write the meaning of each abbreviation listed below.

1. Na — sodium
2. NPO — nothing by mouth
3. reg — regular
4. MN — midnight
5. liq — liquid
6. cal — calorie
7. NSA — no salt added
8. ADA — American Dietetic Association
9. DAT — Diet as tolerated
10. cl — chorides clear
11. chol — cholesteral
12. CHO — carbohydrates
13. gen — general
14. FF — force fluids
15. FS — full strenght
16. TRA — to run at
17. PEG — percutaneous endoscopic gastrostomy
18. NAS — no salt added
19. RD — registered dietitian

## COMMUNICATION WITH THE DIETARY DEPARTMENT

The procedure for ordering a new diet or a change/modification to an existing diet requires the health unit coordinator to communicate the order by computer to the dietary department. The health unit coordinator would choose the correct patient from the unit census screen on the computer, choose dietary from the department ordering screen, then choose the ordered diet from the options on the dietary screen along with other items that apply (e.g., admission, hold for one tray) (Fig. 12–1). There is also a "write-in" option for additional comments. The ordered diet would then be sent to the dietary department.

If the computer is down or the health care facility is not on a computer system, a **diet change sheet** is used. The diet change sheet contains the patient's name, room number, and diet. (Fig. 12–2). To order a new diet, the information on the diet change sheet is simply updated. A copy of the sheet is sent to the dietary department prior to the preparation of each meal.

Most health care facilities provide each patient with the next day's menu of items that are allowed for the particular diet they have been placed on. The patient checks what foods they would like from the menu. The menu is then sent to the dietary department (Figs. 12–3 and 12–4). Some facilities have initiated a new system to save the cost of printing the menus that involves the dietitian interviewing each patient upon admission to obtain and record their food preferences, dislikes, and any allergies they may have. This information is used to prepare that patient's food.

All dietary information must be sent to the dietary department including orders for nothing by mouth, tube feedings, allergies, limit fluids, force fluids, calorie count, etc., so the necessary adjustments will be made when preparing the patient's trays. The dietitian also maintains a Kardex or record on each patient that will be updated with each order received (Fig. 12–5).

### HIGHLIGHT

It is essential that all dietary information be sent to the dietary department, including orders for nothing by mouth, tube feedings, allergies, limit fluids, force fluids, calorie count, etc., so the necessary adjustments will be made when preparing the patient's tray. The dietitian also maintains a record or Kardex on each patient that will be updated with each order received.

## Background Information

During hospitalization, the doctor orders the type of diet the client is to receive. The food is prepared by the dietary department and is designed to attain or maintain the health of the patient. Diets for the hospitalized patient can be divided into three groups: standard diets, therapeutic diets, and tube feedings (Table 12–1).

## Standard Diets

Standard hospital diets consist of a regular diet and diets that vary in consistency or texture of foods. A **regular diet**, also called general, house, routine, and full, is planned to provide good nutrition and consists of all items in the four basic food groups. This diet is ordered for hospitalized patients who do not require restrictions or modifications

F I G U R E  12–1 • A computer screen for ordering from the dietary department.

**DIET CHANGE SHEET**

DAY *Monday*   DATE  8-20-00   UNIT  7E

| Room | Name | Diet Order | Breakfast | Lunch | Dinner |
|------|------|-----------|-----------|-------|--------|
| 701-1 | Hicks Martha | soft | ✓ | ✓ | |
| 701-2 | Haist Sarah | NPO | ✓ | cl liq | |
| 702-1 | James Rick | 2500 mg Na | ✓ | ✓ | |
| 703-1 | Harris Joy | 1000 cal | ✓ | ✓ | |
| 703-2 | Jenkins Pat | full liq | ✓ | soft | |

F I G U R E   12–2 • A diet change sheet with the patient's room number, name, and diet filled in. The breakfast and lunch diets have been ordered, and the changes have been recorded. To order dinner diets, the health unit coordinator fills in the dinner column.

of their diets. Liquid, full liquid, soft, mechanical soft, and bland are types of diets that vary in food texture or consistency.

## Doctors' Orders for Standard Diets

### ■ Regular diet

This diet is nutritionally adequate and includes all the foods a healthy person should eat.

### ■ Soft or light diet

This diet is used in the progression from a full liquid diet to a general diet. It consists of nonirritating, easily digestible foods and modified fiber content, such as broiled chicken and boiled vegetables. It may be ordered postsurgically, for acute infections, or for gastrointestinal disorders.

### ■ Full liquid diet

A full liquid diet is often ordered as a transitional step between a clear liquid diet and a soft diet. Some of the foods included in this diet are milk, creamed soup, custards, ice cream, and fruit and vegetable juices. It is ordered for patients who have difficulty chewing or swallowing, who are acutely ill, or who have just had surgery.

### ■ Clear liquid diet

This diet is used for patients who cannot tolerate solid foods, such as those suffering an acute illness or who have just had surgery. It includes clear liquids only, such as tea, coffee, soda, broth, water, jello, and clear juices.

### ■ Mechanical soft diet

This is a normal diet that changes to meet the needs of patients who have difficulty chewing. The meat is ground and vegetables are diced or chopped. Variations may in-

clude mechanical soft, ground, or pureed depending on a patient's ability to chew food.

### ■ Diet as tolerated

When this dietary order is given, the nurse selects a clear liquid, full liquid, soft, or regular diet for the patient, according to his or her tolerance of food. For example, immediately following surgery the nurse may select a clear liquid diet for the patient. Normally, the patient is advanced to full liquid, soft, and then regular diet, according to the stage of recovery.

### ■ Bland diet

Bland numbers 1, 2, and 3 may be ordered. The diet consists of smooth foods. For example, number 2 includes no meat, whereas number 3 includes chopped meats.

---

**HIGHLIGHT**

When the physician writes an order for diet as tolerated (DAT), the nurse may select from the standard (consistency) diets such as clear liquid, full liquid, soft, or regular. Variations may include mechanical soft, ground, or pureed depending on the patient's ability to chew. The health unit coordinator would then send the selection to the dietary department. **The dietary department cannot make the evaluation of what the patient can tolerate.**

---

TO THE STUDENT

To practice transcribing standard diet orders, complete **Activity 12–1** in the Skills Practice Manual.

disphagia - thicket

## Breakfast

REGULAR · PLEASE (CIRCLE) SELECTIONS · SUNDAY

### Continental Breakfast

🌿 Fresh Baked Fruit Muffin
*with seasonal fruit*

### Or You May Prefer

Scrambled Eggs
🌿 Low Cholesterol Eggs
**French Toast with Syrup**
Bacon
Sausage
Hash Browns
Fruit Muffin
Biscuit
Cinnamon Raisin Bagel
*with Lite Cream Cheese*
Tortilla

Oatmeal
Cream of Wheat
Raisin Bran
Shredded Mini Wheat
Cheerios
Corn Flakes
Frosted Flakes
🌿 Fruited Yogurt
🌿 Fresh Banana
🌿 Fresh Orange
Picante Sauce

### Beverages

**Orange Juice**
Apple Juice
Prune Juice
Grapefruit Juice
**2% Milk**
🌿 Skim Milk

**Coffee**
Decaf. Coffee
Hot Tea
Decaf. Tea
Hot Cocoa
Sugar Sub.

🌿 Designates Pro-health Dining Selections.
*These foods are limited in calories, fat, salt and sugar.*

NAME _____ ROOM _____

---

## Lunch

REGULAR · PLEASE (CIRCLE) SELECTIONS · SUNDAY

### Special of the Day

🌿 CHICKEN BREAST WITH JULIENNE VEGETABLES
*served with*
🌿 *rice pilaf and* 🌿 *steamed broccoli*

### Or You May Prefer

Cream of Tomato Soup
*with turkey sandwich*
🌿 Cottage Cheese &
Fruit Plate *with banana bread*
Steamed Rice
🌿 Pinto Beans
🌿 Steamed Zucchini
Deluxe Hamburger
*with potato chips*
🌿 Chicken Fajita

### On the Side

Orange Juice
Cream of Tomato Soup
🌿 Garden Green Salad
*with Dressing*
French  Ranch  Italian
**Fruited Gelatin Salad**

**Dinner Roll**
Cornbread
Tortilla
Crackers
Picante Sauce

### Finishing Touch

**Home Style Cookies**
🌿 Chilled Fruit Cup
🌿 Seasonal Fresh Fruit
Ice Cream
Gelatin Cubes
Sherbet

### Beverages

**Iced Tea**
Coffee
Decaf. Tea
Decaf. Coffee

Iced Water
Hot Tea
🌿 **2% Milk**
🌿 Skim Milk
Sugar Sub.

🌿 Designates Pro-health Dining Selections.
*These foods are limited in calories, fat, salt and sugar.*

NAME _____ ROOM _____

---

## Dinner

REGULAR · PLEASE (CIRCLE) SELECTIONS · SUNDAY

### Special of the Day

**BRAISED TIPS OF BEEF**
*served in a hearty vegetable sauce
with a roll*

### Or You May Prefer

Vegetable Soup
*with ham sandwich*
🌿 Cottage Cheese & Fruit
Plate *with banana bread*
Steamed Rice
🌿 Vegetable Medley
Glazed Beets
Deluxe Hamburger
*with potato chips*
Fried Chicken with
*coleslaw and a roll*

### On the Side

Apple Juice
Vegetable Soup
🌿 Garden Green Salad
*with Dressing*
French  Ranch  Italian
🌿 **Cucumber &
Tomato Salad**

Dinner Roll
Cornbread
Tortilla
Crackers
Picante Sauce

### Finishing Touch

**Strawberry Shortcake**
🌿 Chilled Pears
🌿 Seasonal Fresh Fruit
Ice Cream
Gelatin Cubes
Sherbet

### Beverages

**Iced Tea**
Coffee
Decaf. Tea
Decaf. Coffee

Iced Water
Hot Tea
🌿 **2% Milk**
🌿 Skim Milk
Sugar Sub.

🌿 Designates Pro-health Dining Selections.
*These foods are limited in calories, fat, salt and sugar.*

NAME _____ ROOM _____

FIGURE 12–3 • A sample patient menu for a standard diet.

## Breakfast

SODIUM RESTRICTED                                    SUNDAY

PLEASE (CIRCLE) SELECTIONS

### Continental Breakfast

Cinnamon Raisin Bagel served with
Lite Cream Cheese and seasonal fruit

### Or You May Prefer

Scrambled Eggs                          **Oatmeal**
🐷 Low Cholesterol Eggs          Cream of Wheat
**French Toast with Syrup**      Shredded Mini Wheat
Hash Browns                              Fruit Loops
Wheat Toast                          🐷 Fruited Yogurt
White Toast                          🐷 Fresh Banana
Cinnamon Raisin Bagel          🐷 Fresh Orange
*with Lite Cream Cheese*
Tortilla

### Beverages

**Orange Juice**                          **Coffee**
Apple Juice                          Decaf. Coffee
Prune Juice                          Hot Tea
Grapefruit Juice                     Decaf. Tea
🐷 **2% Milk**                           Hot Cocoa
🐷 Skim Milk                          Sugar Sub.

*SR = Sodium Restricted*

🐷 *Designates Pro-health Dining Selections.*
*These foods are limited in calories, fat, salt and sugar.*

**NO SALT**

17-699220

NAME _____ ROOM _____

---

## Lunch

SODIUM RESTRICTED                                    SUNDAY

PLEASE (CIRCLE) SELECTIONS

### Special of the Day

🐷 **CHICKEN BREAST WITH JULIENNE VEGETABLES**
*served with*
🐷 *rice pilaf and* 🐷 *steamed broccoli*

### Or You May Prefer          ### On the Side

SR Tomato Soup                          Orange Juice
*with SR turkey sandwich*          SR Tomato Soup
🐷 Cottage Cheese & Fruit Plate   🐷 Garden Green Salad
Steamed Rice                              *with Dressing*
🐷 Pinto Beans                          French Ranch Italian
🐷 Steamed Zucchini               **Fruited Gelatin Salad**
Deluxe Hamburger
🐷 Chicken Fajita                      **Dinner Roll**
                                              Tortilla
                                              SR Crackers

### Beverages          ### Finishing Touch

**Iced Tea**    Iced Water          🐷 **Chilled Fruit Cup**
Coffee          Hot Tea             🐷 Seasonal Fresh Fruit
Decaf. Tea      Sugar Sub.          Ice Cream
Decaf. Coffee                       Gelatin Cubes
                                    Sherbet

*SR = Sodium Restricted*

🐷 *Designates Pro-health Dining Selections.*
*These foods are limited in calories, fat, salt and sugar.*

**NO SALT**

NAME _____ ROOM _____

---

## Dinner

SODIUM RESTRICTED                                    SUNDAY

PLEASE (CIRCLE) SELECTIONS

### Special of the Day

**SR BRAISED TIPS OF BEEF**
*served in a hearty vegetable sauce
with a roll*

### Or You May Prefer          ### On the Side

SR Vegetable Soup                     Apple Juice
*with roast beef sandwich*            SR Vegetable Soup
🐷 Cottage Cheese & Fruit Plate   🐷 Garden Green Salad
Steamed Rice                              *with Dressing*
🐷 Vegetable Medley               French Ranch Italian
Glazed Beets                          🐷 **Cucumber &**
Deluxe Hamburger                      **Tomato Salad**
Oven Fried Chicken *with*
*coleslaw and a roll*                 Dinner Roll
                                              Tortilla
                                              SR Crackers

### Beverages          ### Finishing Touch

**Iced Tea**    Iced Water          🐷 **Strawberry Shortcake**
Coffee          Hot Tea             🐷 Chilled Pears
Decaf. Tea      🐷 **2% Milk**          🐷 Seasonal Fresh Fruit
Decaf. Coffee   🐷 Skim Milk          Ice Cream
                Sugar Sub.          Gelatin Cubes
                                    Sherbet

*SR = Sodium Restricted*

🐷 *Designates Pro-health Dining Selections.*
*These foods are limited in calories, fat, salt and sugar.*

**NO SALT**

NAME _____ ROOM _____

F I G U R E  12–4 • A sample patient menu for a sodium-restricted diet.

| DATE | DIET ORDERS | DIAGNOSIS AND SIGNIFICANT NOTES | LIKES | DISLIKES |
|------|-------------|--------------------------------|-------|----------|
|      |             |                                |       |          |

| | AGE | REL. | BEV. | |
|---|---|---|---|---|

DR.                                         NOURISH.                          INSTR.

| ROOM NO. | FULL NAME |
|----------|-----------|
| A—6—10   |           |

DIET

F I G U R E  12–5 • A dietary Kardex form used by the dietitian.

## Therapeutic Diet Orders

The diets in the following list differ from the regular diet in that the foods served are modified to vary in caloric content, level of one or more nutrients, bulk, or flavor. Some therapeutic diets are still named after disease conditions (such as **ulcer diet**), but the modern trend is toward naming the diet according to the modification (such as **60–80 g protein diet**, or **250 mg Na diet**). This provides for a specific and accurate communication between the doctor, the hospital personnel, and the patient. The following list contains therapeutic diets named according to the modification; however, as a health unit coordinator, you may still encounter other names used to designate specific types of diets orderd by the doctor.

Low-cholesterol diet
Low cholesterol, no free sugar
Modified fat diet
High-carbohydrate diet
Hypoglycemic diet
Sodium-restricted diets:
  Regular no salt added
  2.5 g Na diet (mild restrictions)
  1.0 g Na diet (moderate restrictions)
  250 mg Na diet (severe restrictions)
High-fiber diet
Prudent (low cholesterol/saturated fat/4 g sodium)
Potassium-modified diets: ) fruits + veg
  Potassium restricted
  High potassium

**COMMUNICATION AND IMPLEMENTATION OF DIETARY ORDERS**

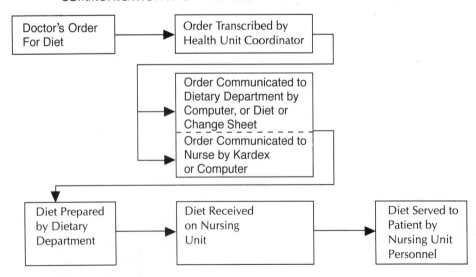

Doctor's Order For Diet → Order Transcribed by Health Unit Coordinator

Order Communicated to Dietary Department by Computer, or Diet or Change Sheet

Order Communicated to Nurse by Kardex or Computer

Diet Prepared by Dietary Department → Diet Received on Nursing Unit → Diet Served to Patient by Nursing Unit Personnel

| TABLE 12-1 | DESCRIPTION AND PURPOSE OF COMMON HOSPITAL DIETS | | |
|---|---|---|---|
| **Type** | **Description** | **Purpose** | **Tray Condiments** |
| Bland diet | May be used for patients who experience stomach irritation. Spicy foods containing black or red pepper and chilli powder are omitted. Beverages that contain caffeine, cola, coffee, cocoa, and tea are omitted. Chocolate is also omitted. Any foods known to cause discomfort. | For patients with ulcers and other problems. | Salt, sugar |
| Prudent—low-cholesterol/ reduced sodium | Controls the type of fat in the diet. Limits saturated fat and cholesterol found in foods from animal sources like eggs, dairy products, meat, and fish. Limits salt added to foods and on tray. | For patients who have high levels of blood cholesterol. | Pepper, sugar, salt substitute or herbal seasoning mix. |
| Sodium-controlled diet | Controls the amount of sodium in the diet. Salt and foods containing salt are high in sodium and are limited. The sodium-controlled diet will vary according to the amount of sodium allowed. | For patients with heart disease, high blood pressure, kidney disease, or who are using certain drugs. | Sugar, pepper, salt substitute, if ordered. |
| Diabetic diet | Total amount of food (calories) is carefully planned. Diabetics cannot receive too much or too little food; therefore, portion sizes must be followed. Concentrated sweets, like syrup, jelly, sweet desserts, and sugar are omitted. Snacks may be planned in between meals to keep blood sugar levels balanced. | For patients who cannot take enough insulin. Insulin is a substance important in helping sugar enter body cells. When there is not enough insulin made, sugar will build up in the blood. | Salt, pepper, sugar substitute |
| Renal | Based on individual needs, diet is controlled in one or more of the following: protein, sodium, potassium, total fluid, phosphorous. | For patients with renal disease. | Sugar, pepper No salt substitutes |
| Neutropenic—no fresh fruits/vegetables low bacteria | No fresh fruits or vegetables allowed. | Reduce the number of bacteria entering the stomach for patients on chemotherapy or those with immune deficiency diseases. | Sugar No pepper or salt |
| Lactose controlled | Limits intake of milk and milk products. | For patients who experience stomach disturbances after drinking/eating milk-containing foods. | Salt, pepper, sugar |
| NPO—nothing by mouth | Patient cannot receive fluids or solid foods. | Presurgery, procedures, test, or as indicated. | None |
| Clear liquid | Foods which are liquid or become liquid at room or body temperatures. Includes foods like tea, coffee, clear broth, gelatin, carbonated beverages. Foods you can see through (i.e., apple, cranberry, grape juice). | For patients who are very sick and cannot eat anything else. For patients before or after surgery. | Sugar |
| Full-liquid diet | Includes food from the clear-liquid diet, with the addition of juices with pulp, such as orange. Includes milk, ice cream, puddings, refined cooked cereals, strained cream soups, and egg nog. | For patients who cannot eat solid foods. For patients after surgery, following the clear-liquid diet. | Salt, pepper, sugar |
| Regular diet/DAT | All foods and beverages are allowed. | For patients who have no dietary restrictions. | Salt, pepper, sugar |
| GI soft diet | Limits raw, highly seasoned, and fried foods. | For patients with nausea and distention in the postsurgical patient. | Salt, pepper, sugar |
| Mechanical soft diet | Any diet made soft with ground meats, soft canned fruits, and well-cooked vegetables. | For patients who have trouble chewing or swallowing. | Salt, pepper, sugar |
| Puree | Mechanically altered foods and full liquids allowed. | For patients with problems in chewing and swallowing. | Salt, pepper, sugar |
| No thin liquids/thick liquids only | No milk (except milk shakes), juice (except nectars), broth soups (only cream soups), no coffee, tea, or soda pop. | To prevent choking. | Salt, pepper, sugar. |

Protein-modified diets:
   60–80 g protein
   40 g protein
   no protein
Gluten-free diet
Low-triglyceride diet
Diabetic diet (ADA)
Liberal diabetic
Calorie-restricted diets:
   1200 calorie diet
   1400 calorie diet
Vegetarian (usually patient request)

> ### HIGHLIGHT
>
> An order modifying a nutrient or number of calories would not change the consistency of a patient's diet. *Example*: If a patient is on a "soft diet" and the doctor then wrote an order for "low fat" the patient's diet would be "soft, low fat."

## Tube Feedings

**Tube feeding**, also called **gavage**, is the administration of liquified foods into the stomach, duodenum, or jejunum through a tube inserted either through the nose (a nasogastric or nasoenteral tube [Fig. 12–6]) or through an opening in the abdominal wall (gastrostomy or jejunostomy [Fig. 12–7]). Tube feedings are ordered for patients who have difficulty swallowing, who are unable to eat sufficient nutrients, or who cannot absorb the nutrients from the food they eat.

Administration of tube feedings may be by gravity, bolus, or a feeding infusion pump:

- **Bolus** consists of infusing a small amount of formula over a short time.
- **Gravity** allows the formula to run in by gravity by attaching a bag or bottle to the nasogastric tube.
- **Infusion pumps** also called enteral feeding pumps, or Kangaroo pump control the rate of administration (Fig. 12–8).

Types of nasogastric or nasoenteral tubes used for feedings include Entron, Dobbhoff, and Levin. A blenderized formula prepared in the dietary department or commercialized defined diets such as Vivonex TEN, Sustacal, Osmolite, Jevity, Pediasure, Pulmocare, or Ensure Plus may be ordered for tube feedings. To transcribe a tube feeding order, the health unit coordinator may need to order a nasogastric tube, formula, and feeding infusion pump.

### Doctors' Orders for Tube Feeding

Three types of preparation are used for tube feedings: standard, blenderized (pureed), and commercial. Examples of a typical doctor's order for each type is written below.

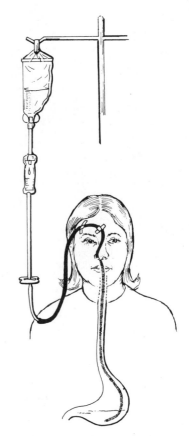

**F I G U R E   12–6 •** Feeding tube. (Courtesy of Baxter Travenol Laboratories, Inc.)

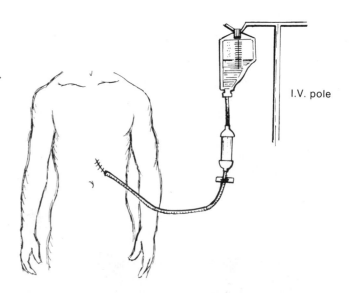

I.V. pole

**F I G U R E   12–7 •** Gastrostomy feeding. (Modified from Wood, L.A. and Ambo, B.J.: *Nursing for Allied Health Services.* Philadelphia, W.B. Saunders Co., 1977, with permission.)

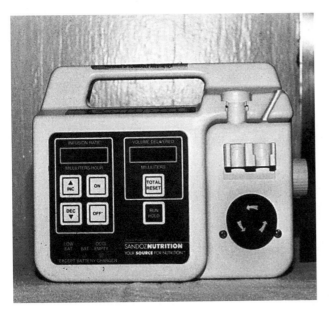

F I G U R E  12–8 • Feeding infusion pump, also referred to as an enteral feeding pump or Kangaroo pump.

■ *Tube feeding 1200 cal in 1200 cc standard formula for 24 h. TRA 200 cc q2h*

This formula contains a milk base with egg powder and vitamins added. The doctor indicates the caloric value, the amount of fluid, and the frequency over a 24-hour period.

■ *Tube feeding 1200 cal in 1200 cc blenderized formula. TRA 200 cc q2h*

Blenderized formula is a variety of basic foods mixed in the blender and strained. Once again, the doctor indicates the caloric value, the amount of fluid, and the frequency over a 24-hour period.

■ *Ensure Plus via Bolus feeding 400 cc q6h*

■ *Insert Dobbhoff, X-ray for placement. When in proper position, begin via pump Jevity ½ strength dilute c̄ water TRA 40 cc/h for 8 h, then 50 cc/h for 8 h, then FS Jevity at 50 cc/h.*

In this order for tube feedings, the doctor is requesting an x-ray to determine the correct placement of the tube before the administration of the formula.

TO THE STUDENT

To practice transcribing therapeutic diet orders, complete **Activity 12–2** in the Skills Practice Manual.

## Other Dietary Orders

The following orders pertain to the patient's intake of foods and liquids but are not orders for a type of diet.

■ *Force fluids*

This order is probably written in addition to the patient's dietary order. The doctor wants the patient to drink more

fluids. The health unit coordinator would send this order to the dietary department so more fluids could be included on the patient's trays.

■ *Limit fluids to 1000 cc per day*

This order is also written in addition to the diet order. The patient's fluid intake is to be restricted to *1000 cc per day*. A restriction of fluids is usually ordered for patients who are retaining fluids (a condition known as **edema**) because of a disease process. The dietary department should be notified of this order so fluids would be limited on the patient's trays and the dietitian would also become involved.

■ *NPO*

This order means the patient is to have *nothing by mouth*. This is usually ordered following major surgery or during a critical illness. This information is sent to the dietary department to update the patient's dietary record so a tray would not be prepared for the patient.

■ *NPO midnight*

The patient is to have *nothing by mouth after midnight*. This is ordered to prepare a patient for surgery, treatment, or a diagnostic procedure. The dietary department is notified so that a tray would not be sent to the patient.

■ *Sips and chips*

The patient may have only sips of water and ice chips. This order would also be sent to the dietary department to update the patient's dietary record.

■ *Have dietitian see patient*

The doctor is requesting the dietitian to discuss the diet with the patient or teach the patient about his or her diet. This order may require a phone call in addition to sending a requisition to the dietary department.

■ *Calorie count today and tomorrow*

This is usually ordered to document amount and types of food consumed by the patient for further nutritional evaluation by the dietitian. Send this information to the dietary department and notify the nurse caring for the patient. You may be required to prepare a form to record the patient's caloric intake.

TO THE STUDENT

To practice transcribing a review set of doctors' orders, complete **Activity 12–3** in the Skills Practice Manual.

To practice recording telephone physicians' orders and telephone messages, complete **Activities 12–4** and **12–5** in the Skills Practice Manual.

## SUMMARY

Accuracy is essential in the transcription of dietary orders, because an error could result in serious consequences. Imagine, for example, a patient who is NPO for surgery receiving breakfast, or a severely diabetic patient receiving a regular diet.

Hospitalized patients are dependent upon the hospital personnel to meet their dietary likes and needs. The diet ordered by the doctor for the patient may be an integral part of the treatment plan, or it may be ordered to maintain health. In either case, mealtime is an important time for many patients, and for some it may be the most pos-

itive experience of the day. The health unit coordinator is responsible for ordering late trays when a patient has missed their meal because of a test or procedure. It is important that the tray is ordered and delivered to the patient promptly. The dietary and nursing departments must work closely together to provide the patient with proper and pleasant meals. Thorough and prompt communication by the health unit coordinator facilitates this tremendously.

## REVIEW QUESTIONS

1. Identify two methods of sending dietary orders to the dietary department.

    a. ___by computer___

    b. ___by diet change sheet___

2. Rewrite the following doctors' orders using symbols and/or abbreviations. Or, to practice writing doctors' orders, have someone read the orders to you, while you record them. Again, practice using symbols and abbreviations while you do this.

    a. nothing per mouth after midnight ___NOP MN___

    b. clear liquid breakfast, then nothing by mouth

    ___cl liq break, then NPO___

    c. one-thousand-calorie American Diabetic Association diet

    ___1000 cal ADA diet___

    d. low-cholesterol diet ___low-~~chest~~ chol diet___

    e. diet as tolerated ___DAT___

    f. regular diet ___reg diet___

    g. low-sodium diet ___low NA diet___

    h. no salt added ___NAS___

3. Define the terms listed below in the space provided.

    a. therapeutic, or special, diet.

    ___a normal diet with modifications or restriction___

    b. regular diet

    ___a diet that provides good nutrition___

    c. tube feeding

    ___administration of liquids through a tube in the stomach___

    d. nothing by mouth

    ___no food or liquids by mouth___

4. List three methods of administering tube feedings.

    a. ___gravity___        c. ___bolus___

    b. ___infusion pump___

5. Below is a list of diets the doctor may order for the patient. Underline those that provide for change of consistency of food from the regular diet, and place a check mark beside those that are special diets.

a. soft diet
b. potassium-restricted diet ✓
c. 800-cal diet ✓
d. full-liquid diet

e. 250-mg Na diet ✓
f. mechanical soft diet ✓
g. hypoglycemic diet ✓
h. low-triglyceride diet ✓

6. For the doctors' order *diet as tolerated* (DAT), list four diets that may be selected for the patient.

a. _clear-liquid_          c. _soft diet_

b. _full liquid_           d. _regular_

7. Explain why a physician's order for DAT requires the health unit coordinator to ask the nurse what diet to order from the dietary department.

_the dietician or dietary dept cant decide what the patient can tolerate_

8. What is the meaning of NPO MN? Why would a doctor order the patient NPO MN?

_Nothing by mouth after midnight prepare pt surgury th the morning, diagnostic procedures, treatment_

9. Write the names of three tubes that may be used to administer tube feedings.

a. _entron_

b. _dobhoff_

c. _Levine_

10. Write the names of five formulas that may be used for tube feedings.

a. _vivonex 10_     c. _Osmolite_     e. _ensure plus_

b. _Sustacal_       d. _Jevity_

## References

Davis Ratcliff, Judi and Sherer, Kim: *Applied Nutrition and Diet Therapy for Nurses*, 2nd ed. Philadelphia, W.B. Saunders Co., 1994.

Kerschner, Velma L.: *Nutrition and Diet Therapy*, 3rd ed. Philadelphia, F. A. Davis Co., 1983.

Long, Barbara C. and Phipps, Wilma J.: *Medical-Surgical Nursing*. St. Louis, The C. V. Mosby Co., 1989.

O'Toole, Marie (ed.): *Miller-Keane Encyclopedia & Dictionary of Medicine, Nursing, & Allied Health*, 6th ed. Philadelphia, W.B. Saunders Co., 1997.

Sundberg, Mary C.: *Fundamentals of Nursing*, 2nd ed. Boston, Jones and Bartlett Publishers, 1989.

# MEDICATION ORDERS

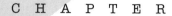
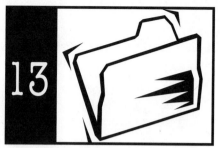

## CHAPTER OBJECTIVES

*Upon completion of this chapter, you will be able to:*

1. Define the terms in the vocabulary list.
2. Write the meaning of each abbreviation in the abbreviations list.
3. Define standing, standing prn, stat, one-time, and short-order series medication orders.
4. List the five components of a medication order.
5. List four groups of drugs that usually have automatic "stop dates."
6. Name two reference books for medications.
7. Name two weight and measure systems used in medication orders and identify the symbols used in each.
8. List four routes by which medications are administered.
9. List four parenteral routes of administration.
10. Describe the purpose of each of the drug groups listed in the text.
11. Spell the name of the most commonly used drugs, marked with an asterisk, and name the drug group to which each belongs.
12. Name a skin test for tuberculosis.
13. Differentiate between IV push, piggy-back, IV admixture, and TPN.
14. Write the usual adult dosages for drugs listed in this chapter.
15. Demonstrate the procedure for using the PDR.
16. List the advantages and disadvantages of computerized medication dispensing.

## VOCABULARY

**Admixture** • The result of adding a medication to a container of intravenous solution

**Ampoule (Ampule)** • A small glass vial sealed to keep contents sterile, used for subcutaneous, intramuscular, and intravenous medications

**Apothecary System** • An ancient system of weight and volume measurements used to measure drugs and solutions

**Automatic Stop Date** • The date on which specific categories of medications must be discontinued unless renewed by the doctor

**Bolus** • A concentrated dose of medication given intravenously, usually by IV push    *ambian*

**Capsule** • A gelatinous container in which a drug is enclosed

**Hypnotic** • A drug that produces sleep

**Intramuscular Injection** • An injection of a medication into a muscle

**Intravenous** • Pertains to within the vein

**Intravenous Hyperalimentation (Total Parenteral Nutrition)** • A method used to administer calories, proteins, vitamins, and other nutrients into the bloodstream of a patient who is unable to eat or whose bowels need time to heal    *central cath.*   *Crohns disease*   *Cancer HIV, Colon surgery*

**IV Push** • A method of giving concentrated doses of medication intravenously

**Lozenge** • A medicated tablet or disk that dissolves in the mouth

**Medication Administration Record** • A form containing the list of medications that each patient is currently taking; it is used by the nurse to administer the medications

**Medication Nurse** • The registered nurse or licensed practical nurse who is licensed to administer medications to patients

**Metric System** • A decimal system of weights and measures based on multiples of 10

**Narcotic** • A controlled drug that relieves pain or produces sleep

**Oral** • By mouth

**Parenteral** • Routes other than by mouth for giving fluids or medications, i.e., injections or intravenously

**Patient-Controlled Analgesia** • Narcotics administered intravenously by means of a special infusion pump controlled by the patient

**Piggyback** • A method by which drugs are usually administered intravenously in 50 to 100 mL of fluid

**Skin Tests** • Tests in which the reactive materials are placed on the skin or just beneath the skin to determine the presence of certain antibodies within the body

**Subcutaneous Injection** • Introduction of a medication under the skin into fatty or connective tissue

**Suppository** • A medicated substance mixed in a solid base that melts when placed in a body opening; suppositories are used in the rectum, vagina, or urethra

**Suspension** • A fine-particle drug suspended in a suitable liquid

**Tablet** • A solid dosage of a drug in a disk form

**Topical** • The direct application of medication to the skin, eye, ear, or other parts of the body

## ABBREVIATIONS

| Abbreviation | Meaning | Example of Usage on a Doctors' Order Sheet |
|---|---|---|
| ā | before | Give Compazine 10 mg IM 30 min ā x-ray |
| āā (ana) | of each | MOM } āā mineral oil } 15 cc |
| amp | ampoule (ampule) | Add 1 amp multivitamins to IV q24h |
| ASA | acetylsalicyclic acid (aspirin) | ASA 325 mg PO q4h prn |
| cap | capsule | ampillicin 500 mg cap 1 q6h |
| CPZ | Compazine | CPZ 10 mg 1M q4h prn N/V |
| dr or ʒ | dram | elixir of phenobarb ʒ 11 PO tid |
| DSS | dioctyl sodium sulfosuccinate (Colace) | DSS 50 mg daily |
| 5-Fu | 5-fluorouracil | 5-Fu 800 mg IV daily × 3 days |
| g | gram | Cefadyl 1 g IVPB q6h |

| | | |
|---|---|---|
| gr | grain | chloral hydrate gr XV PO hs prn |
| HCTZ | hydrochlorothiazide | HCTZ 25 mg PO daily |
| IM | intramuscular | vitamin B$_{12}$ 1000 µg IM tomorrow |
| IVPB | intravenous piggyback | Keflin 0.5 g IVPB q8h |
| KCl | potassium chloride | Add 40 mEq KCl in each IV |
| | liter | 1 L 5% D/W to run @ 125 mL/h |
| µg or mcg | microgram | vitamin B$_{12}$ 1000 mcg IM |
| mEq | milliequivalent | 40 mEq KCl Tab 1̄ PO qid c̄ 1 glass of H$_2$O |
| mg | milligram | Achromycin 250 mg PO qid |
| MgSO$_4$ | magnesium sulfate (epsom salts) | gr xv MgSO$_4$ in glass H$_2$O tonight |
| mL | milliliter | 1000 mL 5% D/W @ KO rate |
| MOM | milk of magnesia | MOM 30 cc hs prn |
| MS or MSO$_4$ | morphine sulfate | MS 10 mg IM q4h prn pain |
| | | MSO$_4$ 4 mg 1M q4h for postop pain |
| noc | night | Offer laxative q noc |
| NTG | nitroglycerin | May leave NTG tablets @ bedside |
| N/V | nausea & vomiting | Compazine 10 mg 1M q6h prn N/V |
| OD | oculus dexter (right eye) | Aureomycin ophth ung OD tid |
| OS | oculus sinister (left eye) | Garamycin ophth sol gtt 1̄ OS tid |
| OU | oculus unitas (both eyes) | Neosporin ophth sol gtts 11̄ OU bid |
| oz or ʒ | ounce | MOM ʒ 1 hs prn constipation |
| PBZ | Pyribenzamine | PBZ 25 mg PO q4h prn nasal congestion |
| pc | post cibum (after meals | Maalox 15 cc tid pc |
| PCA | patient-controlled analgesia | PCA MS 2 mg q10 min |
| PCN | penicillin | PCN 250 mg PO q6h |
| PO | per os (by mouth) | Librium 5 mg PO tid |
| pr | per rectum | Dulcolax 10 mg now pr |
| SC, sq, or sub-q | subcutaneous | heparin 5000 U SC qd |
| SO$_4$ | sulfate | iron SO$_4$ tab 1̄ tid |
| s̄s̄ | semis (one-half) | Amphojel ʒ s̄s̄ prn gastric distress |
| stat | immediately | regular insulin 50 U IV stat |

| subling, SL | sublingual (under tongue) | nitrogenglycerin tab 1 subling prn anginal pain |
| supp | suppository | acetaminophen supp 1 prn for temp ↑ 100⁸⁽ᴿ⁾ |
| syr | syrup | ipecac syr dr 11 now |
| tab | tablets | prednisone 25 mg PO tab 1 bid |
| tinct or tr | tincture | tinct belladonna gtts 111 ac |
| TPN | total parenteral nutrition | ↑ TPN rate of infusion to 100 cc/hr |
| U | unit | NPH insulin 25 U qd |
| ung | unguent (ointment) | Neosporin ung tid to (R) elbow |
| WA | while awake | Hycodan 5 cc PO q4h WA |

## E X E R C I S E  **1**

Write the abbreviation for each term listed below.

1. liter — _L_
2. sulfate — _SO4_
3. aspirin — _ASA_
4. immediately — _stat_
5. capsule — _cap_
6. Compazine — _CPZ_
7. tablet — _tub_
8. milk of magnesia — _MOM_
9. unit — _U_
10. right eye — _OD_
11. milligram — _mg_
12. Colace — _DSS_
13. potassium chloride — _KCl_
14. gram — _G_
15. both eyes — _OU_
16. one-half — _ss̄_
17. morphine sulfate — _MS_
18. milliliter — _~~5 ml~~ ML_
19. 5-fluorouracil — _5-FU_
20. milliequivalent — _mEq_

21. after meals — _pc_
22. ointment — _ung_
23. while awake — _wA_
24. nausea and vomiting — _N+A_
25. of each — _āā_
26. grain — _gr_
27. intramuscular — _IM_
28. sublingual — _SL_
29. tincture — _tinct_
30. by mouth — _PO_
31. ounce — _oz_  _ʒ_
32. left eye — _OS_
33. ampoule — _amp_
34. dram — _dr_
35. suppository — _~~NTG~~_
36. nitroglycerin — _NTG_  _~~subc~~_
37. subcutaneous — _subq_  _SC_  _Sq_
38. microgram — _mcg_  _μg_
39. night — _noc_
40. hydrochlorothiazide — _HCTZ_
41. syrup — _syr_
42. intravenous piggyback — _IVPB_
43. before — _ā_
44. epsom salts — _MgSO4_
45. Pyribenzamine — _PBZ_
46. penicillin — _PCN_
47. per rectum — _pr_
48. total parenteral nutrition — _TPN_
49. patient-controlled analgesia — _PCA_

## E X E R C I S E  **2**

Write the meaning of each abbreviation listed below.

1. KCl — _potassium chloride_
2. OS — _Left eye_
3. amp — _ampule_

4. syr — syrup

5. dr or ℨ — dram

6. noc — night

7. µg, mcg — microgram

8. oz or ℨ — ounce

9. SC — subcutaneous

10. stat — immediatly

11. 5-Fu — 5-fluorouracil

12. mEq — milliequivalent

13. pc — after meals

14. ung — ointment

15. CPZ — Compazine

16. mL — milliliter

17. PO — by mouth

18. tinct — tincture

19. IM — Intramuscular

20. gr — grain

21. mg — milligram

22. HCTZ — Hydroclorothiazide

23. supp — suppository

24. g — gram

25. OU — both eyes

26. āā — of each

27. N/V — nausea and vomiting

28. WA — while awake

29. s̄s̄ — one half

30. MS, MSO₄ — morphine sulfate

31. NTG — nitroglycerin

32. ASA — Aspirin

33. cap — capsule

34. mgSO₄ — epsom salts

35. tab — tablets

36. MOM — milk of magnesia

37. L — liter

38. SO₄ — sulfate

39. U — unit

40. OD — right eye

41. subling — sublingual

42. IVPB — intravenous piggyback

43. ā — before

44. PBZ — Pyrabenzamine

45. PCN — Penakillen

46. DSS — colace

47. TPN — Total parenteral nutrition

48. PCA — patient controlled analgesia

49. pr — per rectum

50. SL — sublingual

## E X E R C I S E  3

The following is a list of medication orders typical of those you may see on the patient's chart. Write the meanings of the *italicized* abbreviations in the space provided.

*MS* $gr\frac{1}{4}$ *IM q3h prn* severe pain

a. morphine Sulfate grain 1/4 intramuscular every 3 hours as needed for severe pain

Keflin 0.5 *g IVPB q8h*

b. Keflin 0.5 grams Intravenous Piggyback

Librium 10 *mg PO qid*

c. 10 milligrams by mouth four times a day

Neosporin ophthalmic *gtts* ii *OU bid*

d. 2 drops both eyed twice a day

Nitroglycerin 0.4 mg *subling prn* chest pain

e. under tongue

*MOM* 30 *cc hs prn* constipation

f. cubic centimeters at bedtime as needed

NPH insulin 25 *U qd*

g. 25 Units every day

*ASA* 325 *mg PO q4h prn* for fever > than 101 ®

h. milligrams by mouth every 4 hours as needed

Donnagel ℨ s̄s̄ *PO tid ac*

i. one half oz by mouth three times a day before meals

## BACKGROUND INFORMATION

### Communicating with the Pharmacy

All medications are ordered by the doctor. Part of the transcription procedure for medication orders is to communicate the order to the pharmacy. Three methods of doing this are to send a direct copy of the doctor's order, to enter the order into a computer, and send a copy by fax machine. Use of requisitions for transcribing medication orders may be practiced in some facilities.

The direct copy is a noncarbon-reproducible copy of the doctors' order sheet. To order medications under this system, the health unit coordinator removes the direct copy from the patient's chart and sends it to the pharmacy. The pharmacist who fills the medication order reads the order directly from the doctor's order on the copy, thus reducing the possibility of transcription error.

For the computer order-entry system, the health unit coordinator enters the order into the computer. The third method of communicating the order to the pharmacy is to fax the original physicians' order sheet. After the sheet is faxed the original is replaced in the patient's chart. The pharmacist who fills the medication order reads the order directly from a copy of the doctors' order sheet; the pharmacists fills the medication order and labels the medication with the patient's name, room and bed number; and the name, dosage, and frequency of administration. The medication is then sent back to the nursing unit, where it is placed in either a medicine room (med room) or on a medication chart.

The medicine cart is a vehicle in which the patient's medications are stored in separate drawers or bins labeled for each patient. The medication cart can be wheeled to the patient's bedside for the administration of the medication (Fig. 13–1.) Some facilities now use a computerized medication cart which requires the user to enter a user ID and password to unlock the cart. The medication cart computer asks the user to verify the name of the medication, the dose, and the patient's name before removing the medication.

### Filling Out the Medication Administration Record

Transcribing medication orders may require the health unit coordinator to write the order on a medication administration record (MAR), or enter the order into the computer. A registered nurse or a licensed practical nurse may be assigned to give the medications. The "med nurse" (as he or she is called) uses the medication administration record as a reference while preparing the medications for administration and also while giving the medications. Utmost accuracy in copying the order from the doctors' order sheet onto the medication administration record or entering it into the computer is absolutely essential.

### *Medication Administration Record*

In hospitals where the MAR is used, the health unit coordinator initiates the record on the patient's admission. Since the medications are ordered by the doctor, the health unit coordinator enters the information on the record. The record varies in the number of days that medications may be entered. When the last date of the dated period on the MAR is reached, a new record with new dates is prepared and all medications still in use are copied onto the new form. The MAR is a part of the patient's chart and is a legal document that is written in ink.

To discontinue medications on the MAR, indicate DC on the correct day and time and draw a line through the days not used (Fig. 13–2).

Facilities utilizing computerized charting for patient care require the nurse to document medication administration in the computer rather than a written MAR. When

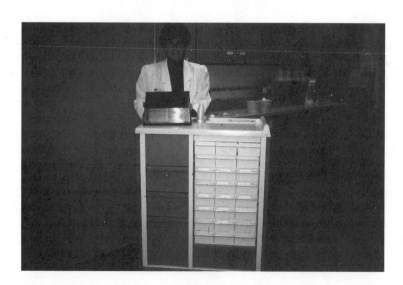

FIGURE  13–1 • A medication cart.

UC Recopy:_____

| Date / Exp. | MEDICATION ADMINISTRATION RECORD SCHEDULED: A | 24 01 02 03 | 04 05 06 07 | 08 09 10 11 | 12 13 14 15 | 16 17 18 19 | 20 21 22 23 | RN ✓ | Date 9-16-00 | | | Date 9-17-00 | | | Date 9-18-00 | | | Injection Code |
|---|---|---|---|---|---|---|---|---|---|---|---|---|---|---|---|---|---|---|
| | | | | | | | | | 23 | 07 | 15 | 23 | 07 | 15 | 23 | 07 | 15 | |
| 9/16 | Theragram tabs Ī qd | | | 09 | | | | | | JR | | | JR | | | JR | | **RU:** RUQ |
| 9/16 | Monopril 10 mg P.O. bid | | | 09 | | 17 | | | | JR | SW | | JR DC | | | | | **LU:** LUQ |
| 9/16 9/23 | Dalmane 15 mg P.O. qH.S. | | | | | | 21 | | | | SW | | | SW | | | SW | **LA:** Left Arm |
| | | | | | | | | | | | | | | | | | | **RA:** Right Arm |
| | | | | | | | | | | | | | | | | | | **LT:** Left Thigh |
| | | | | | | | | | | | | | | | | | | **RT:** Right Thigh |
| | | | | | | | | | | | | | | | | | | **OU:** Both Eyes |
| | | | | | | | | | | | | | | | | | | **ABD:** Abdomen |
| | | | | | | | | | | | | | | | | | | **OD:** Right Eye |
| | | | | | | | | | | | | | | | | | | **OS:** Left Eye |

IV MEDS

Allergies ___ *Dairy Products* ___   Recopy Check

Diagnosis ___ Hypertension ___   Age _51_

Name ___ Smith, John ___   MD _Clark_

FIGURE 13-2 • A medication administration record showing a method of discontinuing medications. *Illustration continued on following page*

the patient is discharged, an MAR with all computer entries should be printed to place on the patient's chart.

## Medication Reference Books

Reference books usually kept on nursing units that are most helpful to doctors, nurses, and allied health personnel are *The American Hospital Formulary* (published by the American Society of Hospital Pharmacists) and the *Physicians' Desk Reference* (PDR) (published yearly by Medical Economics Inc.). The individual hospital pharmacy frequently supplies each nursing unit with a listing of medications and dosage forms available in that particular pharmacy. The listing is the specific formulary compiled for that health care facility. Some units may also have a nurses' drug handbook for nurses to use for reference when passing medications. It is generally a compact paperback, which is more convenient to use.

The *Physicians' Desk Reference* has different sections listed under the table of contents. Each section is printed on a different color paper. The "Product Name" and the "Generic and Chemical Name Index" are the two sections that are most useful to the health unit coordinator.

## Use of the PDR

The following exercises will introduce you to the use of the PDR. Your instructor will assist you, if necessary. It is recommended that during transcription of medication orders you use the PDR for spelling, drug category names, or other information you may need to know in order to transcribe the order accurately.

| | Date | MEDICATION ADMINISTRATION RECORD PRN-ONE TIME & STAT: B | RN ✓ | Date 9-16-00 | | | Date 9-17-00 | | | Date 9-18-00 | | |
|---|---|---|---|---|---|---|---|---|---|---|---|---|
| | Exp. | | | 23 | 07 | 15 | 23 | 07 | 15 | 23 | 07 | 15 |
| PRN | | | | | | | | | | | | |
| | | | | | | | | | | | | |
| | | | | | | | | | | | | |
| | | | | | | | | | | | | |
| | | | | | | | | | | | | |
| | | | | | | | | | | | | |
| | | | | | | | | | | | | |
| | | | | | | | | | | | | |
| | | | | | | | | | | | | |
| ONE-TIME | | | | | | | | | | | | |
| | | | | | | | | | | | | |
| | | | | | | | | | | | | |

PATIENT  Smith, John    ALLERGIES  *Dairy Products*

F I G U R E  13–2 • *Continued*

## EXERCISE 4

Using the PDR, in the section titled "Product Name Index," locate the following drugs in the "Product Information Section,"* and briefly state the purpose of each. (Read the paragraph titled "Indications and Usage" under the drug name to locate the purpose.)

**Example:**

Amesec—given for asthma _____

1. Soma compound w/codeine _____

2. Kay Ceil oral solution _____

3. Indocin SR capsules _____

4. Senokot tablets _____

5. Decadron elixir _____

_____

*Ignore entries listed in the "Product Identification" section. This section shows pictures of the drugs and dosages only.

Using the "Generic and Chemical Names Index," locate the following:

6. furosemide _____

7. meperidine hydrochloride _____

## Naming Medications

Most medications have several names. They are:

1. *Official name*: The name under which the drug is listed in official government publications of drug standards. This name may be followed by the initials U.S.P. (United States Pharmacopia) or N.F. (National Formulary). These are the two official volumes in which drug standards are published.
2. *Chemical name*: This name describes the chemical composition of the drug.
3. *Generic name*: A shortened name given to the drug by the developer so that the longer chemical name does not have to be used. Many states require the pharmacist to use the generic name on the label. Generic names are not capitalized.

4. *Brand name, trade name, or proprietary name*: The name given to and registered by the manufacturer. The general public often knows the drug best by this name. *The brand name is always capitalized and may have a trademark symbol (™ or ®).* Each company that manufactures a drug of the same chemical composition may assign it a brand name. For example, Tylenol, the brand name under which McNeil Laboratories manufactures acetaminophen (its generic name) is named Datril by Bristol Laboratories. *A drug has only one generic name but may have many trade names, depending on how many companies manufacture it.*

Some hospitals have a substitution rule. Under this rule the pharmacist may substitute a different brand from the one that is prescribed or the pharmacist may substitute the generic equivalent. It is good practice for the pharmacist to put an "equivalent" label on the container to decrease confusion on the nursing unit.

## COMPONENTS OF A MEDICATION ORDER

### Introduction

The doctor writes each medication order using specific components that include directions for the person giving the drug.

**Example:**

| Tylenol | 325 mg | PO | q4h | WA |
|---------|--------|-----|-----|-----|
| 1 | 2 | 3 | 4 | 5 |

The numbered portions of this drug order are:

| Number | Component | Example |
|--------|-----------|---------|
| 1 | Name of drug | Tylenol |
| 2 | Dose of drug (amount) | 325 mg |
| 3 | Route of administration | PO (by mouth) |
| 4 | Time of administration (frequency) | q4h (every 4 hours) |
| 5 | Qualifying phrase | WA (while awake) |

### Component One—Name of the Drug

It is impossible for you to learn the names of all the drugs on the market, therefore, *as a beginning or new health unit coordinator you may wish to keep a small notebook with an alphabetical index to jot down names of drugs that you encounter frequently.* Periodic reviewing will help you to become more familiar with medication names.

Many medications are prepared in different forms, depending on their use. The form is often included with the name of the drug, such as Neosporin *ointment.* For example, ointments are used on the skin or the mucous membranes of the body. Other medications may include a letter as shown in 2 and 3 below.

## COMMUNICATION AND IMPLEMENTATION OF MEDICATION ORDERS

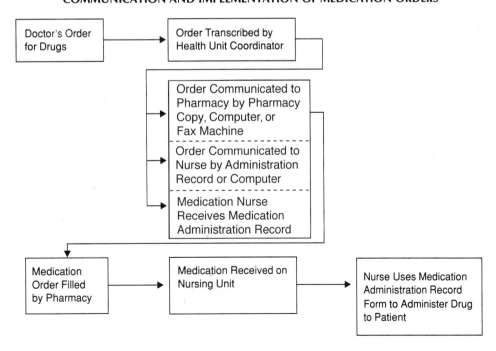

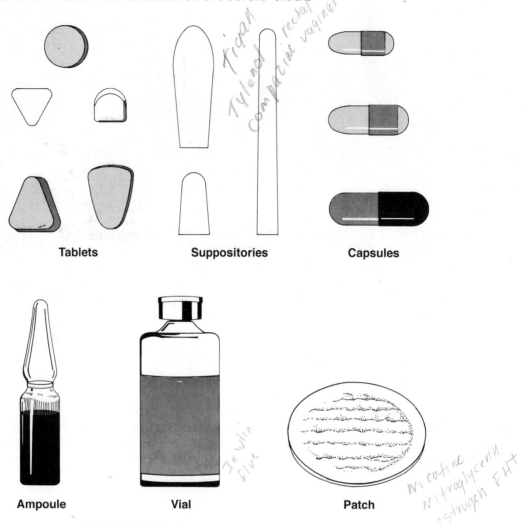

**Tablets**          **Suppositories**          **Capsules**

**Ampoule**          **Vial**          **Patch**

F I G U R E  13–3 • Common forms of medication.

**Examples of Doctors' Medication Orders that Indicate a Specific Form of Medication**

■ *Neosporin ung ophthalmic OD bid*
*Ophthalmic* indicates that this ointment is to be used in the eye only.

■ *Aspirin EC tab ī q3h prn*
The *enteric-coated* (EC) aspirin dissolves only in the small intestine.

■ *Aspirin T-R 650 mg PO q hs*
*Time released* (T-R) aspirin has a longer lasting effect.

■ *Aspirin supp 325 mg q3h for temp 101 (R)*
Aspirin is contained in *suppository* (supp) form for insertion into the rectum.

## Component Two—Dosage of Drugs

The apothecary system and the metric system are the two methods of weights and measures in present-day hospital use. The **metric system**, which is based on multiples of 10, is the system of choice in scientific fields and is gradually replacing the apothecary system. However, until the apothecary system is completely phased out, the health unit coordinator must continue to be knowledgeable about both systems.

### Apothecary System

The **apothecary system** for weighing and measuring drugs and solutions is an ancient system that was brought to the United States from England during the colonial period. Only those terms still used frequently today are listed below.

**Terms relating to weight (solid or powder)**

Grain (gr)
Dram (dr or ʒ)
Ounce (oz or ʒ)

**Terms relating to volume (liquid)**

Minim (m)
Fluid dram (fl dr or ʒ)
Fluid ounce (fl oz or ʒ)

The abbreviation fl is not always used.

Measurements in this system are written in lowercase Roman numerals. These numerals have a line over them and may be dotted to avoid confusion with similar-appearing letters or numerals. Also the unit of measure precedes the numeral.

**Example:** one grain—gr ī.
five grains—gr v̄.

A medication dosage that is less than 1 is written as a fraction.

**Example:** one sixth grain—gr $\frac{1}{6}$.

Remembering that one-half may also be written as s̄s̄, it is proper to write one and one-half grains as īss and one-half ounce as s̄s̄.

## Metric System

The metric system is used everywhere except the United States. The weight, volume, and measurement units are used in other hospital departments as well as in the pharmacy. These basic units are:

Weight = gram (g)
Volume = liter (L)
Length = meter (M)

Smaller and larger units in the metric system can be indicated by attaching prefixes to the basic units. This text will not cover all the prefixes used in the metric system because not all are used in doctors' orders.

To enlarge the basic unit 1000 times, the prefix *kilo* is added.

**Example:** kilogram (kg) = 1000 g.

To diminish the basic unit by 100, the prefix *centi* is added. The prefix *milli* diminishes the basic unit by 1000. A milligram (mg), milliliter (mL), millimeter (mm) represent 1/1000 of the basic unit. The symbol μ represents the prefix *micro*.

**Example:** 1 μ = 1 micrometer or 0.001 millimeter.

The terms *milliliter* (mL) and *cubic centimeter* (cc) are used interchangeably, although milliliter is preferred.

**Example:** 1 L = 1000 cc or 1000 mL.

The metric system uses the Arabic numerals that we all know—1, 2, 3, and so forth. Abbreviations are placed after the number, as in 50 mg or 500 mL.

Quantities less than 1 and fractions are written in decimal form, for example: 0.25 mg, 1.25 mg, 1.5 g.

Abbreviations used in medication dosages that *do not fall* within the apothecary or metric systems are: gtt (drop), mEq (milliequivalent), and U (unit). Examples of their usage in doctors' orders are:

*Pilocarpine 1% gtts īi OU tid*
*Add 40 mEq KCl to each IV*
*Bicillin 600,000 U bid × 3 days*

Listed below for reference is a table of approximate equivalents between the two systems. There are times when knowledge of the equivalents will prove helpful to the health unit coordinator.

| Weight | |
|---|---|
| **Metric** | **Apothecary** |
| 60 or 65 mg | gr ī |
| 100 mg | gr īss |
| 300 or 325 mg | gr v̄ |
| 500 mg or 0.5 g | gr v̄iiss |
| 0.4 mg | gr 1/150 |
| 15 mg | gr $\frac{1}{4}$ |
| 10 mg | gr $\frac{1}{6}$ |
| 32 mg | gr s̄s̄ |

| Volume | |
|---|---|
| 30 cc or 30 mL (mL and cc interchangeable) | fl oz ī or ʒ ī |
| 500 cc or 0.5 L | fl oz xv̄i (pt) |
| 1000 cc or 1 L | fl oz xxxii (qt) |

## EXERCISE 5

Write the following doses in the correct form using the proper abbreviations. (Do not convert to different systems.)

1. Two grains — *gr īi*
2. Five cubic centimeters — *5 cc*
3. Four drams — *4 dr   dr īv*
4. One-half gram — *0.5 g   g s̄s̄*
5. One and one-half grains — *gr īss*
6. Five hundred milligrams — *500 mg*
7. Fifteen grains — *gr XV*
8. One liter — *1 L*
9. One thousand grams — *Kg   1000 g*
10. One-sixth grain — *gr 1/6*
11. One one-hundred-fiftieth grain — *gr 1/150*

## Component Three—Routes of Administration

Medications may be administered to patients using different routes of administration. Also, any one medication may be prepared to be given by several different methods. Doctors should always indicate the route of administration. However, when a medication can be given only by mouth, the route is frequently omitted in the doctor's order. The following list contains the routes most frequently used in medication administration, with an example of each.

### ■ Oral (mouth or PO)

The patient swallows the medication, which may be in the form of a capsule, pill, tablet, spansule, or liquid.

**Example:** Librium 10 mg PO tid.

■ *Sublingual*

The tablet is placed under the tongue, where it is absorbed.

**Example:** nitroglycerin gr 1/150 subling prn anginal pain.

■ *Inhalation*    INH

These liquid medications are most commonly administered by the respiratory care department as part of their treatment procedure (see Chapter 17). albuteral

■ *Topical*

Applied to skin or mucous membrane. Medications in this category may be in the form of lotions, liniments, ointments, powders, sprays, solutions, suppositories, or transdermal preparations.

a. *Applied to the skin*

**Example 1:** apply Neosporin ointment to rt leg ulcer bid.

**Example 2:** Transderm-Nitro 5 ī qd. (The medication is part of a flat disk that is applied to the body, usually the chest; the medication is released over a specified period.)

b. *Spraying onto skin or mucous membrane*

**Example 1:** spray lt ankle wound with Neosporin aerosol tid.

**Example 2:** Chloraseptic throat spray q3h prn for throat irritation.

c. *Instillation*

These liquids are dropped into the eye, ear, or nose.

**Examples:** Eye—Neosporin ophth sol'n gtts ī̄ī OS bid.

Ear—Cortisporin otic suspension gtts ī̄īī in lt ear qid.

Nose—Neo-Synephrine 0.5% nose drops ī̄ī in each nostril q4h prn nasal congestion.

d. *Insertions of drugs into body openings— suppositories*

1. Rectal.

**Example:** Compazine supp 5 mg q4h prn N/V.

2. Vaginal.

**Example:** Mycostatin vag supp ī̄. Insert each AM.

■ *Parenteral*

Fluids or medications given by injection or intravenously.

a. *Intradermal*

Injected between two skin layers. These injections are principally for diagnostic testing.

**Example:** PPD intermediate today. PPD (purified protein derivative) is a tuberculin skin test order. The word "intermediate" indicates the strength of the drug.

b. *Subcutaneous (SC)*

The medication is injected with a syringe under the skin into the fat or connective tissue.

**Example:** heparin 5000 U SC stat.

c. *Intramuscular (IM)*

The medication is injected directly into the muscle (Fig. 13–4).

d. *Intravenous*

i. *Intravenous push (IV push)*—a method of infusing a concentrated dose of medication, commonly called a bolus, that is effective within 1 to 5 minutes. Medication given by IV push can be given by direct penetration of

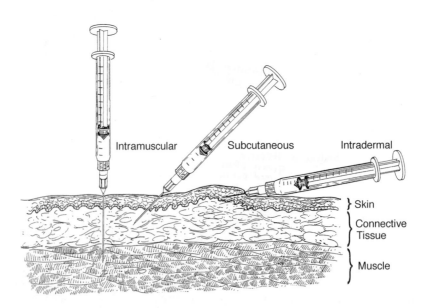

F I G U R E 13–4 • Angle of needle insertion for parenteral injections.

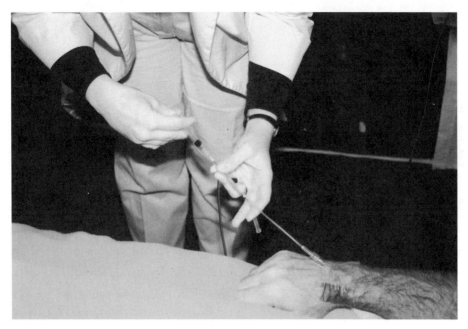

FIGURE 13-5 • Intravenous push (IV push).

a vein or using the low injection port on the primary administration set (Fig. 13–5).

**Example:** *Lanoxin 0.125 mg IV push stat.*

In the example above Lanoxin 0.125 mg is the bolus and IV push is the route of administration.

ii. *Intravenous piggyback (IVPB)*—IVPB is a method of intermittent infusion of medication that has been diluted in 50 to 100 cc of a commercially prepared solution and infused over 30 to 60 minutes through an established IV line (Fig. 13–6). The medication concentration in the IVPB is lower than the medication concentration in the IV push and is administered over a longer period of time.

**Example:** *Keflin 0.5 g IVPB q6h.*

iii. *Admixture*—Admixture is the process of combining one or more medications in a large volume of fluid and infusing it over a prescribed period of time. ~~potassium chloride~~

**Example:** *1000 cc D5W c̄ 20 mEq of KCL TRA 125 cc/h.*

iv. *Heparin lock*—A device used for intermittent intravenous infusion of medication, also used to maintain patent venous access for the infusion of medications in an emergency (see Fig. 11–11). ~~Saline a Heparin given after med put in. Keep open~~

**Example:** *Ampicillin 500 mg q6h via heplock (intermittent); Hyperstat 100 mg via hep lock for diastolic BP > than 100 (emergency).*

### ■ Total parenteral nutrition

Total parenteral nutrition (TPN) or intravenous hyperalimentation is the process of intravenously infusing carbohydrates, proteins, fats, water, electrolytes, vitamins, and minerals. These nutrients are infused through a catheter that is placed directly into a large central vein and advanced into the superior vena cava. The veins most often

used are the jugular and the subclavian veins. It is common procedure for providing nutrients to patients who are unable to receive food via the digestive tract. Some diseases that require TPN intervention are ileitis, bowel obstructions, massive burns, and severe anorexia. Patients receiving TPN require frequent (daily) blood tests for electrolyte and lipid levels.

Total parenteral nutrition is usually a long-term therapy and is administered through central venous catheters (see Chapter 11, p. 186) that are designed for long-term use. Some common types of long-term central venous catheters are Hickman, Boviac, Groshong, and Port-A-Cath. The type of catheter used is dependent on the length of treatment (refer to Chapter 11 for types of catheters). Insertion of a central catheter requires an informal consent and is surgically inserted under local anesthesia and sterile conditions.

The complex composition of TPN solution requires a written doctors' order and is prepared by the pharmacist under sterile conditions using a laminar flow hood. The solution is kept refrigerated until 30 to 40 minutes before infusion. The infusion rate is controlled by an infusion pump and is often referred to as an I-Med (Fig. 13–7). The infusion of TPN is closely monitored by the nurse, since fluid overload is a serious complication for the patient receiving fluids via central venous access. Other complications that may develop are infections, phlebitis, thrombosis, electrolyte imbalance, hyperglycemia, and mechanical trauma to the heart. The nurse will assess the patient for change in status and he or she will use strict aseptic technique when changing dressings, and when handling the administration equipment and solutions.

The order for TPN is a preprinted form that is filled in by the physician (Fig. 13–8). This form takes the place of the regular physicians' order form and a copy is sent to the pharmacy. Because of the length and complexity of the

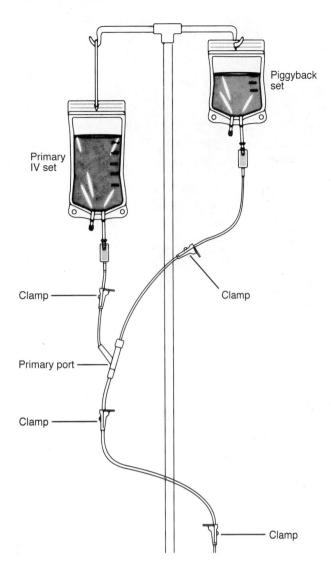

**F I G U R E  13–6** • An intravenous set with piggyback bags.

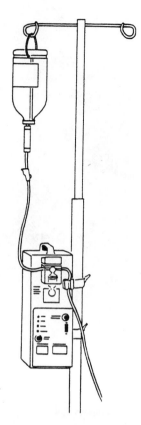

**F I G U R E  13–7** • Example of an intravenous infusion pump. (From deWit Susan C.: *Rambo's Nursing Skills for Clinical Practice*, 4th ed. Philadelphia, W.B. Saunders Co, 1994, with permission.)

TPN order many hospitals transcribe only the date, TPN with rate, and check chart on the medication administration record. The same notation is made on the Kardex form under nutrition heading. When the TPN solution is delivered from the pharmacy, the registered nurse will check it against the physicians' order on the preprinted form. Many times the physician will use the regular physicians' order form to make small changes in the composition of the original order. You must discontinue the original order on the MAR and on the Kardex form and rewrite the order by again noting as above.

**HIGHLIGHT**

Any change in the TPN order must be immediately sent to the pharmacy. The TPN solution is very expensive and is wasted if there is any change in the formula after it has been prepared.

■

## Component Four—Frequency of Administration

Each hospital maintains a schedule of hours for administration of medications. These schedules are set up by the hospital nursing service, and you are required to learn the hours that are standard for your hospital.

Table 13–1 lists examples of time frequencies used to administer medication. Remember that this varies among hospitals. Also, military time may be used in place of standard time. Review military time in Chapter 8. If the schedule does not coincide with the schedule at your hospital, write in the times you will be using.

*Note:* Standard prn orders are never assigned a time, because the drugs are administered as they are needed by the patient.

## Component Five—Qualifying Phrases

There are times when the doctor may wish the drug to be administered only for specific conditions. He or she then includes a phrase to this effect as the fifth part of the medication order. Not all orders contain qualifying phrases; however, when included, they are an important part of the order. Some phrases you may see commonly used are:

# ADULT TPN ORDER FORM

| | Custom | Standard Central | Standard Peripheral |
|---|---|---|---|
| | ☐ | ☐ | ☐ |

**BASE SOLUTION** *amino acids*

| | Custom | Standard Central | Standard Peripheral |
|---|---|---|---|
| gm AA (60-120/d : 4 cal/gm : 10 gm/100 ml) . . . . . . . . . . . . . . . . . | _____gm | 50gm/L | 30gm/L |
| gm Dextrose (200-700/d : 3.4 cal/gm : 70 gm/100 ml) . . . . . . . . . . | _____gm | 200gm/L | 75gm/L |
| gm Lipid (0-100/d : 9 cal/gm : 20 gm/100 ml) . . . . . . . . . . . . . . . . | _____gm | | 40gm/L |

**ADDITIVES**

| | Custom | Standard Central | Standard Peripheral |
|---|---|---|---|
| meq NaCl (60-150/d) . . . . . . . . . . . . . . . . . . . . . . . . . . . . . . . . . | _____/bag | 35/L or ____/L | 35/L or ____/L |
| meq NaAcetate . . . . . . . . . . . . . . . . . . . . . . . . . . . . . . . . . . . . . | _____/bag | _____/L | _____/L |
| meq KCl (30-100/d) . . . . . . . . . . . . . . . . . . . . . . . . . . . . . . . . . . | _____/bag | _____/L | _____/L |
| meq KAcetate . . . . . . . . . . . . . . . . . . . . . . . . . . . . . . . . . . . . . . | _____/bag | 20/L or ____/L | 20/L or ____/L |
| meq KPO4 (15-40/d) . . . . . . . . . . . . . . . . . . . . . . . . . . . . . . . . . | _____/bag | 15/L or ____/L | 15/L or ____/L |
| meq NaPO4 . . . . . . . . . . . . . . . . . . . . . . . . . . . . . . . . . . . . . . . . | _____/bag | _____/L | _____/L |
| meq CaGluconate (9-18/d) . . . . . . . . . . . . . . . . . . . . . . . . . . . . . | _____/bag | 4.5/L or ____/L | 4.5/L or ____/L |
| meq MgSO4 (5-15/d) . . . . . . . . . . . . . . . . . . . . . . . . . . . . . . . . . | _____/bag | 5/L or _____/L | 5/L or _____/L |
| mg ZnSO4 . . . . . . . . . . . . . . . . . . . . . . . . . . . . . . . . . . . . . . . . . | _____/bag | _____/L | _____/L |
| Multivitamin-12 . . . . . . . . . . . . . . . . . . . . . . . . . . . . . . . . . . . . . | _____/bag | Standard | Standard |
| Trace Elements (Zn, Cu, Mn, Cr) . . . . . . . . . . . . . . . . . . . . . . . . . | _____/bag | Standard | Standard |
| *meq* Human Insulin R . . *always IV* . . . . . . . . . . . . . . . . . . . . . . . | _____/bag | _____/L | _____/L |
| Other: _____ | _____ | _____/L | _____/L |
| Other: _____ | _____ | _____/L | _____/L |
| Other: _____ | _____ | _____/L | _____/L |
| **FINAL VOLUME** to be infused over 24 hours . . . . . . . . . . . . . . . . | _____ | _____ | _____ |
| **RATE** ml/hr . . . . . . . . . . . . . . . . . . . . . . . . . . . . . . . . . . . . . . . | _____ | _____ | _____ |

_____ ml Iron Dextran/wk (0.5 ml = 25 mg Fe+ + q wk; incompatible with lipid-containing solutions. Lipids will be omitted from
solution on the day iron is administered.)
_____ mg Vitamin K/wk (5 mg q wk)

IVPB Lipids _____ ml _____% Lipid q _____ . Run over _____ hrs.

**LABORATORY**
Daily: _____ Electrolytes _____ BUN _____ Creat _____ Glucose _____ CBC
Q Mon & Thurs: _____ SMA-20 _____Mg+ + _____ CBC
Q Week: _____ Protime _____Platelets
Other: _____
Other: _____
Other: _____

_____ Fingerstick glucose q _____ hrs.               Weight q _____

**SLIDING SCALE:**

| Glucose | Sub Q Human Insulin R |
|---|---|
| Less than 80 mg% | Call M.D. |
| 80 - 150 mg% | _____ units |
| 151 - 200 mg% | _____ units |
| 201 - 250 mg% | _____ units |
| 251 - 300 mg% | _____ units |
| 301 - 350 mg% | _____ units |
| Greater than 350 mg% | Call M.D. |

Sign. _____

Date _____ Time _____

Phone or pager _____

**IV Pharmacy Phone: X4557**

**ADULT TPN ORDER FORM**

00-2401 REV. (8/91)

F I G U R E   13–8 • Total parenteral nutrition order form.

| TABLE 13–1 | Medication Time Schedule | | |
|---|---|---|---|
| Time Symbols | Meaning | Time Schedule | Military Time |
| qd | Once a day | 9:00 AM | 0900 |
| | | (5:00 PM [daily] for anticoagulants—to allow for results of prothrombin time) | 1700 |
| | | (7:30 AM [daily] for insulin, which must be administered before breakfast) | 0730 |
| bid | Two times a day during waking hours | 9:00 AM and 5:00 PM (9-5) | 0900—1700 |
| tid | Three times a day during waking hours | 9:00 AM—1:00 PM—5:00 PM (9-1-5) | 0900—1300—1700 |
| qid | Four times a day during waking hours | 9:00 AM—1:00 PM—5:00 PM—9:00 PM (9-1-5-9) | 0900—1300—1700—2100 |
| ac | One-half hour before meals. This varies according to when food cart arrives on unit. | | |
| pc | One-half hour after meals. This varies according to when food cart arrives on unit. | | |
| q3h | Every 3 hours | 9:00 AM—12:00 Noon—3:00 PM—6:00 PM—9:00 PM—12:00 Mid—3:00 AM—6:00 AM (9-12-3-6-9-12-3-6) | 0900—1200—1500—1800—2100—0300—2400—0600 |
| q4h | Every 4 hours | 9:00 AM—1:00 PM—5:00 PM—9:00 PM—1:00 AM—5:00 AM (9-1-5-9-1-5) | 0900—1300—1700—2100—0100—0500 |
| q6h | Every 6 hours | 9:00 AM—3:00 PM—9:00 PM—3:00 AM (9-3-9-3) | 0900—1500—2100–0300 |
| q8h | Every 8 hours | 9:00 AM—5:00 PM—9:00 AM (9-5-1) | 0900—1700—0100 |
| q12h | Every 12 hours | 9:00 AM—9:00 PM (9-9) | 0900—2100 |

- For severe pain
- For stomach spasms
- For N/V
- While awake only
- For insomnia

## Examples of Doctors' Orders with a Qualifying Phrase

1. Demerol 75 mg IM q3h prn severe pain

2. Torecan supp q4h for NV

3. Cēpacol lozenges 1̄ q3h prn sore throat

## Exercises for Components of a Medication Order

It is necessary for the health unit coordinator to identify the parts of a medication order quickly, in order to recognize whether the order is complete, and to transcribe it correctly. The following exercise provides you with practice for this task.

EXERCISE 6

Following the example below and using the numbers to indicate each part of a medication order, complete the following exercise.

**Example:**

| Demerol | 50 mg | IM | q4h prn | for severe pain |
|---|---|---|---|---|
| 1 | 2 | 3 | 4 | 5 |

1. List the five parts of a medication order in consecutive order as used in the example above.

   a. 1 _Name_

   b. 2 _dose_

   c. 3 _route_

   d. 4 _Frequency of administration_

   e. 5 _Qualifying phrase_

2. Identify each component of the medication orders below by writing the number of the component below the component part, as shown in the preceding example.

   a. Compazine /10 mg /IM /stat
   
   b. Sodium phenobarbital /gr 1̄1̄ /IM /q3–4h /prn /restlessness

   c. Librium /5 mg /PO /tid & hs

   d. Seconal /100 mg /PO /hs prn

   e. Lomotil /1̄ /PO /after each loose stool

   f. Percodan /Tabs 1̄ /q4h /prn /severe pain

g. *Lente Insulin 25 U/qd*

h. *procaine penicillin 600,000 U/IM/q8h*

i. *Dramamine/50 mg/IM/q4h prn/N/V*

j. *ASA/supp/gr x̄/q3h/ for temp ↑ 102^R*

## E X E R C I S E  7

Test your knowledge of material covered thus far by completing the following exercise. Below you will find a list of doctors' orders for medications written as they would be spoken. Rewrite the orders as they would be written using abbreviations where needed, and use the correct form for the apothecary and metric systems.

**Example:**
Demerol fifty milligrams intramuscularly every four hours whenever necessary for severe pain.

Answer: *Demerol 50 mg IM q4h prn severe pain.*

1. Aspirin grains ten by mouth every four hours when necessary for pain.

   *ASA gr X PO q4h PRN Pain*

2. Ampicillin two hundred fifty milligrams by mouth four times a day.

   *Ampicillin 250 mg PO Qid*

3. Penicillin one million six hundred thousand units intramuscularly every twelve hours.

   *PCN 1,600,000 units IM Q 12 hrs*

4. Nembutal one hundred milligrams at bedtime if necessary for sleep.

   *Nembutal 100 mg hs PRN sleep*

5. Donnatal elixir four milliliters by mouth three times a day before meals.

   *Donnatal elixer 4 mL PO Tid ac*

6. Belladonna and opium suppositories grains one every three to four hours when necessary for rectal spasms.

   *B & O*
   *Belladonna/opium sppp gr I q 3 to 4 hrs PRN Rectal spasm*

7. Neo-Synephrine ophthalmic 10% drops two in right eye twice a day.

   *NeoSynephrine opthalmic 10% gtts II OD Bid*

8. Benadryl fifty milligrams by mouth immediately.

   *Benadryl 50 mg PO stat*

9. Equanil four hundred milligrams by mouth twice a day and at bedtime.

   *Equanil 400 mg PO bid & hs*

10. Coumadin five milligrams by mouth daily.

    *Coumadin 5 mg PO qd*

## CATEGORIES OF DOCTORS' ORDERS RELATED TO MEDICATION ORDERS

Categories of doctors' orders are especially relevant to medication orders. For example, a standing medication order must have times assigned on the medication administration record or medication Kardex form, whereas the standing prn order does not have times assigned. To review, read "Categories of Doctors' Orders," Chapter 9, then read and complete the following unit.

### Standing Orders

Fill in the definition below:

A standing order is _executed as ordered_ _until discontinued by doctor or changed_

### Examples of Standing Medication Orders

■ *Lente Insulin U40 qd*
This medication is administered one time each day, such as 7:30 AM, until discontinued by the doctor.

■ *Penicilin 600,000 U IM q6h*
This medication is administered every 6 hours, such as 9:00 AM, 3:00 PM, 9:00 PM, 3:00 AM until discontinued by the doctor.

■ *Vitamin B₁₂ 1000 µg IM twice a week*
This medication is to be administered twice a week, such as Monday and Thursday at 9:00 AM, until discontinued by the doctor.

+-----------------------------------+
|        T O  T H E  S T U D E N T  |
+-----------------------------------+

To practice transcribing standing medication orders, complete **Activity 13–1** in the Skills Practice Manual.

### Standing PRN Orders

Fill in the definition below:

A standing PRN order is _executed as needed until doctor discontinues_

### Examples of Standing PRN Orders

■ *MS 10 mg IM q4h prn severe pain*
The morphine sulfate may not be given to the patient more often than every 4 hours and then only if needed. In a prn order it is impossible to set up a time sequence.

■ *MOM 30 mL hs prn constipation*
Milk of magnesia, a laxative, is given as needed, usually when the patient communicates to the nurse that he or she is constipated. This order is in effect until discontinued by the doctor. Laxatives are usually administered at bedtime.

- *Vistaril 25 mg IM q3h prn restlessness*

Vistaril may not be given more often than every 3 hours, and only if the patient exhibits restlessness.

---

**TO THE STUDENT**

To practice transcribing standing prn medication orders, complete **Activity 13–2** in the Skills Practice Manual.

---

## One-Time or Short-Series Order

Fill in the definition below:

A one-time or short-series order is __executed__ __immediatly then automatically discontinued__

## Examples of One-Time or Short-Series Order Medication Orders

- *Procaine penicillin 600,000 U IM @ 6 PM today and 6 AM tomorrow*

This medication is given at the two times ordered and then discontinued.

- *Compazine 10 mg IM to be given 1 h before cobalt therapy tomorrow*

This medication is to be administered 1 hour before the patient is sent for cobalt radiation therapy tomorrow, and then the order is discontinued.

- *Give Dulcolax supp tonight*

This medication is to be administered the evening the order was written; then it is discontinued.

---

**TO THE STUDENT**

To practice transcribing one-time medication orders, complete **Activity 13–3** in the Skills Practice Manual.

To practice transcribing short-series order medication orders, complete **Activity 13–4** in the Skills Practice Manual.

---

## Stat Orders

Fill in the definition below.

A stat order is __an order given__ __immediatly then discontinued__

## Examples of Stat Orders

- *Heparin 20,000μ IV push stat*

This order indicates that the heparin should be given immediately. The order then is to be discontinued.

- *Achromycin 500 mg PO stat and q6h*

This medication order is in two parts. The first part calls for the antibiotic Achromycin to be given immediately.

Part 2 of this order contains a standing order for the medication to be given four times a day, such as 9:00 AM, 3:00 PM, 9:00 PM, 3:00 AM. The standing order remains in effect until the doctor discontinues it.

## Communication of Stat Medication Orders

The medication must be ordered immediately from the pharmacy by pharmacy copy, or by the computer. Communicate the medication order to the medication nurse verbally. The medication nurse must then review the order directly from the doctors' order sheet.

---

**TO THE STUDENT**

To practice transcribing and communicating stat medication orders, complete **Activity 13–5** in the Skills Practice Manual.

---

## CONTROLLED SUBSTANCES

In 1971, the Controlled Substances Act updated previous laws that regulated the manufacture, sale, and dispensing of narcotics and drugs having potential for abuse. These drugs are referred to as controlled drugs or controlled substances. **Controlled substances** are classified into five classes, or **schedules**. Each of these classes differs according to its potential for abuse and therefore are controlled to different degrees. The U.S. attorney general has the authority to reschedule the class in which a drug is placed, remove a substance from the controlled list, or assign an unscheduled drug to a controlled category. Therefore, the drugs in particular classes are subject to change. Examples of scheduled drugs follow.

### Schedule I

This group has such a high potential for abuse that they usually are nonexistent in a health care setting except for specific, approved research. Examples are heroin, marijuana, and LSD.

### Schedule II

This group has a high potential for abuse and may lead to severe physical or psychologic dependence. Examples are Percodan, morphine, meperidine (Demerol), amphetamines, codeine, Dilaudid, and cocaine.

### Schedule III

There is moderate or low potential for abuse in this group. Examples are Tylenol with codeine, Phenaphen with codeine, Doriden, Fiorinal, Butisol, Percogesic with codeine, and paregoric.

## Schedule IV

The potential for abuse is lower in this class than in schedule III. Examples are Talwin, Valium, meprobamate, Noctec, Equagesic, and Centrax.

## Schedule V

The abuse potential of these drugs is limited. Examples are Actifed with codeine, Lomotil, Phenergan with codeine, and Triaminic Expectorant with codeine.

As dispensers of controlled substances for medicinal purposes, hospital pharmacies are required to be registered with the Drug Enforcement Administration, which mandates that records be maintained on certain drugs (Fig. 13–9).

Controlled drugs must be kept in a locked cupboard or medication cart on the nursing unit, both because of the potential for theft and because the law requires it. A nurse carries the key to the locked cupboard. If the medication cart is computerized, an ID and password may be utilized to unlock the cart.

Each time a medication from the locked cupboard or cart is given, the nurse who administers the medication is responsible for writing the required information on the disposition sheet. Each drug and each dosage of the drug requires the use of a separate disposition sheet. When the disposition sheet is completed, it is returned to the pharmacy.

Replacement of the drugs in the cupboard or cart is usually under the direction and supervision of pharmacy personnel who deliver the drugs in person to the nursing unit and in return receive a signed delivery slip from the nurse who accepts the drugs. The computerized cart keeps track of the number of medications given, to whom they were given, and the name of the nurse removing the drug.

Technology in some hospitals allows controlled, regularly scheduled, and prn medications to be computer dispensed. The pharmacist receives the doctors' orders by one of the three methods of ordering from the pharmacy department. Using the doctors' orders the pharmacist will then load the computer system with that patient's medication, usually for a 24-hour period.

Each nurse has a password that will allow him or her to access the system. The nurse must input the patient's name, doctor's name, and the drug along with the dosage. The drug will then drop into a receptacle, similar to purchasing a candy bar from a vending machine. Dispensing medication by the computer method significantly decreases medication errors because the system will not dispense the drug if there is a discrepancy in the patient's orders and the drug requisitioned by the nurse.

Two advantages of using the computer dispensing method are a decreased number of errors in medication administration and an increased accuracy in accounting and billing. One disadvantage in this system is that drugs that need to be refrigerated and drugs in breakable containers cannot be loaded into the system. Another disadvantage is that all new and changed medication orders written after the system has been loaded will have to be handled in the regular fashion. The computer system works best on nursing units where changes in orders are not frequent. You are not likely to see the computerized system on intensive care units at this time.

Medications that fall in the category of controlled drugs have an automatic stop date. An **automatic stop date** means that after a certain period, for example 72 hours, the drug may no longer be given to the patient unless renewed by a written doctor's order. Controlled substances usually have a 72-hour limit. Each health care facility develops its own list of automatic stop date drugs.

Although other types of drugs are included under the heading "controlled substances," narcotics and hypnotics probably are the most frequently used.

## DRUG GROUPS

The following are the most commonly used drugs that you will transcribe and order from the pharmacy. The drugs are in specific groups according to function or use, and are listed by their trade names. Generic drugs that are frequently ordered appear in brackets. There are many more drug groups and more drugs in each group than we are able to address in this introduction to drug groups. The asterisk (*) identifies the drugs most often ordered.

## Narcotics

**Narcotics** are ordered to relieve pain. All narcotics have an automatic stop date.

*Codeine
*Demerol (meperidine)
Innovar
*MS Contin
*Morphine sulfate
Pentanyl (oral transmucosal fentanyl citrate: OTFC)
*Percocet
*Percodan
Percodan-demi
Sublimaze
*Vicodin
Cocaine

## Analgesics with Narcotics

Empirin with codeine #1, #2, #3, #4
Fiorinal with codeine #3
Phenaphen with codeine #2, #3, #4

Numbers are assigned to analgesics containing codeine to differentiate the amount of codeine found in the medications. The numbers mean:

#1 contains gr 1/8 (8 mg) codeine
#2 contains gr 1/4 (15 mg) codeine

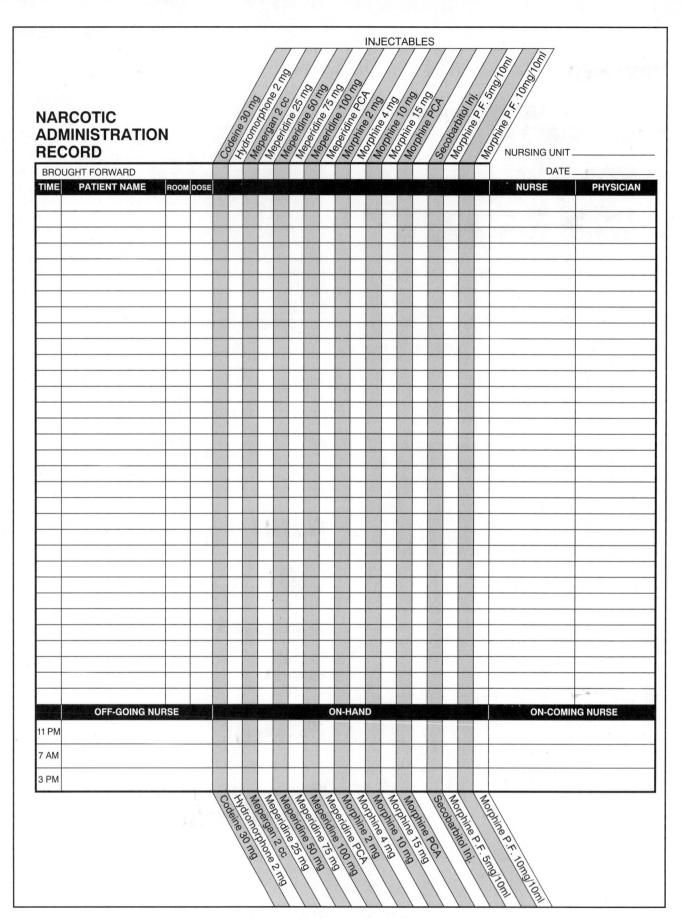

FIGURE 13–9 • Controlled-drug disposition sheet.

#3 contains gr 1/2 (30 mg) codeine
#4 contains gr 1 (60 mg) codeine

## Patient-Controlled Analgesia

**Patient-controlled analgesia (PCA)** allows the client, in some situations, to self-administer small doses of narcotics intravenously. A special IV infusion pump is used (Fig. 13–7). The physician orders the amount of individual doses, the frequency of delivery, and the total dose permitted within a certain period. The nurse fills the infusion pump with the narcotic. An internal system within the PCA unit is programmed and does not permit the patient to overdose or self-administer the medication too frequently. The most common narcotics used in PCA systems are meperidine and morphine. Some conditions for patients using PCAs are severe postoperative pain or the chronic pain of a terminal illness.

## Hypnotics

**Hypnotics** are ordered to induce sleep. All hypnotics have an automatic stop date.

— sleeping pill

Ambien
*Dalmane
Doriden
Halcion (triazolam)
*Nembutal
*Noctec (chloral hydrate)
Noludar
Placidyl
*Restoril
Seconal
Valmid

> **TO THE STUDENT**
>
> To practice transcribing orders for medications with automatic stop dates, complete **Activity 13–6** in the Skills Practice Manual.

## Antianxiety Agents, or Tranquilizers

**Antianxiety agents** are used to relieve tension and anxiety.

*Atarax
*Ativan
BuSpar
*Equagesic (meprobamate with aspirin); *Equanil, Miltown (meprobamate)
*Librium
Serax
Tranxene
*Valium (diazepam)
*Xanax

## Antibiotics

**Antibiotics** are drugs used primarily to treat infection and infectious diseases. They usually have an *automatic stop date*.

*Note*: Many antibiotic names end in *-cillin*, *-statin*, or *-mycin*; this makes identification easier.

Achromycin (*tetracycline); Achromycin V (tetracyline hydrochloride)
Amikin (amikacin)
*Amoxicillin
Amoxil
Ampicillin
Ancef, Kefzol (cefazolin)
Augmentin (amoxicillin trihydrate and clavulanic acid)
Biaxin
*Bicillin
*Ceclor
Cefadyl
Ceftin
*Cipro
Cleocin
Doryx
Duricef
E.E.S., E-Mycin, Ilotycin, (*erythromycin)
*Erythrocin (erythromycin stearate)
*Flagyl (metronidazole)
Floxin
Fortax
Fulvicin
Fungizone (amphotericin B)
*Garamycin (gentamicin)
Geocillin
Geopen
*Ilosone (erythromycin estolate)
kanamycin
Kantrex
*Keflex, Keftab (cephalexin)
*Keflin (cephalothin)
Mefoxin
Neomycin
Noroxin
Panmycin, *Tetrex (tetracycline phosphate)
PCE (an erythromycin base)
*penicillin
Polycillin, Omnipen (*ampicillin)
Primaxin
*Prostaphlin
Staphcillin
Sumycin
Suprax
*Terramycin
tobramycin
Trimox
Unipen
Urobiotic
Vibramycin
Wycillin (procaine penicillin)
Zefazone

### Urinary Antibiotics

These drugs destroy pathogenic microorganisms in the urinary tract.

Azo Gantanol
Azo Gantrisin
*Bactrim, Septra, Gantanol (sulfamethoxazole)
Cirpo
Furadantin
Gastrisin
Macrodantin
Mandelamine
Noroxin
*NegGram

---

**TO THE STUDENT**

To practice transcribing IV medication orders, complete **Activity 13–7** in the Skills Practice Manual.

## Analgesics—Nonnarcotic

**Analgesics** are drugs that relieve or lessen pain. Analgesics *may* have automatic stop dates.

*Advil, Nuprin, Motrin (ibuprofen)
Ascriptin, Bufferin, Ecotrin (enteric-coated aspirin),
    Anacin (aspirin)
Anaprox
Darvon, *Darvon compound (propoxyphene
    hydrochloride)
*Empirin
Fiorinal
Norgesic
Percogesic
Talwin
*Tylenol, Panadol (acetaminophen)

## Antacids

**Antacids** are drugs used to counteract gastric acidity.

AlternaGel, Aludrox, Amphojel (aluminum hydroxide)
Basalgel
*Gaviscon
Gelusil
*Maalox
*Mylanta
*Riopan
Titralac

## Anticonvulsants

**Anticonvulsants** are drugs that prevent or relieve convulsions.

Depakote
Dilantin (phenytoin)
Mysoline (primidone)
phenobarbital
Tegretol

---

**HIGHLIGHT**

List Of Drugs You Need To Know To Meet Objective #11

| Narcotics | Hypnotics | Antianxiety Agents or Tranquilizers |
|---|---|---|
| codeine | Dalmane | Atarax |
| Demerol | Nembutal | Ativan |
| morphine sulfate | Noctec | Librium |
| Percocet | Restoril | Valium |
| Vicodin | | Xanax |

| Antibiotics | Urinary Antibiotics | Analgesics-Nonnarcotic |
|---|---|---|
| amoxicillin | Bactrim | Advil |
| amoxil | NegGram | Empirin |
| Biaxin | | Tylenol |
| Cipro | | |
| Duricef | | |
| Erythrocin | | |
| Garamycin | | |
| Keflex | | |
| penicillin | | |
| Staphcillin | | |
| Sumycin | | |
| Terramycin | | |
| Trimox | | |
| Bicillin | | |
| Ceclor | | |
| Flagyl | | |

## Antidepressants

**Antidepressants** are drugs that relieve depression.

Aventyl, Pamelor (nortriptyline)
*Desyrel
Effexor
*Elavil
Ludiomil
Marplan
Nardil
Norpramin, Pertofrane (desipramine)
Pamelor
Paxil
*Prozac
Serzone
Sinequan (doxepin)
Tofranil
Triavil
Vivactil
Welbutrin
*Zoloft

## Antidiabetics or Hypoglycemics

**Antidiabetics**, or **hypoglycemics** are given to lower blood sugar and are ordered for the diabetic patient.

### Standing Order for Insulin

A standing order for insulin to be administered once a day is commonly scheduled to be given 1/2 h a.c. breakfast. Also, if the doctor is normalizing the amount of insulin required by the patient, the doctor may order insulin to be given on a sliding scale.

**Sliding-Scale Insulin Orders.** The amount of sliding-scale insulin given is dependent upon the results obtained from blood glucose monitoring.

---

**EXAMPLE OF SLIDING-SCALE ORDER**

Using Accu-Check (blood glucose monitoring)

| Blood Sugar Level | Dosage or Action |
|---|---|
| 200–249 | 5 U regular insulin |
| 250–299 | 10 U regular insulin |
| 300–349 | 15 U regular insulin |
| >350 | Call house officer |

---

This insulin may be given in addition to the daily insulin order the doctor has prescribed. Not all diabetic patients have sliding-scale orders.

### Oral Hypoglycemics

*DiaBeta (glyburide)
Diabinese chlorpropamide)
Dymelor
*Glucotrol (glipizide)
*glyburide
Micronase
Orinase (tolbutamide)
Tolinase (tolazimide)

### Subcutaneous Antidiabetics

Humalog
Humulin N, Humulin R, Mixtard, Novolin N (human insulin)
Iletin, Lente
Iletin, NPH
Iletin, Semilente
insulin, regular
insulin, Lente
insulin, Semilente
Isophene insulin (NPH)
Novolin L
Protamine Zinc & Iletin (PZI)
*70/30 insulin (70% NPH and 30% regular insulin)

## Antianemic Agents

**Antianemic drugs** are ordered to build iron in the blood.

Feosol
Fergon
Ferro-Sequels
*ferrous sulfate
folic acid
Imferon
vitamin $B_{12}$

---

**HIGHLIGHT**

List Of Drugs You Need To Know To Meet Objective #11

| Antacids | Anticonvulsants | Antidepressants |
|---|---|---|
| Gaviscon | Depakote | Desyrel |
| Maalox | Dilantin | Elavil |
| Mylanta | phenobarbital | Prozac |
| Riopan | Tegretol | Zoloft |
| Oral Hypoglycemics | Subcutaneous Antidiabetics | Antianemic |
| Glucotrol (glyburide) | insulin, regular insulin, Lente | ferrous sulfate |
| Glyburide | 70/30 insulin | |
| Orinase | (70% NPH and | |
| DiaBeta (glyburide) | 30% regular insulin) | |

---

## Antidiarrheal Drugs

**Antidiarrheal drugs** are drugs that lessen or stop diarrhea.

Donnagel P.G. (atropine sulfate and paregoric)
Donnatal
Lomotil (atropine sulfate)
*Imodium
Kaopectate

## Antihistamines

**Antihistamines** are drugs that prevent or relieve allergic reactions.

Actifed
*Benadryl
Chlor-Trimeton
*Claritin
Dimetane
*Hismanal
Ornade
Periactin
Pyribenzamine

*Seldane
Tavist
Teldrin
Triaminic preparations
Tussionex

## Antiinflammatory Drugs

Antiinflammatory drugs are used to reduce inflammation and relieve pain. They are most commonly used in arthritis and arthritis-like conditions. These drugs are divided into two groups, steroidal and nonsteroidal antiinflammatory drugs (NSAIDs).

### Steroids

Celestone
Cortef
Decadron
Deltasone
Kenalog
prednisolone
*prednisone

### NSAIDs

Anaprox
Ansaid
*Clinoril
Feldene
Indocin
Lodine
*Motrin
*Naprosyn
Orudis
Relafen
Tandearil
Toradol
Voltaren

## Antinauseants

**Antinauseants** are drugs that lessen or help prevent nausea.

Antivert, Bonine (meclizine)
*Compazine (prochlorperazine)
Dramamine (dimenhydrinate)
Emete-Con
*Phenergan
Thorazine
*Tigan
Torecan (thiethylperazine maleate)
Trilafon
Vistaril
*Zofran

## Antineoplastics (Chemotherapy)

**Antineoplastic drugs** are used in the treatment of cancer.

Cisplatin
*Cytoxan
*Fluorouracil
interferon
Leukeran
*methotrexate
Myleran
Oncovin (vincristine)
Paraplatin
thioguanine
Thiotepa
Vinblastine

---

**H I G H L I G H T**

List Of Drugs You Need To Know To Meet Objective #11

| Antidiarrheals | Antihistamines | Antinauseants |
|---|---|---|
| Lomotil | Benadryl | Compazine |
| Kaopectate | Claritin | Phenergan |
| Imodium | Hismanal | Tigan |
| | Seldane | Zofran |
| Antiinflammatory (steroids) | Antiinflammatory (NSAIDs) | Antineoplastics (Chemotherapy) |
| Decadron | Motrin | Cytoxan |
| prednisone | Naprosyn | Fluorouracil |
| | | Methotrexate |

---

## Antipsychotic Agents

**Antipsychotic agents** are used to relieve specific symptoms in psychotic disorders.

Clozaril
*Haldol (haloperidol)
*Mellaril
Navane
*Prolixin
*Risperdal
Serentil
Stelazine
*Thorazine
Lithobid

## Antispasmodics for Gastrointestinal Tract

**Antispasmodics** are drugs that prevent or relieve spasms of the gastrointestinal tract.

*Bentyl
*Donnatal
Librax
Milpath
Pro-Banthine
Robinul
Valpin

## Antiulcer Agents

**Antiulcer agents** are used to relieve ulcer symptoms through a specific chemical action. These drugs are not antacids

*Carafate (sucralfate)
*Cytotec
*Prilosec
Pepcid
*Tagamet (*cimetidine)
*Zantac (ranitidine)

## Cardiovascular Drugs

### Antihypertensives

Diuretics
Diuretics lower blood pressure by removing excess fluid from the body by stimulating the kidneys to secrete urine.

Accupril
Aldactazide
Aldactone (spironolactone)
Bumex
*Diuril (chlorothiazide)
Edecrin
Esidrix, HydroDiuril (hydrochlorothiazide [HCTZ])
*Lasix (furosemide)
Lozol
Maxzide, Dyazide, (hydrochlorothiazide and triamterene)
Metahydrin
Midamor
Proaqua

## Beta Blockers

Beta blockers lower blood pressure by decreasing the heart rate through blocking the absorption of adrenalin. Beta blockers are used not only for hypertension but also for adjusting the rhythm of the heart, to treat angina, and to dilate blood vessels.

Blocadren
Brevibloc (parenteral administration)
Cartrol
Corgard (nadolol)
*Inderal (propranolol)
Kerlone

Levatol
*Lopressor
Normodyne, Trandate (labetalol)
Sectral
Tenormin (atenolol)
Visken (pindolol)

## ACE Inhibitors

ACE inhibitors lower blood pressure by inhibiting angiotensin-converting enzyme (ACE) and are useful in the treatment of congestive heart failure.

*Capoten (captopril)
Monopril
*Prinivil, Zestril (lisinopril)
*Vasotec (enalapril)

## Calcium Channel Blockers

Calcium channel blockers lower blood pressure by blocking calcium and as a result relax the heart muscle and the muscles of the blood vessel walls.

*Calan, Isoptin (verapamil)
Cardene (nicardipine)
Cardizem (diltiazem)
*Procardia (nifedipine)

## Vasodilators

Vasodilators lower blood pressure by relaxing the blood vessel walls.

Apresoline
Cardilate
Hytrin
*Isordil (isosorbide dinitrate)
*Nitro-Bid, Nitro-Dur, Nitrostat, Transderm-Nitro (nitroglycerin)
Peritrate
Vasodilan

## Drugs for Hypertensive Emergencies

These drugs are used to lower blood pressure in crisis situations. They *may* have automatic stop dates.

Arfonad
*Dobutrex
*dopamine
*Hyperstat (diazoxide)
Nipride (sodium nitroprusside)

## Others

These group of medications used as antihypertensive agents do not all act through the same mechanism. They may or may not have automatic stop dates. Check with your facility pharmacy for clear directives.

*Aldomet (methyldopa)
Catapres
Ismelin (guanethidine)
*Minipress
Tenex
Wytensin (guanabene)

## Antiarrhythmics

**Antiarrhythmics** cause the heart to beat more rhythmically.

Adenocard
Bretylol
Cordarone
*Enkaid
Mexitil
Norpace
*Procan-SR, Pronestyl (*procainamide)
Quinidine
Tambocor
Xylocaine (*lidocaine)

## Anticoagulants

**Anticoagulants** slow the blood clotting process.

The physician may monitor the drug dosage of an anticoagulant. Laboratory tests called **PT** (prothrombin time) or **PTT** (partial thromboplastin time) may be ordered. The physician then orders, according to the results of the test, the amount of anticoagulant for the patient to receive that particular day. In this instance, the anticoagulant order is a one-time order. Anticoagulants also are ordered as standing orders. An anticoagulant record is a supplementary chart form added to the patient's chart. Anticoagulants frequently have automatic stop dates.

Anacin, Ascriptin, Bufferin (*aspirin)
*Coumadin (*warfarin)
*Dicumarol
Ecotrin (enteric coated aspirin)
*heparin
Liquamar
Lovenox

## Cardiotonics

**Cardiotonics** strengthen the forcefulness of the heartbeat, thereby slowing the heart rate. There may be facility or physician guidelines for the nurse to withhold the medication if the heart rate is less than a certain rate (e.g., 60 beats per minute). Be advised to identify the particular regulations regarding cardiotonic administration.

amrinone
*Crystodigin (*digitoxin)
Inocor
*Lanoxin (*digoxin)
Primacor

## Antilipemics (Cholesterol-Lowering Drugs)

**Antilipemics** reduce cholesterol formation.

*Atromid-S (clofibrate)
Cholybar, *Questran (cholestyramine resin)
Colestid
*Lopid
*Lorelco
*Mevacor
*niacin
*Zocor

## Hormones

**Hormones** are drugs that are given to replace grandular secretions that are lacking or to reduce inflammation.

Delestrogen
Hydrocortisone
Medrol (methylprednisolone)
Prednisone
Provera (medroxyprogesterone)
*Premarin
*Solu-Cortef
Solu-Medrol
Testrone (testosterone)

## Laxatives and Fecal Softeners

**Laxatives** produce or facilitate bowel movements.

*Colace, Doxinate (docusate sodium)
Dialose
Dialose Plus
Doxidan, Surfak (docusate calcium)
*Dulcolax
Metamucil
*milk of magnesia
mineral oil
Modane
Perdiem
Peri-Colace (docusate sodium and casanthranol)
Senokot

## Muscle Relaxants

**Muscle relaxants** reduce spasms in the muscles.

diazepam
Flexeril
Lioresal
Norflex
*Robaxin
*Soma (carisoprodol)

## Potassium Replacements

**Potassium replacements** replace potassium that has been lost because of the use of diuretics.

*Kaochlor, K-Lor, Klorvess, Micro K, Slow-K (potassium chloride)
*Kaon
K-Lyte (potassium bicarbonate)

<table>
<tr><th colspan="3">HIGHLIGHT</th></tr>
<tr><td colspan="3">List Of Drugs You Need To Know To Meet Objective #11</td></tr>
<tr><td>Anticoagulants</td><td>Antilipemics</td><td>Hormones</td></tr>
<tr><td>Coumadin<br>Dicumarol<br>heparin</td><td>Atromid<br>Lopid<br>Lorelco<br>Mevacor<br>niacin<br>Zocar</td><td>Premarin<br>Solu-Cortef</td></tr>
<tr><td>Laxatives<br>(Fecal Softeners)</td><td>Muscle<br>Relaxants</td><td>Potassium<br>Replacements</td></tr>
<tr><td>Colace<br>Dulcolax<br>Milk of magnesia</td><td>Lioresal<br>Robaxin<br>Soma</td><td>potassium<br>chloride<br>Kaon</td></tr>
</table>

## Respiratory Drugs

**Respiratory drugs** are used to treat pulmonary emphysema, asthma, congestive heart failure, and other respiratory conditions.

*Adrenalin, Sus-Phrine (epinephrine)
*Alupent
*aminophylline
*Atrovent
Brethine, Bricanyl (terbutaline)
*Bronkosol
Elixophyllin
Isuprel
Maxair Inhaler
*Proventil, Ventolin (albuterol)
*Slo-Phyllin, Theo-Dur (theophylline)
*Vanceril Inhaler

## Thyroid Preparations

**Thyroid drugs** are given for thyroid deficiency.

Armour thyroid
Cytomel
Proloid
*Synthroid

## Vitamins

**Vitamins** are organic substances found in food. Occasionally, the body becomes deficient in vitamins, especially during illness.

*Albee c̄ C
AquaMephyton

Berocca
Betalin
Folbesyn
Multicebrin
MVI
Optilets
*Solu B c̄ C
Stresstabs
Stuart Formula
Synkayvite
*Theragran
vitamin B$_{12}$

## Topical Medications

The following preparations are frequently ordered for the eye or the ear or to be applied to the skin.

### Ophthalmic Preparations (for the Eye)

Achromycin ophthalmic ointment
*Cortisporin ophthalmic ointment and suspension
Decadron phosphate ophthalmic ointment and solution
Garamycin ophthalmic ointment
*Neosporin ophthalmic ointment and solution
Polysporin ophthalmic ointment
Propine
Silver nitrate solution
*Timoptic ophthalmic solution
Tobrex

### Otic Preparations (for the Ear)

Auralgen otic solution
*Cortisporin otic solution
VoSol HC otic solution

### Topical Preparations (for the Skin)

Betadine spray
Cortisporin ointment
Furacin topical cream
Garamycin cream
Lotrisone
*Mycolog cream and ointment
*Mycostatin cream and ointment
*Neosporin ointment
*Silvadene cream    Burns

## COMMON DRUG DOSAGES

As the role of the health unit coordinator expands, more knowledge of medication dosages will be needed. The following list contains some frequently ordered medications and their usual adult dosages.

---

**HIGHLIGHT**

List Of Drugs You Need To Know To Meet Objective #11

| Respiratory Drugs | Thyroid Drugs | Vitamins |
|---|---|---|
| Adrenalin | Synthroid | Albee c C |
| Alupent | | Solu B c C |
| aminophylline | | Theragran |
| Atrovent | | |
| Bronkosol | | |
| Proventil | | |
| Slo-Phyllin | | |
| Vanceril | | |

| Ophthalmics | Otics | Topicals |
|---|---|---|
| Cortisporin ointment & suspension | Cortisporin solution | Mycolog Mycostatin Neosporin ointment |
| Neosporin ointment & solution | | |
| Timoptic | | |

---

aspirin: 325–650 mg
codeine: 15–60 mg
Coumadin: 2–10 mg
Dalmane: 30 mg
Demerol: 50–100 mg
Dilaudid: 2–4 mg
heparin: 5000 U
Keflin: 0.5–1.0 g
Lanoxin: 0.125–0.25 mg
morphine sulfate: 10–15 mg
Nembutal: 100 mg
Notec: 0.5 g
Seconal: 100 mg
Percocet: tab 1 or 2
Restoril: 15–20 mg
Tylenol: 325–650 mg

## REAGENTS USED FOR DIAGNOSTIC TESTS

The following diagnostic procedures are performed by the nursing staff. The supplies used to perform the tests are requisitioned from the pharmacy during the transcription procedure.

## Skin Tests

**Skin tests** are administered intradermally or intracutaneously for diagnostic purposes. Types and explanations of common skin tests are written below in the sample doctor's order.

## Doctors' Orders for Skin Tests

- *PPD inter today*

This is a screening test for tuberculosis. The test agent that is administered to the patient is *purified protein derivative (PPD)*. Inter (intermediate) is the dosage strength.

- *Cocci 1:100 now*

This is a diagnostic test for coccidioidomycosis (valley fever). The ratio 1:100 refers to the dilution of the test material. It may also be administered in a 1:10 dilution.

- *Histoplasmin 0.1 mL today*

This skin test is employed as an aid in diagnosing histoplasmosis, a fungal disease.

## MEDICATION STOCK SUPPLY

Hospitals store a supply of medications on nursing units. This supply is often called the medication stock supply, and it includes such drugs as aspirin, acetaminophen, mineral oil, and milk of magnesia. When floor stock medicines are ordered from the pharmacy, they are charged to the unit budget.

## RENEWAL MEDICATION ORDERS

Drugs such as *narcotics, hypnotics,* and other drugs controlled by federal or state laws have an automatic stop date. Hospital medical committees may also set automatic stop dates on *anticoagulants and antibiotics.* Thus, these drugs must be reordered by the doctor before or when the stop date is reached. Your instructor or hospital pharmacist may provide you with a list of medications that have an automatic stop date in your hospital and the number of hours the drugs may be in effect before reordering is necessary.

A renewal stamp is used by some hospitals to remind the doctor of the automatic stop date (Fig. 13–10). This stamp is placed on the doctors' order sheet by nursing personnel shortly before the order is due to expire, and when completed by the doctor, it is regarded as a new order and is transcribed as such. Where permitted, this date may require only changing the dates on the medication Kardex form or medication administration record.

If the doctor wishes to discontinue the medication that is to be renewed, he or she may indicate this by writing "No" on the renewal stamp or by not signing the renewal stamp. This automatically discontinues the medication.

## DISCONTINUING MEDICATION ORDERS

When a doctor discontinues a standing or standing prn order, he or she indicates this by writing an order on the doctors' order sheet.

**Example:** *DC Achromycin 500 mg PO tid*

Occasionally, a physician may order a medication that has the same purpose as another drug the patient is already receiving. For example, Nembutal, a sleeping medication, is ordered while the patient still has an order for Seconal, another sleeping medication. Before transcribing this order, the health unit coordinator should bring it to the nurse's attention. Usually, the second order takes precedence over the first, and the first medication is automatically discontinued. However, you may be asked to contact the doctor to clear up any discrepancy.

> ### TO THE STUDENT
> To practice renewing and discontinuing medication orders, complete **Activities 13–8** and **13–9** in the Skills Practice Manual

## MEDICATION ORDER CHANGES

The doctor may wish to change a patient's medication order for any number of reasons. The doctor may change the dosage, route of administration, and time frequency of a drug already ordered. Whenever this is done, it is considered a new order and should be written as such on the

DOCTOR, THE _____ *Narcotic* _____

HAS EXPIRED.                    **DO YOU**

WISH THE _____ *Demerol* _____

RENEWED?                        **THANK YOU.**

DR's. SIGNATURE _____ *Dr. Starr* _____

F I G U R E   13–10 • Drug renewal stamp.

medication administration record. It is illegal to erase or cross out parts of an order or to write over an order on the MAR because this is a record of what medication has been administered to the patient. This may result in a serious medication error. The old order must be discontinued according to the policy and the new order written. (See also Fig. 13–2 for discontinuing medication on the MAR.)

## Doctors' Orders for Medication Order Changes

■ *Change Demerol 50 mg IM q4h prn to Demerol 50 mg PO q4h prn*
Change in route of administration.

■ *Decrease ampicillin 500 mg PO qid to 250 mg PO qid*
Change in dosage.

■ *Change Librium 5 mg PO tid to 5 mg PO qid*
Change in frequency of administration.

### TO THE STUDENT

To practice transcribing medication order changes, complete **Activity 13–10** in the Skills Practice Manual.

To test your skill in transcribing a review set of medication orders, complete **Activity 13–11** in the Skills Practice Manual.

To test your skill in transcribing a review set of doctor's orders, complete **Activity 13–12** in the Skills Practice Manual.

To practice locating medications in the Physicians' Desk Reference, complete **Activity 13–13** in the Skills Practice Manual.

To practice recording doctor's orders and to practice recording telephoned messages, complete **Activities 13–14** and **13–15** in the Skills Practice Manual.

## SUMMARY

Transcribing medication orders requires extreme accuracy. Errors may result in serious consequences to the patient and liability to the hospital and all involved personnel. The health unit coordinator must also be careful not to omit any orders from the several forms that he or she is responsible for during the transcription procedure. Each order must be transcribed exactly as written by the doctor. Write each order legibly so that it can be easily read by the nurse administering the medication.

An understanding of the type, form, and proper transcription procedure of medication orders should be acquired by all who work with drug orders. As you gain experience, you will learn the more commonly administered medications and the groupings to which they belong, such as laxatives, sedatives, heart medications, and so forth. Highlight boxes containing the most-prescribed drug(s) in each drug group have been provided for a quick and easy reference.

Whenever there is doubt in your mind concerning a medication order or *any* order, *always check* with the nurse. Never hesitate to call the doctor whenever there is a possibility of misinterpreting the medication order or when the order cannot be read.

---

**REVIEW QUESTIONS**

1. Define the following:
   a. standing medication order

   *a medication order that remains in effect and is executed until the doctor DC or changes it.*

   b. standing prn medication order

   *Same as standing order but executed according to the patient needs*

   c. stat medication order

   *order executed immediately, then automatically discontinued*

   d. one-time medication order

   *medication executed according to the qualifying phrase then discontinued*

   e. short-series order for medication

   *same as one time med*

f. IV push

_small amount of drug given directly into a vein_

g. intramuscular injection

_injection of medication directly into muscle_

h. oral medication

_medication given by mouth_

i. automatic stop date

_medication is automatically discontinued unless renewed by MD._

j. capsule

_a geletanous container that encloses a medication_

k. tablet

_solid disk form of a drug_

l. ampoule

_small glass vial to keep contents sterile_

m. total parenteral nutrition

_method of administering vitamins, protiens, calories and other nutrients directly into the blood stream_

n. patient-controlled analgesia

_Method by which narcotics are administered by patient intravenously_

o. bolus

_concentrated dose of medication given by IV-Push_

p. intravenous

_pertains to within the vein_

q. IV push

_a method of giving IV in concentrated doses_

2. Write the abbreviations for each term listed below.

| | | | | | |
|---|---|---|---|---|---|
| 1. syrup | syr | | 13. microgram | ug | mcg |
| 2. one-half | ss | | 14. potassium chloride | | KCl |
| 3. liter | L | | 15. before | | a |
| 4. morphine sulfate | MSO4 | MS | 16. milliequivalent | | mEq |
| 5. patient-controlled analgesia | PCA | | 17. subcutaneous | Sq SC | subq |
| 6. both eyes | OU | | 18. hypodermic | | hypo |
| 7. intravenous piggyback | IVPB | | 19. after meals | | pc |
| 8. milliliter | mL | | 20. immediately | | stat |
| 9. night | noc | | 21. milligram | | mg |
| 10. gram | g | | 22. capsule | | cap |
| 11. aspirin | ASA | | 23. ointment | | ung |
| 12. per rectum | pr | | 24. suppository | | sup |

25. right eye _OD_

26. penicillin _pCN_

27. while awake _WA_

28. dram _3_ _dr_

29. unit _U_

30. tablet _m_

31. milk of magnesia _MOM_

32. nausea and vomiting _N/V_

33. ampoule _amp_

34. of each _āā_

35. grain _gr_

36. left eye _OS_

37. ounce _ʒ_ _oz_

38. intramuscular _IM_

39. sublingual _sub ling_

40. by mouth _PO_

41. tincture _tinc_

42. nitroglycerin _NTG_

3. Writing the meaning of each abbreviation listed below.

1. gr _grain_

2. mg _milligram_

3. IM _Intramuscular_

4. PCN _pennicillin_

5. tinct _tincture_

6. supp _suppository_

7. PO _by mouth_

8. g _gram_

9. OU _both eyes_

10. mL _milliliter_

11. āā _of each_

12. TPN _Total Parenteral Nutrition_

13. ung _ointment_

14. N/V _Nausea + Vomiting_

15. WA _while awake_

16. pc _after meals_

17. s̄s̄ _one half_

18. mEq _milliequivalant_

19. MS, MSO₄ _Morphine Sulphate_

20. PCA _patient controlled Analgesic_

21. stat _Immediatly_

22. IVPB _Intravenous Piggyback_

23. ā _of each_

24. SC, sq, sub-q _subcutaneous_

25. ASA _asprin_

26. oz or ʒ _ounce_

27. cap _capsule_

28. µg, mcg _microgram_

29. CPZ _Compazine_

30. noc _night_

31. tab _tablet_

32. MOM _milk of Magnesia_

33. dr or ʒ _dram_

34. L _Liter_

35. NTG _Nitroglycerin_

36. syr _syrup_

37. U _Unit_

38. amp _ampoule_

39. OD _right eye_

40. OS _left eye_

41. subling _sublingually_

42. KCl _Potassium chloride_

4. The five components of a medication order are:

a. _Name_

b. _dose_

c. _route_

d. _____ Frequency _____

e. _____ Qualifying phrase _____

5. Two reference books on medications that the health unit coordinator may refer to in the hospital are:

a. _____ PDR _____    b. _____ Nursing _____

6. Four groups of drugs that usually have automatic "stop dates" are:

a. _____ Antibiotics _____    c. _____ hypnotics _____

b. _____ narcotics _____    d. _____ anticoagulants _____

7. Two weight and measure systems used in the pharmacy are _____ metric _____

and _____ apothecary _____ .

Identify the symbols belonging to the systems above by writing the first letter of the system in the blank.

a. _A_ gr    e. _A_ ʒ

b. _M_ kg    f. _M_ mg

c. _A_ dr    g. _M_ mL

d. _M_ g    h. _A_ ʒ

8. Four routes by which medications may be administered are:

a. _____ oral _____    c. _____ parenteral _____

b. _____ inhalation _____    d. _____ topical _____

9. List four parenteral routes of administration of medications:

a. _____ intramuscular _____    c. _____ subcutaneous intradermal _____

b. _____ iv push hypodermic _____    d. _____ intravenous _____

10. Describe the purpose for which each of the following drug groups is administered.

a. analgesics _____ relieve lessen pain _____

b. antibiotics _____ treat infection and disease _____

c. anticoagulants _____ slow clotting time of blood _____

d. antihistamines _____ prevent or relieve allergic reaction _____

e. vasodilators _____ lower blood pressure _____

f. antinauseants _____ lessen or help prevent nausea _____

g. antineoplastics _____ treatment of cancer _____

h. antihypertensives _____ lower blood pressure _____

i. diuretics _____ remove excessive fluid from the body _____

j. hypnotics _____ induce sleep _____

k. hypoglycemics _____ lower blood sugar _____

l. laxatives _____ produce + facilitate bowel movements _____

m. narcotics _relieve pain and may induce sleep_

n. tranquilizers _relieve anxiety and tension_

o. antianemics _build iron in blood_

11. The name of a skin test for tuberculosis is _PPD_.

12. Name the drug groups to which the following drugs belong.

| Drug Name | Drug Group | Drug Name | Drug Group |
|---|---|---|---|
| a. codeine | narcotic | m. Demerol | narcotic |
| b. chloral hydrate | hypnotic | n. Unipen | antibiotic |
| c. Achromycin | antibiotic | o. Coumadin | anticoagulant |
| d. Percodan | narcotic | p. Terramycin | antibiotic |
| e. Doriden | hypnotic | q. Percocet | narcotic |
| f. Nembutal | narcotic | r. heparin | anticoagulant |
| g. erythromycin | antibiotic | s. ampicillin | antibiotic |
| h. penicillin | antibiotic | t. Sublimaze | narcotic |
| i. Seconal | hypnotic | u. morphine sulfate | narcotic |
| j. Keflin | antibiotic | v. Phenaphen with codeine | narcotic |
| k. Ilosone | antibiotic | w. Keflex | antibiotic |
| l. Placidyl | hypnotic | | |

13. Match the definitions in the second column with the words in the first column by placing the correct letter in the space provided.

**Column I**

_F_ 1. topical

_I_ 2. metric

_D_ 3. hypnotic

_J_ 4. parenteral

_B_ 5. oral

_H_ 6. total parenteral nutrition

_K_ 7. narcotic

_E_ 8. skin test

_G_ 9. patient-controlled analgesia

_L_ 10. medication nurse

_A_ 11. subcutaneous injection

_C_ 12. capsule

**Column II**

a. an injection given under the skin into connective tissue

b. by mouth

c. a gelatinous container enclosing a drug

d. a drug that produces sleep

e. a test to determine the presence of antibodies within the body

f. direct application of medicine to the skin

g. used to self-administer narcotics

h. also called intravenous hyperalimentation

i. a weight and measure system

j. fluids or medications given by injection

k. a drug that relieves pain and may produce sleep

l. one who administers medications

14. Differentiate between IV push, piggyback, IV admixture, and TPN.

_IV push - small amount of drug given directly into vein. Piggyback - administered IV in 50-100 mL of fluid. IV admixtures - drugs administered in larger quantities of fluid. TPN - used to administer nutrients into the blood stream._

_____

_____

15. Write the generic names of the following drugs.

| Drug | Generic Name |
|------|-------------|
| a. Demerol | meperidine |
| b. Tylenol | acetaminiphen |
| c. Noctec | chloral Hydrate |
| d. Garamycin | Gentamicin |
| e. Coumadin | warfarin |
| f. Tagamet | cimetidine |
| g. Lanoxin | digoxin |
| h. Pronestyl | procainamide |
| i. Hydro-Diuril | Hydrochlorothiazide |
| j. Lasix | furosemide |
| k. Nitrostat | nitroglycerin |
| l. Inderal | propranolol |
| m. Achromycin | tetra cycline |
| n. Advil | Ibuprofen |
| o. Orinase | tolbutamide |

16. Write the usual adult dosages for the following drugs.

| Drug | Usual Adult Dosage |
|------|-------------------|
| a. codeine | 15-60 mg |
| b. Demerol | 50-100 mg |
| c. morphine sulfate | 10-15 mg |
| d. Dalmane | 30 mg |
| e. Restoril | 15-20 mg |
| f. Seconal | 100 mg |
| g. Keflin | 0.5 to 1g |
| h. aspirin | 325 to 500 |
| i. Tylenol | 325 to 500 |
| j. Lanoxin | 0.125 mg to 0.25 mg |

17. List two advantages of computerized medication dispensing.

a. decreased number of errors in medication administration

b. increased accuracy in accounting + billing

18. List two disadvantages of computerized medication dispensing.

a. _Refrigerated + breakable container meds cannot be loaded into the system_

b. _new + changed order have to be handled in reg fashion_

**Rewrite the telephoned doctor's orders using appropriate symbols and abbreviations or have someone read the orders to you for practice in recording physicians' orders.**

19. a. Give one gram of Keflin intravenous piggyback now and one half gram every six hours times seven days. _1g Keflin IVPB now Keflin 0.5 gm q6hr x 7 days_

b. Give fifteen units of regular insulin every morning one half hour before breakfast and ten units of NPH at bedtime. _reg insulin 15 U q am 1/2 hr ac bkf NPH 10 U q HS_

c. Give Haldol ten milligrams intramuscular immediately, ten milligrams by mouth three times a day, and fifty milligrams of Haldol Deconoate every two weeks. _Haldon 10 mg IM stat Haldol 10 mg PO tid, Haldol Deconoate 50 mg IM q 2 wks_

d. Give Vicodin one tablet every four hours for pain if pain is unrelieved after thirty minutes give morphine sulfate ten milligrams intramuscular. _Vicodin 1 tab q4hrs for pain if pain is unrelieved p̄ 30 min give MS 10 mg IM._

## References

Blackburn, Elsa: *Health Unit Coordinator*. Englewood Cliffs, NJ, Prentice-Hall, Brady Division. 1991.

Brown, Meta and Mulholland, Joyce: *Drug Calculations Process and Problems for Clinical Practice*, 5th ed. St. Louis, The CV Mosby Co., 1996.

*Hospital Research and Educational Trust*: *Being a Health Unit Coordinator*. Englewood Cliffs, NJ, Prentice-Hall, Brady Division, 1991.

Loebl, Suzanne, Spratto, George R., and Woods, Adrienne L.: *RN Magazine's The Nurse's Drug Handbook*, 7th ed. Delmar Publishers Inc., 1994.

Phillips, Dianne Lynn: *Manual of I.V. Therapeutics*. Philadelphia, F.A. Davis Co., 1993.

*Physicians' Desk Reference*, 50th ed. Montvale, NJ, Medical Economics Data, 1996.

Terry, Judy, Baranowski, Leslie, Lonsway, Rose Anne, and Hedrick, Carolyn: *Intravenous Therapy Clinical Principles and Practice*. Philadelphia, W.B. Saunders Co., 1993.

Staff Springhouse Corporation: *Nursing Student's Guide To Drugs*. Springhouse, PA, Springhouse, 1993.

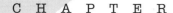
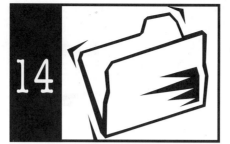

# 14

# LABORATORY ORDERS AND RECORDING TELEPHONED LABORATORY RESULTS

## C H A P T E R  OBJECTIVES

*Upon completion of this chapter, you will be able to:*

1. Define the terms in the vocabulary list.

2. Write the meaning of each abbreviation in the abbreviations list.

3. List the two general purposes of laboratory studies.

4. Name the three major laboratory divisions, briefly state the purpose of each, and name six studies performed in each division.

5. List five specimens that may be studied in the laboratory, and indicate three of these that are usually obtained by the nursing staff personnel. Describe your responsibilities in sending specimens to the laboratory.

6. Name three methods of obtaining urine specimens.

7. List the four tests that are generally performed as part of electrolyte studies.

8. Name the three chemistry tests that are performed on cardiac enzymes.

9. List five laboratory studies that may require a written consent form.

10. Describe the procedure for requisitioning stat blood tests from the laboratory.

11. Name the procedure that must be performed to order blood for transfusion.

12. Describe HUC responsibilities in an order for a 2 h PP.

13. Explain the difference between fasting and NPO.

14. Define serology and name six serologic tests.

15. Name four drugs whose levels are monitored in the blood.

16. Name three urine chemistry tests.

17. Describe how errors may be avoided in recording telephoned laboratory results.

## V O C A B U L A R Y

**Amniocentesis** • A needle puncture into the uterine cavity to remove amniotic fluid, the liquid that surrounds the unborn baby

**Antigen** • Any substance that induces an immune response

**Antibody** • An immunoglobulin (protein) produced by the body that reacts with and neutralizes an antigen (usually a foreign substance)

**Bacteriology** • The study of bacteria and the diseases they produce (abbreviated: bacti)

**Biopsy** • Tissue removed from a living body for examination

**Clean Catch** • A method of obtaining a urine specimen using a special cleansing technique; also called a midstream urine

**Culture and Sensitivity** • The growth of microorganisms in a special media (culture), followed by a test to determine the antibiotic to which they best respond

**Cytology** • The study of cells

**Daily Laboratory Tests** • Tests that are ordered once by the doctor but are ordered every day until the order is discontinued by the doctor

**Differential** • Identification of the types of white cells found in the blood

**Dipstick Urine** • The visual examination of urine using a special chemically treated stick

**Electrolytes** • A group of tests done in chemistry which usually includes sodium, potassium, chloride, and $CO_2$

**Erythrocyte** • A red blood cell

**Fasting** • No solid foods by mouth and no fluids containing nourishment (ie: sugar or milk) ice chips or water

**Guaiac** • A substance for testing for hidden (occult) blood   Positive - blue

**Hemolysis** • Rupture of erythrocytes (red blood cells) with release of hemoglobin and potassium into the plasma

**Lumbar Puncture** • A procedure used to remove cerebrospinal fluid from the spinal canal   fetal position

**Mycology** • The study of fungi and fungal diseases

**Occult Blood** • Blood that is undetectable to the eye

**Pap Smear** • A test performed to detect cancerous cells in the female genital tract; body secretions, excretions, and tissue scrapings can also be studied by the Pap staining method

**Postprandial** • After eating   gastrointestinal

**Paracentesis** • A surgical puncture and drainage of a body cavity

**Pathology** • The study of body changes caused by disease

**Plasma** • The fluid portion of the blood in which the cells are suspended; it contains a clotting factor called *fibrinogen*

**Random Specimen** • A body fluid sample that can be collected at any time

**Reference Range** • Range of normal values for a laboratory test result

**Serology** • The study of blood serum or other body fluids for immune bodies, which are the body's defense when disease occurs

**Serum** • Plasma from which fibrinogen, a clotting factor, has been removed

**Sputum** • The mucous secretion from lungs, bronchi, or trachea

**Sternal Puncture** • The procedure to remove bone marrow from the breast bone cavity for diagnostic purposes; also called a bone marrow biopsy

**Thoracentesis** • A needle puncture into the pleural space in the chest cavity to remove pleural fluid for diagnostic or therapeutic reasons

**Tissue Typing** • Identification of tissue types in order to predict acceptance or rejection of tissue and organ transplants

**Titer** • The quantity of substance needed to react with a given amount of another substance—used to detect and quantify antibody levels

**Type and Crossmatch** • The patient's blood is typed, then tested for compatibility with blood from a donor of the same blood type and Rh factor

**Type and Screen** • The patient's blood type and Rh factor are determined, and a general antibody screen is performed

**Urinalysis** • The physical, chemical, and microscopic examination of the urine

## ABBREVIATIONS

Most of the abbreviations listed on pp. 250 to 252 are for laboratory tests. The words in parentheses indicate in which division of the laboratory the test is performed.

| Abbreviation | Meaning | Example of Usage on a Doctors' Order Sheet |
|---|---|---|
| AFB | acid-fast bacillus Tb | *Note:* Many doctors' orders |
| Ab | antibody | for laboratory tests are written on the doctors' order sheet as the abbreviation appears here; for example, CBC is the doctor's written order for complete blood count. Examples of doctors' orders are given only for those orders that require more than the abbreviation. |
| Ag | antigen | HIV B24 Ag |
| APTT | activated partial thromboplastin time (coagulation) | |
| bili | bilirubin (chemistry) | |
| BS | blood sugar (chemistry) | |
| BT | bleeding time (coagulation) | |
| Bx | biopsy (cytology) | |
| Ca or Ca++ | calcium (chemistry) | |
| CBC | complete blood count (hematology) | |
| CC | colony count (bacti) | |

| Abbreviation | Meaning | Example of Usage on a Doctors' Order Sheet | Abbreviation | Meaning | Example of Usage on a Doctors' Order Sheet |
|---|---|---|---|---|---|
| Cl or Cl⁻ | chlorides (chemistry) | | LDL | low-density lipoproteins (chemistry) | |
| CMV | cytomegalovirus (microbiology, serology) | | LP | lumbar puncture | LP in AM; obtain tray and consent |
| creat | creatinine (chemistry) | | lytes | electrolytes (chemistry) | |
| CRP | C-reactive protein (serology) | *auto-immune diseases test* | Na | sodium (chemistry) | |
| C&S | culture and sensitivity (bacti) | Sputum for C&S | NP | nasopharynx (smears from this area studied in bacti) | NP smear for C&S |
| CSF | cerebrospinal fluid | CSF for serology | O&P | ova and parasites (parasitology) | Stool for O&P × 3 |
| Cx | culture (microbiology) | | OSMO | osmolality | |
| DAT | direct antiglobulin test (blood bank) | | P | phosphorus (chemistry) | |
| Diff | differential (hematology) | | PAP | prostatic acid phosphatase | |
| Dig | digoxin (chemistry) | Dig level now | PC | packed cells (blood bank) | Give 2 U PC now |
| EBV | Epstein-Barr virus (serology) | | POCT | point-of-care testing | |
| ESR | erythrocyte sedimentation rate | *auto-immune disease test* | PSA | prostatic specific antigen | *test for male problems* |
| FBS | fasting blood sugar (chemistry) | | PCV | packed-cell volume (hematology; same as hematocrit) | |
| Fe | iron (chemistry) | | | | |
| fib | fibrinogen (coagulation) | | PP | postprandial (chemistry) | 2 h PP BS |
| FS | frozen section (cytology) | | PT | prothrombin time (coagulation) | |
| gluc | glucose (chemistry) | *drink sugar and test* | PTT | partial thromboplastin time (coagulation) | |
| GTT | glucose tolerance test (chemistry) | | RBC | red blood cell count (hematology) | |
| HCO₃⁻ | bicarbonate (may be reported as carbon dioxide—CO₂) (chemistry) | | RDW | red cell distribution width (hematology) | |
| | | | Retics | reticulocytes (hematology) | |
| HBₛAg | hepatitis B surface antigen (serology) | | R&M | routine and microscopic (chemistry) | Urine, R&M |
| HCG | human chorionic gonadotropin (test for pregnancy; special chemistry) | | RPR | rapid plasma reagin (serology) | |
| Hgb | hemoglobin (hematology) | | RSV | respiratory syncytial virus (microbiology) | *infants strep throat* |
| Hct | hematocrit (hematology) | | SMA | sequential multiple analysis (one of many automated chemistry profiles) (chemistry) | |
| HDL | high-density lipoproteins (chemistry) | | | | |
| H&H | hemoglobin and hematocrit (hematology) | | | | |
| HIV | human immunodeficiency virus screen (serology) | | T₃, T₄, T₇ | thyroid tests (chemistry) | |
| | | | TBD | to be done | CBC TBD in AM |
| K | potassium (chemistry) | | TBT | template bleeding time | |

$HCO_3^-$

$CO_2$

$HB_sAg$

$T_3, T_4, T_7$

| Abbreviation | Meaning | Example of Usage on a Doctors' Order Sheet |
|---|---|---|
| T&C | type and crossmatch | T&C for 2 U of packed red cells |
| TCT or TT | thrombin-clotting time or thrombin time (coagulation) | |
| TIBC | total iron-binding capacity (chemistry) | |
| T&S | type and screen (blood bank) | |
| TSH | thyroid-stimulating hormone (chemistry) | *Hypo thyroid* |
| UA or U/A | urinalysis | |
| VDRL | Venereal Disease Research Laboratories (serology) | *Syphillis test* |
| VMA | vanillylmandelic acid (chemistry) test for epinephrine metabolism | |
| WBC | white blood cell count (hematology) | |
| X-match | crossmatch (blood bank) | T&X-match for 1 U packed red cells |
| Zn | zinc | |

# E X E R C I S E  1

Write the abbreviation for each term listed below.

1. fasting blood sugar — FBS
2. ova and parasites — O&P
3. hemoglobin — Hgb
4. erythrocyte sedimentation rate — ~~ESR~~
5. potassium — K
6. acid-fast bacilli — AFB
7. red blood cells — RBC
8. postprandial — PP
9. cerebrospinal fluid — CSF
10. iron — Fe
11. culture and sensitivity — C&S
12. type and crossmatch — T&C ~~X-match~~
13. complete blood count — CBC

14. activated partial thromboplastin time — APTT
15. glucose tolerance test — GTT
16. packed cells — PC
17. prothrombin time — PT
18. urinalysis — UA
19. C-reactive protein — CRP
20. direct antiglobulin test — DAT
21. frozen section — FS
22. hepatitis B surface antigen — Hb₅Ag
23. high-density lipoprotein — HDL
24. human immunodeficiency virus — HIV
25. low-density lipoprotein — LDL
26. routine and microscopic — R&M
27. red cell distribution width — RDW
28. to be done — TBD
29. template bleeding time — TBT
30. thrombin time — TT or TCT
31. thyroid tests — T₃ T₄ T₇
32. thyroid-stimulating hormone — TSH
33. vanillylmandelic acid — VMA
34. bilirubin — bili
35. antigen — Ag
36. human chorionic gonadotropin — HCG
37. glucose — gluc
38. creatinine — creat
39. fibrinogen — fib
40. bleeding time — BT
41. cytomegalovirus — CMV
42. osmolality — osmo
43. type and screen — T&S
44. digoxin — dig
45. culture — C
46. respiratory syncytial virus — RSV

47. zinc — _Zn_

48. electrolytes — _lytes_

49. Epstein-Barr virus — _EBV_

50. biopsy — _bx_

51. point-of-care testing — _POCT_

## EXERCISE 2

Write the meaning of each abbreviation listed below.

1. BS — _Blood sugar_
2. $HCO_3^-$ — _CO2 or Bicarbonate_
3. H&H — _Hematocrit and hemoglobin_
4. LP — _Lumbar puncture_
5. VDRL — _Veneral Disease Research lab_
6. WBC — _white Blood cell count_
7. UA — _Urinalysis_
8. TCT — _Thrombo Clotting time_
9. NP — _nasopharynx_
10. Ca — _Calcium_
11. Cl — _Chlorides_
12. TIBC — _total Iron Binding Capacity_
13. SMA — _Sysquential multiple Analysis_
14. Diff — _Differential_
15. Na — _Natacin sodium_
16. PCV — _Packed cell volume_
17. Hct — _Hematocrit_
18. P — _Pulse_
19. LDL — _Low Density lipo_
20. CRP — _C-Reactive protien_
21. R&M — _Range + motion_
22. RDW — _red cell distribution weldh_
23. DAT — _Direct Antiglobin Test_
24. TT — _Thrombin Time_
25. $T_3, T_4, T_7$ — _Thyroid tests_
26. FS — _frozen section_
27. TSH — _thyroid stymulating Hormone_
28. VMA — _vandilly maddelic Acid_

29. HB$_s$Ag — _Hepatitis B / Surface Antigen_
30. HDL — _High Density Lipo protiens_
31. TBT — _template bleeding time_
32. HIV — _Human Immunodificiency virus_
33. TBD — _Total Binding to be done_
34. Cx — _culture_
35. Zn — _Zinc_
36. BT — _bleeding time_
37. HCG — _Human Chorionic Gonadotropin_
38. creat — _creatinine_
39. Fib — _fibrinogen_
40. lytes — _Electrolytes_
41. gluc — _glucose_
42. Ag — _antigen_
43. Dig — _digoxin_
44. CMV — _Cytomegalovirus_
45. Ab — _antibody_
46. RSV — _Respiratory syncytial virus_
47. bili — _bilirubin_
48. osmo — _osmolality_
49. T&S — _type+screen_
50. Bx — _Biopsy_
51. POCT — _point of care testing_

## INTRODUCTION TO LABORATORY PROCEDURE

Tests performed by the laboratory are ordered for diagnostic purposes and for the evaluation of a prescribed treatment. See Appendix F for a comprehensive list of the studies that are performed in a laboratory.

Hospital size determines the number of divisions within the laboratory and the kinds of tests performed in each division. For example, a large hospital may have a microbiology division with subdivisions such as bacteriology, serology, parasitology, virology, and mycology. In smaller hospitals all the tests performed in the divisions mentioned above may be done in the microbiology division or sent to outside laboratories. (Figure 14–1 is a laboratory divisional chart.) Also, you may find in your hospital that the division and some test names vary from those used in this book.

In this chapter we will discuss three major laboratory divisions: hematology, chemistry, and microbiology; and

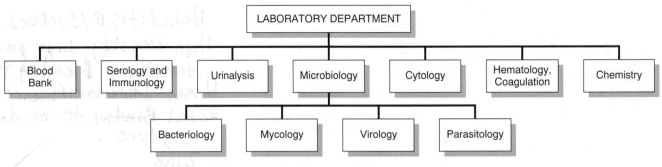

FIGURE 14–1 • A laboratory divisional chart.

five other divisions: blood bank, urinalysis, cerebrospinal studies, cytology, and serology. Tests related to nuclear medicine and gastroenterology may also be performed by the clinical laboratory when a hospital is not of sufficient size to maintain a separate nuclear medicine or gastroenterology department.

It is necessary for the health unit coordinator to interpret terms the doctor may use to write laboratory orders. The word *routine*, when used in a written laboratory order, may indicate that the test is to be done within the regular laboratory workday, because there is no urgency for the test results. For example, the doctor may write the order *Routine CBC*, meaning that the blood specimen for the complete blood count may be drawn according to the laboratory routine. The laboratory normally draws all the blood samples early in the morning. Once again the word *routine* has no special meaning to the transcription procedure, and the steps of transcription are followed as outlined.

The doctor may also use the word *daily*, as in the order *daily Hgb*; this means that the test is ordered once by the doctor, but requisitioned every day by the health unit coordinator until the order is discontinued. In some health care facilities, the computer may accept multiple dates for daily labs on each patient.

The word *stat*, as you recall, means to be done immediately. Because of the urgency of a stat order, a different communication procedure is used. The procedure is to notify the laboratory by phone; supply the name of the patient, the unit, the room number, and the test requested. The requisition is completed immediately and retained at the nursing unit for the technician to pick up prior to obtaining the specimen. Stat orders sent by computer may or may not require a telephone call. Write *stat* on the order. If the stat order requires the nurse to collect the specimen, the health unit coordinator verbally notifies the nursing staff of the stat order, immediately completes the requisition, and inputs the order into the computer.

## Specimens

*All laboratory tests require a specimen.* Blood is the most common specimen used and is most often obtained by the laboratory personnel through venipuncture (puncture into the vein) or fingerstick (puncture into a capillary) (Fig.

14–2). Currently, in some health care facilities, blood specimens are being collected by nursing personnel on the unit and sent to the laboratory for testing.

Blood specimens may need to be collected in different containers depending on the test ordered. For example, coagulation studies and chemistry studies must be in different tubes. Cultures performed on blood for different types of organisms (aerobic vs. anaerobic bacteria) may also require different tubes. Clear and complete information on all tests to be collected reduces the need for the patient to be redrawn for additional blood specimens.

Some other specimens tested are *urine, stool, sputum, sweat, wound drainage, discharge from body openings,* and *gastric washings (lavage).* These specimens are obtained by the nursing staff (Fig. 14–3).

Specimens collected *by entering parts of the body* or a *body cavity* are obtained by the *doctor.* Types of specimens and the names of the procedures used to obtain them are listed below. It is usually hospital policy to request written consent from the patient prior to performing these procedures, except for pelvic examination. (Review "Preparing a Consent Form," Chapter 8.) It may be your responsibility to order trays, such as a lumbar puncture tray, or other equipment from the CSD for the doctor to use to perform these procedures.

| Specimen | Procedure |
|---|---|
| ■ Spinal fluid | Lumbar puncture; also called spinal tap |
| ■ Bone marrow | Sternal puncture; also called bone marrow biopsy   *Hip Illiac crest* |
| ■ Abdominal cavity fluid | Abdominal paracentesis |
| ■ Pleural fluid | Thoracentesis |
| ■ Amniotic fluid | Amniocentesis |
| ■ Biopsy specimen | Biopsy of a part of the body |
| ■ Cervical smear | Pelvic examination |

All specimens obtained by the nursing staff or doctor must be labeled. It is sometimes the health unit coordinator's responsibility to prepare the label. This is done by imprinting the patient's name and pertinent information on a self-adhering label or providing a preprinted computer label for the patient. Requisitions for laboratory tests of specimens obtained by the nursing staff or doctor are kept on the nursing unit until the specimen is collected. The requisition is attached to the specimen container, which has been placed in a sealed plastic bag, and then sent to the laboratory. When using a computer, enter the order just

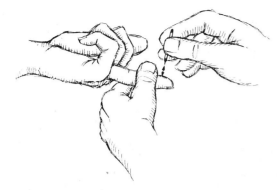

a. Finger stick

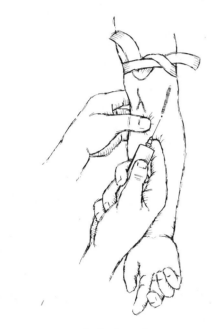

b. Venipuncture

F I G U R E  14–2 • Methods of obtaining blood specimens.

analyzed on the hospital unit by nursing personnel is called a **point-of-care** lab test. Because of point-of-care testing, the procedure for ordering a test may change.

Results are obtained by utilizing several methodologies. These include analysis by portable automated analyzers, the use of reagents (chemicals), and microscopic visualization.

Portable automated analyzers may be used in departments that require immediate results, and they decrease the need for stat specimens to be sent to the laboratory. Some tests that may be done on the unit by this method are **electrolytes, blood glucose, BUN, hemoglobin**, and **hematocrit**. A pulmonary function test (see Chapter 16), **arterial blood gases (ABGs)**, may also be run on an automated analyzer in the unit.

Reagent-based tests may include a test for pregnancy or **human chorionic gonadotropin (HCG), automatic clotting time (ACT)**, and a test for *Helicobacter pylori* (CLO test), a bacterium that has been indicated in ulcers of the gastrointestinal system. The CLO test actually uses a biopsy specimen obtained in the endoscopy department (see Chapter 16) and may give positive results within 2 hours.

Some of the reagent-based tests that are considered point-of-care lab tests are those traditionally carried out by nursing personnel, and include blood and urine monitoring for the presence of ketones and the levels of glucose. A common brand of machine used for blood glucose monitoring is the **Accu-Chek**. These tests are discussed in Chapter 11. **Gastroccults** and **hemoccults**, which use slides and reagents to detect hidden blood in gastric and stool specimens, are also considered point-of-care tests in some health care facilities. Another common reagent used to test for hidden blood in stool is **guaiac**.

A test that uses both a reagent and microscopic visualization is the **fern test**, which is used to indicate the presence of amniotic fluid (due to the rupture of the amnion). The reagent portion utilizes a strip of paper that indicates acidity (pH paper), and the microscopic portion detects the characteristic fern pattern of crystallized amniotic sodium chloride (salt).

before sending the specimen. The computer printout of the order may be attached to the labeled specimen.

It is often your responsibility to take the specimen and requisition to the laboratory. This should be done as soon as possible. In many health care facilities, most specimens may be sent by the pneumatic tube system, especially when results are needed quickly (emergency department and surgery). Specimens that should *not* be sent by the pneumatic tube system are those that are not easily retrievable, such as cerebrospinal and amniotic fluids.

## Point-of-Care Testing

Many laboratory tests that were once only drawn and analyzed in the laboratory department may now be performed on the nursing unit; this is a recent trend in many health care facilities. A laboratory test that is collected and

## Communication with the Laboratory Department

All laboratory tests are communicated to the laboratory department by the ordering step of transcription.

## DIVISIONS WITHIN THE LABORATORY

## Hematology

The **hematology division** performs tests related to physical properties of the blood (including blood cells and their appearance), tests related to clotting and bleeding disor-

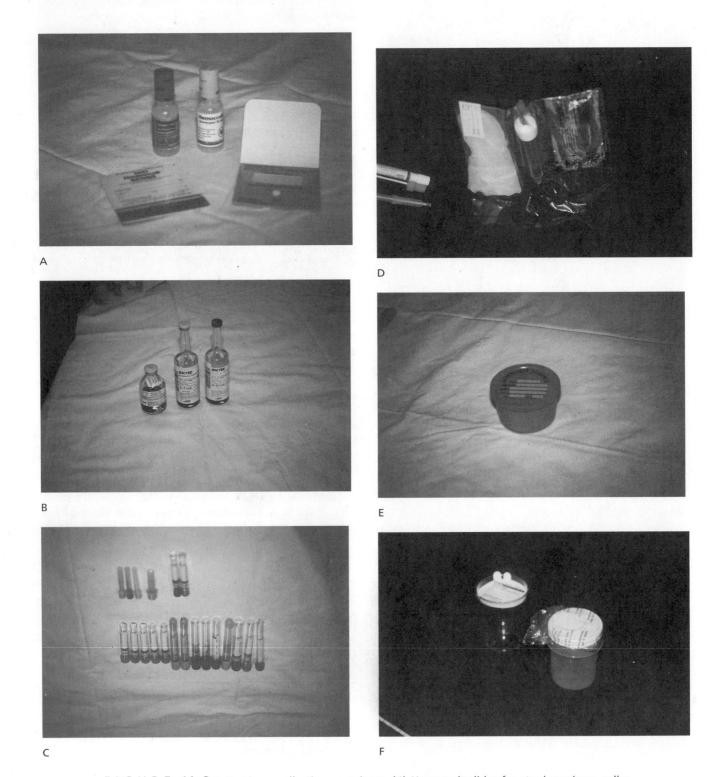

**FIGURE 14–3** • Specimen collection containers. (*A*) Hemoccult slides for stool specimen collection. (*B*) Containers for blood culture specimen. (*C*) Various containers for blood specimen. (*D*) Cath urine specimen container kit. (*E*) Stool specimen container. (*F*) Urine specimen containers: left for voided specimen, right for midstream specimen. *Illustration continued on opposite page*

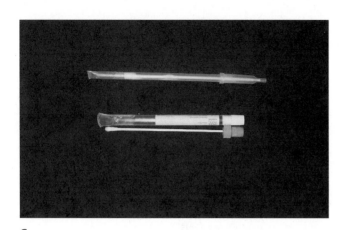

G

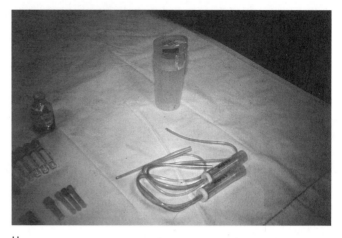

H

FIGURE 14-3 • *Continued* (*G*) Culturette and container for throat culture. (*H*) Types of sputum collection containers.

ders, and coagulation (clotting) studies to monitor patients on anticoagulant therapy.

### Specimen

The majority of these tests are done on a blood specimen. However, bone marrow and spinal fluid may also be studied in the hematology division.

### Fasting

Fasting is generally not required for tests performed in the hematology division of the laboratory.

### Communication with the Laboratory

Hematology studies are ordered by computer or by completing a general laboratory requisition form (Fig. 14-4).

### Doctors' Orders for Hematology Studies

It is impossible to list all doctors' orders relating to this division of the laboratory. However, we have listed the more common ones in their abbreviated forms with an interpretation for reference. Refer to the abbreviations list at the beginning of the chapter if necessary. *Note:* All of the following tests are performed on blood specimens; therefore, as mentioned earlier, the laboratory personnel obtain the specimen or by POCT.

### ■ APTT and PTT

**Activated partial thromboplastin time** and **partial thromboplastin time** are coagulation studies. They are performed individually and are commonly used to monitor heparin dosage.

## COMMUNICATION AND IMPLEMENTATION OF LABORATORY ORDERS

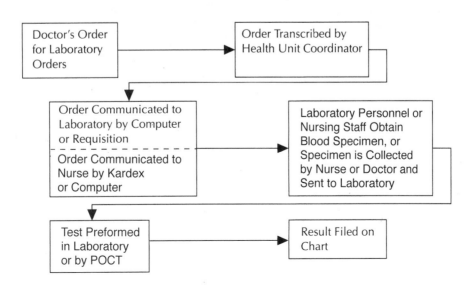

| DR. ORDERING _____ | SURGERY | |
|---|---|---|
| DIAGNOSIS _____ | DATE _____ | |
| DRAW AT _____ TIME _____ DATE _____ | TIME _____ | |
| REQUEST BY _____ | ☐ STAT | |
| DATE _____ | ☐ ROUTINE | |

| CHEMISTRY | | |
|---|---|---|
| ☐ Acetone | ☐ Cholesterol | ☐ Lactic Acid |
| ☐ Acid Phos. | ☐ Creatinine, Serum | ☐ Lipase |
| ☐ Albumin | ☐ Creatinine Clearance | ☐ Magnesium |
| ☐ Alk. Phos. | ☐ Drug Screen | ☐ Osmolality, Serum |
| ☐ Bilirubin, Total | ☐ Electrolytes | ☐ Phosphorus |
|    ☐ Direct |    ☐ Sodium | ☐ Protein, Total |
|    ☐ Indirect |    ☐ Potassium | ☐ SGPT (ALT) |
| ☐ BUN |    ☐ Chloride | ☐ SMA 6 |
| ☐ Calcium |    ☐ Carbon Dioxide | ☐ SMA 12 |
| ☐ Cardiac Enzymes | ☐ Glucose, Random | ☐ SMA 20 (SMAC) |
|    ☐ CPK (CK) | ☐ Glucose, Fasting | ☐ TIBC |
|    ☐ LDH | ☐ Glucose, _____ hr PP | ☐ Triglycerides |
|    ☐ SGOT (AST) | ☐ Glucose Tolerance _____ hr | ☐ Troponin |
| | ☐ Iron | ☐ Uric Acid |

| SPECIAL CHEMISTRY | SEROLOGY | OTHER |
|---|---|---|
| ☐ ACTH | ☐ ANA | |
| ☐ Cortisol | ☐ ASO Titer | |
| ☐ Folate | ☐ CEA | |
| ☐ FSH | ☐ CMV | |
| ☐ LH |    ☐ IgG | |
| ☐ TBG |    ☐ IgM | |
| ☐ TSH | ☐ Cocci Screen | |
| ☐ $T_3$ | ☐ EBV Panel | |
| ☐ $T_4$ | ☐ Histoplasma | |
| | ☐ HIV | |
| | ☐ Monospot | |
| | ☐ Rq Factor | |
| | ☐ RPR | |
| | ☐ RSV | |
| | ☐ Rubella Screen | |
| | ☐ Streptozyme | |
| | ☐ VDRL | |

| HEMATOLOGY | COAGULATION | Special Instructions |
|---|---|---|
| ☐ CBC | ☐ Platelet Count | |
| ☐ HGB | ☐ APTT (PTT) | |
| ☐ HCT | ☐ PT | |
| ☐ WBC | ☐ Fibrinogen | |
| ☐ DIFF | ☐ Bleeding Time | |
| ☐ RBC | ☐ Factor VIII | |
| ☐ RBC Indices | | Drawn by _____ |
| ☐ Reticulocyte Count | | Date _____ |
| ☐ ESR | | Time _____ |
| ☐ Sickle Cell Prep. | | Spec. # _____ |

| GENERAL LABORATORY REQUISITION |
|---|

A

F I G U R E  14–4 • General laboratory requisition. (A) Chemistry, special chemistry, serology, hematology, and coagulation. *Illustration continued on opposite page*

DR. ORDERING _____

DIAGNOSIS _____

COLLECTED BY _____

Time _____ Date _____

REQUESTED BY _____

SURGERY

Time _____

Date _____

☐ STAT
☐ ROUTINE

## ANTIBIOTICS BEING GIVEN

### MICROBIOLOGY

| SPEC. SOURCE | TEST REQUESTED |
|---|---|
| ☐ Abcess | ☐ AFB Culture (TB) |
|    Source _____ | ☐ AFB Stain |
| ☐ Blood | ☐ Cult. & Sens. |
| ☐ Body Cavity | ☐ Cult. & Sens. |
|    Source _____ |    Anaerobic |
| ☐ Ear | ☐ Fungal Culture |
| ☐ Eye | ☐ GC Screen |
| ☐ Nose | ☐ Strep Screen |
| ☐ Spinal Fluid | ☐ Viral Culture |
| ☐ Sputum | ☐ Other _____ |
| ☐ Stool | |
| ☐ Throat | |
| ☐ Tissue | |
| ☐ Urine | |
|   ☐ Clean Catch | |
|   ☐ Cath, St. | |
|   ☐ Cath, Foley | |
| ☐ Wound | |
| ☐ Other _____ | |

### FLUIDS

| SPEC. SOURCE | TEST REQUESTED |
|---|---|
| ☐ Abdominal | ☐ Cell Count |
| ☐ Amniotic | ☐ Glucose |
| ☐ Pericardial | ☐ LDH |
| ☐ Peritoneal | ☐ Occult Blood |
| ☐ Pleural | ☐ Protein |
| ☐ Spinal Fluid | ☐ Sp. Gravity |
| ☐ Synovial | ☐ VDRL (CSF) |
| | ☐ # of Tubes |
| | ☐ _____ |
| | ☐ _____ |

### STOOL

| | |
|---|---|
| ☐ Fat | |
| ☐ Fiber | |
| ☐ Occult Blood | |
| ☐ Ova & Parasites | |

### CYTOLOGY

| SPEC. SOURCE | TEST REQUESTED |
|---|---|
| ☐ Amniotic | ☐ Pap |
| ☐ Breast | ☐ Fungal |
| ☐ Bronchial Asp. | ☐ Buccal |
| ☐ Cervical | ☐ Maturation Index |
| ☐ Colon | |
| ☐ Gastric | |
| ☐ Lung Asp. | |
| ☐ Pleural | |
| ☐ Pericardial | |
| ☐ Peritoneal | |
| ☐ Spinal Fluid | |
| ☐ Sputum | |
| ☐ Urine | |
| ☐ Vaginal | |

### URINALYSIS/URINE CHEMISTRY

| | |
|---|---|
| ☐ Routine | ☐ Occult Blood |
| ☐ Amylase (2 hr) | ☐ Osmolality |
| ☐ Bilirubin | ☐ Phosphorus |
| ☐ Calcium | ☐ Potassium |
| ☐ Chloride | ☐ Pregnancy |
| ☐ Creatinine | ☐ Protein |
|    Clearance | ☐ Sodium |
| ☐ Glucose | ☐ Sp. Gravity |
|    Tolerance | ☐ Uric Acid |
| ☐ Nitrogen | |

### OTHER TESTS

SPEC. INSTRUCTIONS

SPEC #

## GENERAL LABORATORY REQUISITION II

B

F I G U R E  14–4 • *Continued* (*B*) Microbiology, fluids, stool, urinalysis, and cytology.

■ *Bleeding time*

The measurement of the time it takes a standardized incision to cease bleeding. It differs from clotting time in that this test involves constriction of the smaller blood vessels. A standardized incision is an incision of specific length and depth. Several methods may be used, but the **template bleeding time (TBT)** is preferred, as the incision is standardized by the use of a cutting device called a template (Fig. 14–5).

■ *Clotting time*

A determination of the time it takes blood to clot.

■ *CBC*

A **complete blood count** comprises a number of tests, including Hgb, Hct, WBC, and Diff. These tests may also be ordered separately. (An RBC, RBC indices, and RDW may be part of this study if done on automated instruments.)

■ *Diff*

A **differential** reports the various types of WBCs (or leukocytes) found in the blood specimen. Some of the types are lymphocytes (lymphs), monocytes (monos), neutrophils (neutros), eosinophils (eos), and basophils (basos).

■ *ESR*

Also called **sed rate**. An **erythrocyte sedimentation rate** determines the rate at which RBCs settle out of the liquid portion of the blood. The test is used to determine the progress of inflammatory diseases.

■ *Hct*

Also called **PCV (packed-cell volume)**. **Hematocrit** is a measurement of the volume percentage of red blood cells in whole blood.

■ *Hgb*

Hemoglobin is the oxygen-carrying pigment of blood that gives it its red color. This test may determine the need for additional blood, or it may aid in diagnosing types of anemia.

■ *LE cell prep*

A diagnostic study for lupus erythematosus, an inflammatory disease

■ *Platelets*

The count of cells (platelets) that are essential for the coagulation process to take place

■ *PT (prothrombin time)*

**Prothrombin time** measures the clotting ability of blood. This test assists the doctor in determining the dosage of the drugs—usually Coumadin—prescribed in anticoagulant therapy. The health unit coordinator may be required to telephone the test results to the doctor. How the results are reported depends on the testing method used, such as patient/control in seconds (Example: 17 sec/13 sec); or, patient/% of prothrombin activity (Example: 14 sec/70% activity).   INR ~ Standardize pro time

In addition to the PT result, an additional result called the INR may be included. This is a calculation using the patient's PT result, the normal control result, and a coefficient factor that depends on the reagent used. The INR calculation is an attempt to standardize PT results.

■ *RBC*

The measurement of **red blood cells** (erythrocytes) per cubic millimeter of blood

■ *RBC indices*   diagnoses certain type anemia

A method for determining the characteristics of red blood cells. The measurements are reported as MCH (content of hemoglobin in average individual red cell), MCHC (average hemoglobin concentration per 100 mL of packed red cells), and MCV (average volume of individual red cells).

■ *RDW*

The **red cell distribution width** is included on most instruments as part of a CBC. It measures the distribution of red cell volume.

■ *Retics*

The count of **reticulocytes** (immature red blood cells), which determines bone marrow activity. It is often used in the diagnosis of anemia.

■ *Thrombin-clotting time (TCT)* or *thrombin time (TT)*

May be performed to monitor heparin therapy.

■ *WBC*

The count of the number of **white blood cells** (leukocytes) that are present in the blood to fight disease-causing organisms often used in the diagnosis of infection.

Refer to the Appendix F for other tests performed in the hematology division.

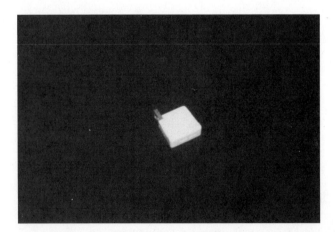

F I G U R E  14–5 • A type of cutting device used to perform bleeding time.

---

### TO THE STUDENT

To practice transcribing hematology and coagulation orders, complete **Activity 14–1** in the Skills Practice Manual.

To practice transcribing daily laboratory orders, complete **Activity 14–2** in the Skills Practice Manual.

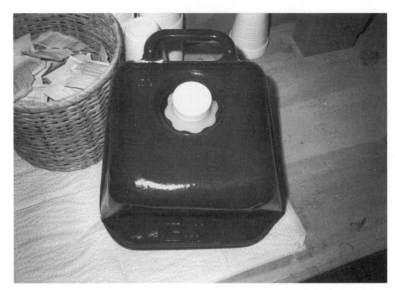

**FIGURE 14–6 •** A 24-hour urine specimen container.

## Chemistry or Biochemistry

The chemistry division performs tests related to the study of chemical reactions occurring in living organisms. When a disease process occurs, the chemicals within the body fluids vary from the normal. Any variance permits a diagnosis or evaluation of the patient's health status to be made.

### Specimens

Blood and urine are the specimens most commonly collected for study in this division of the laboratory. Whole blood, plasma, or serum may be used for chemistry tests. Many tests of the same name can be done on either blood or urine; therefore, often the doctor uses the word *serum* to indicate that the test is to be performed on blood and uses the term *urine* if the test is to be done on a urine specimen.

Specimens for urine chemistries may require the urine to be collected over a period, such as 24 hours. This is often referred to as a **24-hour urine specimen** (Fig. 14–6). It may be the health unit coordinator's responsibility to obtain the receptacle from the laboratory to be used for the collection of the specimen. Some specimens that are to be kept for a period have a preservative added to the collection bottle before it is sent to the unit. Other 24-hour specimens may have to be iced in the patient's bathroom until the collection is completed. See "Chemistry Tests that Require a 24-Hour Urine Specimen," below.

### Fasting

Many of the blood chemistry tests require the patient to fast or to be NPO. **Fasting** means that the patient has nothing to eat for 8 to 10 hours prior to the collection of the specimen to be tested; the patient may have water. **NPO** means **nothing by mouth**—food *or* fluid—after midnight. It may be your responsibility to notify the dietary department, or you may be asked to obtain bedside signs to be posted to remind personnel that the patient is being pre-pared for a test. Table 14–1 lists chemistry and other laboratory tests that require the patient to fast or be NPO. (Since some of these tests are not considered fasting by all laboratories, check with your instructor for their correct classification in your hospital.)

### Communication with the Laboratory

Chemistry tests are requisitioned by using the computer or completing a requisition form (Fig. 14–4).

The development of automated equipment permits many tests to be performed on a small sample of blood and in a short time. One requisition (or computer-entered laboratory request) is used to request a number of tests. The name of the automated instrument used is followed by the number of tests ordered. Some of the automated instruments used are the Ektachem, Paramax, Colter, and Dacos. The SMA (sequential multiple analyzer) may also be used. For example, 20 tests performed with SMA instrumentation would be ordered as $SMA_{20}$. It is possible that the panel with the same name can have different numbers depending on how the automated instrument is programmed in a particular lab. These automated multicomponent studies are called **profiles**, **panels**, or **surveys**.

### Doctors' Orders for Blood Chemistry Studies

Below are listed frequently ordered blood chemistry tests,[*] written in abbreviated form as the doctor would write them on the doctors' order sheet. The full name of each test is given in parentheses. Normal values for common blood chemistry studies are given below and p. 263.

▪ *Acid phos* (acid phosphatase)
Used in diagnosing metastatic carcinomas of the prostate gland and breast, among other uses.

---

*Note:* Unless otherwise indicated, the specimen used for the following tests is serum, which is collected by the laboratory personnel.

## CHEMISTRY TESTS THAT REQUIRE A 24-HOUR URINE SPECIMEN*

Epinephrine-norepinephrine
Albumin, quantitative & qualitative
Aldosterone
Amino acids, quantitative-fractionated
Arsenic, quantitative
Calcium, quantitative
Catecholamines
Chlorides
Chorionic gonadotropin (HCG)
Coproporphyrin, qualitative & quantitative
Cortisol
Creatine
Creatinine
Epinephrine
Estrogens, total
FIGLU (N-formiminoglutamic acid)
Flouoride
Follicle-stimulating hormone (FSH)
Glucose, quantitative

Homovanillic acid (HVA)
17-Hydroxycorticosteroids
5-Hydroxyindoleacetic acid, quantitative (5-HIAA)
17-Ketogenic steroids
17-Ketosteroids
Lactose
Lead
Metanephrines
Phosphorus
Porphobilinogen, quantitative
Potassium
Pregnanetriol
Protein, total
Sodium clearance
Uric acid
Uroporphyrins, qualitative & quantitative
Vanillylmandelic acid (VMA)
Zinc

*Note: Check with you laboratory concerning these tests. The methods used may vary from hospital to hospital.

## TABLE 14-1  Fasting and/or NPO List for Laboratory Studies

| Procedure | Fasting | NPO | Laboratory Division |
|---|---|---|---|
| Bromsulphalein (BSP) | Yes | No | Chemistry |
| Cholesterol | Yes | No | Chemistry |
| Chromosomes | Yes | No | Blood bank |
| Deoxycorticosterone | Yes | No | Chemistry or nuclear medicine |
| D-Xylose (blood or urine) | Yes | Yes | Chemistry |
| Electrophoresis, lipids | Yes | No | Chemistry |
| Electrophoresis, lipoprotein | Yes | No | Chemistry |
| Factor VIII assay | Yes | Yes | Coagulation |
| Fasting blood sugar (FBS) | Yes | No | Chemistry |
| Gastrin (serum) | Yes | Yes | Chemistry or nuclear medicine |
| Glucose, fasting (FBS) | Yes | No | Chemistry |
| Glucose tolerance test (GTT) | Yes | Yes | Chemistry |
| Insulin tolerance test (ITT) | Yes | Yes | Chemistry |
| Iron (Fe) | Yes | Yes | Chemistry |
| Iron-binding capacity (IBC) | Yes | Yes | Chemistry |
| Lipids | Yes | Yes | Chemistry or GI lab |
| Neutral fat (lipid profile fractionization) | Yes | Yes | Chemistry or GI lab |
| Orinase tolerance test | Yes | Yes | Chemistry |
| Parathyroid hormone (PTH) | Yes | Yes | Chemistry or nuclear medicine |
| Phenolsulfonphthalein (PSP) urine | Yes | Yes | Chemistry |
| Phospholipids | Yes | Yes | Chemistry or GI lab |
| Plasma cortisol | Yes | Yes | Chemistry or nuclear medicine |
| Renin | Yes | Yes | Chemistry or nuclear medicine |
| Schilling test | No | Yes | Chemistry or nuclear medicine |
| Serum lipids | Yes | Yes | Chemistry or GI lab |
| SMA | Yes | Yes | Chemistry |
| Testosterone | Yes | Yes | Chemistry or nuclear medicine |
| Total iron-binding capacity (TIBC) | Yes | Yes | Chemistry |
| Triglycerides | Yes | Yes | Chemistry |

■ *Alk phos* (alkaline phosphatase)
Used to evaluate bone and liver disease, among other uses.

■ *Amylase* (serum)
The level of amylase is elevated in acute pancreatitis, as well as some other illnesses.

■ *AST (SGOT), CPK (CK), and LDH*
These are known as **cardiac enzymes**. These tests are ordered when a myocardial infarction (heart attack) is suspected.

■ *Bili* (bilirubin)
This test measures liver function. Bilirubin is the result of red blood cells that have broken down and are excreted by the liver. In diseases in which a large number of red blood cells are destroyed (such as in liver disease and obstruction of the common bile duct), a high concentration of bilirubin is found in the blood serum. The physician may order this test as **total bilirubin**, using the **direct** or **indirect** method of testing.

■ *BS* (blood sugar)
A test to determine the amount of sugar in the blood. It is usually ordered at a specific time, such as 4 PM BS. The patient is not fasting when this test is performed.

■ *BUN* (blood urea nitrogen)
Useful in diagnosing diseases that affect kidney function.

■ *Cholesterol*
The client is in a fasting state for this test, which may be used to measure the function of the liver. It is believed that cholesterol may sometimes be responsible for causing high blood pressure and hardening of the arteries (atherosclerosis). It is also important that the "good" cholesterol, or **high-density lipoproteins (HDL)**, be measured in relationship to total cholesterol.

■ *CPK or CK* (creatine phosphokinase or creatine kinase)
An enzyme found in heart, brain, or skeletal muscle, which is released when there is damage from a disease process.

■ *Creatinine clearance test*
This test is done to study kidney function. It requires testing of the blood and urine.

NORMAL VALUES FOR FREQUENTLY
PERFORMED HEMATOLOGY-COAGULATION
STUDIES AND BLOOD CHEMISTRY STUDIES

Hematocrit (Hct)   Male 45–50 vol/dL
                   Female 40–45 vol/dL
Hemoglobin (Hgb) Male 14.5–16.0 g/dL
                   Female 13.0–15.5 g/dL
White blood count (WBC) 6000–9000/mm³  5-10
Prothrombin time (PT) 12–15 sec
Sodium (Na) 132–142 mEq/L
Potassium (K) 3.5–5.0 mEq/L
Fasting blood sugar (FBS) 70–120 mg/dL

■ *Electrophoresis*
This is a procedure performed to determine protein or fatty acid levels. The doctor may order any of three tests that result in a serum protein pattern. The tests are **protein electrophoresis, lipoprotein electrophoresis, immuno-electrophoresis**.

■ *FBS* (fasting blood sugar)
Also called **fasting glucose**. As the name indicates, the patient must be in a fasting state. The test determines the amount of sugar in the bloodstream after the patient has not eaten for 8 to 10 hours. This test is used in the diagnosis of and monitoring of treatment of diabetes.

■ *Gentamicin level* (peak and trough)
When the physician wants to check the levels of certain medications the client is receiving, he or she orders peak-and-trough levels. Sometimes, toxic blood levels accumulate instead of being excreted. Antibiotics (such as amikacin, gentamicin, kanamycin, and tobramycin) are examples of types of medication ordered to be done in peak-and-trough levels. Other medication levels may include Dilantin (random), digoxin (random), and cyclosporine (trough level). For peak levels, the blood is usually collected 15 minutes after IV infusion and 30 to 60 minutes after IM injection. Trough levels usually require that blood be drawn 15 minutes before the next dose of the medication is given to the patient. For peak-and-trough orders, the health unit coordinator needs to work closely with the laboratory and nursing staff to assure proper scheduling of collections (Fig. 14–7).

**HIGHLIGHT**

Peak and/or trough, or random blood levels are commonly drawn for these medications:

- amikacin
- cyclosporine
- digoxin
- Dilantin
- gentamicin
- kanamycin
- tobramycin

■ *GTT* (glucose tolerance test)
A test performed to determine abnormalities in glucose metabolism. The patient is in a fasting state. The test may be performed over several hours—usually 3 to 6. The patient has an FBS drawn to establish baseline data and then is given a large amount of glucose solution to drink. Timed blood and urine specimens are taken. The urine specimens, collected by the nursing staff, must be carefully labeled with the time the urine was collected. At the completion of the test, all urine is sent to the laboratory. (The order has been communicated to the laboratory by requisition or computer to alert the laboratory personnel to perform a fasting blood sugar test before administering the sugar solution.)

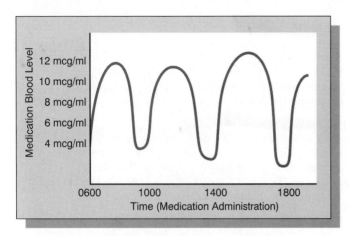

FIGURE 14–7 • A graphic example of peak-and-trough levels of a medication.

■ *HbA_{lc}* (glycosylated hemoglobin)
This test is a reflection of the blood glucose on the red blood cells during the past 3 months. This test is sometimes used to replace the GTT.

■ *HDL* (high-density lipoprotein)
The "good" cholesterol, which is thought to be important in the total cholesterol profile.

■ *Isoenzymes* (also called isozymes)
This test determines the source (body part enzymes) responsible for the elevation of enzymes such as LDH, CPK, or CK by determining the variations in these enzymes, such as CK-MB.

■ *LDH* (lactate dehydrogenase)
An enzyme released into the circulation after tissue damage to heart, liver, kidney, brain, or skeletal muscle.

■ *Lytes* (electrolytes)
Consists of four tests: sodium (Na), potassium (K), chlorides (Cl), and bicarbonate ($HCO_3$). These four tests may be performed separately.

■ *PAP*
Prostatic acid phosphatase is an enzyme produced by prostate tissue; it increases as prostate disease becomes more severe. PAP may be used to monitor prostate cancer patients.

■ *PSA*
This test measures the body's level of prostatic specific antigen. Increased PSA levels may indicate the presence of prostate cancer.

■ *Serum creatinine*
This test is performed to diagnose kidney diseases. It studies the creatinine in the blood serum.

■ *SGOT* (serum glutamic-oxaloacetic transaminase)
Another name for this test is **aspartate aminotransferase (AST)**. This enzyme is released into the circulation from destroyed skeletal or cardiac muscle or the liver. The AST level is elevated in myocardial infarction, liver diseases, acute pancreatitis, acute renal diseases, and severe burns.

■ *SGPT* (serum glutamic-pyruvic transaminase)
The new name for this test is **alanine aminotransferase (ALT)**. This enzyme is released into the circulation from destroyed liver cells.

■ *SMA*
This is an example for a chemistry profile panel or survey. Several tests are performed at the same time by an automated analyzer on a single blood sample, Other types of automated instruments are the Ektachem, Paramax, Colter, Astro, and Dacos. Also, a group of tests may be named for a particular organ (liver profile = SGPT, GGTP, and T. bili). The number of tests is determined by how the instrument is programmed and can vary even within the same instrument. For example, an $SMA_{20}$ analyzes 20 chemicals in the serum, while an $SMA_{12}$ analyzes 12 chemicals in the serum.

■ *TIBC* (total iron-binding capacity)
This test is useful in diagnosing anemia, some infections, and cirrhosis of the liver.

■ *Troponin*
This test is performed to diagnose acute myocardial infarction (AMI) from a few hours onset to as long as 120 hours. It is more sensitive in detecting unstable angina with minor myocardial cell damage than CK-MB.

■ *2 h PP BS* (2 hours postprandial blood sugar)
A test performed to determine the patient's response to carbohydrate intake. It is the health unit coordinator's responsibility to *notify the laboratory* when the patient *has finished eating*. The blood for this test may be drawn 2 hours after any meal.

■ *Triglycerides*
Triglycerides are the principal lipid (greasy organic substances) in the blood. The patient is in a fasting state for this study, which is important in diagnosing heart disease, hypertension, and diabetes.

■ *Uric acid*
This test is used principally to diagnose gout. painful toe

## Nuclear Chemistry Studies or Special Chemistry Studies

Many of the tests previously included in the nuclear chemistry division of the clinical laboratory or the nuclear medicine laboratory may now be performed using a non–radioisotope-based method, and may be included in the chemistry division as a **special chemistry** study. The following studies are examples of tests that may be performed by these divisions (see Appendix F):

ACTH (adrenocorticotropic hormone)
Cortisol
Folate
FSH-urine (follicle-stimulating hormone)
LH (luteinizing hormone)
Schilling test
TBG (thyroxine-binding globulin)

TSH (thyroid-simulating hormone)
$T_3$ (triiodothyronine)
$T_4$ (thyroxine)
$T_7$ (free thyroxine index)

### Doctors' Orders for Urine Chemistry Studies

Below are listed a few urine chemistry tests. Refer to the list presented earlier for the tests that require a 24-hour urine collection.

■ *Urine glucose*
Ordered in conjunction with the blood glucose for a glucose tolerance test. Determines the amount of glucose in the urine.

■ *Urine creatinine*
Usually ordered in conjunction with the blood chemistry portion of the creatinine clearance test but may be ordered separately.

■ *Urine protein*
An elevated urine protein is found in inflammatory diseases of the urinary system and prostate gland.

■ *Urine osmolality*
Determines the diluting and concentrating ability of the kidneys.

---

**HIGHLIGHT**

Laboratory Divisions

- **Hematology:** Study of **physical properties** of blood, including blood cell studies and coagulation
- **Chemistry:** Study of **chemicals** of the blood and other body fluids
- **Microbiology:** Study of the **organisms** that cause disease; includes bacteriology, mycology, virology, and parasitology
- **Blood Bank: Blood typing** and crossmatching, storing blood and blood components for **transfusion**
- **Urinalysis:** Study of **urine**
- **Cytology:** Study of **cells** obtained from body tissues and fluid
- **Serology:** Study of **immunologic** substances

---

## Microbiology

The terms *microbiology* and *bacteriology* are sometimes used interchangeably. However, large laboratories may use the broader term *microbiology* as a division name within the hospital, with areas in that division designated for bacteriology, parasitology, mycology, and virology, to name a few.

**Bacteriology**, commonly abbreviated as bacti, is the study of bacteria that produce disease. Specimens are cultured, grown in a reproducing medium, identified using biochemical tests, and then tested for antibiotic sensitivity.

This process is known as a **culture and sensitivity test**. Gram's stains, tests for the causative organism of tuberculosis, and colony counts are also performed in this division.

**Parasites**, organisms that live off other living organisms, are dealt with in **parasitology**. Fecal specimens are studied here for ova and parasites.

In **mycology**, cultures are set up to isolate and identify **fungi**. Since the plants must grow to produce spores, these cultures may take several weeks.

**Virology** is the study of viruses that cause disease. Identification of the exact virus or bacterium that is the causative organism of a specific disease is important, since isolation procedures are based upon the methods by which organisms are spread.

### Specimen

Almost any type of specimen may be studied in the microbiology division.

### Fasting

Fasting is not required for tests performed in the microbiology division of the laboratory.

### Communication with the Laboratory

To order a microbiology/bacteriology study, a requisition form (see Fig. 14–4) or the computer is used.

As mentioned earlier, if the specimen is obtained by the nurse or doctor, the requisition form remains on the unit until the specimen is obtained. The health unit coordinator may then transport the properly labeled specimen and completed requisition form to the laboratory. When a computer is used, the test order is typed in when the specimen is obtained.

### Doctors' Orders for Bacteriology Studies

Below are listed the frequently ordered tests performed in the bacteriology laboratory, with an interpretation relating to the health unit coordinator's role. For assistance with abbreviations, check the abbreviations list at the beginning of the chapter.

## Bacteriology

### ■ Culture and sensitivity

A specimen is placed on an appropriate medium for growth. If organisms grow, they are tested for antibiotic sensitivity, which determines those antibiotics that should be effective for treatment. The nursing staff is responsible for the collection of the specimen. Culture and sensitivity tests can be ordered on blood, urine, sputum, wound drainage, and nose and throat specimens.

### ■ AFB culture

This test is done to determine the presence of such acid-fast bacilli as *Mycobacterium tuberculosis*, which causes tuberculosis. The nursing staff is responsible for the collection of the specimen (usually sputum). A special stain may also be performed.

### ■ Urine for CC (colony count)

A test done to determine the number of bacteria present in a urine specimen.

### ■ Gram's stain

Gram's stains classify bacteria into gram-negative or gram-positive groupings, thus allowing for differential diagnosis of the causative agent. Treatment can begin immediately, while awaiting the results of cultures.

### ■ Blood cultures × 2, 15 min apart

Blood specimens may be collected as multiple specimens (different times or different sites) in order to ensure accurate isolation and identification of the causative organism.

The following studies are also performed in the microbiology division.

## Parasitology

### ■ Stool spec × 3 for O&P

This order requires three different stool specimens (three requisition forms must be prepared) to determine the presence of ova (eggs) or parasites in the stool. The nursing staff is responsible for the collection of the stool specimens.

## Mycology

### ■ Mycology cultures

A test designed to determine the presence of fungi. It may be performed on blood or spinal fluid specimens. The results may take several weeks to determine. Studies may be performed to determine the presence of fungi such as *Histoplasma*, *Coccidioides*, and *Candida*.

Coccidio mycosis

## Virology

### ■ Virus culture and virus serology

Virus cultures may be done on any specimen, and virus serology is done on a blood specimen to determine the presence of viruses or antibodies to viruses.

### ■ CMV cultures

Buffy coat, urine, and throat. Viral cultures for cytomegalovirus are often done on blood (buffy coat), urine, and throat specimens in immunocompromised patients (AIDs and transplantation).

---

**TO THE STUDENT**

To practice transcribing microbiology/bacteriology orders, complete **Activity 14–7** in the Skills Practice Manual.

## Serology

The study of antibodies and antigens can be useful in detecting the presence and intensity of a current infection. It may also be useful in identifying a previous infection or exposure to an organism. Autoimmune diseases may be studied, as well as pre- and posttransplant evaluations and treatment. Tests for syphilis, rheumatoid arthritis, HIV, some influenzas and tissue typing are a few of the studies done in this area.

## Immunology

The response of the body to a foreign substance may include mobilization of leukocytes (white blood cells) against the foreign substance as well as the production of certain proteins that neutralize the substance. These proteins are **immunoglobulins** (or more commonly **antibodies**) and circulate in the blood. There are five main types of immunoglobulins: IgG, IgM, IgA, IgD, and IgE.

An important characteristic of antibodies is that much of the time they are produced specifically against a particular foreign substance, and are ordered in reference to that substance. Any substance that elicits an immune response is called an **antigen**. The measurement of the antibody level may be ordered as a **titer**. Many serologic tests are done in order to detect antibody levels, since the antibodies are usually in the serum portion of the blood. Serologic tests can also detect the presence of antigens.

### Specimen

The majority of these tests are done on the serum portion of a blood specimen. However, other body fluids such as spinal fluid may be tested, as well as biopsy specimens and secretions from wounds.

### Fasting

Fasting is not required for tests performed in the serology division of the laboratory.

### Communication with the Laboratory

Serology studies are ordered by computer or by completing a general laboratory requisition form (see Fig. 14–4).

## Doctors' Orders for Serology

### ■ *ANA* (antinuclear antibody)
This test determines the presence of certain autoimmune diseases such as SLE (systemic lupus erythematosus).

### ■ *ASO titer* (antistreptolysin O titer)
An elevated titer usually indicates the presence of a streptococcal infection, such as acute rheumatic fever.

### ■ *CEA* (carcinoembryonic antigen)
An elevated level of the antigen indicates liver, colon, or pancreatic cancer. It is also used to assess the treatment of these conditions.

### ■ *CMV IgG and IgM*   *cause birth defects*
This test determines the levels of different types of antibodies (immunoglobulins) against cytomegalovirus. The presence of these antibodies may indicate exposure to or possible infection with cytomegalovirus.
*tells if you've had infection*

### ■ *Complement fixation titers*
These tests are done to detect various viral, fungal, and parasitic diseases.

### ■ *EBV panel*
This test determines various levels of antibodies (IgG and IgM) produced and directed against specific parts of the Epstein-Barr virus, such as viral capsid antigen (VCA) and Epstein-Barr virus nuclear antigen (EBNA). This can determine whether the patient has had a recent or previous EBV infection.

### ■ *ELISA (enzyme-linked immunosorbent assay)*
EIA (enzyme immunoassay) and RIA (radioimmunoassay) are additional methods used for detection of antibody levels.

### ■ *FTA* (fluorescent treponemal antibody)
This is a serology test for syphilis.

### ■ *HB$_s$Ag*
This is a serum study to determine the presence of hepatitis B in the blood.

### ■ *HIV* (human immunodeficiency virus)
This is the test used to detect the virus that causes AIDS (acquired immunodeficiency syndrome).

### ■ *Heterophil agglutination test*
This is a diagnostic study for infectious mononucleosis.

### ■ *RA factor*
This is a specific test for rheumatoid arthritis.

### ■ *VDRL or RPR*
These tests, which are performed on blood, are screening tests for syphilis.

### ■ *Anti-OKT$_3$ antibody level*
Many substances can cause an immune response. This test detects the presence of antibodies against a medication (OKT$_3$).

Refer to Appendix F for other tests performed in the microbiology division and the serology division.

---

### TO THE STUDENT

To practice transcribing immunology and serology orders, complete **Activity 14–8** in the Skills Practice Manual.

## Blood Bank

The **blood bank**, which is usually a part of the clinical laboratory, has the responsibilities of typing and crossmatching patient blood, obtaining blood for transfusions, storing blood and blood components, and keeping records of transfusions and blood donors.

Prior to the administration of whole blood, packed cells, and some other blood components, the patient must have a **type and crossmatch** done. This is a test that determines the patient's blood type and compatibility. The four major blood groups are A, B, AB, and O.

- Patients with type A blood may receive transfusions of types A and O.
- Patients with type B may receive types B and O.
- Patients with type AB may receive types A, B, AB, and O.
- Patients with type O may receive only type O blood transfusions.

The order for blood transfusion or transfusion of blood components automatically indicates that the blood will be typed and crossmatched.

This laboratory division also performs several other blood studies, including the Coombs' tests. The **DAT (direct antiglobulin test)** is a synonym for the Coombs' test. In a direct Coombs' test, a positive result is found in hemolytic disease of the newborn, hemolytic transfusion reactions, and acquired hemolytic anemia. The indirect Coombs' test detects the presence of antibodies to red blood cell antigens. This test is valuable in detecting the presence of anti-Rh antibodies in the serum of a pregnant woman before delivery.

Since the transfusion of blood and blood components is a treatment administered by nursing personnel, additional information on various types of blood transfusions (autologous, donor directed, and autotransfusion) is discussed in Chapter 11.

### Specimen
A specimen of blood is used for type and crossmatch.

### Fasting
Fasting is not required for this procedure.

### Communication with the Laboratory
A blood bank requisition form (Fig. 14–8) or a computer is used to order a type and crossmatch. The number of units to be given and the name of the blood components are items included on this requisition.

DR. ORDERING _____

DIAGNOSIS _____

DRAW AT _____ TIME _____ DATE

REQUESTED BY _____

---

□ ROUTINE          □ ASAP          □ STAT          □ FOR HOLD

DATE OF SURGERY _____     DATE/TIME of TRANSFUSION _____

---

□ CROSSMATCH     □ SCREEN          # of Units _____

□ WHOLE BLOOD                      Other Tests

□ PACKED CELLS                     SPECIAL INSTRUCTIONS

□ WASHED CELLS

□ FROZEN CELLS                     Spec. Collected by _____

□ FRESH FROZEN PLASMA             Date Collected _____

□ PLATELET CONCENTRATE            Time Collected _____

BLOOD BANK REQUISITION

**F I G U R E   14–8 •** Blood bank requisition.

## Doctors' Orders for Blood Bank

Below are listed examples of doctors' orders for blood component administration. Refer to Chapter 11, pp. 188–189 for examples of blood, blood components, and plasma substitutes.

- *T&C for 2 U packed cells* (need type and crossmatching)

- *Packed cells, 1 U* (need type and crossmatching)

- *Plasma, 3 U stat*

- *Give washed cells 1 U* (need type and crossmatching)

- *Cryoprecipitates 1 U*

- *Give 2 U of platelets* (no crossmatching needed, but donor plasma and recipient RBCs should be ABO compatible)

- *Normal serum albumin 5%* (no crossmatching)

- *T&C 6 U pc—hold for surgery in* AM

---

**T O   T H E   S T U D E N T**

To practice transcribing blood bank orders, complete **Activity 14–9** in the Skills Practice Manual.

---

## Urinalysis

In this laboratory division, urine specimens are studied for color, clarity, pH (degree of acidity or alkalinity), specific gravity (degree of concentration), protein (albumin), glucose (sugar), blood, bilirubin, and urobilinogen. The sediment is viewed microscopically for organisms, intact cells, and crystals.

### Specimen

Urine is the specimen used for this test; however, the doctor may indicate that the nursing staff should follow a special procedure to obtain the specimen.

**Procedures for Obtaining Urine Specimens**
- **Voided urine specimen:** The patient voids into a clean container.
- **Clean catch**, or **midstream, urine specimen:** The nursing staff uses a special cleansing technique to obtain this type of specimen.
- **Catheterized urine specimen:** This specimen is obtained by catheterizing the patient. This procedure is usually done for culture and sensitivity testing, which is performed by microbiology.

Urine specimens that are collected at an unspecified time are called **random specimens**. However, the preferred collection time for a urine specimen is in the early morning upon rising.

## Fasting

Fasting is not required for a urinalysis.

## Communication with the Laboratory

A requisition form (see Fig. 14–4) or computer is used to order this test. Once again the requisition is held on the nursing unit until the specimen is collected. When it has been obtained, the carefully labeled specimen and the requisition are transported to the laboratory. Where computers are in use, the order is entered on the computer when the specimen is obtained.

## Doctors' Orders for Urinalysis

Below are listed examples of doctors' orders for urinalysis.

- *UA or R&M*
  *Routine and microscopic*

- *Cath UA*

- *Clean catch UA*

- *Dipstick urine for ketones*

A urine specimen is sent to the laboratory. All regular urinalysis studies are performed, except the specimen is not examined microscopically.

---

**HIGHLIGHT**

Points to Remember When Ordering Laboratory Studies:

- Determine if a test is a point of care test, or needs to be sent to the laboratory.
- All tests ordered require a specimen.
- Each specimen sent to the lab requires a requisition and must be labeled.
- Include date and time of collection on the requisition, as well as the name of the person collecting specimens obtained by unit personnel.
- Order tests as efficiently as possible in order to avoid the necessity for the patient to be redrawn (i.e., routines with stats).
- Communicate stat laboratory tests immediately to the lab and/or nursing personnel, and include all pertinent information.

---

**TO THE STUDENT**

To practice transcribing urinalysis/urine chemistry orders, complete **Activity 14–10** in the Skills Practice Manual.

## Studies Performed on Pleural Fluid

Studies are performed on pleural fluid to determine the cause and nature of pleural effusion, including hypertension, CHF, cirrhosis, infections, and neoplasms.

## Specimen

A thoracentesis is done by the doctor to obtain the pleural fluid specimen for testing. The patient must sign a consent form for this procedure.

## Fasting

Fasting is not required for tests performed on pleural fluid.

## Communication with the Laboratory

The doctor orders the tests to be done on the specimen and the health unit coordinator orders the tests on the pleural fluid requisition (see Fig. 14–4) or on the computer. As with any nonretrievable specimen obtained by invasive procedures it should be transported to the laboratory immediately, and should not be sent through a pneumatic-tube system.

## Doctors' Orders for Pleural Fluid

Below are listed examples of doctors' orders performed on pleural fluid.

- *Thoracentesis, pleural fluid to lab for LDH, glucose, and amylase. R/O CA*

- *Pleural fluid for cell count, diff and culture*

## Studies Performed on Cerebrospinal Fluid

Studies are performed on cerebrospinal fluid to determine various brain diseases or injuries.

## Specimen

A lumbar puncture is done by the doctor to obtain the cerebrospinal fluid specimen for these tests. The patient must sign a consent form for this procedure.

## Fasting

Fasting is not required for tests performed on cerebrospinal fluid.

## Communication with the Laboratory

The doctor orders the tests to be done on each specimen, of which there may be three or four. The health unit coordinator orders the respective tests on the cerebrospinal fluid requisition (see Fig. 14–4) or on the computer. A separate requisition may be required for each tube. It is sometimes the health unit coordinator's responsibility to transport these specimens to the laboratory. It is important to transport cerebrospinal fluid specimens to the laboratory *immediately*. Because they are difficult to obtain, *never* send the specimens via pneumatic tube.

## Doctors' Orders for Cerebrospinal Fluid

Below are listed examples of doctors' orders performed on cerebrospinal fluid.

■ *Lumbar puncture, fluid to lab for cell count and diff*

■ *Cerebrospinal fluid for serology*

■ *Spinal fluid to lab for:*
   tube #1—cell count, protein and glucose
   tube #2—AFB and fungal culture
   tube #3—Gram's stain
The requisitions are to be marked #1, #2, and #3, and the specified tests should be noted on each requisition.

---

### TO THE STUDENT

To practice transcribing cerebrospinal fluid orders, complete **Activity 14–11** in the Skills Practice Manual.

## Cytology

**Cytology** is the study of cells obtained from body tissues and fluid to determine cell type and to detect cancer or a precancerous condition. Although it is not common for the health unit coordinator who works on the nursing unit to requisition cytology tests, two types of specimens studied in this division deserve mention in this chapter. One is the **Pap smear**, a staining method developed by Dr. George Nicolas Papanicolaou that can be performed on various types of specimens to determine the presence of cancer. However, cells from the cervix are the specimens most frequently studied (cervical smear). During a pelvic examination the doctor may remove cells from the cervix for study.

The other specimens studied in the cytology division are biopsy specimens obtained from procedures, such as ster-

---

**TELEPHONED LABORATORY RESULTS**

Patient's Name _____  Report called by _____
Room Number _____  Report taken by _____
Date _____ Time _____

| **HEMATOLOGY** | **CHEMISTRY** | **URINE** |
|---|---|---|
| RBC_____ | GLUCOSE | COLOR_____ |
| Hgb_____ |   Random _____ | APPEARANCE_____ |
| Hct_____ |   FBS _____ | PH_____ |
| WBC_____ | E'LYTES | SP. GRAVITY_____ |
|   lymphs_____ |   Na _____ | ACETONE_____ |
|   monos_____ |   K _____ | GLUCOSE_____ |
|   neutros_____ |   C1 _____ | BACTERIA_____ |
|   eos_____ |   $CO_2$ _____ | WBC_____ |
|   basos_____ | CARDIAC ENZYMES | RBC_____ |
| PLATELETS_____ |   SGOT_____ | CASTS_____ |
| RETICS_____ |   LDH_____ | OCCULT BLOOD_____ |
| SED RATE_____ |   CPK_____ | OTHER |
| OTHER | CALCIUM_____ | |
| | PHOS_____ | |
| | BUN_____ | |
| | CREATININE_____ | |
| | OTHER | |

| **COAGULATION** | **TELEPHONED BLOOD GAS REPORT** |
|---|---|
| BLEEDING TIME_____ | Patient's Name_____ |
| COAGULATION TIME_____ | Room Number_____ |
| PROTIME_____ | Date _____ Time_____ |
|   Patient_____ | Report called by_____ |
|   Control_____ | Report taken by_____ |
|   %_____ | |
| PT | $O_2$ CONCENTRATION_____ |
|   Patient_____ | $O_2$ TENSION_____ |
|   Control_____ | $CO_2$ TENSION_____ |
|   INR_____ | PH_____ |
| PTT_____ | ACT BICARB_____ |
| | BASE EXCESS_____ |
| | $O_2$ SAT_____ |

F I G U R E  14–9 • Telephoned laboratory tests result form.

```
  COLLEGE HOSPITAL                              PAGE 1
  A. MELZER MD & D. RUDOLPH MD PATHOLOGISTS

                  *** RESULT INQUIRY ***
PATIENT NAME: WADSWORTH, JENNIFER        PATIENT #: 437592
  LOC: 4W    AGE: 20   SEX: F   ADM PHY: PAYNE, IMA    ADM DATE: 10/9/96
-----------------------------------------------------------------------
CHEMISTRY PANEL         RESULT          UNITS       REFERENCE VALUES
----------------        ----------      -------     ----------------
  SODIUM              L    134          MMOL/L      (135-145
  POTASSIUM           H    5.4          MMOL/L      (3.6-5.0
  CHLORIDE                 96           MMOL/L      (96-110)
  CO2                      29           MMOL/L      (21-31       )
  GLUCOSE                  103          MG/DL       (70-110)
  BUN                 H    33           MG/DL       (6-20        )
  CREATININE               1.2          MG/DL       (0.5-1.2
  CALCIUM                  10.4         MG/DL       (8.5-10)5
  URIC ACID                4.8          MG/DL       (3.9-7.8
  CHOLESTEROL              166          MG/DL       (140-200
  T. BILIRUBIN             1.0          MG/DL       (0.0-1.2
  T. PROTEIN               6.9          GM/DL       (6.1-8.0
  ALBUMIN             L    2.4          GM/DL       (3.5-4.8
  ALK PHOS            H    132          U/L         (30-107)
  GGTP                H    195          U/L         (8-69        )
  ALT (SGPT)               29           U/L         (0-55        )
  LDH                 H    398          U/L         (94-172)
  AST (SGOT)               29           U/L         (8-42        )
  CPK                 L    27           U/L         (38-224)
  TRIGLYCERIDES            154          MG/DL       (30-64       )
  PHOSPHORUS               3.1          MG/DL       (2.4-4.8

  COMPLETE BLOOD COUNT
  --------------------
  WHITE BLOOD CELL COUNT  H   14.9      X10^3       (4.8-10)8
  RED BLOOD CELL COUNT    L   4.29      X10^6       (4.7-6.10
  HEMOGLOBIN              L   12.6       GM/DL       (14.0-18.0
  HEMATOCRIT             L   37.3        %           (42.0-52.0
  MCV                        87.0       U3          (80-94       )
  MCH                        29.4       PG          (27-32       )
  MCHC                       33.8       %           (33-37       )
  RDW                    H   17.6        %           (11.5-14.5
  POLYSEGMENTED NEUTROPHIL H  82         %           (50-70       )
  BAND                       6          %           (0-10        )
  LYMPHOCYTE             L   4           %           (20-40       )
  MONOCYTE                   1          %           (0-10        )
  METAMYELOCYTE         H   6           %           (0           )
  ATYPICAL LYMPHOCYTE   H   1           %           (0           )
  PLATELET ESTIMATE          ADEQ
  RBC MORPHOLOGY             SLT ANISO
                             SLT POLYC
  PLATELET COUNT             220        X1000       (130-400
```

F I G U R E   14–10 • Computerized laboratory result sheet.

nal puncture or biopsy of other body parts. Biopsy specimens are also obtained by the doctor. Amniotic fluid and cerebrospinal fluid may also be studied (see Fig. 14–4).

## Transplantation

Many health care facilities are involved in tissue and whole-organ transplantation. Pretransplant evaluation and posttransplant care of the transplant recipient may include many laboratory tests, some of which may be specialized or sent to various outside reference labs. It is important for the health unit coordinator to follow special directions of protocols as closely as possible when ordering all tests.

A major concern for transplant patients is the potential for **rejection** of the transplanted organ. In order to prevent rejection the patient is required to take immunosuppressive medication. Another major concern for transplant patients is the potential for **infection** due to this medication because it suppresses the immune system. Because of these potential complications, tests ordered from the serology and microbiology divisions are numerous. An additional pretransplant laboratory test included in some evaluations is human leukocyte antigen (HLA) typing (more commonly known as **tissue typing**). This test identifies major antigens (proteins) of the potential transplant recipient, and is used to match the donor organs with the appropriate patient. Additional tests may include **lymphocytotoxic antibody screening** (antibodies against the antigens in the general population), and the **HLA crossmatch** test (antibodies against specific donor antigens).

## RECORDING LABORATORY RESULTS

The results of laboratory tests are a valuable tool to the doctor in the diagnosis and treatment of patients; therefore, the test result values are often communicated to the doctor before the computer report can be placed on the patient's chart. Stat and/or abnormal laboratory test results are communicated verbally or by telephone to the doctor by the health unit coordinator or nurse. Also, the doctor may request on the physicians' order sheet that the laboratory test results be communicated to him or her by telephone immediately upon their completion.

To verbally communicate laboratory results, the laboratory personnel telephones them to the health unit coordinator on the nursing unit, who records them on a telephone laboratory report sheet (Fig. 14–9). Where computers are in use, the results may reach the unit via the computer printer. Also, the results may be faxed to the nursing unit. The printed results also include the reference range, or range of normal values for each lab test (Fig. 14–10). The health unit coordinator in turn telephones the laboratory results to the physician's office. Although the task may appear simple to perform, it is a very responsible task, since the doctor may prescribe treatment according to the laboratory values. Consider for a moment what the consequences could be should the value be recorded inaccurately. To avoid errors, *always* read the laboratory values you have recorded back to the person in the laboratory. *Always* have the person you are communicating to in the doctor's office repeat his or her recorded values back to you. The written report should be placed on the patient's chart in a timely manner. Accuracy in the selection of the correct patient's chart as well as the appropriate location in the chart is very important.

## SUMMARY

Laboratory studies are very useful diagnostic tools, and therefore they are frequently ordered. Accuracy in ordering is of utmost importance, because an error could result in the wrong test being performed or the wrong patient being tested. It is imperative that all specimens are properly labeled according to hospital policy and with the correct patient information. Prompt delivery of properly labeled specimens to the laboratory is also important.

One of your challenges as a health unit coordinator is to become familiar with the particular hospital's process of requisitioning laboratory orders. You should be able, after time, to process orders quickly and efficiently. Where a computer is in use, familiarize yourself with the various laboratory screens. Whether the hospital uses the computer or a requisition, it is important to know from which laboratory department a particular test is requisitioned.

As diagnostic procedures from other departments are added to your medical knowledge, you may find that they may conflict with some laboratory tests, or vice versa. Coordinating laboratory studies with x-ray, nuclear medicine, or GI studies (to name a few) is one of the tasks you learn as you proceed with this program.

If your hospital does not have a written laboratory procedure manual, call your hospital laboratory to get your questions answered.

**REVIEW QUESTIONS**

1. List two general purposes of laboratory studies.
   a. _diagnostic_
   b. _evaluate treatment prescribed_

2. State the purpose of the microbiology, chemistry, and hematology divisions of the laboratory.
   Microbiology: _studies specimens to determine disease causing organisms._
   Chemistry: _performs tests related to chemical reaction occuring in living organisms_
   Hematology: _performs test related to the physical properties of blood_

3. Name three methods used by the nursing staff to collect urine specimens.
   a. _clean catch, midstream_
   b. _voiding_
   c. _catheterization_

4. List five types of specimens collected for laboratory study.
   a. _blood serum_          d. _urine_
   b. _pleural fluid sputum_  e. _stool_
   c. _cerebro spinal fluid_

5. What is the procedure for ordering stat blood tests from the laboratory?
   _call the order to lab give patients name, unit, rm no. and the test requested. Prepare the requisition immediatly so that the technician can pick it up on arrival to the unit to draw the specimen. On the computer type stat when ordering_

6. What are the health unit coordinator's responsibilities for an order for a 2 h PP BS?
   _Prepare requisition and send to Lab, on the day that the test is to be done notify the Lab of the time the patient finished eating._

7. List three specimens usually collected by nursing personnel.
   a. _urine_
   b. _sputum_
   c. _stool_

8. What is the difference between a stat and a routine laboratory order?
   _stat is done immediatly and routine is done any time of the day as per hospital procedure_

9. List five procedures that require a consent form that are performed by the doctor to obtain specimens for study.

a. _____ lumbar puncture _____

b. _____ biopsies _____

c. _____ centesis (para, amnio, thora) _____

d. _____ C&U smears _____

e. _____ sternal puncture _____

10. What procedure must be performed before some blood components, such as packed red cells, can be ordered for a patient for a transfusion? _____ type & crossmatch _____

11. What is the health unit coordinator's responsibility concerning specimens collected on the unit to be sent to or delivered to the laboratory? _____ make sure it is properly labeled and carried to the lab as soon as possible, never send by tube _____ with the requisition

12. What four laboratory studies make up the test called electrolytes?

a. _____ NA _____    c. _____ Cl _____

b. _____ K _____    d. _____ $HCO_3$ _____

13. Write the abbreviations for the three cardiac enzyme studies.

a. _____ CK / CPK _____

b. _____ SGOT (AST) _____

c. _____ LDH _____

14. Write the meaning of each abbreviation listed below.

a. T&C _____ Type & crossmatch _____    g. CSF _____ Cerebro Spinal fluid _____

b. O&P _____ Ova & Parasite _____    h. FBS _____ Fasting Blood sugar _____

c. LP _____ Lumbar Puncture _____    i. AFB _____ Acid-Fast Bacillus _____

d. Na _____ sodium _____    j. CBC _____ complete blood count _____

e. K _____ potassium _____    k. P _____ Phosphorus _____

f. C&S _____ Culture & Sensitivity _____    l. UA _____ Urinalysis _____

15. Name six microbiology and six chemistry studies.

| Microbiology | Chemistry |
|---|---|
| 1. Culture & Sensitivity | 1. Amylase serum |
| 2. AFB culture | 2. Cardiac enzymes |
| 3. gram stain | 3. (BS) Blood sugar |
| 4. Cmv culture | 4. (BUN) Blood Urea Nitrogen |
| 5. urine colony count | 5. FBS Fasting Blood sugar |
| 6. Stool specimen for O&P | 6. Lytes |

16. Name six hematology studies.
   a. _RBC indices_
   b. _CBC c diff_
   c. ~~Hct Hgb coagulation profile~~ coagulation profile
   d. bleeding time  Fibrinogen Level
   e. coagulation time, clotting time, TC T&T
   f. _WBC_

17. Explain the difference between fasting and NPO.  or non sugared drink
   fasting — allowed water only  breakfast held till test
   NPO — nothing by mouth  food or liquid  completed

18. Define the following:
   a. biopsy _tissue removed from a living body for examination_
   b. clean catch _one method by which a urine specimen is obtained_
   c. fasting _no solid food or liquids containing sugar→may allow tea or coffee_
   d. lumbar puncture _procedure to remove spinal fluid from the spinal cord_
   e. midstream _a method of obtaining a urine specimen_
   f. occult blood _hidden blood — undetectible to the eye_
   g. postprandial ~~before~~ after _a meal or eating_
   h. sputum _mucus excreation from the lungs_
   i. sternal puncture _procedure to remove bone marrow from the sternum_
   j. urinalysis _analysis of urine (physical, chemical, microscopic)_
   k. voided specimen _a specimen obtained by urinating_
   l. dipstick urine _visual examination of urine using a commercially treated stick_

19. In the space provided, write in the laboratory division that performs each of the following tests:

   a. FBS          chemistry       j. triglycerides   micro biology
   b. urine for C&S microbiology    k. RA factor       hematology
   c. lytes         chemistry       l. sputum for AFB  microbiology
   d. CBC           hematology      m. RBC indices     hematology
   e. FE & TIBC     chemistry       n. T₃              chemistry
   f. APTT          hematology      o. GTT             chemistry
   g. unit of PC    ~~hematology~~ blood bank   p. Retics   hematology
   h. Hct & Hgb     hematology      q. WBC & diff      hematology
   i. VDRL          serology        r. 2 h PP BS       ~~chemistry~~

s.  PT                          _hematology_           v.  TCT            _hematology_

t.  protein electrophoresis     _chemistry_            w.  Na & K         _Chemistry_

u.  T&C                         _bloodbank_            x.  stool for O&P   _microbiology_

20. a. Serologic studies are studies of body fluids for immune bodies that are the body's
       ___defense___ when ___disease___
       occurs.

    b. In the following orders, underline those that are serologic studies.

       1. ANA                    6. VDRL
       2. BUN                    7. retics
       3. T$_3$                  8. TIBC
       4. RA factor             9. ASO titer
       5. PT                    10. HIV

21. Underline the studies that require the specimen to be sent to the urine chemistry laboratory.

    1. creatinine clearance      5. urine for C&S
    2. CBC                       6. urine for protein
    3. PCV                       7. urine for AFB
    4. GTT                       8. FSH

22. Three drugs studied for their therapeutic drug levels in the chemistry laboratory are:

    a. ___gentamycin___          c. ___digoxin___

    b. ___tobramycin___

23. How may errors be avoided in recording of telephoned laboratory results?
    ___alway read back the laboratory values___
    ___recorded to the person in the Lab___

24. Rewrite the following doctors' orders using symbols and abbreviations. Or, to practice
    writing doctors' orders, have someone read the orders to you while you record them. Again,
    practice using symbols and abbreviations.

    a. complete blood count and electrolytes every morning ___CBC & Lytes every AM___

    b. hemoglobin and hematocrit immediately ___H&H stat___

    c. type and crossmatch for six units of packed (red blood) cells—hold for surgery in the
       morning ___T&C 6 U PRB Hold for surgery in am___

    d. sputum specimen for culture and sensitivity for acid-fast bacillus ___Sputum spec for___
       ___C&S for AFB___

    e. lumbar puncture for cerebrospinal fluid: on tube number one, do protein and glucose
       ___LP for CSF: #1 proteins + glucose___
       ___#2 CX for CMV + Fungus___ levels; on tube number two, do cultures
       ___#3 AFB stain___
       for cytomegalovirus and fungus; on tube number three, do an acid fast bacillus
       stain _____

    f. sequential multiple analysis for 20 serum chemicals in the morning ___SMA$_{20}$ in AM___

# References

Bennington, James L.: *Saunders Dictionary & Encyclopedia of Laboratory Medicine and Technology*. Philadelphia, W. B. Saunders Co., 1984.

Blackburn, Elsa: *Health Unit Coordinator*. Englewood Cliffs, NJ, Prentice-Hall, Inc., Brady Division, 1991.

*Dorland's Pocket Medical Dictionary*, 25th ed. Philadelphia, W. B. Saunders Co., 1995.

Fischbach, Frances Talaska: *A Manual of Laboratory Diagnostic Tests*. Philadelphia, J. B. Lippincott Co., 1980.

Good Samaritan Hospital, Department of Pathology: *A Nursing Guide to Laboratory Procedures*. Phoenix, AZ, 1977.

McFarland, Mary Brambilla and Grant, Marcia Moeller: *Nursing Implications of Laboratory Tests*. New York, John Wiley & Sons, 1982.

St. Joseph's Hospital and Medical Center, Laboratory Department: *Laboratory Requisition Guide Book*. Phoenix, AZ.

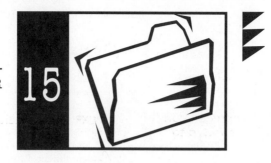

CHAPTER 15

# DIAGNOSTIC IMAGING ORDERS

## X-Rays, Ultrasound, CT Scans, Magnetic Resonance Imaging, and Nuclear Medicine

---

### CHAPTER OBJECTIVES

*Upon completion of this chapter, you will be able to:*

1. Define the terms in the vocabulary list.

2. Write the meaning of each abbreviation in the abbreviations list.

3. Name five patient positions that may be included in an x-ray order.

4. Identify those x-ray orders that require no preparation and those that require a preparation.

5. Name five x-ray orders that require a signed patient consent form.

6. List, in order, the four x-rays that should be performed in sequence.

7. List six studies performed by the nuclear medicine department.

8. List seven special instructions about the client that the health unit coordinator is to include when ordering tests from the diagnostic imaging department.

---

### VOCABULARY

**Clinical Indications** • Notations recorded when ordering diagnostic imaging to indicate the reason for doing the procedure

**Computed Tomography** • The study performed using a device that records views of selected levels of the body (body section radiography) onto a computer; sometimes referred to as a CT or CAT scan

**Contrast Media** • Substances (solids, liquids, or gases) used in diagnostic imaging procedures that permit the radiologist to distinguish between the different body densities; they may be injected, swallowed, or introduced by rectum

**C-Arm** • A mobile fluoroscopy unit used in surgery or at the bedside

**Fluoroscopy** • The observation of deep body structures made visible by use of a television screen instead of film; a contrast medium is required for this procedure

**Magnetic Resonance Imaging** • A technique used for computer imaging of the interior of the body using magnetic fields

**"On Call" Medication** • Medications prescribed by the doctor to be given prior to the diagnostic imaging procedure; the department notifies the nursing unit of the time the medication is to be administered to the patient

**Portable X-ray** • An x-ray taken by a mobile x-ray machine, which is moved to the patient's bedside

**Position** • An alignment of the body on the x-ray table favorable for taking the best view of the part of the body to be radiographed

**Reinforcing Dose Study** • A repeat x-ray study done because the initial cholecystogram (x-ray of the gallbladder) results were poor or did not outline the gallbladder

**Routine Preparation** • The standard preparation suggested by the radiologist to be followed to prepare the patient for an ordered diagnostic imaging study

**Scan** • a. The image produced when the concentration of radionuclide in an organ is photographed (nuclear medicine)

b. The radiograph produced of selected body levels when using computed tomography (CT)

**Ultrasonography** • A procedure performed to examine body structures by the use of ultrasound; a device used to record the echoes of sound waves striking body tissues of different densities; procedures using this method may also be referred to as sonography or echography

## ABBREVIATIONS

| Abbreviation | Meaning | Example of Usage on a Doctors' Order Sheet |
|---|---|---|
| AP | anteroposterior | AP view of abd |
| BE | barium enema | BE tomorrow |
| CI | clinical indications | BE-CI: R/O tumor |
| CT | computed tomography | CT scan of abd |
| CXR | chest x-ray | CXR today |
| DSA | digital subtraction angiography | cerebral DSA |
| f/u | follow-up | f/u KUB in AM |
| Fx | fracture | x-ray lt femur CI: R/O Fx |
| GB series | gallbladder | GB tomorrow |
| GI | gastrointestinal | GI study tomorrow |
| h/o | history of | UGI CI: h/o ulcers |
| IVP | intravenous pyelogram | IVP c̄ Rt prep |
| IVU | intravenous urogram; synonymous with IVP | IVU |
| KUB | kidneys, ureters, and bladder | KUB today |
| lat | lateral | PA & lat chest |
| LLQ | left lower quadrant | Abd x-ray special attention to LUQ & LLQ |
| LUQ | left upper quadrant | |
| L&S | Liver and spleen | L&S scan tomorrow (nuclear medicine) |
| LS | lumbosacral | X-ray LS spine (x-ray) |
| MRI | magnetic resonance imaging | MRI of brain |
| OCG | oral cholecystogram | OCG routine prep |

| Abbreviation | Meaning | Example of Usage on a Doctors' Order Sheet |
|---|---|---|
| PA | posteroanterior | PA chest x-ray |
| PCXR | portable chest x-ray | PCXR stat |
| PET | positron emission tomography | PET tomorrow AM |
| PTC | percutaneous transhepatic cholangiography | PTC tomorrow |
| R/O | rule out | UGI to R/O ulcers |
| RLQ | right lower quadrant | X-ray of abd Compare c̄ x-ray of 12/2/xx. Check RUQ and RLQ |
| RUQ | right upper quadrant | |
| SBFT | small bowel follow-through | UGI c̄ SBFT |
| UGI | upper gastrointestinal | UGI p̄ GB |
| US | ultrasound | US of GB |

## EXERCISE 1

Write the abbreviation for each term listed below.

1. intravenous pyelogram _IVP_
2. right lower quadrant _RLQ_
3. kidneys, ureters, and bladder _KUB_
4. barium enema _BE_
5. posteroanterior _PA_
6. upper gastrointestinal _UGI_
7. lateral _Lat_
8. lumbosacral _LS_
9. left upper quadrant _LUQ_
10. anteroposterior _AP_
11. gastrointestinal _GI_
12. right upper quadrant _RUQ_
13. computed axial tomography _CAT_
14. left lower quadrant _LLQ_
15. gallbladder _GB_
16. magnetic resonance imaging _MIR_
17. small bowel follow-through _SBFT_
18. chest x-ray _CXR_
19. digital subtraction angiography _DSA_
20. oral cholecystogram _OCG_

21. portable chest x-ray _____ PCXR
22. percutaneous transhepatic cholangiography _____ PTC
23. fracture _____ FX
24. history of _____ h/o
25. follow-up _____ F/U
26. clinical indications _____ CI
27. intravenous urogram _____ IVU

## E X E R C I S E  2

The following is a list of orders for imaging procedures that may appear on patients' charts. Write the meaning of each underlined abbreviation.

1. <u>BE</u> tomorrow p̄ sigmoidoscopy — Barium Enema

2. Stat <u>LS</u> spine x-ray — Lumbar Spinal

3. <u>KUB</u> this AM — Kidney Ureter Bladder

4. <u>US</u> for fetal age — Ultra Sound

5. Abdominal x-ray c̄ attention to <u>RLQ</u> & <u>LUQ</u> — Right Lower Quadrant / Left Upper Quadrant

6. <u>IVU</u> & <u>UGI</u> tomorrow. Check with radiologist for prep — Intravenous Urogram / Upper Gastro intestenal

7. <u>CT</u> scan of brain — Computed Tomography

8. <u>GI</u> study c̄ barium swallow — Gastro Intestinal

9. <u>PA</u> & <u>lat</u> chest now — Posterior/Antererior lateral

10. <u>MRI</u> of brain — Magnetic Resonance Imaging

11. <u>PCXR</u> — Portable Chest X Ray

12. <u>UGI</u> c̄ <u>SBFT</u> — Upper Gastro intestinal Small Bowel Follow through

## COMMUNICATION WITH THE DIAGNOSTIC IMAGING DEPARTMENT

Orders for the diagnostic imaging department are communicated by the ordering step of transcription by using a computer or requisition form (Fig. 15–1). Since the patient usually is transported to the diagnostic imaging department for the procedure, it is important to indicate the mode of transportation—wheelchair or gurney (stretcher). The patient is transported by the nursing staff, diagnostic imaging department staff, or transport service.

A portable or mobile x-ray is an exception to the standard transportation procedure. A request for a portable x-ray necessitates the radiographer taking the portable equipment to the patient's room. A portable x-ray is ordered when movement might be detrimental to the patient's condition.

When ordering the diagnostic procedure indicate the following **information** about the client:

■ Is receiving intravenous fluids
■ Has a seizure disorder
■ Is receiving oxygen
■ Needs isolation precautions
■ Does not speak English
■ Is a diabetic
■ Is sight or hearing impaired

This information will assist personnel in the diagnostic imaging department provide better care for the patient (see Fig. 15–1). **Clinical indications**, the reason the doctor is ordering the procedure must also be recorded by the health unit coordinator. Since this information is often required by insurance companies before they will provide reimbursement to the health care facilities, many diagnostic imaging departments will not perform procedures until they have the clinical indications recorded.

## BACKGROUND INFORMATION FOR RADIOLOGY

In 1895, Wilhelm Roentgen discovered a strange phenomenon that produced a photograph of the bones of his wife's hand. The exact mechanism for the production of the rays was unknown to Roentgen; therefore, he used the algebraic symbol for the unknown, "x," to title his discovery.

The x-ray studies performed in the radiology area of the diagnostic imaging department are carried out by a **radiographer**, a person with special education in the area of radiography. The x-ray films are developed in the department and are interpreted by a radiologist, a physician who has specialized in this field. Some studies are done by observing the path of contrast media in the body by means of a fluoroscope.

It should be noted that doctors' orders for radiology do not always have the term "x-ray" in them. An order for "Chest, PA and lat" is an order for a chest x-ray taken from posterior to anterior and laterally. Some studies are also called CT sans and others are identified by the suffix "gram" as in carotid arteriogram.

The new trend in diagnostic imaging is a computerized radiology system, which will be filmless. In filmless radiology there will be no x-ray films, only images, stored in computer systems.

As you learn more about diagnostic procedures, you will find that the tests scheduled in the radiology area must be carried out in specific sequences so as not to interfere with one another.

F I G U R E  15–1 • (A) General requisition for diagnostic imaging. (B) Diagnostic imaging computer order screen.

## PATIENT POSITIONING

The doctor may wish x-rays to be taken while the patient is placed in a specific position on the x-ray table to allow the best view of the area to be exposed. The health unit coordinator must be careful to include all of the x-ray order without making any changes, and to be absolutely accurate when transcribing such orders. For example: the health unit coordinator should be sure not to write AP (anteroposterior) when the order calls for PA (posteroanterior) positioning. The wrong abbreviation can cause the radiographer to film a different view, which may obscure an abnormality.

Following is a list of the positions used most frequently in writing x-ray orders.

■ *AP position (anteroposterior):* This view may be taken while the patient is either standing or lying on his back (supine); the machine is placed in front of the patient.
■ *PA position (posteroanterior):* this view may be taken while the patient is either standing or lying on his stomach (prone) with the x-ray machine aimed at his back.
■ *Lateral position:* This view is taken from the side.
■ *Oblique position:* This picture is taken with the patient lying halfway on his side in either the AP or PA position.
■ *Decubitus position:* In this view, the patient is lying on his side with the x-ray beam positioned horizontally.

## CONSENT FORMS

Diagnostic imaging procedures that are invasive, those requiring the injection of contrast medium, require the patient to sign a consent form. It is the responsibility of the health unit coordinator to prepare the consent form for the patient's signature. Diagnostic imaging procedures that require a consent form may vary among health care facilities. As a beginning health unit coordinator, keep a list of those procedures requiring a consent form to assist you until you have this information committed to memory.

## RADIOGRAPHIC (X-RAY) PROCEDURES

### X-Rays that Do Not Require Preparation

X-rays can penetrate solid material, such as bone, which in turn produces a shadow that is recorded on film. Procedures that require the filming of bone structures or that are ordered to determine the position of other organs in relation to these structures can be performed by qualified x-ray personnel without any preparation for the procedure by the nursing or x-ray staff.

Below are listed some x-ray studies as they are commonly written on a doctors' order sheet.

**COMMUNICATION AND IMPLEMENTATION OF DIAGNOSTIC IMAGING ORDERS**

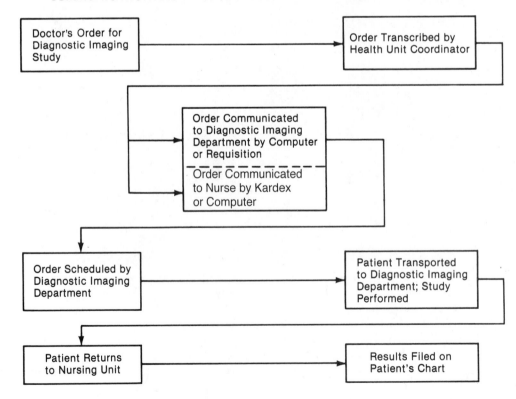

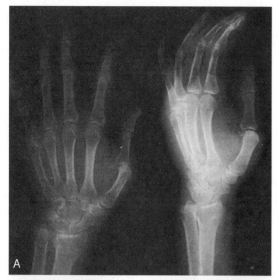

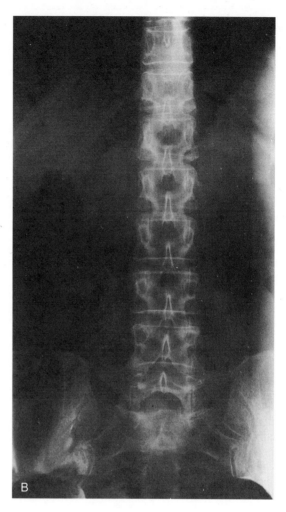

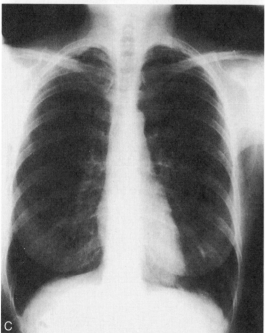

F I G U R E   15–2 • Chest x-ray film. (From Dowd, Stephen B. and Wilson, Betty G.: *Encyclopedia of Radiographic Positioning*, vols. I and II. Philadelphia, W. B. Saunders Co., 1995, with permission.)

## Doctors' Orders for X-Rays that Do Not Require Preparation

■ *Sinus series CI: R/O sinusitis*
An order for an x-ray of the paranasal sinus structures.

### a. Purpose
Used to determine infection, trauma, or disease in the paranasal sinuses.

■ *PA and lat chest CI: R/O pneumonia*
An order for a chest x-ray. Frequently the word *x-ray* is not written on the order because some terms in the order are recognized as directions used only in radiography. The terms *PA* and *lat* indicate the angles at which the doctor wishes the film to be taken (Fig. 15–2).

### a. Purpose
Used to diagnose or assess patients with pneumonia, pneumothorax, or atelectasis. Also used to determine the size and position of the heart or for the placement of invasive lines or tubes.

■ *LS spine CI: R/O fracture*
The doctor requests an x-ray of the lumbosacral area of the spine. Used to determine abnormalities of the lumbosacral region.

■ *Mammogram CI: hmp 10° lt br*
The doctor requests an x-ray of the breast.
### a. Purpose
Used to detect cancer or cysts located in the soft tissue of the breast.

■ *X-ray of the tibia with close attention to the distal portion CI: R/O fracture*

An order of an x-ray of the bone in the patient's lower leg. The word *distal* indicates that the radiologist is to observe a particular portion of the bone. Remember to include the entire order on the requisition. Used to determine fractures.

■ *KUB CI: hydronephrosis*

A request for an x-ray of the abdomen.

    *a. Purpose*

Used to determine male or female reproductive system disorders such as masses, tumors, or fibroids.

■ *Portable film of rt femur CI: R/O Fx*

A radiographer takes a portable x-ray machine to the patient's bedside to film the right upper leg of the patient. It is important for the health unit coordinator to write the word *portable* or *mobile* on the requisition form.

    *a. Purpose*

Used to determine fractures.

■ *Tomogram of lt lung, upper lobe CI: Eval chest lesion*

A tomogram is a type of x-ray picture that studies selected levels of the body, in this case levels of the left lung. This order is not a request for computerized tomography.

    *a. Purpose*

Used only for further evaluation of a chest lesion.

■ *Postreduction study of the forearm*

    *a. Purpose*

Used to evaluate the alignment of a fracture after intervention.

■ *AP and lat rt hip*

    *a. Purpose*

Used to evaluate prosthetic replacement of the hip. Done at the bedside.

---

### TO THE STUDENT

To practice transcribing radiology (x-ray) orders that require no preparation, complete **Activity 15–1** in the Skills Practice Manual.

---

## X-Rays that Require Preparation and Contrast Media

When an x-ray is made, images of varying density appear on the exposed film. The differences in density are due to the degree of absorption offered by different tissues and air to the radiation. It is easy to differentiate bony structures, because the bones offer resistance and therefore appear light on film. The lungs, however, which contain air, do not offer much resistance to radiation and appear black on film.

Certain organs and blood vessels within the body are difficult for the radiologist to see because there is little difference in density between them and their surroundings parts. In order to increase the contrast, it is necessary for a **contrast medium** to be given to the patient.

The most common types of contrast media are organic iodine compounds and barium preparations. Organic iodine compounds may be injected or taken into the body by mouth, rectum, or other approaches.

Contraindications to the use of iodine dye includes allergy to shellfish.

For the contrast medium to prove most effective, the nursing unit prepares the patient by the method suggested by the diagnostic imaging department. This is known as a **routine preparation**.

The attending physician may change the routine preparation if the patient's condition does not permit it. Specific preparation orders must be written on the doctors' order sheet by the patient's doctor.

Sometimes a contrast medium used for one test may interfere with results obtained in another scheduled test. Therefore, if multiple x-ray tests are ordered, proper sequencing is necessary to obtain clear results. Sequencing is outlined by the diagnostic imaging department and may vary among hospitals.

### Sequencing

The following are typical guidelines for scheduling x-ray studies.

1. X-ray studies of the lower spine and pelvis should be ordered first, before a barium enema or an upper gastrointestinal study is done. The presence of barium in specific parts of the body may obscure the portion of the body that is being studied.
2. Abdominal studies using ultrasound or CT should precede studies using barium.
3. Liver and bone scans performed by nuclear medicine may also conflict with barium studies and should be done first.
4. Four x-ray studies that require contrast media are frequently ordered at the same time for diagnostic reasons. Only one or sometimes two can be done on the same day; thus, the studies may have to be scheduled 3 or more days in advance. The order of scheduling is listed below.
   1. Intravenous pyelogram (IVU)
   2. Gallbladder (GB), oral cholecystogram (OCG)
   3. Barium enema (BE), colon enema
   4. Upper gastrointestinal (UGI), small bowel

### Preparation Procedure

To visualize internal organs by the use of contrast media, preparation is usually required. Most of the preparation is done by the nursing staff and may begin the day before the x-ray study is scheduled.

Below are examples of doctors' orders for x-rays that require the patient to have some type of preparation. Each procedure and preparation is explained to help you understand its relationship to the others and to your role as a health unit coordinator.

Many hospitals have preparation cards—cards listing the tasks to be done to prepare the patient for the x-ray

(Fig. 15–3). When a patient is scheduled for one of the x-rays requiring preparation, a preparation card is usually placed in the patient's Kardex form holder to remind the nursing staff of the tasks they need to perform.

*Note:* It is possible for the preparation procedures to vary among hospitals.

---

**HIGHLIGHT**

When transcribing diagnostic imaging orders, the health unit coordinator should:

- Record the clinical indication on the requisition
- Record patient information on the requisition
- Check if a consent form is necessary; if so, prepare one for signature
- Check if patient preparation is required; if so, carry out the communication
- Check if scheduling is required; if so, schedule the procedure for the proper day and/or time

Accuracy in performing these steps is vital to reach the expected outcome.

---

## Doctors' Orders for X-Rays that Require Preparation and Contrast Media

■ *IVU CI: R/O ureterolithiasis* (synonymous with IVP; IVU is becoming the more common usage)

A procedure performed to outline the kidney, particularly the renal pelvis, ureters, and urinary bladder (Fig. 15–4). This is carried out in radiology by injecting an iodinated contrast medium into the vein.

---

**Preparation for IVP**

1 PM Rt. cathartic — 2 oz. Castor Oil

Limit fluids po 600 cc for 18 hrs

Low residue evening meal

NPO 8–12 hours

**F I G U R E 15–3** • Example of an x-ray preparation card.

*a. Purpose*

Used to determine the size and location of the kidneys, ureters, and bladder and to determine the presence of abnormalities such as tumors or strictures.

*b. Patient preparation*

- 2 oz castor oil day before test
- Low-residue evening meal
- NPO 8 to 12 hours
- Limit fluids to 600 cc PO for 18 hours
- Sign a consent form

*c. Transcribing the order*

In addition to transcribing this order, the health unit coordinator may initiate the diet changes and alert the nurse to administer enemas and/or cathartics. Prepare a consent form.

■ *OCG CI: R/O cholelithiasis* (synonymous with GB series or gallbladder series)

This study is performed to determine the ability of the gallbladder to function properly (Fig. 15–5).

*a. Purpose*

Used to identify obstruction, such as stones.

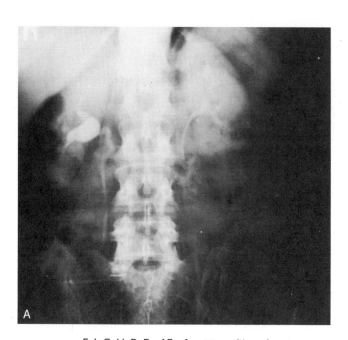

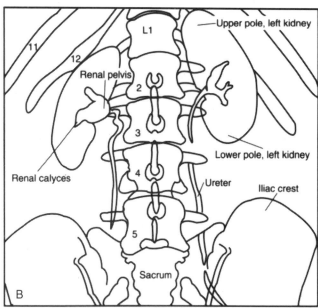

**F I G U R E 15–4** • X-ray film of an intravenous urogram. (From Dowd, Stephen B. and Wilson, Betty G.: *Encyclopedia of Radiographic Positioning*, vols. I and II. Philadelphia, W. B. Saunders Co., 1995, with permission.)

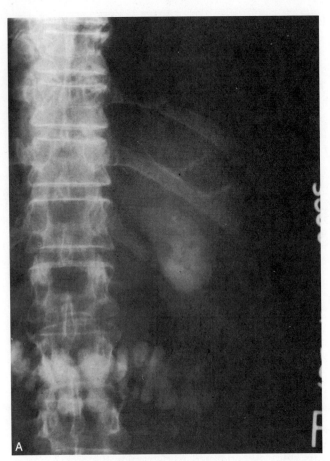
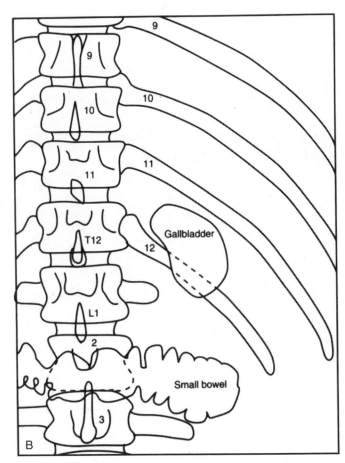

**FIGURE 15–5** • X-ray film of a gallbladder. (From Dowd, Stephen B. and Wilson, Betty G.: *Encyclopedia of Radiographic Positioning*, vols. I and II. Philadelphia, W. B. Saunders Co., 1995, with permission.)

b. *Patient preparation*
- Give oral contrast medium evening before test
- Light, fat-free evening meal
- NPO 8 to 12 hours

c. *Transcribing the order*

In addition to transcribing this order, the health unit coordinator initiates diet changes and alerts the nurse to administer the oral contrast medium, usually after the evening meal. There are times when the structure of the gallbladder does not appear (visualize) on the radiograph. The diagnostic imaging department notifies the nursing unit that a **reinforcing dose study** is indicated. This requires the procedure to be done again the next day, with the preparation repeated as for the first gallbladder study.

*Note:* The oral cholecystogram is being replaced by ultrasound studies of the gallbladder; however, since the oral cholecystogram is more cost effective, it is continuing to be required by some reimbursement programs.

■ *PIC CI: R/O obstruction of the bile ducts*

Using an iodine dye, this diagnostic x-ray visualizes the biliary duct system of the liver.

a. *Purpose*

Usually done to determine the cause of jaundice or persistent upper abdominal pain after cholecystectomy.

b. *Patient preparation*

Special prep orders may or may not be ordered.

■ *BE CI: R/O lesion of the colon*

This procedure is performed to visualize the large intestine (Fig. 15–6). In the diagnostic imaging department the patient is given an enema using a barium contrast medium.

a. *Purpose*

Used to identify diseases of the large intestine such as diverticula, cancer, or ulcerative colitis.

b. *Patient preparation*
- Castor oil 2 oz 2 PM day before test
- Clear liquid evening meal
- Tap water enema evening before test
- Tap water enemas until clear day of test
- Clear liquids only after midnight

c. *Transcribing the order*

In addition to transcribing the order for a barium enema, the health unit coordinator may initiate diet changes and alert the medication nurse concerning any medications to be given as preparation. The doctor may wish to order an air contrast barium enema, which requires the same preparation as a barium enema but uses air as well as barium for the contrast medium.

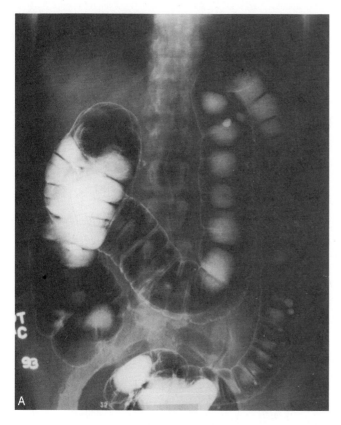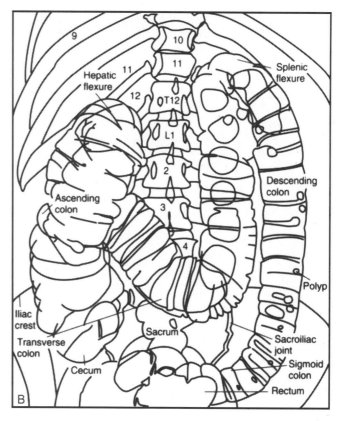

F I G U R E  15–6 • X-ray film of barium enema with air contrast. (From Dowd, Stephen B. and Wilson, Betty G.: *Encyclopedia of Radiographic Positioning*, vols. I and II. Philadelphia, W. B. Saunders Co., 1995, with permission.)

■ *UGI c̄ SBFT CI: R/O peptic ulcer*

An upper gastrointestinal study utilizes the fluoroscope, television, and x-ray machine as the means to examine the upper portion of the esophagus, stomach, and small intestines (Fig. 15–7).

   *a. Purpose*

Used to detect hiatal hernia, strictures, ulcers, or tumors.

   *b. Patient preparation*

The patient is usually NPO after supper until the procedure is completed

   • NPO 8 to 12 hours
   • No smoking or gum chewing

   *c. Transcribing the order*

The health unit coordinator transcribes the order and initiates the diet change.

> ### T O  T H E  S T U D E N T
>
> To practice transcribing radiology (x-ray) orders that require preparation, complete **Activity 15–2** in the Skills Practice Manual.

## Special X-ray Procedures

These procedures are performed under the direction of the radiologist alone or the surgeon with a radiologist present.

A request for the use of a special x-ray room or operating room must be submitted by the doctor in advance, or the procedure may be scheduled by telephone as part of the transcription procedure. *Before the procedure is done, the patient is requested to sign a patient consent form.* (See Chapter 8 for use and preparation of a consent form.)

These special x-ray procedures may be performed with or without a general anesthetic. When a general anesthetic is used, the nursing staff follows a preoperative routine (see Chapter 19). Preparations for these studies vary with each hospital.

The radiologist and/or surgeon may prescribe preprocedure medications to be given at a specific time or "on call." When medications are ordered **on call**, the doctor or department personnel, at the request of the radiologist and/or surgeon, notify the nursing unit to administer the medication that has been previously ordered for the procedure. *A consent form is required for all of the following procedures.*

### Doctors' Orders for Special X-ray Procedures

■ *Cerebral angiogram CI: R/O aneurysm*

A picture of vascular structures within the body after injection of a contrast medium (Fig. 15–8). The specific name given to the study is determined by the vascular structure

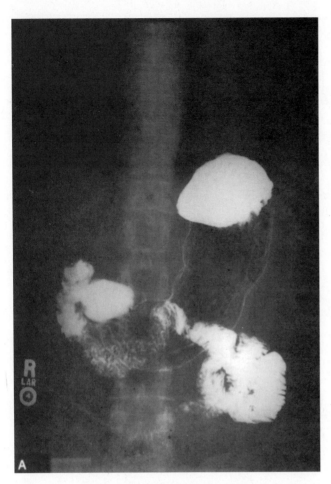
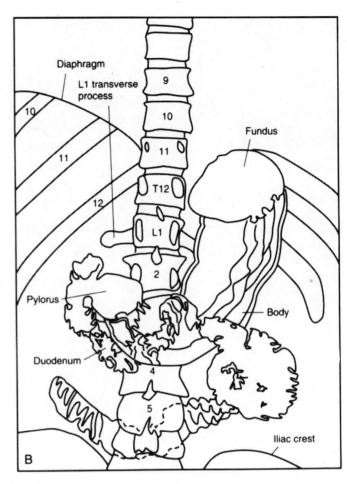

F I G U R E 15–7 • X-ray film of an upper gastrointestinal study. (From Dowd, Stephen B. and Wilson, Betty G.: *Encyclopedia of Radiographic Positioning*, vols. I and II. Philadelphia, W. B. Saunders Co., 1995, with permission.)

to be studied (such as renal angiogram or cerebral angiogram).

*a. Purpose*

Used to diagnose vascular aneurysms, malformations, and occluded or leaking blood vessels.

■ *Abdominal arteriogram CI: R/O angiodysplasia*

An x-ray picture of an artery after injection of a contrast medium. An arteriogram may be identified according to the anatomic location (such as femoral arteriogram).

*a. Purpose*

Used to detect obstruction or narrowing of an artery or aneurysm.

■ *Arthrogram of the left knee CI: R/O torn ligament*

An x-ray of a joint after injection of contrast medium.

*a. Purpose*

Used to determine trauma, such as bone chips or torn ligament, from an injury.

■ *Cholangiogram, postoperative (T-tube cholangiogram) CI: R/O retained stones*

An x-ray taken 6 to 9 days after a cholecystectomy to examine the bile ducts. Examination is done after injection of a contrast medium through T-tube.

*a. Purpose*

Used to rule out residual stones in the biliary tract following a cholecystectomy. It is called a T-tube cholangiogram because the catheter placed in the biliary ducts during surgery is called a T-tube.

■ *Hysterosalpingogram CI: R/O obstruction of fallopian tubes*

An x-ray of the uterus and fallopian tubes made after injection of a contrast medium (Fig. 15–9).

*a. Purpose*

Used in fertility studies and also to confirm abnormalities such as adhesions, fistulas, and so forth.

■ *Lymphangiogram left leg CI: R/O lymphatic obstruction*

An x-ray of the lymph channels and lymph nodes made after injection of a contrast medium.

*a. Purpose*

Used to identify metastatic cancer in the lymph nodes and to evaluate the effectiveness of chemotherapy.

■ *Spinal myelogram CI: R/O cord compression*

An x-ray of the spinal cord after a contrast medium has been injected between lumbar vertebrae into the spinal canal (Fig. 15–10).

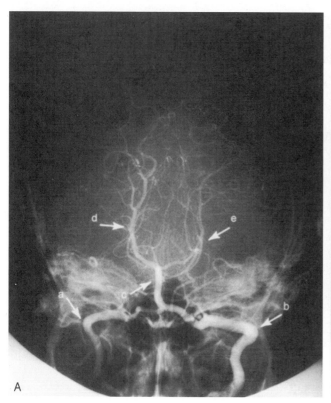 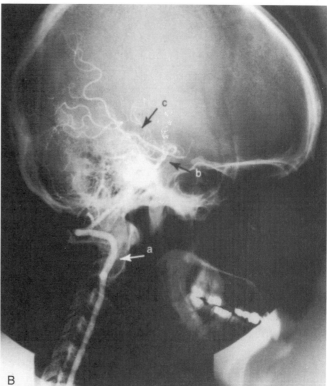

**F I G U R E  15–8 •** Cerebral arteriograms. (From Dowd, Stephen B. and Wilson, Betty G.: *Encyclopedia of Radiographic Positioning*, vols. I and II. Philadelphia, W. B. Saunders Co., 1995, with permission.)

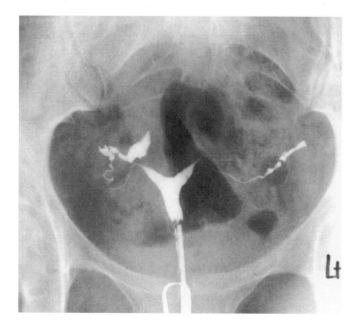

**F I G U R E  15–9 •** Hysterosalpingogram. (From Dowd, Stephen B. and Wilson, Betty G.: *Encyclopedia of Radiographic Positioning*, vols. I and II. Philadelphia, W. B. Saunders Co., 1995, with permission.)

*a. Purpose*

Used to detect herniated disks, tumors, and spinal nerve root injuries.

■ *Venogram of left leg CI: R/O DVT*

An x-ray of a vein, usually lower extremities, made after injection of a contrast medium.

*a. Purpose*

Used to evaluate veins before and after bypass surgery and to investigate venous function when obstruction is suspected.

■ *Voiding cystourethrogram CI: R/O bladder dysfunction*

X-ray films are taken to demonstrate the bladder filling then emptying as the patient voids.

*a. Purpose*

Used to demonstrate bladder dysfunction and uretheral strictures.

*Note:* Endoscopies including ERCP are covered in Chapter 16.

| TO THE STUDENT |
| --- |

To practice transcribing orders for special radiology (x-ray) procedures, complete **Activity 15–3** in the Skills Practice Manual.

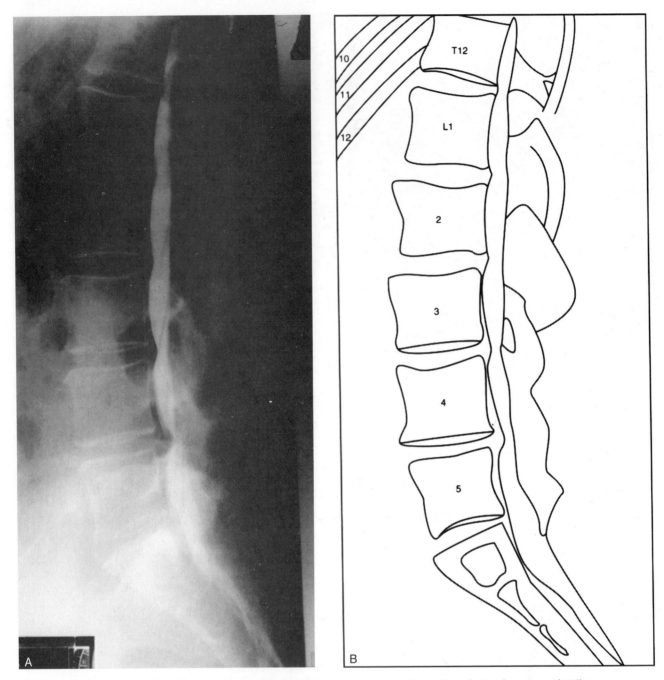

F I G U R E  15–10 • Myelogram showing the lumbar spine. (From Dowd, Stephen B. and Wilson, Betty G.: *Encyclopedia of Radiographic Positioning*, vols. I and II. Philadelphia, W. B. Saunders Co., 1995, with permission.)

## COMPUTED TOMOGRAPHY

Computed tomography (CT) scan provides a computerized image that reproduces a section of a body part as if sliced from front to back horizontally (Fig. 15–11). Contrast medium is not used unless specified.

### Doctors' Orders for CT Scans

■ *CT scan of the head c̄ DSA CI: R/O aneurysm*

Digital subtraction angiography (DSA) combines angiography, fluoroscopy, and computer technology to visualize the cardiovascular system without the interference of the bone and soft tissue structure to obscure the image.

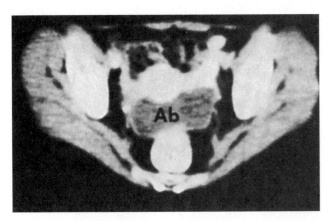

F I G U R E 15–11 • A CT scan showing a tuboovarian abscess (Ab). (From Chinn, D. H. and Callen, P. W.: Ultrasound of the acutely ill obstetrics and gynecology patient. *Radiologic Clinics of North America* 21[3]:585–594, 1983, with permission.)

a. *Purpose*
Used to evaluate postoperatively, such as endarterectomies, and to detect any cerebrovascular abnormalities.

■ *CT scan of the brain CI: headaches, R/O tumor*
a. *Purpose*
Used to diagnose lesions or abnormalities or to monitor the effects of surgery or chemotherapy.
b. *Patient preparation*
The patient is usually NPO for several hours before the test.

■ *CT scan of abdomen and pelvis CI: R/O retroperitoneal lesion*
a. *Purpose*
Used to determine malignancy or source of infection, abscess, and so forth.
b. *Patient preparation*
Patient is usually NPO for 4 hours. These studies should be performed before studies that require barium.

■ *CT of LS spine CI: R/O spinal stenosis*
The scan studies the lumbrosacral area of the spine.
a. *Purpose*
Often ordered after myelogram. Used to confirm spinal stenosis, changes in the disk and vertebrae, and to confirm spinal infection.

■ *CT of the neck CI: R/O tumor*
a. *Purpose*
Used to identify soft tissue masses and/or to evaluate the larynx.

■ *CT of the sinus CI: sinus infection*
a. *Purpose*
Used to diagnose infectious processes.

■ *CT guided liver biopsies*
CT is used to identify the location of tissue to be biopsied so needle placement is precise.
a. *Purpose*

Used to obtain tissue of the liver for diagnostic purposes. CT-guided lung and breast biopsies are also performed.

## ULTRASONOGRAPHY

These noninvasive studies are also called *sonograms* or echograms. Images are produced on a screen from body surface echoes when sound waves produced by an electrical device come in contact with structures in the body (Fig. 15–12).

### Doctors' Orders for Ultrasonography Studies

■ *Ultrasound abd*
a. *Purpose*
Used to detect liver cysts, abscesses, hematomas, and tumors.
b. *Patient preparation*
  • NPO 8 to 12 hours
  • Full bladder, drink fluids—do not void
  • No smoking AM of exam

■ *Ultrasound pelvis*
a. *Purpose*
Used during pregnancy to identify ectopic pregnancy, multiple births, and fetal abnormality. Used otherwise to identify ovarian cancer and other disorders.
b. *Patient preparation*
  • Full bladder—drink fluids, do not void
  • May require water enema

■ *Ultrasound GB*
a. *Purpose*
Used to diagnose cholelithiasis, cholecystitis, and to identify obstructive jaundice.

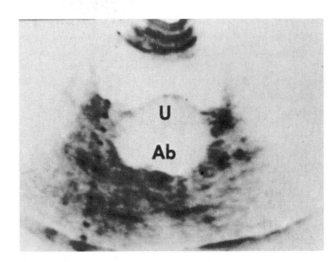

F I G U R E 15–12 • An ultrasound study showing the same tubo-ovarian abscess (Ab) as in Figure 15–11. (From Chinn, D. H. and Callen, P. W.: Ultrasound of the acutely ill obstetrics and gynecology patient. *Radiologic Clinics of North America* 21[3]:585–594, 1983, with permission.)

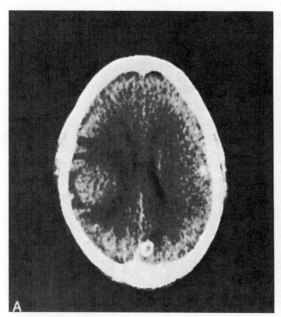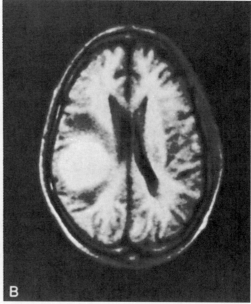

FIGURE 15–13 • An example of magnetic resonance imaging (MRI). (*A*) CT scan of brain. (*B*) Same patient's brain with round tumor on left side. (From Bydder, G. M.: Magnetic resonance imaging of the brain. *Radiologic Clinics of North America* 22[4]:779–793, 1984, with permission.)

*b. Patient preparation*
- Fat-free evening meal
- Fast 8 to 10 hours
- No smoking AM of exam

*Note:* Doppler studies are covered in Chapter 16.

## MAGNETIC RESONANCE IMAGING

**Magnetic resonance imaging (MRI),** is a technique for viewing the interior of the body using a powerful magnetic field that lines up the protons in the nuclei of the body's cells. The protons spin when a radio frequency is turned on. The protons return to their normal position when the radio signal is discontinued. During proton movement, a computer records cross-sectional images of the part being studied. Bones do not obscure the image as they do in x-rays. Studies are done on selected areas of the body, such as the brain, spinal cord, and bone (Fig. 15–13). MRI can distinguish between benign and malignant tumors.

Due to the strength of the magnet and the radiofrequency waves, MRI contraindications exist for patients with the following:

- Pacemakers
- Cerebral aneurysm clips
- Any electrically, magnetically, or mechanically activated implants
- Ferrous-based prosthetic devices
- Pregnancy

Dental bridge work may need to be removed prior to the scan but permanent fillings and inlays are acceptable because they are not made of ferrous metals. Prior to the exam, the patient is asked to remove metallic jewelry, wristwatches, eyeglasses, hairpins, or wigs if metal clips are present. Credit cards, bank cards, and similar devices with magnetically coded strips should be removed as well. This is especially important to remember in an outpatient diagnostic setting.

### Doctors' Orders for Magnetic Resonance Imaging

- *MRI of brain and spinal cord CI: R/O malignancy*
- *MRI rt shoulder CI: R/O rotator cuff injury*
- *MRI lt knee CI: R/O posterior cruciate ligament tear*

---

TO THE STUDENT

To practice transcribing orders for computerized tomography scans, ultrasound, and magnetic resonance imaging, complete **Activity 15–4** in the Skills Practice Manual.

---

## NUCLEAR MEDICINE

### Background Information

Nuclear medicine utilizes radioactive materials called *radiopharmaceuticals* to determine the functioning capacity of organs. Radioactive materials are used in diagnostic studies because of their ability to give off radiation in the form of gamma rays, which can be traced.

Depending upon the study to be made, the patient may take the radiopharmaceutical by mouth or it may be injected within a vein. A gamma scintillation camera is the instrument used to form an image of the concentration of the radioactive material in a specific organ of the body, thus producing a picture called a **scan**. It is possible to perform organ scans on the following body parts: bone, brain, thyroid, spleen, liver, heart, lungs, kidneys, gallbladder, and pancreas (Fig. 15–14).

Some diseases may be treated by the use of therapeutic doses of radiopharmaceuticals. Cancer of the thyroid and a blood condition called polycythemia vera respond to this treatment.

Radioactivity used in nuclear medicine differs from x-rays in that gamma radiation is from an outside source that passes the radiation through the body. In nuclear medicine, the radioactive material is taken internally by mouth or intravenously and emits gamma radiation from the specific organ being studied.

To communicate the doctors' order to nuclear medicine, the health unit coordinator must complete a nuclear medicine requisition or order on the computer.

Preparation may be required prior to the test. Check with your health care facility about preparation prior to scheduling the test.

## Doctors' Orders for Nuclear Medicine Studies

■ *Bone scan—total body CI: cancer, prostate R/O mets*
   *a. Purpose*
Performed to determine the presence of tumors, arthritis, or osteoporosis.

■ *Bone scan—limited CI: R/O cervical Fx*
   *a. Purpose*
Done when the doctor wishes to study a particular area of the body, such as vertebral compression fractures or unexplained bone pain.

■ *L&S (liver and spleen) scan CI: R/O cirrhosis*
   *a. Purpose*
Performed to evaluate injury to the spleen, chronic hepatitis, and metastatic processes. It should be done before barium studies. Other body scans may be performed on the brain, heart, lungs, kidneys, gallbladder, and pancreas.

■ *Gallium scan—total body CI: R/O abscess*
Also may be ordered regionally.
   *a. Purpose*
It is performed to locate the primary site of cancer, as well as to detect an abscess. May be used to examine the brain, liver, and breast tissue if disease is suspected.

■ *Thyroid uptake and scan CI: check for cold nodules*
   *a. Purpose*
A diagnostic study for thyroid gland performance. It demonstrates the ability of the thyroid gland to "take up" radioactive iodine.

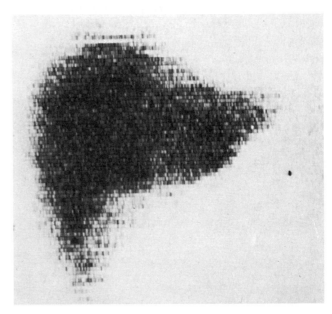

F I G U R E  15–14 • Nuclear scan of the liver.

■ *Lung perfusion/ventilation study CI: R/O embolism*
A diagnostic study for pulmonary embolism.

■ *DISIDA scan (formerly PIPIDA scan, also called hepatobiliary scan)*
A scan of the biliary tract (gallbladder).
   *a. Purpose*
Used to identify blockage or abnormal function.

■ *PET (positron emission tomography) scan*
   *a. Purpose*
Used to obtain information about blood flow to the myocardium, metabolism, glucose utilization, and schizophrenia. Isotopes are used.
   *b. Patient preparation*
Diet and medication adjustments are required before this procedure.

## Doctors' Orders for Nuclear Cardiology Tests

■ *MUGA scan CI: R/O CHF*
   *a. Purpose*
Used to study the function of the heart muscle, especially the left ventricle.

■ *Thallium stress scan CI: evaluate for CAD*
Stress is induced by using the treadmill or, if the patient cannot use the treadmill, medications are given to the patient to simulate the effects of exercise in the body. Drugs that simulate the effects of exercise are Persantine, adenosine, and dipyridamole.
   *a. Purpose*
Used to determine the blood flow to the myocardium while at rest or after normal stress to diagnose coronary

artery disease or to evaluate blood flow after a coronary bypass operation.

■ *Adenosine/thallium scan or Persantine/thallium scan*
An example of an order for a thallium scan using medication to simulate the effects of exercise.

■ *Sestamibi stress test or Persantine/sestamibi*
This is the same test as in thallium stress scan above using sestamibi as a radionuclide instead of thallium.

---

### TO THE STUDENT

To practice transcribing nuclear medicine orders, complete **Activity 15–5** in the Skills Practice Manual.

To practice transcribing a review set of doctors' orders, complete **Activity 15–6** in the Skills Practice Manual.

To practice recording doctors' orders and to practice recording telephoned messages, complete **Activities 15–7** and **15–8** in the Skills Practice Manual.

---

## SUMMARY

### HIGHLIGHT

Overview of diagnostic imaging procedures discussed in Chapter 15

| X-rays Not Requiring Prep | X-rays Requiring Prep |
| --- | --- |
| chest | IVU |
| bones | GB series |
| mammmogram | PTC |
| sinus | BE |
| tomogram of lung | UGI |

---

| Special X-ray Procedures Requiring a Consent Form | CT Scans |
| --- | --- |
| angiogram | brain |
| arteriogram | abdomen |
| arthrogram | LS spine |
| cholangiogram | neck |
| hysterosalpingogram | sinus |
| lymphangiogram | CT guided liver, lung, or breast biopsy |
| pyelogram | |
| venogram | |
| voiding cystourethrogram | CT of head c̄ DSA |

| Ultrasound | MRI | Nuclear Medicine Scans |
| --- | --- | --- |
| abdomen | brain | bone |
| pelvis | shoulder | liver and spleen |
| gallbladder | knee | gallium |
| | | thyroid uptake |
| | | lung perfusion/ventilation study |
| | | PET |
| | | DISIDA |
| | | MUGA |
| | | thallium |
| | | sestamibi |

Many imaging procedures can be carried out without any advance patient preparation; however, others require preparation before the body organ can be visualized.

The prime responsibility of the health unit coordinator in the transcription of diagnostic imaging orders, beyond ordering the requested study, is the communication to the nursing staff concerning preparation and the communication to the dietary department regarding diet changes. Accurate communication of the preparation procedure is *vital* to the expected outcome. An error may cause a procedure to be postponed or result in an unclear or nonvisible diagnostic image, each costly to the patient and hospital in both time and money. It is important to indicate, as part of the requisitioning process, the date the procedure is to be done (TBD).

## REVIEW QUESTIONS

1. Write the meaning of each abbreviation listed below.

   a. PA _____Postero Anterior_____    n. MRI _____Magnetic Resonance Imaging_____

   b. Lat _____Lateral_____    o. L&S _____Liver & Spleen_____
   (nuclear medicine)

   c. BE _____Barium Enema_____    p. SBFT _____Smaall bowel follow-through_____

   d. IVP _____Intravenous Pyelogram_____    q. US _____Ultra Sound_____

   e. IVU _____Intravenous Urogram_____    r. LLQ _____Lower Left Quadrant_____

   f. AP _____Antero posterior_____    s. CXR _____Chest X Ray_____

   g. KUB _____Kidneys,Ureters,Bladder_____    t. DSA _____digital subtraction angiography_____

   h. CT _____Computed Tomography_____    u. PCXR _____Portable Chest X Ray_____

   i. LS _____Lumbo sacral_____    v. OCG _____oral cholecystogram_____
   (x-ray)

   j. UGI _____Upper Gastro intestinal_____    w. PTHC _____Percutaneous transhepatic Choleangiogram_____

   k. GB _____Gallbladder_____    x. PET _____Positron emission tomography_____

   l. RUQ _____Right Upper Quadrant_____    y. Fx _____fracture_____

   m. R/O _____Rule Out_____

2. A substance used in x-ray procedures that helps the radiologist to distinguish between various body densities is called a _____Contrast medium_____

3. An x-ray taken at the patient's bedside is called a _____portable x ray_____

4. A study of deep body structures recorded on a fluorescent screen instead of on film is called a _____Fluoroscopy_____

5. A technique used for computer imaging of the interior of the body using magnetic fields is called _____MRI_____

6. A procedure that produces a record of echoes made by sound waves that strike different body densities is called _____Echo Ultrasonography_____

7. Preparation of patients for x-rays that are performed according to procedures set forth by the radiology department is called _____routine prep_____

8. Medications given to a patient by the nursing personnel when notified by the diagnostic department are called _____on Call_____ medications.

9. List five positions that may be included in a doctors' order for x-rays:

a. _AP -Lat_        d. _Lateral_

b. _PA -LAT_        e. _decubitus_

c. _Oblique_

10. In the event the doctor ordered the following x-rays for the same patient, in what sequence would they be scheduled? GB, BE, IVP, UGI

a. _IVP_        c. _BE_

b. _GB_        d. _UGI_

11. Five x-ray procedures that may require a signed consent form before they may be done are:

a. _Cerebral Angiogram_        d. _Cholangiogram_

b. _Spinal myelogram_        e. _venogram_

c. _arthrogram of Lt knee_

12. Seven diagnostic procedures performed by nuclear medicine are:

a. _bone scan_        e. _Lung perfusion ventilation study_

b. _Thyroid uptake & scan_        f. _Pet scan_

c. _L+S scan_        g. _MUGA scan_

d. _Gallium scan_

13. Place a check mark in the proper space after obtaining preparation information and consent form requirements for diagnostic imaging in your hospital from your instructor.

| Procedure | Preparation | | Patient Consent Form | |
|---|---|---|---|---|
| | Yes | No | Yes | No |
| a. KUB | | | | |
| b. IVU | | | | |
| c. CT-guided liver biopsy | | | | |
| d. femoral arteriogram | | | | |
| e. gallium scan | | | | |
| f. air contrast BE | | | | |
| g. tomogram rt lung | | | | |
| h. mammogram | | | | |
| i. UGI | | | | |
| j. bronchogram | | | | |
| k. BE | | | | |
| l. bone scan | | | | |
| m. GB | | | | |
| n. lymphangiogram | | | | |
| o. thallium stress scan | | | | |

14. Rewrite the following doctors' orders using abbreviations. Or, to practice writing doctors' orders, have someone read the orders to you while you record them.

a. lumbosacral spine, rule out fracture _LSpinR/O FX_

b. posterioanterior and lateral chest x-ray, rule out pneumonia _PA + Lat CXR R/O pneumonia_

c. upper gastrointestinal, intravenous urogram, gallbladder series, and barium enema _____

_UGI, IVU, GB Series, BE_

d. myelogram tomorrow _____ myelogram in AM

e. magnetic resonance imaging of the right shoulder rule out rotator cuff injury _____

MRI R shoulder R/O rotator cuff injury

15. When ordering diagnostic procedures, the clinical indication, or the the reason for the test must be recorded. Other information about the patient to be noted is:

a. _____ seizure _____        e. _____ oxygen _____

b. _____ language ~~barrier~~ _____        f. _____ isolation precautions _____

c. _____ blindness or hearing loss _____        g. _____ diabetic _____

d. _____ IV fluids _____

## References

Blackburn, Elsa: *Health Unit Coordinator.* Englewood Cliffs, NJ, Prentice-Hall, 1991.

Chabner, Davi-Ellen: *The Language of Medicine,* 5th ed. Philadelphia, W. B. Saunders Co., 1996.

*Dorland's Illustrated Medical Dictionary,* 28th ed. Philadelphia, W. B. Saunders Co., 1994.

Dowd, Steven B. and Wilson, Bettye G.: *Encyclopedia of Radiographic Positioning,* vols. I and II. Philadelphia, W. B. Saunders Co., 1995.

Good Samaritan Hospital, Department of Radiology: *Radiology Procedures and Patient Preparation.* Phoenix, AZ, 1977.

Ignatavicius, Donna D. and Bayne, Marilyn Varner: *Medical-Surgical Nursing.* Philadelphia, W. B. Saunders Co., 1991.

Miller, Benjamin F. and Keane, Claire Brackman: *Encyclopedia and Dictionary of Medicine and Nursing,* 3rd ed. Philadelphia, W. B. Saunders Co., 1983.

*Nurse's Reference Library Diagnostics,* 2nd ed. Springhouse, PA, Springhouse Corporation, 1989.

Schultz, Susan J., Foley, Carol R. and Gordon, Donald G. Preparing Your Patient for a Cardiac PET Scan. *Nursing 91.* September 1991, p. 63.

Tri-County Magnetic Imaging Associates, Ltd., *MRI: Contraindications.* Mt. Pleasant, PA, 1990.

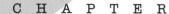

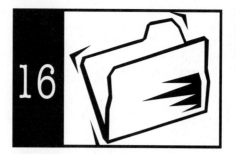

# CHAPTER 16

## OTHER DIAGNOSTIC STUDIES

### Cardiovascular Diagnostics, Neurodiagnostics, Endoscopy, Gastroenterology, and Pulmonary Function

---

**CHAPTER OBJECTIVES**

*Upon completion of this chapter, you will be able to:*

1. Identify tests performed by the following diagnostic departments: cardiovascular diagnostics, endoscopy, neurodiagnostics, gastroenterology, and pulmonary function.

2. State the meaning of each abbreviation in the abbreviations list.

3. Define the terms in the vocabulary list.

4. Name four diagnostic studies related to the heart.

5. Name three drugs that should be noted on an electrocardiogram requisition.

6. State the purpose of an electroencephalogram.

7. Name six endoscopies and the parts of the body visualized by each.

8. Describe the purpose of the gastroenterology department.

9. List five studies that may be performed by the gastroenterology department.

10. Describe the purpose of the pulmonary function department and name two tests performed there.

11. Name two medications that should be noted on requisitions for arterial blood gases.

12. Name two studies performed to diagnose vascular diseases.

---

**VOCABULARY**

**Blood Gases** • A diagnostic study to determine the exchange of gases in the blood

**Echoencephalogram** • A graphic recording that indicates (by sound waves) the position of the brain within the skull

**Electrocardiogram** • A graphic recording produced by the electric impulses of the heart

**Electroencephalogram** • A graphic recording of the electric impulses of the brain

**Electromyogram** • A record of muscle contraction produced by electrical stimulation

**Endoscopy** • The visualization of a body cavity or hollow organ by means of an endoscope

**Gastroenterology** • The study of the stomach, the intestines, and the accessory digestive organs, such as the esophagus, the liver, the gallbladder, and the pancreas

**GI Study** • A diagnostic study related to the gastrointestinal system

---

**Invasive Cardiac Study** • A method of studying the heart by making an entry into the body, such as by placing a cardiac catheter into a blood vessel

**Noninvasive Cardiac Study** • A method of studying the heart without entering the body to perform the procedure

**Pacemaker** • An electronic device, either temporary or permanent, that regulates the pace of the heart when the heart is incapable of doing it

**Plethysmography** • The recording of the changes in the size of a part as altered by the circulation of blood in it

**Radiopaque Catheter** • A catheter coated with a substance that does not allow the passage of x-rays, thus allowing the movement of the catheter to be followed on the television screen

**Rhythm Strip** • A cardiac study that demonstrates the waveform produced by electric impulses from one lead   *usually Lead 2*

**Spirometry** • A study to measure the body's lung capacity and function

## A B B R E V I A T I O N S

| Abbreviation | Meaning | Example of Usage on a Doctors' Order Sheet |
|---|---|---|
| ABG | arterial blood gases | ABG on RA |
| CBG | capillary blood gases | CBG @ 10 AM |
| ECG, EKG | electrocardiogram | ECG before surgery; EKG today |
| EchoEG | echoencephalogram | Schedule EchoEG |
| EEG | electroencephalogram | Schedule EEG |
| EGD | esophagogastro-duodenoscopy | EGD |
| EMG | electromyogram | EMG tomorrow |
| ERCP | endoscopic retrograde cholangiopancrea-tography | ERCP |
| IPG | impedance plethysmography | IPG today |
| LOC | leave on chart (when it follows ECG or EKG) | ECG, LOC |
| RA | room air | ABG on RA |

## E X E R C I S E  1

Write the abbreviation for each term listed below.

1. electroencephalogram  *EEG*
2. electrocardiogram (2)  *ECG*
3. electromyogram  *EMG*
4. room air  *RA*
5. leave on chart  *LOC*

6. impedance plethysmography  *IPG*
7. arterial blood gases  *ABG*
8. capillary blood gases  *CBG*
9. echoencephalogram  *EchoEG*
10. endoscopic retrograde cholangiopancreatography  *ERCP*
11. esophagogastroduodenoscopy  *EGD*

## E X E R C I S E  2

Write the meaning of each abbreviation listed below.

1. ABG   *Arterial blood Gases*
2. ECG   *Electrocardiogram*
3. EEG   *Electro encephalogram*
4. EKG   *Electro cardiogram*
5. CBG   *Capillary blood gasses*
6. LOC   *Leave on chart*
7. EMG   *Electro myogram*
8. RA   *Room air*
9. IPG   *Impedence plethysmography*
10. EchoEG   *echo encephalo gram*
11. EGD   *Esophago gastro duodenoscopy*
12. ERCP   *endoscopic retrograde cholangio pancreatography*

## CARDIOVASCULAR DIAGNOSTICS

## Background Information

The procedures carried out by this department are related to the performance of the heart and the vascular system. The results of these studies aid the physician in making a diagnosis and effecting a treatment.

In the following paragraphs the types of tests performed by the cardiovascular studies department are described. They are categorized as either invasive or noninvasive studies. **Invasive procedures** are those that require entry into the body by some means (such as a catheter into a blood vessel in cardiac catheterization); **noninvasive procedures** are those that are performed without entering into any body part (such as electrocardiogram).

The role of the health unit coordinator is to communicate the order to the cardiovascular diagnostics department by completing a *cardiovascular diagnostics requisition* (Fig. 16–1) or by using the computer.

| DR. ORDERING_____ | | |
|---|---|---|
| DIAGNOSIS_____ | | |
| REASON FOR TEST_____ | | |
| DATE ORDERED_____ | | |
| DATE/TIME OF TEST_____ | | |
| REQUESTED BY_____ | | |
| CARDIAC MEDICATIONS: | WT | ☐ EKG        LAST EKG _____ |
| | HT | ☐ ROUTINE |
| | | ☐ STAT |
| ☐ ECHOCARDIOGRAM | | ☐ PRE-SURGICAL |
| ☐ TREADMILL STRESS TEST | | ☐ PACEMAKER EVALUATION |
| ☐ HOLTER MONITOR   ☐ 12 hr ☐ 24 hr | | OTHER |
| ☐ DOPPLER FLOW STUDIES | | |
| ☐ CAROTID | | |
| ☐ LOWER EXTREMITIES | | |
| ☐ IMPEDANCE PLETHYSMOGRAPHY | | |
| ☐ CAROTID PHONOONGIOGRAPHY | | |
| **CARDIOVASCULAR DIAGNOSTICS REQUISITION** | | |

F I G U R E  16–1 • Cardiovascular diagnostics requisition.

## Doctors' Orders for Cardiac Studies (Noninvasive)

### ■ EKG, LOC

An **electrocardiogram (EKG)** measures the electrical activity of the heart to detect specific cardiac abnormalities. The electric impulses are picked up and conveyed to the electrocardiograph by electrodes or leads that are placed on various points of the body. A regular EKG has 12 leads. The doctor may also use the abbreviation ECG to order this study, which is performed at the bedside. LOC is a request to the EKG technician to leave a copy of the cardiac tracing on the patient's chart (Fig. 16–2). Restructuring taking place in many health care facilities involves the reorganization of labor. As a result, it may now be the role of the patient care technician to perform the EKG. If this is so, a requisition would not be forwarded to cardiovascular diagnostics but the information would be communicated to the patient care technician on the unit.

When ordering an EKG, the health unit coordinator should indicate if the client is on a specific cardiac medication, such as digitoxin, nitroglycerin, quinidine, Lanoxin, or beta blockers.

A **rhythm strip**, when ordered, shows the waveform produced by electric impulses from lead II. (Only one lead is used.)

### ■ Echocardiogram or ultrasonic cardiogram

The **echocardiogram** is a graphic recording of the internal structure of the heart and the position and motion of the cardiac walls and valves. This study is made by sending ultra-high-frequency sound waves through the chest wall. This test can also be ordered as M-mode or two-dimensional (2D) mode. The **echo M-mode**, or **motion**, uses a narrow beam of sound producing an "icepick" view of the cardiac structures. The **2D mode** uses a wider sound beam, and images showing both motion and shape are produced.

### ■ Exercise electrocardiogram (also called treadmill stress test)  *n medications*

A treadmill or stationary bicycle is used to increase the heartbeat and to place the heart in a stress condition.

### ■ Holter monitor for 24 h  *recording of ht beat*

This diagnostic study is an ambulatory ECG. It may be used to evaluate chest pain, abnormal heart rhythm, and drug effectiveness. Electrodes are attached to the chest, and the heart sounds are recorded on a cassette tape recorder. The ECG tape recorder is worn in a sling or holder around the chest or waist. The patient usually keeps a 24-hour diary of activities performed while wearing the recorder. A microcomputer analyzes the tape correlating the record of heart activity with the patient's daily activity.

A **telemetry unit** is a patient care area where the activity of Holter monitors worn by patients are registered at the nurses' station. If a nurse detects an abnormality or if the patient complains of chest pain or discomfort, the nurse can print a strip of the continuous electrocardiogram for study and interpretation of the occurrence.

### ■ Transesophageal electrocardiogram

Examines cardiac function and structure with an ultrasound transducer placed in the esophagus. The transducer provides views of the heart structure.

## Doctors' Orders for Vascular Studies (Noninvasive)

### ■ Carotid Doppler flow analysis

A directional Doppler probe is used to detect the flow of blood in the major neck artery.

COLLEGE HOSPITAL

| Otis Hart | 60 | M | 123-456 | 3:15 am |
| PATIENT'S NAME | AGE | SEX | HOSP. Number | TIME |
| | Poss Pancreatitis | | | |
| ADDRESS | CLINICAL DIAGNOSIS | | | |
| | 9876 | | 12-11-XX | |
| DIGITALIS QUINIDINE POTASSIUM ETC. | ECG Number | | DATE | |

Abnormal electrocardiogram. Sinus rhythm. Low voltage of the T wave in several leads is a nonspecific finding.

A.P. Valve, M.D.

*A.P. Valve, M.D.*

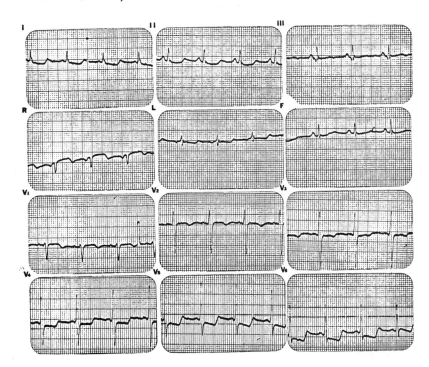

F I G U R E   16–2 • Electrocardiogram report.

## COMMUNICATION AND IMPLEMENTATION OF CARDIOVASCULAR DIAGNOSTICS

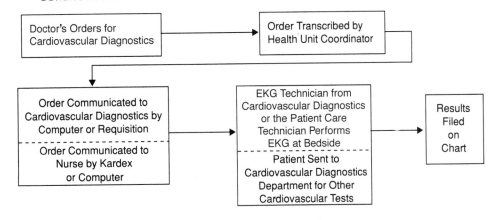

■ *Carotid phonoangiography*

The lumen (opening) of the carotid artery can be measured by placing an electronic microphone over this artery.

■ *Doppler flow studies on lower extremities*

In this procedure, an ultrasound probe is placed over the major leg veins or arteries. A graphic tracing is produced, showing flow changes caused by changes within the blood vessels.

■ *Impedance plethysmography studies— right leg (IPG)*

Changes in the blood volume are shown when electrodes are applied to the leg and electric resistance changes are recorded.

---

**HIGHLIGHT**

Cardiovascular Diagnostics Tests

- Electrocardiogram (EKG)
- Echocardiogram
- Holter monitor
- Doppler flow studies
- Impedance plethysmography (IPG)
- Carotid phonoangiography
- Cardiac catheterization

---

### Doctors' Orders for Cardiac Studies (Invasive)

■ *Cardiac catheterization at 8 AM tomorrow. Have permit signed*

In this study, a long, flexible radiopaque catheter is passed through a vein in the arm or leg into the heart cavities. The use of a **radiopaque catheter** (a catheter coated with a substance that does not permit the passage of x-rays) allows the catheter to be followed on a television screen. This procedure is performed to detect cardiac disease or defects, and to study the results of heart surgery.

Cardiac catheterization is performed under surgical conditions. It may be performed in the cardiac diagnostics, in a catheterization lab, or in the diagnostic imaging department. A surgical consent form must be signed.

■ *Insertion of a pacemaker*

In some heart disorders, the heart is incapable of regulating its own pace. An electronic device called a **pacemaker** jolts the heart into a normal rate and rhythm. Permanent pacemakers are implanted under a chest muscle in surgery (Fig. 16–3). Temporary pacemakers have wires from outside of the body leading into the heart. *transvenous-temporary pacemaker*

■ *Swan-Ganz catheter insertion*

This is a special procedure performed by a physician in a critical care unit. A balloon-tipped catheter is inserted through the subclavian vein into the right side of the heart. The catheter goes through the right ventricle past the pulmonic valve and into a branch of the pulmonary artery.

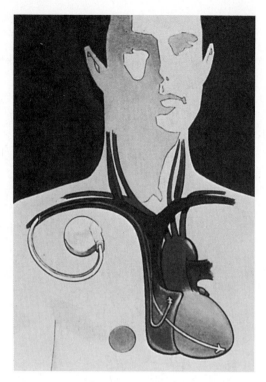

**FIGURE 16–3** • Dual-chamber pacemaker implant. (Courtesy of Medtronic Inc., Minneapolis, MN.)

The measurements revealed by this procedure are used to guide and evaluate therapy.

---

**TO THE STUDENT**

To practice transcribing cardiovascular diagnostics orders, complete **Activity 16–1** in the Skills Practice Manual.

---

## NEURODIAGNOSTICS

Neurodiagnostics may include several tests related to the function of the nervous system. In smaller facilities, the electroencephalography may be the only neurodiagnostic test performed.

### Electroencephalography

An **electroencephalogram** is a recording of a patient's brain waves. The procedure is performed to study brain function. The results of the study may be used to diagnose brain tumors, epilepsy, other brain diseases or injuries, and to confirm "brain death" (Fig. 16–4).

The role of the health unit coordinator is to communicate the order to the EEG department by completing the *neurodiagnostics requisition* (Fig. 16–5) or by using the computer.

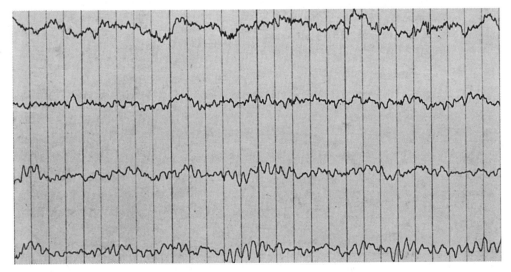

F I G U R E 16–4 • An electroencephalogram.

Preparation of the patient by the nursing staff is usually required. The patient's hair is washed the night before the test is to be done. The use of cola drinks, coffee, or tea may be restricted because they may act as stimulants; however, food and other fluids are permitted. Some hospitals have special preparation cards that contain information for the preparation of the patient for an EEG. The health unit coordinator places the preparation card in the patient's Kardex holder during the transcription procedure.

The patient is transported to the neurodiagnostic department for the test, which is performed by the EEG technician.

In hospitals that do not have a neurodiagnostic department, you may need to call a neurologist to arrange for a portable EEG to be brought to the hospital.

To order an electroencephalogram, the doctor usually writes "EEG" on the doctors' order sheet.

## Echoencephalography

**Echoencephalography (EchoEG)** uses ultrasound to produce an image of the brain. It is being replaced in some instances by computerized tomography.

## Evoked Potentials

**Evoked potentials (EP)** are a group of diagnostic tests that measure changes in various parts of the brain produced

---

| DR. ORDERING_____ | |
| DIAGNOSIS_____ | |
| REASON FOR TEST_____ | |
| DATE ORDERED_____ | |
| APPOINTMENT TIME/DATE_____ | |
| REQUESTED BY_____ | |
| ANTICONVULSIVE MEDICATIONS: | TRANSPORTATION: |
| MEDICATION FOR SEDATION: | □ EEG<br>□ PORTABLE EEG<br>□ ECHOENCEPHALOGRAPH<br>□ PORTABLE ECHO |
| PREVIOUS EEG?  □ YES  □ NO | □ EMG |
| OTHER | |
| **NEURODIAGNOSTICS REQUISITION** | |

F I G U R E 16–5 • Electroencephalography requisition.

## COMMUNICATION AND IMPLEMENTATION OF NEURODIAGNOSTIC ORDERS

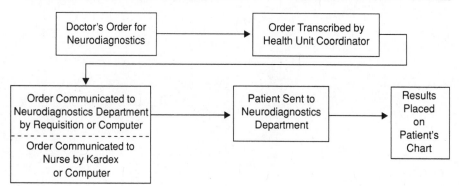

by visual, auditory, or somatosensory stimuli. Examples of EPs follow.

### Visual Evoked Response

The **visual evoked response (VER)** is a response to visual stimuli. It can also be called **visual evoked potentials (VEP)**. It is sometimes used to confirm cerebral silence (brain death).

### Auditory Evoked Response

The **auditory evoked response (AER)** is related to hearing (an auditory stimulus); it is also called the **brainstem auditory evoked response (BAER)**.

### Somatosensory Evoked Potential

The **somatosensory evoked potentials (SEP)** are done to record a response to a painless stimulation of a peripheral nerve.

### HIGHLIGHT

Neurodiagnostics Tests
- Electroencephalogram (EEG)
- Echoencephalogram (EchEG)
- Electronystagmography (ENG)
- Electromyography (EMG)
- Evoked potentials
- Visual evoked response
- Auditory evoked response
- Somatosensory evoked potential

## Electronystagmography

**Electronystagmography (ENG)** is done by placing electrodes near the patient's eyes and records involuntary eye movements.

## Electromyography

An electromyogram (EMG) is a diagnostic study that records muscle contraction produced by electrical stimulation.

### Doctors' Orders for Neurodiagnostics

- *EEG tomorrow*
- *Schedule for ENG*
- *Echoencephalogram today*
- *EMG tomorrow* AM

### TO THE STUDENT

To practice transcribing a neurodiagnostics order, complete **Activity 16–2** in the Skills Practice Manual.

## ENDOSCOPY

The word *endoscopy* is a general term used to indicate the visual examination of a body cavity or hollow organ. It is a diagnostic procedure performed by a doctor. Hospitals have a designated area for these studies. During some endoscopic procedures, biopsies are performed.

To transcribe an endoscopy order, the health unit coordinator schedules the procedure with the responsible department. Requisitions or computers may be used to order the study. Endoscopies usually require a patient consent form to be signed. Some endoscopies require preparation. The doctor writes any preprocedure preparation orders on the doctors' order sheet.

## Types of Endoscopies

There are many types of endoscopic examinations. The name of the procedure and the instruments used depend upon the organ to be examined.

The following is a list of endoscopic examinations commonly performed in a hospital either on an inpatient or outpatient basis.

**Bronchoscopy:** The visual inspection of the bronchi by means of a bronchoscope

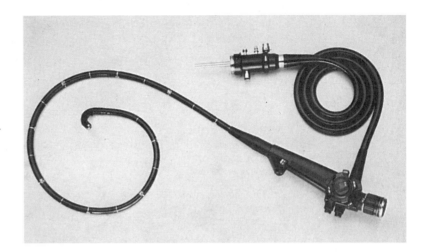

**FIGURE 16–6** • Fiberoptic gastroscope. (Courtesy of Olympus Corp., Lake Success, NY.)

**Colonoscopy:** The visual examination of the large intestine from the anus to the cecum by means of a fiberoptic colonoscope

**Esophagoscopy:** The visual examination of the esophagus by means of an esophagoscope

**Gastroscopy:** The visual examination of the interior of the stomach by means of a gastroscope (Fig. 16–6).

**Proctoscopy:** The visual inspection of the rectum by means of a proctoscope

**Sigmoidoscopy:** The visual examination of the sigmoid portion of the large intestine by means of a sigmoidoscope

*Note:* When a barium enema (BE) is ordered for the same day, note when ordering that the patient is also having a sigmoidoscopy done. The sigmoidoscopy must be done before the BE. It may be the policy of some health care facilities not to perform a sigmoidoscopy and a BE on the same day.

Some other diagnostic procedures related to endoscopy are the following:

**Anoscopy:** Visual inspection of the anal canal

**Endoscopic retrograde cholangiopancreatography (ERCP):** This diagnostic procedure is an inspection of the common bile duct, biliary tract, and pancreatic duct; it is done by insertion of a catheter through an endoscope

**Esophagogastroduodenoscopy (EGD):** Visual inspection of the esophagus, stomach, and duodenum (Fig. 16–7).

## Doctors' Orders for Endoscopies

■ *Sigmoidoscopy tomorrow* AM. *Fleet enema* × 2, 1 h prior procedure

■ *Schedule for gastroscopy tomorrow* AM. *NPO p̄ MN*

■ *Schedule ERCP for tomorrow. NPO p̄ MN*

■ *Bronchoscopy tomorrow* @ 9:30 AM. *Have consent form signed*

  *Demerol 50 mg* ⎫
  *Atropine 0.8 mg* ⎭ *IM @ 8:30* AM

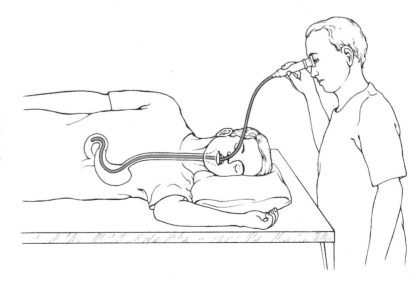

**FIGURE 16–7** • Esophagogastroduodenoscopy (EGD) is the visualization of the esophagus, stomach, and duodenum. (From Ignatavicius, Donna D., Workman, M. Linda, and Mishler, Mary A.: *Medical-Surgical Nursing: A Nursing Process Approach*, 2nd ed. Philadelphia, W. B. Saunders Co., 1995, with permission.)

## COMMUNICATION AND IMPLEMENTATION OF ENDOSCOPY ORDERS

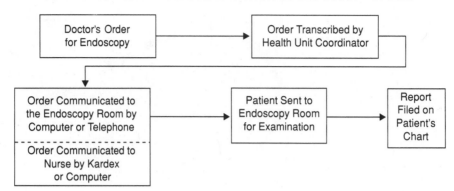

■ *Schedule colonoscopy for 8 AM on Wednesday. Permit, clear liquids, NPO p̄ MN, Fleet prep kit #2 today*

**HIGHLIGHT**

| Types of Endoscopies | Organ Examination |
| --- | --- |
| Bronchoscopy | Bronchi |
| Colonoscopy | Large intestine |
| Esophagoscopy | Esophagus |
| Proctoscopy | Rectum |
| Sigmoidoscopy | Sigmoid colon |
| Anoscopy | Anal canal |
| Endoscopic retrograde cholangiopancreatography (ERCP) | Biliary and pancreatic ducts |
| Esophagogastroduodenoscopy (EGD) | Gastrointestinal tract |

**TO THE STUDENT**

To practice transcribing endoscopy orders, complete **Activity 16–3** in the Skills Practice Manual.

## GASTROENTEROLOGY

### Background Information

The gastroenterology department (usually shortened to GI lab) performs diagnostic tests related to problems of the gastrointestinal system.

In hospitals where a GI lab does not exist, a few of these tests may be performed by the nurse at the bedside. You may then be asked to requisition the necessary equipment from the central service department. Specimens collected by the nurse are sent to the hospital clinical laboratory for study, or they may be sent to a private laboratory.

To communicate the doctor's order to the gastroenterology department, complete a *gastroenterology requisition* (Fig. 16–8) or order the study by computer.

If the study requires an appointment time for the client, the department notifies the nursing unit of the time the patient is expected. This time should be noted on the client's Kardex form.

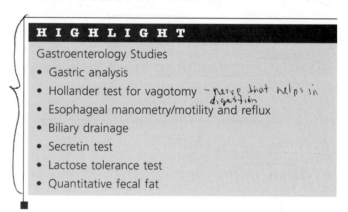

**HIGHLIGHT**

Gastroenterology Studies
- Gastric analysis
- Hollander test for vagotomy — *nerve that helps in digestion*
- Esophageal manometry/motility and reflux
- Biliary drainage
- Secretin test
- Lactose tolerance test
- Quantitative fecal fat

### Doctors' Orders for Gastroenterology Studies

Below are listed doctors' orders for some diagnostic studies performed by a gastroenterology department.

■ *Gastric analysis*
A study performed to measure the stomach's secretion of hydrochloric acid and pepsin as well as for the evaluation of stomach and duodenal ulcers. This test takes approximately 2½ hours.

■ *Hollander test for vagotomy*
A test performed to determine the amount of hydrochloric acid in the patient's gastric juice after a vagotomy. A vagotomy reduces the secretion of gastric juices. This test takes approximately 3½ hours.

■ *Esophageal mamometry or esophageal motility and reflux study*
The motility portion of this test studies esophageal function. The reflux study is performed to determine the rea-

DR. ORDERING_____

DIAGNOSIS_____

DATE ORDERED   _____

COLLECTED BY_____

Date _____ Time _____

REQUESTED BY_____

TRANSPORTATION:

**TEST/STUDIES**

☐ GASTRIC ANALYSIS

☐ HOLLANDER TEST FOR VAGOTOMY

OTHER:

☐ ESOPHAGEAL MOTILITY AND REFLUX STUDY

☐ BILIARY DRAINAGE

☐ SECRETIN TEST

☐ LACTOSE TOLERANCE TEST

☐ QUALITATIVE FECAL FAT

**GASTROENTEROLOGY REQUISITION**

F I G U R E  16–8 • Example of gastroenterology requisition.

son for food and gastric juices flowing back into the esophagus. This test takes approximately 1 hour.

■ *Biliary drainage*
A procedure to obtain duodenal fluids to study for cholesterol crystals, which indicate gallstone formation. This test, which takes approximately 2 hours, also is performed to determine the presence of parasites.

■ *Secretin test*
A test of pancreatic function, this takes approximately 3 hours.

■ *Lactose tolerance test*
A test to determine intolerance to lactose, the sugar in milk. This test takes approximately 2 hours.

■ *Quantitative fecal fat*   *measure numbers*
A study to determine the malabsorption of fat by a client. The patient's stools are collected for 48 to 72 hours after the patient has eaten a 100-g fat diet for 2 to 3 days.
*how much fat is left in stool*

**TO THE STUDENT**

To practice transcribing a gastroenterology order, complete **Activity 16–4** in the Skills Practice Manual.

## PULMONARY FUNCTION

### Background Information

The pulmonary (respiratory) function performs diagnostic tests to determine lung function. The results are used to diagnose and treat respiratory diseases. In many health care facilities, pulmonary function tests are performed by the respiratory care department.

The health unit coordinator communicates the doctors' order to the pulmonary function or respiratory care de-

**COMMUNICATION AND IMPLEMENTATION OF GASTROENTEROLOGY ORDERS**

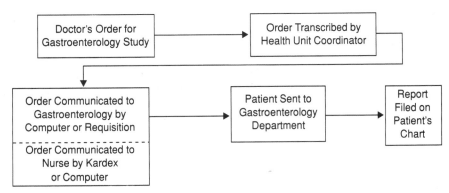

DR. ORDERING _____

DIAGNOSIS _____

REASON FOR TEST _____

DATE ORDERED _____

DATE/TIME OF TEST _____ STAT

REQUESTED BY

| BLOOD GAS STUDIES | PULMONARY FUNCTION TESTS |
|---|---|

**BLOOD GAS STUDIES**

☐ ARTERIAL

☐ VENOUS

☐ CAPILLARY

> INDICATE IF PATIENT
> ON ANTICOAGULANTS
> ☐ YES ☐ NO

☐ ROOM AIR      O₂_____% in

O₂_____L/M N.P.      ISOLETTE, HOOD,
O₂_____% MASK      MASK

☐ TRACH      ☐ IPPB

**PULMONARY FUNCTION TESTS**

☐ LUNG VOLUME STUDY

☐ SPIROMETRY STUDY
(before bronchodilator)

☐ SPIROMETRY STUDY
(before & after bronchodilator)

☐ BEDSIDE SPIROMETRY STUDY

OTHER/SPECIAL INSTRUCTIONS

PULMONARY FUNCTION REQUISITION

F I G U R E  16–9 • Pulmonary function requisition.

partment by completing a *pulmonary function requisition* (Fig. 16–9) or by using the computer.

No preparation is required for pulmonary tests unless the doctor has included special instructions with the order. For example, the doctor may want the amount of oxygen adjusted or turned off before a study on the patient's blood gases is done, as in the following orders: *DC O₂ at 10 AM ABG at 11 AM*. The instruction to DC (disconnect) the O₂ is carried out by the nursing staff; thus the communication of the instructions by the health unit coordinator to the nurse is necessary.

It is important on any requisition form or with a computer order for arterial blood gases (the test done most frequently by this department) to note whether the patient is taking an anticoagulant drug, such as Coumadin or heparin. These medications, which lengthen the time it takes for blood to clot, cause the patient to bleed excessively when the artery is punctured for this test. Capillary blood may also be used for blood gas determination upon request by the doctor.

## Doctors' Orders for Pulmonary Function

Below are listed examples of doctors' orders for pulmonary function studies.

### ■ Room air ABGs

The blood sample for this diagnostic study is obtained from the patient's artery by the pulmonary function technician while the patient is breathing room air (which is 21% oxygen). The blood is then analyzed in the pulmonary function department (Table 16–1).

### ■ ABG on O₂ @ 2 L/min

The blood sample for this test is to be drawn while the patient is breathing oxygen (O₂), which is being delivered at a rate of 2 liters per minute.

### ■ Bedside spirometry study

Certain aspects of lung function are determined by measuring and recording the patient's lung capacity for air. The patient is transported to the pulmonary function department for this test. *may take bronchodialator before test.*

### ■ Pulse oximetry

This study measures the oxygen saturation of the arterial blood. A probe is attached to either the ear or the finger. This is a noninvasive procedure (Fig. 16–10). It may also be performed by the nursing staff. If performed by the nursing staff the ordering step of transcription is not necessary.

| T A B L E  16–1 | Arterial Blood Gas Values—Normal Ranges |
|---|---|
| $Pa_{O_2}$ | 80–100 mm Hg |
| $Pc_{CO_2}$ | 35–45 mm Hg |
| pH | 7.35–7.45 |
| O₂ sat | 94–100% |
| $HCO_3^-$ | 22–26 mEq/L |

## COMMUNICATION AND IMPLEMENTATION OF PULMONARY FUNCTION ORDERS

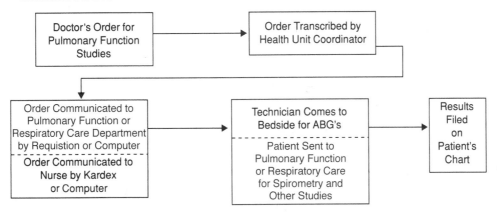

### ■ *Pre and post spirometry*

Done at the bedside before bronchodilator treatment and is repeated after the treatment. If the current treatment order does not exist, contact the physician for a bronchodilator treatment order.

### TO THE STUDENT

To practice transcribing pulmonary function orders, complete **Activity 16–5** in the Skills Practice Manual.

To practice transcribing a review set of doctor's orders, complete **Activity 16–6** in the Skills Practice Manual.

To practice recording doctors' orders and to practice recording telephoned messages, complete **Activities 16–7** and **16–8** in the Skills Practice Manual.

## SUMMARY

The recognition and proper scheduling of all diagnostic studies are of utmost importance to the patient, the physician(s), and the hospital. Both the patient who is as yet undiagnosed and the patient awaiting test results that hopefully will show improvement are dependent upon the knowledge and communication skills of the individual performing the clerical duties. The health unit coordinator who can identify and order correctly all diagnostic studies is an asset to the unit.

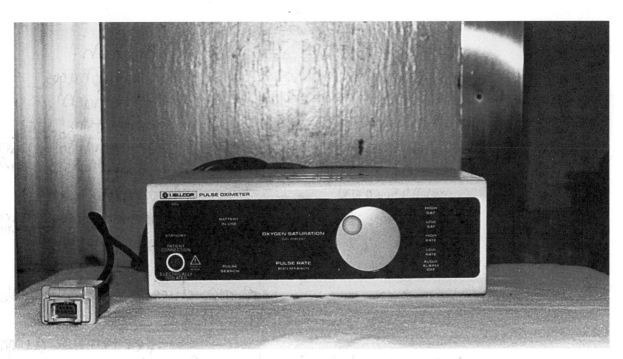

FIGURE 16–10 • Pulse oximeter.

**REVIEW QUESTIONS**

1. Write out the meaning of each underlined abbreviation appearing in the following sets of doctors' orders.

   a. <u>EMG</u> tomorrow AM.

   _Electro myography tomorrow morning_

   b. <u>EKG</u> stat

   _Electro cardiograph immediatly_

   c. <u>ABG</u> on <u>RA</u> @ 4 PM today

   _Arterial Blood Gas on Right atrium at 4pm today_

   d. EKG today, <u>LOC</u>

   _Electrocardiograph today, Leave on chart_

   e. Schedule <u>EEG</u> tomorrow

   _schedule Electro Encephalograph tomorrow_

   f. <u>CBG</u> @ 6 AM

   _capillary blood gases at 6 am_

2. Four cardiac studies the doctor may request to diagnose cardiac abnormalities are:

   a. _electro cardiogram_    c. _Cardiac Catherization_

   b. _echo cardiogram_    d. _exercise electro cardiogram_

3. Four medications affecting the heart which should be noted on an EKG requisition are:

   a. _digitoxin_    c. _quinidine_

   b. _nitroglycerin_    d. _Lanoxin_

4. Name nine endoscopic procedures and name the portion of the body that is studied by each procedure.

|   | Procedure | Organ(s) Studied |
|---|---|---|
| a. | bronchoscopy | bronchi |
| b. | esophagoscopy | esophagus |
| c. | gastroscopy | stomach |
| d. | proctoscopy | rectum |
| e. | sigmoidscopy | sigmoid colon, portion of large intestine |
| f. | colonoscopy | secum to anus |
| g. | anoscopy | anal canal |
| h. | ERCP | common bile duct, billary tract, pancreatic duct |
| i. | EGD | upper GI tract |

5. Describe the purpose of:

   a. the gastroenterology department _performs diagnostic tests related to problems of the GI tract_

   b. the pulmonary (respiratory) function department _performs diagnostic tests to determine lung function_

c. neurodiagnostics _used to study brain function_

6. Two medications that lengthen clotting time and that should be noted on an arterial blood gas requisition are

a. _Coumadin_  b. _Heparin_

7. Define the following:

a. GI study _diagnostic study related to gastro intestinal tract_

b. noninvasive cardiac study _method of studying the heart without entering the body_

c. pacemaker _electronic device implanted in the chest eithe temp or permanent that regulated the heart_

d. blood gases _a diagnostic study to determine the change or gases in the blood._

e. endoscopy _the visualization of a Hollow organ or body cavity using a endoscope_

f. electroencephalogram _graphic recording of or electrical impulses of thebrain_

g. plethysmography _the recording of the changes in the size of a part as altered by blood circulation in it._

8. Five studies performed by the gastroenterology department are:

a. _gastric Analysis_  d. _secreation test_

b. _esophageal motility oreflux_  e. _lactose tolerance test_

c. _biliary drainage_

9. Using the list in the left-hand column below for reference, identify the department that performs the studies indicated in the following sets of doctors' orders.

| Reference List | Doctors' Orders |
|---|---|
| a. cardiovascular diagnostics | _C_ 1. electromyogram |
| b. endoscopies | _A_ 2. pre and post spirometry |
| c. neurodiagnostics department | _E_ 3. ABG on RA |
| d. gastroenterology department | _B_ 4. sigmoidoscopy at 8 AM in clinic |
| e. pulmonary function | _C_ 5. EEG tomorrow |
|  | _B_ 6. colonoscopy |
|  | _A_ 7. EKG, LOC |
|  | _A_ 8. echocardiogram |
|  | _A_ 9. Doppler flow studies |

_D_ 10. secretin test

_A_ 11. treadmill stress test

_E_ 12. schedule for spirometry study tomorrow

_A_ 13. rhythm strip

_D_ 14. gastric analysis

_B_ 15. schedule esophagoscopy for Monday

_A_ 16. Holter monitor for 24 hours

_A_ 17. IPG—left leg

_B_ 18. ERCP tomorrow

10. Rewrite the following doctors' orders using abbreviations. Or, to practice writing doctors' orders, have someone read the orders to you, while you record them. Again practice using abbreviations while you do this.

a. impedance plethysmography this morning ___IPG this AM___

b. electrocardiogram now ___EKG stat___

c. endoscopic retrograde cholangiopancreatography tomorrow morning ___
___ERCP in AM___

d. arterial blood gases on oxygen at two liters per minute ___
___ABG on $O_2$ at 2L/min___

## References

Blackburn, Elsa: *Health Unit Coordinator*. Englewood Cliffs, NJ, Prentice-Hall, Brady Division, 1991.

Chabner, Davi-Ellen: *The Language of Medicine*, 5th ed. Philadelphia, W. B. Saunders Co., 1996.

Hamilton, Helen K: *Diagnostics*, 2nd ed. Springhouse, PA, Springhouse, 1989.

Ignatavicius, Donna D., Workman, M. Linda, and Mishler, Mary A.: *Medical-Surgical Nursing: A Nursing Process Approach*, 2nd ed. Philadelphia, W. B. Saunders Co., 1995.

*Nurses' Reference Library*. Springhouse, PA, Intermed Communications Inc., 1986.

*Peripheral Vascular Laboratory Manual*. Good Samaritan Medical Center, Phoenix, AZ, 1983.

Sloan, Robert M. and Sloan, Beverly LeBov: *A Guide to Health Facilities*, 2nd ed. St. Louis, The C. V. Mosby Co., 1977.

Know what controlled substance is

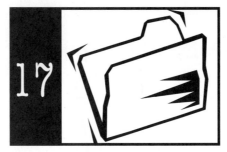

# TREATMENT ORDERS

Traction, Respiratory Care,
Physical Medicine, Rehabilitation,
Dialysis, and Radiation Therapy

## C H A P T E R   OBJECTIVES

*Upon completion of this chapter, you will be able to:*

1. Write the meaning of each abbreviation in the abbreviations list.

2. List three items that may be ordered from the central service department for traction.

3. List three types of traction used to treat bone fractures and two types of traction used to treat ailments other than bone fractures.

4. Name the traction set-up used by patients to assist them to move in bed.

5. List three treatments performed by the respiratory care department.

6. List three types of treatments performed by the physical medicine department and give an example of each.

7. List the two main types of dialysis.

## V O C A B U L A R Y

**Aerosol** • Liquid suspension of particles in a gas stream for inhalation purposes

**Dialysis** • The removal of wastes in the blood usually excreted by the kidneys

**Diathermy** • The application of deep heat to the body *PT* by use of electric current

**Extubation** • Removal of a previously inserted tube (as in an endotracheal tube)

**Hydrotherapy** • Treatment with water

**Hypertonic** • Concentrated salt solution (>0.9%) *above normal saline*

**Hypotonic** • Dilute salt solution (<0.9%)

**Infrared** • A treatment using infrared rays

**Intervention** • Synonymous with treatment

**Intubation** • Insertion and placement of a tube (within the trachea may be endotracheal or tracheostomy)

**Nebulizer** • A gas-driven device that produces an *RT* aerosol

**Positive Pressure** • Pressure above atmospheric *RT* pressure

**Reduction** • The correction of a deformity in a bone fracture or dislocation *ORIF*

**Titrate** • To adjust the amount of treatment to maintain a specific physiologic response

**Traction** • A mechanical pull to part of the body to maintain alignment and facilitate healing; traction may be static (continuous) or intermittent

**Unit Dose** • Any premixed or prespecified dose; often administered with SVN or IPPB treatments

## ABBREVIATIONS

| Abbreviation | Meaning | Example of Usage on a Doctors' Order Sheet |
|---|---|---|
| AA | active assistance | AA exer bilat LE |
| ADL | activities of daily living | OT for ADL *small motor skills* |
| AKA | above-the-knee amputation | AKA protocol |
| Bilat, B, Ⓑ | bilateral, both | ROM B LE |
| BiW | twice a week | PT BiW |
| BKA | below-the-knee amputation | consent for BKA |
| CP | cold packs | CP L arm |
| CPM | continuous passive motion | CPM |
| CPT | chest physiotherapy | DC CPT |
| EPC | electronic pain control | EPC |
| ET | endotracheal tube | CXR for ET tube placement *nc a movth* |
| ES | electrical stimulation | ES |
| HA | heated aerosol | HA T-piece @ 60% |
| HD | hemodialysis | HD BiW × 3 h |
| HP | hot packs | HP to neck |
| IPPB | intermittent positive-pressure breathing *own machm* | IPPB q4h c̄ 0.5 cc Ventolin in 2 cc NS |
| IS | incentive spirometry | IS tid *forced into lungs over IS to 20 mm period* |
| ISOM | isometric | |
| lb, # | pounds | pelvic traction c̄ 15 lb |
| LE | lower extremities | |
| LLL | left lower lobe | CPT-LLL only |
| L/min | liters per minute | ↑ O₂ to 4 L/min |
| LUL | left upper lobe | CPT to LUL |
| MDI | metered dose inhaler | MDI c̄ Ventolin ii puffs qid |
| NWB | nonweight-bearing | Crutchwalking NWB |
| O₂ | oxygen | O₂ 5 L/min by mask |
| ORIF | open reduction, internal fixation | |
| OT | occupational therapy | OT for ADL |
| PD | peritoneal dialysis | Tenckhoff cath for PD |
| PEP | positive expiratory pressure | IS c̄ PEP |
| PT | physical therapy | To PT for crutchwalking |
| P&PD | percussion and postural drainage | P&PD to LUL |
| RLL | right lower lobe | CPT RLL |
| RML | right middle lobe | CPT RML |
| ROM | range of motion | ROM to upper extremities bid |
| RUL | right upper lobe | P&PD RUL p̄ IPPB |
| Sa$_{O_2}$ | oxygen saturation (on pulse oximetry, not ABGs) | Titrate O₂ flow to Sa$_{O_2}$ >95% |
| STM, STW | soft tissue massage/work | |
| SVN | small volume nebulizer | ΔSVN to bid |
| TENS | transcutaneous electrical nerve stimulation *pain management clinic* | Postop TENS |
| TT | tilt table | Tilt table for PT |

| | | |
|---|---|---|
| THR, THA | total hip replacement/arthroplasty | |
| TKR, TKA | total knee replacement/arthroplasty | |
| Tx | traction | Buck's Tx |
| UD | unit dose | UD Ventolin now |
| USN | ultrasonic nebulizer | USN 15 min tid |
| WP | whirlpool | WP to L leg bid |
| > | greater than | |
| < | less than | |

## EXERCISE 1

Write the abbreviation for each term listed below.

1. left upper lobe — *LUL*
2. occupational therapy — *OT*
3. physical therapy — *PT*
4. liter per minute — *L/min*
5. oxygen — *O₂*
6. intermittent positive-pressure breathing — *IPPB*
7. right upper lobe — *RUL*
8. range of motion — *ROM*
9. right lower lobe — *RLL*
10. activities of daily living — *ADL*
11. electromyogram — *EMG*
12. right middle lobe — *RML*
13. ultrasonic nebulizer — *USN*
14. small volume nebulizer — *SVN*
15. left lower lobe — *LLL*
16. vibration and percussion — *V&P*
17. pounds — *p# lb #*
18. nonweight-bearing — *NWB*
19. whirlpool — *WP*
20. hot packs — *HP*
21. transcutaneous electrical nerve stimulation — *TENS*
22. electronic pain control — *EPC*
23. electrical stimulation — *ES*
24. continuous passive motion — *CPM*
25. incentive spirometry — *IS*
26. metered dose inhaler — *MDI*
27. chest physiotherapy — *CPT*

28. active assistance — AA

29. twice a week — B̶T̶W

30. ultraviolet — UV

31. bilateral, both — Bilat B Ⓑ

32. above-the-knee amputation — A̶K̶A̶ amp

33. exercise — ex

34. soft tissue massage/work — STM STW

35. lower extremities — LE

36. hemodialysis — HD

37. total hip relacement/arthroplasty — THR, THA

38. open reduction, internal fixation — ORIF

39. traction — tx

40. tilt table — TT

41. isometric — ISOM

42. below-the-knee amputation — BKA

43. endotracheal — ET

44. heated aerosol — HA

45. positive expiratory pressure — PEP

46. percussion and postural drainage — P & PD

47. oxygen saturation — SaO₂

48. unit dose — US

49. greater than — >

50. total knee replacement/arthroplasty — TKA

51. less than — <

52. cold packs — CP

## EXERCISE 2

Write the meaning of each abbreviation listed below.

1. O₂ — oxeyen

2. LUL — Left upper Lobe

3. RLL — Right Lower Loble

4. OT — Occupational therapy

5. PT — Physical therapy

6. EMG — Electromyogram

7. ADL — Activities of Daily Living

8. lb — lb #

9. RUL — Right upper Lobe

10. RML — Right middle Lobe

11. NWB — Non weight bearing

12. ROM — Range of Motion

13. L/min — Liters per minute

14. SVN — Small volume nebulizer

15. Vib & perc — vibration + percussion

16. LLL — Left Lower Lobe

17. IPPB — intermittent positive pressure Breathing

18. USN — Ultra sonic nebulizer

19. HP — hot packs

20. WP — wirl pool

21. CPM — continuous passive motion

22. ES — electrical stimulation

23. EPC — electronic pain control

24. TENS — Transcutaneous electric nerve sTimulation

25. IS — incentive Spirometry

26. CPT — chest physio therapy

27. MDI — metered dose inhaler

28. bilat, B, Ⓑ — bilateral

29. ex, exer — exercise

30. ORIF — open reduction Internal fixat

31. TT — tilt table

32. SaO₂ — oxegen saturation

33. AKA — Above the Knee amputation

34. UD — unit dose

35. HA — H̶e̶a̶t̶e̶d̶ ̶a̶e̶rosol

36. isom — isometric

37. LE — lower extremities

38. STM/STW — soft tissue massage work

39. HD — hemo dialysis

40. Tx — traction

41. P&PD — percussion + postural drainage

42. > — increase greater than

| 43. | TKR, TKA | *total knee replacement* |
| 44. | UV | *ultra violet* |
| 45. | THR, THA | *total hip replacement* |
| 46. | ET | *endo tracheal* |
| 47. | PD | *peritoneal dialysis* |
| 48. | < | *less than* |
| 49. | BiW | *twice a week* |
| 50. | PEP | *positive expiratory pressure* |
| 51. | CP | *cold pack* |
| 52. | AA | *active assistance* |

# TRACTION

**Traction** is the mechanical pull applied to a part of the body. The pull is achieved by connecting an apparatus attached to a bed to an apparatus attached to the patient (Fig. 17–1).

Traction is ordered by the doctor to restore alignment to a fractured bone and facilitate proper healing or to maintain the patient in an anatomically correct position prior to surgery and after surgery. Traction is also ordered to overcome muscle spasms resulting from a slipped disk, strained muscle, or various other conditions.

## Apparatus Set-Up

### Bed

The apparatus attached to the client's bed may include pulleys, rope, weights, and metal bars. The weights (metal disks or sandbags) provide the "pull" to a part of the body. The pulleys, rope, and metal bars are assembled to suspend the weights. Each type of traction requires a different assemblage of these parts; thus a skilled person must perform this task. It is usually the responsibility of the orthopedic technician to attach the traction apparatus to the bed. The health unit coordinator communicates a traction order to the person responsible for assembling the bed apparatus by telephone, by computer, or by a requisition form (Fig. 17–2).

### Patient

The apparatus that is attached to the patient may be an internal attachment, such as a pin, tongs, or wires placed directly into the bone by the surgeon; or an external attachment, such as a halter, belt, or boot. The external apparatus is applied to the patient by the nursing staff, and it sometimes requires the health unit coordinator to order the necessary supplies from the central service department.

Although the kinds of supplies the health unit coordinator orders varies among hospitals, the head halter, the

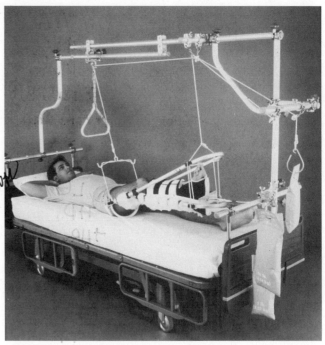

F I G U R E  17–1 • Thomas leg splint with a Pearson attachment. (Courtesy of Zimmer USA.)

pelvic sling, and the pelvic belt are three items commonly requisitioned from the central service department.

## Doctors' Orders for Traction

### Traction Orders for Treatment of Bone Fractures

Below are examples of doctors' orders for traction that include the types of traction frequently used in the hospital. Illustrations and explanations are provided to assist you in interpreting the orders.

■ *Bryant's traction*
Bryant's traction is used to treat fractured femurs in children under the age of 3 (Fig. 17–3). *pediatric*

■ *Traction on the humerus*
This type of traction is used to treat a fracture of the humerus (Fig. 17–4).

■ *Pelvic sling*
A set-up used in the treatment of fractures of the pelvic bone (Fig. 17–5). It is usually the responsibility of the health unit coordinator to order a pelvic sling from the central service department when transcribing this order. Recent advances in the management of pelvic fractures includes open reduction (surgical) and internal fixation (internal devices for stabilization). An advantage is the ability to mobilize the patient immediately after surgery.

■ *Thomas' leg splint c̄ Steinmann pin 20 lb of traction*
This set-up is used in the treatment of a fractured hip, femur, or lower leg (see Fig. 17–1). Steinmann pin is

```
DR. ORDERING _____

DIAGNOSIS _____

DATE ORDERED _____

REQUESTED BY _____
```

TRACTION                          □ OVERHEAD FRAME AND TRAPEZE

□ BUCKS

□ CERVICAL                        SPECIAL INSTRUCTIONS

□ PELVIC

□ OTHER _____

F I G U R E  17–2 • Orthopedic equipment requisition.

driven through the femur or tibia during surgery, and the traction apparatus is applied to the pin. A Thomas splint is frequently used with a Pearson attachment. The physicians' order for these types of external fixator pins may also include nursing treatment orders for care of the pin sites.

■ *Russell's traction*
Russell's traction is used in the treatment of a fractured hip or femur (Fig. 17–6).

■ *Cervical traction c̄ Crutchfield tongs*
Traction used in the treatment of fractures of the cervical vertebrae. Crutchfield tongs are inserted into the skull bone, and the traction apparatus is applied to the tongs. Other devices used for cervical traction are Gardner-Wells

tongs and Vinke tongs. A special bed or Stryker frame may need to be obtained for the patient.

■ *Left unilateral Buck's traction 5 lb*
A traction set-up used as temporary treatment of a fractured hip, for sciatica, or for other knee and hip disorders. *Unilateral* indicates that the traction is to be applied to one leg only; *bilateral leg traction* indicates that the traction is to be applied to both legs (Fig. 17–7). A buck's boot is applied to the leg, and the traction apparatus is attached to the boot. Buck's traction may also be referred to as straight or running traction. *doctor decides weight*

■ *Dunlop's traction*
This traction is ordered for treatment of the upper extremities.

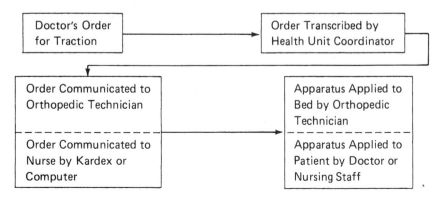

COMMUNICATION AND IMPLEMENTATION OF TRACTION ORDERS

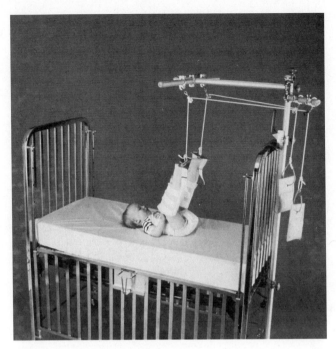

**FIGURE 17–3** • Bryant's traction. (Courtesy of Zimmer USA.)

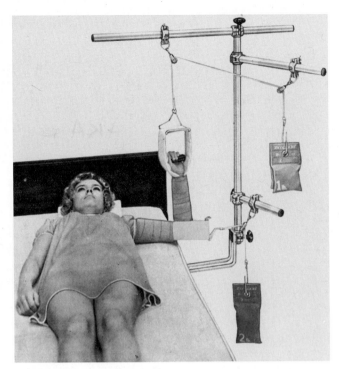

**FIGURE 17–4** • Side arm traction on humerus. (Courtesy of Zimmer USA.)

■ *Milwaukee brace*
This device is used to treat scoliosis.

■ *Consent for Ilizarov external fixator application with corticotomy*

### Traction Orders for Treatment of Muscle Spasms

■ *Pelvic traction 20 lb release prn*
Pelvic traction is ordered for treatment of muscle spasm, sciatica, or muscle sprain (Fig. 17–8). It is usually the health unit coordinator's responsibility to order a pelvic traction belt from the central service department when transcribing this order. The amount of weight that the doctor may order usually varies from 15 to 30 lb.

■ *Cervical traction 5 lb according to patient's tolerance*
Cervical traction is ordered for the treatment of muscle spasm or dislocation of the cervical area of the spinal column (Fig. 17–9). It is usually the health unit coordinator's responsibility to order a *head halter* from the central service department when transcribing this order. The amount of weight the doctor may order usually varies from 2 to 20 lb.

### Other Traction Orders

■ *Overhead frame and trapeze*
The overhead frame and trapeze is used by the patient for assistance in moving while in bed (Fig. 17–7).

*Used for the patient to move around*

---

### TO THE STUDENT

To practice transcribing traction orders, complete **Activity 17–1** in the Skills Practice Manual.

## RESPIRATORY CARE

### Background Information

Respiratory care is the department within the hospital that performs treatments ordered by the doctor that are related to respiratory function. The task of the health unit coordinator is to communicate these orders to the respiratory care department. The treatments are performed at the patient's bedside by a respiratory technician or therapist. If the doctor orders medication as a part of the treatment, it may be the health unit coordinator's task to order medications from the pharmacy. Upon completion of the treatment, the therapist records the type of treatment and other pertinent data on a record sheet on the patient's chart.

To communicate the doctor's order to the respiratory care department, use the computer or complete a respiratory care requisition (Fig. 17–10). Usually there is only one requisition form for the respiratory care department.

In many health care facilities, much of the diagnostic testing previously done in the pulmonary functions department is now performed in the respiratory care department. In some facilities, the departments may be combined.

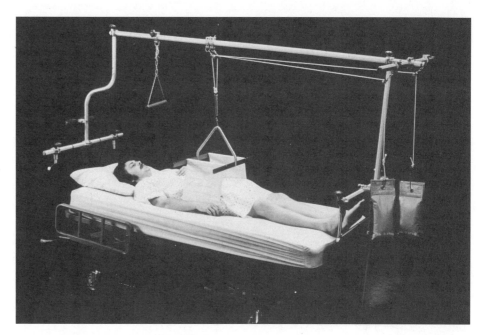

FIGURE 17–5 • Pelvic sling. (Courtesy of Zimmer USA.)

## Doctors' Orders for Respiratory Care

Below are listed examples of doctors' orders for the types of treatments performed by the respiratory care department. Because of staff reorganization, more common respiratory treatments may be performed by the nurse on the unit rather than by the respiratory care department. Explanations and illustrations are provided to promote your familiarity with an interpretation of the orders. The orders are written as you may find them on the doctors' order sheet.

### ■ O₂ 4 L/min nasal cannula continuously

Oxygen is either piped into the patient's room (wall outlet) or brought to the patient's room in a steel cylinder.

Oxygen is administered under pressure and may have a drying effect upon the respiratory tract; therefore, oxygen is commonly humidified during administration. Oxygen supports combustion; therefore, no smoking is allowed in the room while oxygen is being administered. Signs must be posted to this effect. In some locations the entire health care facility may be designated a nonsmoking area, and signs may not be required.

An oxygen order contains the amount of oxygen (flow rate or concentration) the patient is to receive and the type of delivery device (mode of delivery). The flow rate is ordered in liters per minute. In the above order, the flow rate is 4 L/min.

*Nasal cannula*, frequently referred to as nasal prongs, is a popular method used for oxygen administration. *Nasal catheter* and *mask* are two other methods also used for the administration of oxygen (Fig. 17–11).

Plastic tubing is used to carry the oxygen from the oxygen tank or wall outlet to the patient. Although the respiratory care department personnel usually set up, take down, and handle the equipment for oxygen administration, the nursing staff also monitors this treatment.

*Might order foam pads for ears*

### ■ Oxygen tent 40% O₂

The oxygen tent is another method used for administration of oxygen to the patient. It is used mostly for pediatric patients. *Kids need a lot of lining. Babys.*

### ■ IPPB c̄ 3 cc saline qid

An IPPB machine is used to administer this treatment order. This treatment is used to improve ventilation, to help remove secretions from the lungs, to administer aerosol medications, and for various other reasons (Fig. 17–12).

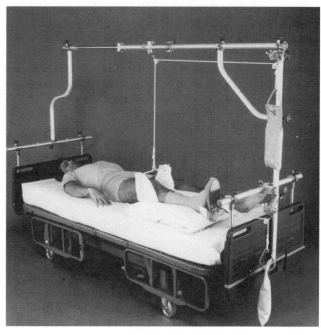

FIGURE 17–6 • Russell's traction. (Courtesy of Zimmer USA.)

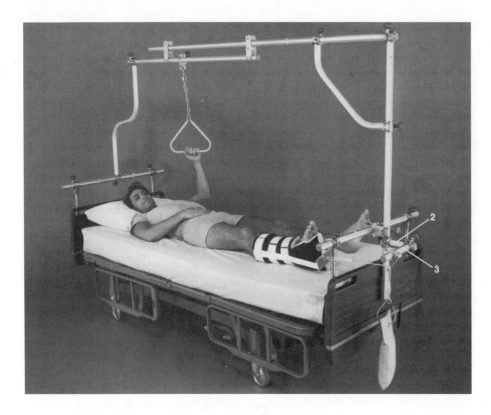

F I G U R E  17–7 • Unilateral Buck's traction with overhead frame and trapeze. Note the Buck's boot on the right leg. (Courtesy of Zimmer USA.)

The above order includes many instructions for the respiratory therapist. It is very important to be accurate in copying the order onto the respiratory therapy requisition or entering it into the computer.

■ *IPPB 0.5 mL Ventolin & 3 mL NS tid*
This IPPB order includes medication Ventolin and dosage (0.5 mL). IPPB orders must include frequency and medication; duration and pressure used may be optional.

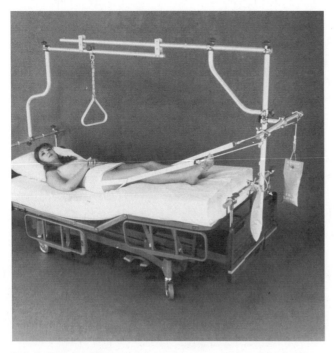

F I G U R E  17–8 • Pelvic traction with pelvic belt. (Courtesy of Zimmer USA.)

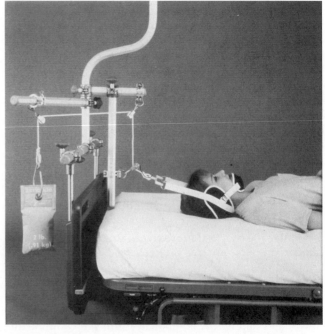

F I G U R E  17–9 • Cervical traction with head halter.

```
┌─────────────────────────────────────┬───────────────────────────────┐
│ DR. ORDERING_____ │                               │
│ DIAGNOSIS_____ │                               │
│ DATE ORDERED _____ │                               │
│ REQUESTED BY_____ │                               │
├─────────────────────────────────────┼───────────────────────────────┤
│ OXYGEN THERAPY                      │ RESPIRATORY CARE TREATMENTS   │
│ O₂_____ L/M    PRN_____ │ ☐ CPT                         │
│ ☐ NP                                │ ☐ SVN                         │
│ ☐ MASK                              │ ☐ USN                         │
│ ☐ AEROSOL                           │ ☐ IPPB                        │
│ ☐ TENT                              │ ☐ IS                          │
│ ☐ OTHER_____ │ ☐ HA                          │
│                                     │ ☐ B. PAP                      │
│                                     │ ☐ CPAP                        │
│                                     │ ☐ OTHER                       │
├─────────────────────────────────────┴───────────────────────────────┤
│              RESPIRATORY CARE REQUISITION                            │
└─────────────────────────────────────────────────────────────────────┘
```

F I G U R E  17–10 • Respiratory care requisition.

**HIGHLIGHT**

Orders for oxygen therapy include the **amount of oxygen** (flow rate or concentration) and the **type of delivery device**.

It is important to recognize a new order for oxygen or a change in a previous order. An ABG on O₂ @ 4 L/min is **NOT** a new order for oxygen, but is an arterial blood gas drawn while the patient's oxygen flow rate is at 4 liters per minute. It may be necessary to notify nursing staff or respiratory care of the oxygen flow rate.

As mentioned before, it may be your responsibility to order the medication from the pharmacy, although in most facilities, the respiratory care department provides any medication used during treatment. The names of other medications commonly used for IPPB treatments are Vaponephrin, Mucomyst, Bronkosol, terbutaline (Monovent),

Alupent, albuterol (Ventolin), and Atrovent. Figure 17–12 shows a Bennett machine used for IPPB treatments.

■ *SVN with UD Ventolin tid*
This SVN order includes a unit dose of Ventolin.
*Home care nurses are giving treat ment*

■ *SVN 0.5 cc Bronkosol with 2.5 cc NS qid*
This treatment is a simple device that produces an aerosol from liquid medication to be inhaled into the lungs.

■ *Hypertonic USN for sputum inducement*
An ultrasonic nebulizer is used for this treatment. It produces an aerosol that carries further into the airways of the lung in order to loosen secretions so that the patient may produce a sputum specimen. The solution used is a hypertonic (concentrated) salt solution of 5% NaCl.

■ *CPT*
Chest physiotherapy includes vibration and percussion, which are hand or mechanical techniques used to loosen secretions within the lung. This treatment is performed in

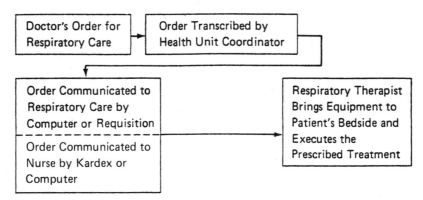

**COMMUNICATION AND IMPLEMENTATION OF RESPIRATORY THERAPY ORDERS**

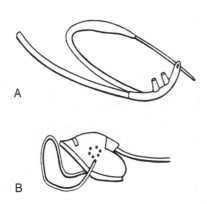

**F I G U R E  17–11** • Apparatus used to administer oxygen. (*A*) Cannula. (*B*) Mask.

conjunction with postural drainage, a treatment of patient positioning designed to remove secretions from the lung.

■ *Mechanical ventilator $O_2$ concentration ($Fi_{O_2}$) 30%, tidal volume (Vt) 800, SIMV-14, PSV of 10, Pe − 5*

This is an example of a doctors' order to place the patient on a ventilator, or gives parameters for a patient already placed on a ventilator. The respirator assists or replaces

*Respiratory therapy & nursing staff*
*oxygen is get order breath*

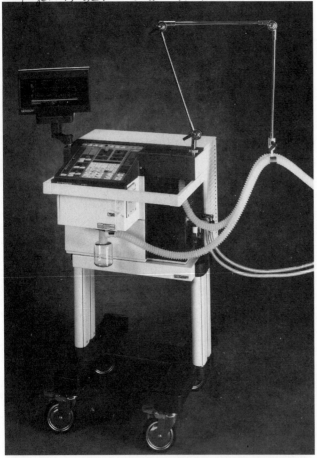

**F I G U R E  17–12** • Bennett machine, used to administer IPPB treatments. (Courtesy of Puritan Bennett.)

respiration of the patient. Servo, Bennet 7200 and Bear 5 are types of ventilators that may be used for this purpose. You may see these terms included in a doctors' order for mechanical ventilation (Fig. 17–13). Weaning is a term to describe the gradual removal of mechanical ventilation from a patient.

■ *HA @ 60% via T-piece*

A heated mist (heated aerosol) is produced for the patient to breathe in. It may be ordered for patients who are breathing through a tracheostomy or endotracheal tube.

■ *Incentive spirometry tid (IS)*

This technique is often used postoperatively to encourage patients to breathe deeply. Various devices are used (Fig. 17–14). *Used before surgery*

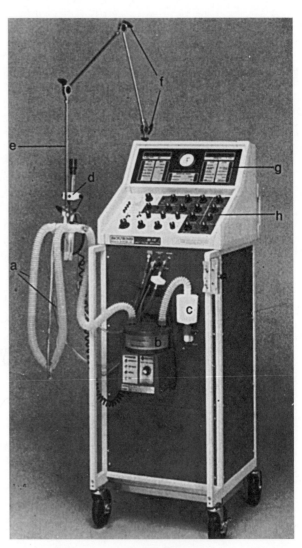

**F I G U R E  17–13** • A ventilator. (From Ignatavicius, Donna D., Workman, M. Linda, and Mishler, Mary A.: Medical-Surgical Nursing: A Nursing Process Approach, 2nd ed. Philadelphia, W. B. Saunders Co., 1995, with permission.)

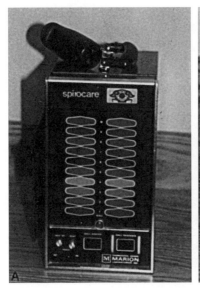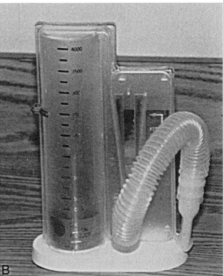

FIGURE 17–14 • Examples of incentive spirometry. (From Ignatavicius, Donna D., Workman, M. Linda, and Mishler, Mary A.: Medical-Surgical Nursing: A Nursing Process Approach, 2nd ed. Philadelphia, W. B. Saunders Co., 1995, with permission.)

■ *IS c̄ PEP @ 5 cm H₂O*

This incentive spirometry treatment includes positive expiratory pressure (PEP), which supplies resistance against exhalation (keeps air from coming out) in order to reinflate the alveoli in patients with atelectasis. PEP may also be ordered with SVN treatments.

■ *BiPAP I:10 E:5*

Biphasic positive airway pressure is a treatment that uses a machine to push air into the lungs during inspiration (like an IPPB) and expiration (like CPAP) in order to treat severe atelectasis or sleep apnea (Fig. 17–15).

■ *CPAP 5 cm H₂O*

This positive airway pressure treatment provides positive pressure in the airway continuously throughout the entire respiratory cycle. This prevents the lungs from completely returning to the resting level, and may be used to treat sleep apnea and other respiratory syndromes. It also can be used in weaning patients from a mechanical ventilator.

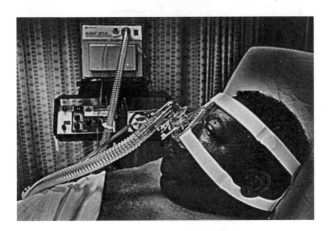

FIGURE 17–15 • BiPAP. (From Ignatavicius, Donna D., Workman, M. Linda, and Mishler, Mary A.: Medical-Surgical Nursing: A Nursing Process Approach, 2nd ed. Philadelphia, W. B. Saunders Co., 1995, with permission.)

■ *MDI c̄ Ventolin qid ⃛iii puffs*

MDI is a metered dose inhaler in which the medication is premeasured in the pharmacy.

> **HIGHLIGHT**
>
> Common medications administered via the respiratory tract are Vaponephrin, Mucomyst, Bronkosol, terbutaline (Monovent), Alupent, albuterol (Ventolin), and Atrovent.

## Other Terms and Abbreviations Used in Respiratory Care Orders

The following list includes some terms and abbreviations that have not been included in the vocabulary or abbreviations list, but which you may see included in a respiratory care order.

Compressed air (CA)
Intermittent mandatory ventilation (IMV)
Positive end expiratory pressure (PEEP)

> **TO THE STUDENT**
>
> To practice transcribing respiratory care orders, complete **Activity 17–2** in the Skills Practice Manual.

## PHYSICAL MEDICINE AND REHABILITATION

Larger hospitals usually have a physical medicine department, which comprises physical therapy, occupational therapy, and electromyography, along with other areas of treatment. In a smaller hospital, each of the above departments may be a separate department or perhaps there will be only a physical therapy department.

## PHYSICAL THERAPY

### Background Information

Physical therapy is the division within the hospital that treats patients to improve their bodily function by methods such as gait training, exercise, water therapy, and heat and ice treatments. Patients include those injured during sports and work-related activities. Children affected by cerebral palsy and muscular dystrophy are assisted towards normal physical development through physical therapy. Individuals who suffer strokes, spinal cord injuries, and amputations are assisted back to their highest level of physical function through therapy. The physical therapist, a person licensed to practice in this field, performs the treatment on the patient. Most treatments are performed in the physical therapy department; therefore, transportation of the patient is usually necessary. Following treatment, the physical therapist records the treatment and other pertinent data to be included in the patient's chart.

To communicate the order to the physical therapy department, complete a physical therapy or physical medicine requisition form or use the computer (Fig. 17–16). Because physical therapy involves rehabilitation, which is frequently a lengthy process, it may also be necessary to schedule the patient's treatments with the department.

### Doctors' Orders for Physical Therapy

Below are examples of doctors' orders for physical therapy. Brief descriptions and illustrations are included to assist you with the interpretation of the orders.

> **HIGHLIGHT**
>
> A commonly made mistake is in interpreting the abbreviation "PT." It may be an order for physical therapy, or an order for a prothrombin time, which is a coagulation study (see Chapter 14). It is important to fully understand physicians' orders during transcription.

**Hydrotherapy Orders**

■ *Hubbard tank 30 min qd T 100° F, active underwater exercises to elbows and knees c̄ débridement*

This treatment is used for underwater exercises and for cleansing wounds and burns (Fig. 17–17). Hydrotherapy treatments may be ordered to be done with a sterile solution. The physical therapy department will select an appropriate substance to use.

■ *Whirlpool bath left leg bid*

The whirlpool is smaller than the Hubbard tank. It is used for the same purposes (Fig. 17–18).

DR. ORDERING _____

DIAGNOSIS _____

DATE ORDERING _____

REQUESTED BY _____

REQUEST FOR      ☐ EMG      ☐ PHYSIATRIST CONSULT/THERAPY

☐ PHYSICAL THERAPY      ☐ OCCUPATIONAL THERAPY

☐ OTHER _____

PHYSICIAN ORDER

**PHYSICAL MEDICINE AND REHABILITATION REQUISITION**

F I G U R E   17–16 • Physical medicine and rehabilitation requisition.

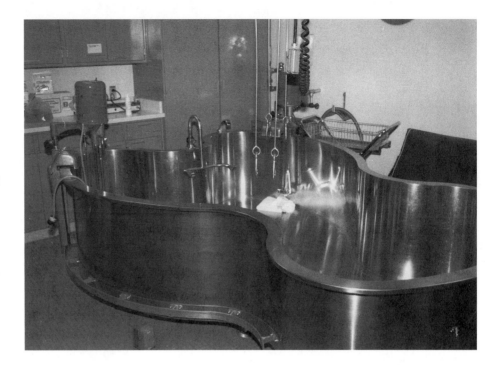

FIGURE 17–17 • Hubbard tank.

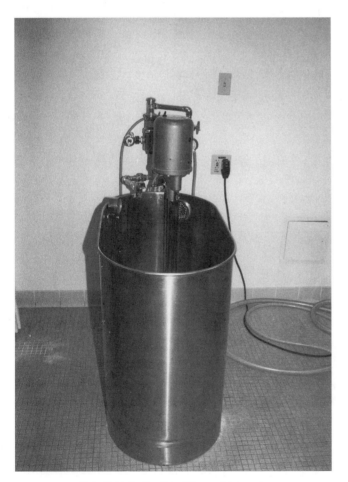

FIGURE 17–18 • Whirlpool.

### Exercise Orders

■ *Active assistive exercise left shoulder and elbow daily bid*
*Passive, active, resistive, reeducation, coordination,* and *relaxation* are other types of exercises that may be ordered by the doctor.

■ *ROM bid to upper extremities*
Range-of-motion exercises are frequently ordered for bedridden patients and therefore are usually performed in the patient's room. These exercises involve moving each joint of the upper extremities to the maximum in each direction.

■ *PT to ambulate patient with walker as tolerated*
The physical therapy department often decides which equipment is best suited for the patient.

■ *PT to evaluate and treat*

■ *ACL protocol per Dr. Melzer*
Many physicians have preprinted courses of treatment (protocols) on file with the physical therapy department which are implemented throughout the patient's stay (precluding any complications). These programs of treatment include critical pathways and goals, and are often named after the orthopedic surgery performed on the patient. Familiarity with orthopedic surgical procedures and abbreviations is helpful. An ACL protocol would follow an anterior cruciate ligament (ACL) repair.

■ *Dr. Jen's BKA protocol*
This preprinted protocol is for rehabilatation after a below-the-knee amputation. Another physician's protocol may be different.

■ *Transfer training, wheelchair mobility*
The physical therapist teaches the patient how to transfer from the bed to the wheelchair and how to use the wheel-

## COMMUNICATION AND IMPLEMENTATION OF PHYSICAL MEDICINE ORDERS

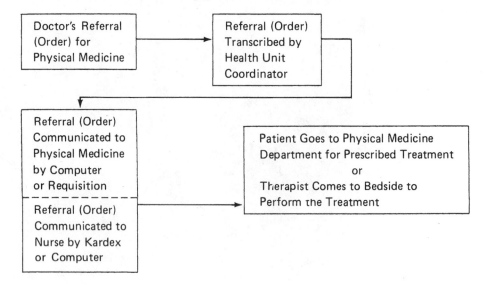

chair. Usually ordered for patients who have had an amputation, stroke, or other physical disability.

■ *Gait training with a walker, partial wt bearing lt leg*
The physical therapist teaches the patient to walk with an appropriate device, such as a walker. Additional devices used in patient ambulation are the large base quad cane (LBQC) and the short arc quad (SAQ).

■ *Crutch walking NWB daily*
The physical therapist instructs the patient to walk with crutches. Variations to this order may be noted regarding the amount of weight bearing (such as *full weight*), any precautions to take, or the type of crutch walking to teach the patient (such as *4-point gait*). Additional variations in the amount of weight bearing may include the following: full weight bearing (FWB), partial weight bearing (PWB), touchdown weight bearing (TDWB), toe touch weight bearing (TTWB), and weight bearing as tolerated (WBAT).

*can cause nerve damage in not instructed properly in usage*

■ *CPM*
Continuous passive motion machine is used after joint replacement. It may be monitored by the physical therapist or by the nursing staff (Fig. 17–19). Additional motion orders may include active assistive range of motion (AAROM), active range of motion (AROM), and passive range of motion (PROM) (Fig. 17–19).

■ *T-band exercises*
These are exercises using a band of rubber, or a "theraband" for resistance.

■ *Codman's exercises R shoulder*
These exercises for the shoulder are also called pendulum exercises.

■ *Isometrics bilat upper extremities*
Isometric exercises flex muscles without allowing actual movement of the limb.

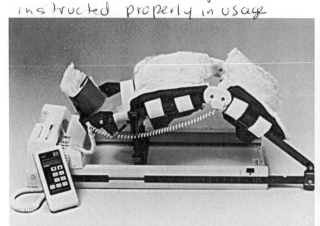
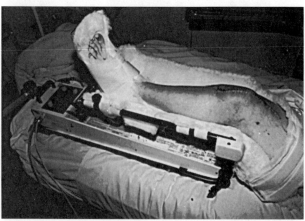

**F I G U R E   17–19** • Examples of continuous passive motion (CPM) machine. (From Ignatavicius, Donna D., Workman, M. Linda, and Mishler, Mary A.: Medical-Surgical Nursing: A Nursing Process Approach, 2nd ed. Philadelphia, W. B. Saunders Co., 1995, with permission.)

### Heat and Cold Orders

- *Shortwave diathermy to lower back daily*   US *treatment*

Diathermy generates heat deep within the body tissues. Ultrasonic and microwave diathermy may also be ordered by the doctor. If a physician writes "may substitute PRN," the physical therapist may change the mode of heat delivery to one that is more effective. The therapist may also select a different mode if the written one is contraindicated.

- *Infrared lamp daily*

This is heat treatment given by use of infrared rays.

- *Ultrasound and massage to lower back*

- *Hydrocollator packs or hot packs to back bid*

- *Ice or cold packs to left leg bid*

### Pain Relief Orders

- *Postop TENS*

Transcutaneous electrical nerve stimulation is used to control pain by blocking transmission of pain impulses to the brain. Electrodes are applied to the skin surrounding the incision during surgery. Thin wires lead from the elec-

trodes to a powered stimulator with a control. Usually the patient is taught how to use the device prior to surgery. For nonsurgical use, the physical therapist attaches the external electrodes to the skin (Fig. 17–20).

- *EPC*

Electronic pain control is another way of ordering TENS.

- *ES*

Electrical stimulation may be used to reduce pain or swelling, promote healing, or assist in exercising muscles. Different types of machines are used to deliver this treatment. A variation is functional electrical stimulation (FES).

## Occupational Therapy

Occupational therapy is the department within the hospital that works toward rehabilitation of patients, in conjunction with other health team members, to return the patient to the greatest possible independence. Creative, manual, recreational, and prevocational assessment are examples of activities used in rehabilitation of the patient. Occupational therapy activities are ordered by the doctor and administered by a qualified occupational therapist.

---

**HIGHLIGHT**

Examples of basic skills to be achieved as a result of occupational therapy include toileting, bathing, dressing, cooking, and feeding oneself.

---

### Doctors' Orders for Occupational Therapy

- *OT for evaluation and treatment if nec daily*

- *ADL*

- *Supply and train in adaptive equipment use ADL button hooks and feeding utensils*

- *OT to increase mobility*

- *Fabricate cock-up splint for left upper extremity*

---

TO THE STUDENT

To practice transcribing physical medicine and rehabilitation orders, complete **Activity 17–3** in the Skills Practice Manual.

---

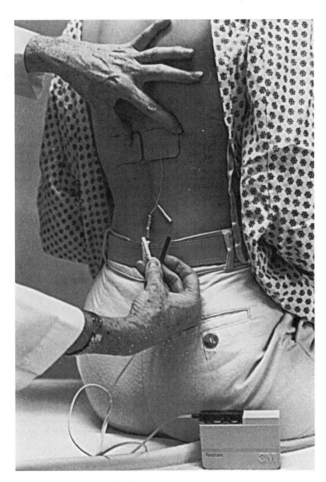

F I G U R E  17–20 • TENS unit for pain control. (From Ignatavicius, Donna D., Workman, M. Linda, and Mishler, Mary A.: Medical-Surgical Nursing: A Nursing Process Approach, 2nd ed. Philadelphia, W. B. Saunders Co., 1995, with permission.)

## DIALYSIS

The kidneys are essential organs in the removal of toxic wastes from the blood. When the kidneys fail to remove those wastes, medical intervention is necessary to sustain life. The kidneys may fail temporarily (acute renal failure), or they may be permanently damaged and become nonfunctional (chronic renal failure and end-stage renal disease [ESRD]). There are two main types of dialysis: **hemodialysis** and **peritoneal dialysis**.

Hemodialysis (also called extracorporeal dialysis) is the removal of waste products from the blood by the utilization of a machine through which the blood flows. This is regularly performed in a special outpatient dialysis facility, and is commonly done for 3- to 4-hour periods 3 days a week. For the hospitalized patient, hemodialysis is usually performed in a special unit in the hospital. If the patient is too ill to be moved, a portable hemodialysis machine may be used.

Peritoneal dialysis is the introduction of a fluid (dialyzing fluid) into the abdominal cavity that then absorbs the wastes from the blood through the lining of the abdominal cavity, or peritoneum. The dialysate is then emptied from the abdominal cavity. This type of dialysis allows for a greater level of freedom for the patient, as they may perform this fluid transfer outside of any health care facility. Some variations of peritoneal dialysis include continuous ambulatory peritoneal dialysis (CAPD), continuous cycling peritoneal dialysis (CCPD), and intermittent peritoneal dialysis (IPD).

### Doctors' Orders for Dialysis

■ *Hemodialysis three times per week for 2 hours*
The patient will have hemodialysis for 2 hours per session three times a week.

■ *Consent for Tenckhoff catheter placement for peritoneal dialysis*
This procedure is surgical placement of a long-term catheter or tube into the patient's abdomen so that they are able to perform peritoneal dialysis.

■ *Consent for A-V shunt creation*
Hemodialysis requires vascular access. This surgical procedure inserts a cannula into an artery, as well as one into a vein. These are both then connected to tubing that allows for easier needle insertion necessary for hemodialysis.

## RADIATION TREATMENTS

The area in the hospital where radiation therapy is performed may be a division of the diagnostic imaging department, or it may be a totally separate department.

Many of those undergoing radiation therapy are outpatients. However, the health unit coordinator may be called upon to schedule an appointment for an inpatient who requires treatment for a malignant neoplasm (cancer). Many hospitals require the units to use a requisition form, and others may schedule an appointment by telephone. After the initial visit, radiation therapy usually notifies the nursing unit of the patient's treatment schedule.

TO THE STUDENT

To practice recording a review set of doctors' orders and to practice recording telephone doctors' orders, complete **Activities 17–4** and **17–5** in the Skills Practice Manual.

To practice recording telephone messages, complete **Activity 17–6** in the Skills Practice Manual.

## SUMMARY

The transcription of treatment orders involves the communication of the order to the necessary department by requisition form or by computer, and the communication of the order to the nursing staff by the kardexing step of the transcription procedure. The orders are then executed by professionals in their respective departments.

**REVIEW QUESTIONS**

1. Write the meaning of the following abbreviations in the space provided.

   a. ROM _Range of Motion_          d. SVN _Small Volume Nebulizer_

   b. EMG _Electro myogram_          e. IPPB _Intermettent Possitive Pressure Breathing_

   c. MDI _Metered dose inhaler_     f. ADL _Activities of Daily Living_

2. Circle the items listed below which the health unit coordinator may order from the CSD as part of the transcription procedure of a traction order.

   nebulizer
   (head halter)
   oxygen mask
   (moleskin and elastic bandage)

   (pelvic belt)
   hydrotherapy
   (pelvic sling)

3. Below are listed eight types of traction:

   pelvic traction
   (Bryant's traction)
   (cervical traction with Crutchfield tongs)
   (pelvic sling)

   (Russell's traction)
   cervical traction
   (Thomas splint)
   (overhead frame and trapeze)

   a. Underline the traction set-up used to treat bone fractures.
   b. Circle the traction set-up used to assist patients to move in bed.

4. Below are listed various types of treatments, including treatments performed by the nursing staff. Indicate the treatment performed by the physical medicine department by writing PM in the space provided, and indicate the treatment performed by the respiratory care department by writing RC in the space provided.

   a. IPPB ___RC___                   j. cath _____

   b. SSE _____                      k. ROM ___PM___

   c. USN ___RC___                    l. K-pad ___PM___

   d. diathermy ___PM___             m. whirlpool ___PM___

   e. O₂ ___Oxegen RC___             n. infrared ___PM___

   f. SVN ___RC___                    o. TENS ___PM___

   g. P&PD ___RC___                   p. MDI ___RC___

   h. ADL ___PM Activities Daily Living___   q. gait training ___PM___

   i. IV _____                       r. CPT ___RC___

5. Define dialysis.
   _removal of wastes in the blood, usually excreated by the Kidneys_

6. Two types of dialysis are:

   a. _hemodialysis_

   b. _peritoneal Dialysis_

## References

Cahill, Matthew: *Treatments (Nurses Reference Library)*. Springhouse, PA, Springhouse, 1988.

Johnson, Laura: Operative management of unstable pelvic fractures. *Orthopaedic Nursing* 8:21–25, 1989.

Jones-Walton, Peggy: Clinical standards in skeletal traction pin site care. *Orthopaedic Nursing* 10:12–16, 1991.

Kottke, Frederic J. and Lehmann, Justus F: *Krusen's Handbook of Physical Medicine and Rehabilitation*, 4th ed. Philadelphia, W. B. Saunders Co., 1990.

Monahan, Frances D., Drake, Tanya, and Neighbors, Marianne: *Nursing Care of Adults*. Philadelphia, W. B. Saunders Co., 1994.

Newschwander, Gregg E. and Dunst, Regina M.: Limb lengthening with the Ilizarov external fixator. *Orthopaedic Nursing* 8:15–21, 1989.

Wood, Lucille A. and Rambo, Beverly J.: *Nursing Skills for Allied Health Services*, vol. 2, 2nd ed. Philadelphia, W. B. Saunders Co., 1977.

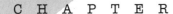
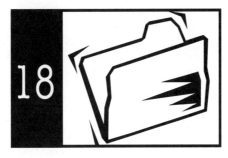

# 18

# MISCELLANEOUS ORDERS

Consultation, Health Records, Home Care, Scheduling, Social Service, Temporary Absence, Discharge/ Transfer, and Other Orders

---

## CHAPTER OBJECTIVES

*Upon completion of this chapter, you will be able to:*

1. Define the terms in the vocabulary list.
2. List five points of information that should be communicated to the consulting physician's office when transcribing a consultation order.
3. List three reasons why a doctor may wish to transfer a patient to another hospital room.
4. Write the meaning of each abbreviation in the abbreviations list.
5. List six tasks the health unit coordinator may have to perform when arranging for a patient to leave the hospital on a pass.
6. Name two services rendered by the home care department and four services rendered by the social service department.

## VOCABULARY

**Consultation Order** • A request by the patient's attending physician for the opinion of a second physician with respect to diagnosis and treatment of the patient

**Discharge Order** • A doctor's order that states the patient may leave the hospital. A doctor's order is necessary for a patient to be discharged from the hospital

**Transfer Order** • A doctor's order that requests a patient to be transferred to another hospital room

---

## ABBREVIATIONS

| Abbreviation | Meaning | Example of Usage on a Doctors' Order Sheet |
|---|---|---|
| appt | appointment | Make appt with dental clinic |
| disch | discharge | Disch today |
| DME | durable medical equipment | Contact DME supplier |
| DNR | do not resuscitate | DNR |
| wk | week | Disch see me next wk |
| Rx | take (treatment, medication, etc.) | Disch c̄ Rx |
| NINP | no information, no publication | Pt. requests NINP |

## CONSULTATION ORDERS

### Background Information

The attending physician may want to have the opinion of another doctor regarding the diagnosis and treatment of a client. The request for the opinion of another doctor is written on the doctors' order sheet by the patient's doctor and is called a **consultation order** (Fig. 18–1).

The transcription process for consultation orders requires the health unit coordinator to notify the consulting doctor's office of the order.

The following information should be communicated to the consulting doctor's office:

- Hospital name
- Patient's name
- Patient's location
- Name of the doctor requesting the consultation
- Patient's diagnosis

### Doctors' Orders for Consultation

Doctors' orders for consultation may be expressed in writing on the doctors' order sheet as follows:

- *Have Dr. Avery see in consult*
- *Call Dr. Reidy for consultation*
- *Call Dr. Casey to see patient re radiation therapy*
- *Have Dr. Williams see patient today please*

> ### TO THE STUDENT
>
> To practice transcribing consultation orders, complete **Activity 18–1** in the Skills Practice Manual.

## HEALTH RECORD ORDERS

### Background Information

The health records department, also called health information management department, stores the charts of patients who have been treated at the health care facility in the past. Frequently, upon readmission of a patient to the hospital, the doctor may request the records of the patient's previous hospital stay (old charts) to be brought from the health records department to the nursing unit. The request is put in writing on the doctors' order sheet by the patient's doctor and is called a health record order.

The order for the old chart is communicated by the health unit coordinator to the health records department either by telephone, computer, or by the ordering step for transcription. See Figure 18–2 for a typical example of a health record requisition.

While the old chart is on the nursing unit, it is usually stored in a specially designed area rather than in the current patient's chart holder.

**COMMUNICATION AND IMPLEMENTATION OF CONSULTATION ORDERS**

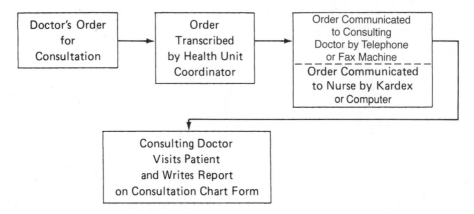

**CONSULTATION ORDER AND REPORT**

I have authorized Dr. *Ossie Goldven* to
examine my patient *June Bugg*
and

☒ CONSULT AND MAKE RECOMMENDATIONS

☐ WRITE ORDERS

☐ CONSULT AND ASSUME CARE OF PATIENT

*12/01/xx*
DATE

*Oscar Gold, M.D.*
SIGNATURE ATTENDING PHYSICIAN

Reason for Consultation: *Recently developed a dermatitis that is spreading over body. Vesicles and pustules become infected causing severe pain which now affects sleep and appetite*

FINDINGS AND RECOMMENDATIONS:

Date of Consultation _____ Signature _____
(CONSULTANT)

00-0569

**CONSULTATION ORDER AND REPORT**

F I G U R E   18–1 • Consultation order and report form.

F I G U R E  18–2 • Health records (medical records) requisition.

The doctor may also request records of diagnostic studies from the patient's previous stay in another hospital. Since this information is confidential, the patient must give written permission for release of the information from one hospital to another. To transcribe a doctor's order to obtain old health records from another hospital, the health unit coordinator initiates a consent form (Fig. 18–3): when signed by the patient, this form is forwarded to the health records department of the health care facility. The personnel in the health records department assume the task of obtaining the records from the indicated hospital and delivering them to the nursing unit.

It may be the practice of some facilities for the health records department to automatically send records of the patient's past hospitalizations to the nursing unit.

### Doctors' Orders for Health Records

Doctors' orders for health records may be expressed in writing on the doctors' order sheet as follows:

- *Old charts to floor*
- *Obtain old charts from health records*
- *Obtain report on total body CT scan from St. Joseph's Hospital (done 2/28/xx)*

---

### TO THE STUDENT

To practice transcribing a health records order, complete **Activity 18–2** in the Skills Practice Manual.

## HOME HEALTH CARE DEPARTMENT ORDERS

### Background Information

This department plans with the patient and/or family for the patient's care in the home with outside agency personnel and assists in obtaining necessary medical equipment. The patient makes the choice of a home health care agency when one is ordered by the physician, or in some instances the home care agency is defined by the health care insurance carrier. Many hospitals have a home health care component within their system. Other home care agencies (Visiting Nurse Associations) are independent and not affiliated with a particular hospital. Discharge planners or home health care coordinators have offices in the hospital and help make arrangements to have home health care services started when the patient is discharged. Home health care can include skilled nursing, home health aide services, physical therapy, occupational therapy, respiratory care, speech therapy, and medical social work. The discharged patient may also need durable medical equipment (DME), such as a hospital bed, oxygen, a walker, or wheelchair. A separate company (a DME company) usually supplies these patient care items and delivers them to the patient's home.

When a patient is being discharged and home health care services are being ordered and planned, the case management department may become involved. Case management acts as a patient's advocate in getting the home health care services that best suit the patient's needs and

## AUTHORIZATION TO OBTAIN MEDICAL INFORMATION

DATE _1/11/XX_

TO: _Memorial Hospital_  RE. _Marilee Owens_
(NAME OF PATIENT)

_1100 Ash St._
(ADDRESS)

_Phoenix_

_7/7/XX_
(BIRTHDATE)

THE ABOVE NAMED PERSON IS NOW A PATIENT IN THIS HOSPITAL UNDER THE CARE OF

DR. _Roosevelt Conklin_

WE WERE INFORMED THAT THIS PATIENT WAS IN YOUR INSTITUTION ON OR ABOUT

_March 10-15 19XX_

WOULD YOU PLEASE SEND US A TRANSCRIPT OF  _HER_  MEDICAL RECORD AS SOON AS POSSIBLE?  WE ARE PARTICULARLY INTERESTED IN THE FOLLOWING REPORTS.

_____ HISTORY AND PHYSICAL EXAMINATION

_____ OPERATION REPORTS

_____ CONSULTATIONS

_____ X-RAY REPORTS

THANK YOU FOR YOUR COOPERATION

_____ LABORATORY REPORTS

_____ PATHOLOGY REPORTS

__X__ DISCHARGE SUMMARY

__X__ OTHER REPORTS

_CT Brain_

SINCERELY YOURS,

| KINDLY ADDRESS YOUR REPLY |
| ATTENTION OF |
| MEDICOLEGAL SECRETARY |
| MEDICAL RECORD DEPARTMENT |

DIRECTOR
HEALTH RECORDS SERVICES

I HEREBY AUTHORIZE _Memorial Hospital_ TO GIVE TO THIS HOSPITAL A COPY OF MY HOSPITAL RECORDS OR ANY INFORMATION WHICH MAY HAVE BEEN ACQUIRED IN THE COURSE OF MY EXAMINATION OR TREATMENT.

_Marilee Owens_
(SIGNATURE OF PATIENT)

_1/11/XX_
(DATE)

F I G U R E  18–3 • Consent form to obtain records from another hospital.

## COMMUNICATION AND IMPLEMENTATION OF HEALTH RECORD ORDERS

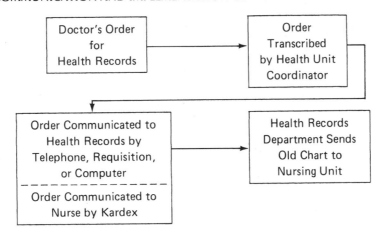

335

**COMMUNICATION AND IMPLEMENTATION OF A DOCTOR'S ORDER THAT REQUIRES SCHEDULING**

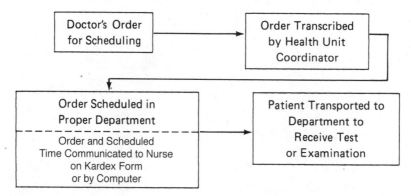

coordinates financial coverage through private insurers, Medicare, and so forth.

When a patient has a life-limiting illness, they can frequently benefit from the services of hospice. Hospice is a multidisciplined organization which stresses a holistic approach to care of the patient during their final stage of life. The team comprises a physician, nurses, certified nursing assistants, social workers, a chaplain, and volunteers. Most hospice care can be rendered in the patient's home.

### Doctors' Orders for Home Health Care

- *Contact home health care to plan for discharge next week*

- *Have home health care plan with patient's family for discharge in 2 days*

- *Have hospice see pt*

## SCHEDULING ORDERS

## Background Information

Frequently, while the patient is in a health care facility, the doctor may write an order to schedule the patient for var-

ious types of tests or examinations performed in specialized departments or outside of the health care facility.

It is the health unit coordinator's task to notify the department or facility that performs the test or examination and schedule a time convenient to both the involved department and the patient. It is important to record the scheduled time on the patient's Kardex form.

┌─────────────────────────────────────┐
│          TO THE STUDENT              │
└─────────────────────────────────────┘

To practice transcribing an order to schedule an examination, complete **Activity 18–3** in the Skills Practice Manual.

### Doctors' Orders that Require Scheduling

Below are examples of doctors' orders that require scheduling. These vary greatly among health care facilities, according to the services available.

- *Schedule pt in outpatient department for vaginal examination*

- *Schedule pt for psychological testing*

- *Schedule pt for diabetic classes*

- *Schedule client for hearing evaluation test*

- *Schedule in dental clinic for evaluation and care*

**COMMUNICATION AND IMPLEMENTATION OF SOCIAL SERVICE ORDERS**

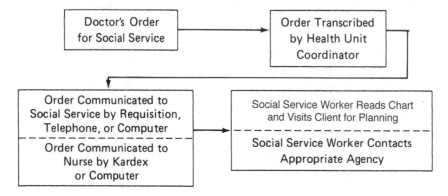

## SOCIAL SERVICE DEPARTMENT ORDERS

### Background Information

Social service provides much needed information concerning resources available to the patient and their families as they transition from the health care facility back to their home. Financial considerations, transportation, meals, and other support services are some areas with which social service can assist.

### *Doctors' Orders for the Social Services Department*

- *Contact family re: plans to place in custodial care facility*

- *Arrange for home-bound teacher for 1 month*

- *Have social worker arrange for CNA to assist pt at home*

- *Have social worker order hospital bed for pt upon discharge*

- *Have social worker see pt for discharge planning*

## TEMPORARY ABSENCES (PASSES TO LEAVE THE HEALTH CARE FACILITY)

Some clients may be allowed to leave the health care facility for several hours, and other clients who have been confined for a long time may be allowed to leave for several days. Long-term care clients receive many benefits from visiting their homes or experiencing a recreational outing. A gradual return to society has therapeutic value for rehabilitating clients.

A temporary pass requires the health unit coordinator to do the following:

- arrange with the pharmacy for medications the patient is taking

- note on the census when the patient leaves and returns
- cancel all meals for the length of the absence
- cancel any hospital treatments for the length of the absence
- arrange for any special equipment that the patient may need
- have the patient sign a temporary absence release (Fig. 18–4)

### *Doctors' Orders for Temporary Absence*

- *May have pass for tomorrow from 9 AM to 7 PM*

- *Temporary hospital absence from 3 PM Friday to 3 PM Sunday; arrange for rental of wheelchair*

- *May leave hospital from 10 AM to 1 PM today; have patient sign permit*

## TRANSFER AND DISCHARGE ORDERS

If the doctor plans to transfer the patient to another room or to another unit, or plans to discharge the patient to his or her home or to another facility, he or she writes an order for such on the doctors' order sheet.

To transcribe a transfer or discharge order, the health unit coordinator must notify the hospital admitting department (or discharge department) by telephone or computer, or by completing a discharge or transfer slip.

**Discharge orders** may include information such as instructions for the patient to follow after he or she leaves the hospital, requests for appointments for the patient, and so forth.

The doctor may request a **transfer** of a patient for various reasons, such as for a different type of room accommodation (ward to private), or for more intense nursing care (regular unit to ICU). Another reason for a transfer is if the patient's condition requires that he or she be placed in an isolation unit.

Later on in the text we will cover the procedures for transferring and discharging a patient. Here we have dealt only with the transcription procedures for a transfer or discharge order.

**COMMUNICATION AND IMPLEMENTATION OF TEMPORARY ABSENCE ORDERS**

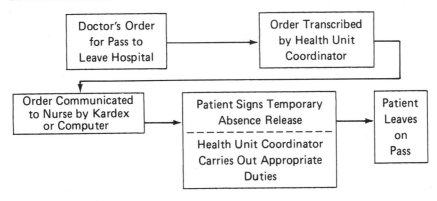

**TEMPORARY ABSENCE RELEASE**

The undersigned, being a patient of The Above Named Hospital, hereby confirms his (or her) agreement and understanding that neither the hospital, its employees, nor the attending physicians shall be responsible for his (or her) care or condition during any absences of the undersigned from the building or resulting from such absences.

Signed _____
          PATIENT / PARENT / GUARDIAN

Date _____

Hour _____

Witness _____

09-0366                                    **TEMPORARY ABSENCE RELEASE**

F I G U R E  18–4 • Temporary absence release form.

**COMMUNICATION AND IMPLEMENTATION OF TRANSFER AND DISCHARGE ORDERS**

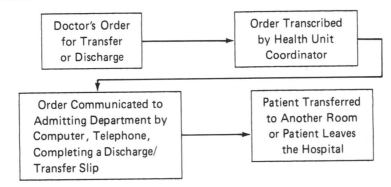

## Doctors' Orders for Transfer or Discharge of a Patient

Below are examples of how discharge or transfer orders may be expressed by the doctor on the doctors' order sheet.

### Transfer

■ *Transfer patient to 3E please*

■ *Transfer patient to a private room*

■ *Transfer patient to ICU after surgery*

■ *Transfer patient out of ICU to semiprivate room*

### Discharge

■ *Home today*

■ *Discharge*

■ *Home c̄ Rx*

■ *Home make appt to see me in 2 wk*

■ *Home c̄ crutches*

## MISCELLANEOUS ORDERS

There are orders that do not relate to any department that are nevertheless deserving of mention. All should be kardexed in their appropriate places. A few of the orders appear below.

■ *No visitors, limited number of visitors, or have visitors ck c̄ nurse before seeing pt*
A sign should be posted on the patient's door to see the nurse for further explanation. The switchboard and information desk should also be notified.

■ *DNR (do not resuscitate) or no code*
This order means that no resuscitative measures are to be performed. Some facilities have defined "code-related"

categories. An example is "all but CPR." The category of the patient's code status (if one is established) may be required to be indicated on the patient's identification bracelet at the time the admission is being processed. If a code status order is written by the physician, the order should be visible on the Kardex and on the patient's chart.

■ *NINP (no information, no publication)*
Your hospital may use a different abbreviation, but whatever words or abbreviation is used, this order means that the unit denies having the patient and no news concerning the patient is to be given to the press or friends. This order may also be extended to include family members.

■ *Notify Dr. Avery of patient's admission to the hospital*
This order is to inform the patient's primary physician of their admission to the unit when another physician has admitted the patient to the health care facility.

■ *Notify HO if systolic pressure above 200*
House officer is the name given to the resident on call.

┌─────────────────────────────────────┐
│        TO THE STUDENT                │
└─────────────────────────────────────┘

To practice transcribing a review set of doctors' orders, complete **Activity 18–4** in the Skills Practice Manual.

## SUMMARY

This chapter has discussed a variety of doctors' orders. It concludes the transcription practice for all classifications of doctors' orders. Transcribing doctors' orders is a major health unit coordinator task. Repeated performance is necessary to gain expertise in this area.

As you begin transcribing doctors' orders on the nursing unit of the hospital, you will find it helpful to use the transcription procedures presented in this textbook as a reference.

**REVIEW QUESTIONS**

1. Define the following terms:

   a. transfer order _doctors order requesting the patient be moved to another Unit or Rm_

   b. discharge order _doctors order for patient to leave hospital_

   c. consultation order _doctors order to consult with a 2nd physician on diagnosis + treatment of a certain patient_

2. You are planning to call a doctor's office to notify him or her of a consultation request. You must first gather five points of information to communicate to the consulting physician's office. These five points of information are:

   a. _the physicians name requesting consult_    d. _hospitals name_

   b. _the patients name_    e. _patients location_

   c. _the diagnosis_

3. The doctor may request to transfer a patient to another hospital room because:

   a. _the patient requires more intensive nursing care_

   b. _to obtain a different room accomodation_

   c. _need of an isolation room_

4. Write the meaning of each of the following abbreviations.

   a. Rx _take treatment_    e. NINP _No information No Publication_

   b. wk _week_    f. DNR _Do NOT Rescusitate_

   c. Disch _Discharge_    g. DME _Durable medical Equiptment_

   d. Appt _Appointment_

5. List six tasks the health unit coordinator may need to perform for a patient having a weekend pass.

   a. _cancel meals for length of pass_

   b. _note on census when the patient leaust returns_

   c. _cancel hospital treatments for lengthof Absence_

   d. _Arrange for medication the patient must take with pharmacy_

   e. _arrange for special equiptment the patient might need_

   f. _have patient sign a temporary absence release_

6. Two services that the home health care department may perform for the hospitalized patient are

   a. _assist in getting home nursing services from outside agencies_

   b. _assist in obtaining necessary medical equiptment_

7. To help lessen anxiety caused by hospitalization, the social service department may assist the patient by

   a. _obtain child care_

   b. _assists with money problems_

   c. _arrange transfers to nursing care facilities_

   d. _obtain tutors for hospital bound students_

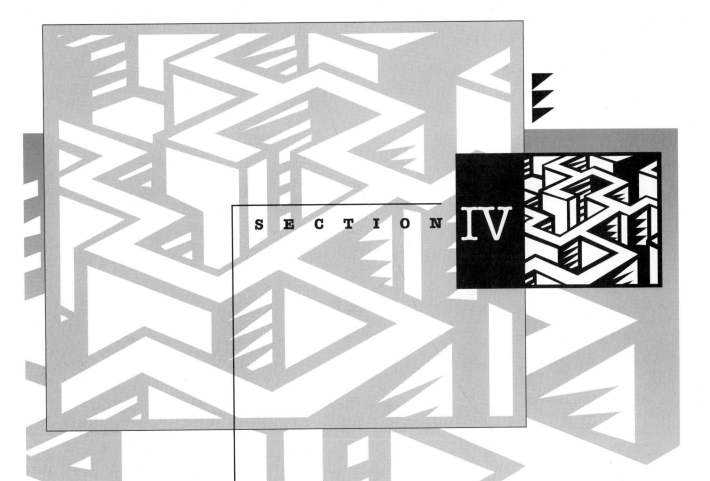

SECTION **IV**

# HEALTH UNIT COORDINATOR PROCEDURES

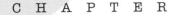

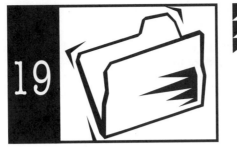

# 19

# ADMISSION, PREOPERATIVE, AND POSTOPERATIVE PROCEDURES

## VOCABULARY

**Admission Agreement** • A form signed upon the patient's admission that sets forth the general services that the hospital will provide; it may also be called the condition of admission, contract for services, or treatment consent.

**Admission Day Surgery** • Surgery in which the patient enters the hospital the day of surgery; it may be called same-day surgery or AM Admission (AMAD)

**Admission Orders** • Written directions by the doctor for the care and treatment of the patient upon entry into the hospital

**Advance Directives** • Instructions given by the patient in advance regarding his or her preference about future medical treatment

**Allergy Identification Bracelet** • A plastic band with a cardboard insert on which allergy information is printed and that the patient wears throughout the hospitalization

**Allergy Information** • Information obtained from the patient concerning his or her sensitivity to medications and/or food

**Blood Consent** • A patient's written permission to receive or refuse blood or blood products

**Census** • A list of all occupied and unoccupied hospital beds

**Direct Admission** • A patient who bypasses the admitting office and the emergency room and goes directly to a hospital bed on the nursing unit

**Elective Surgery** • Surgery which is not emergency or mandatory and can be planned at a time of convenience

**Emergency Admission** • An admission necessitated by accident or a medical emergency; such an admission is processed through the emergency department

**Facesheet** • The first page of the inpatient medical record containing personal (demographic information); usually computer generated at the time of admission

**Health Records Number** • The number assigned to the patient on admission; it is used for identification

**Identification Bracelet** • A plastic band with a cardboard insert on which the identification information is printed; it is worn throughout the patient's hospitalization

**Informed Consent** • The duty to inform a patient prior to obtaining their permission

**Information Sheet** • A form that contains information obtained from the patient or family during the registration process; it may include the patient's name, address, and telephone number; employer's name and address; insurance carrier; doctor's name; diagnosis; and so forth—may also be called the admission data form, face sheet, or summary sheet

**Living Will** • A declaration made by the patient to family, medical staff, and all concerned with the patient's care stating what is to be done in the event of a terminal illness; it directs the withholding or withdrawing of life-sustaining procedures

**Observation Patient** • A patient who is assigned to a bed on the nursing unit to receive care for a period of less than 24 hours; may also be referred to as a medical short stay or ambulatory patient

**Outpatient** • A patient receiving care in a hospital, but not admitted or staying overnight

**Postoperative Orders** • Orders written immediately after surgery; postoperative orders cancel preoperative orders

**Power of Attorney for Health Care** • The patient appoints a person (called a proxy or agent) to make health care decisions should the patient be unable to do so

**Preadmit** • The process of obtaining information and partially preparing admitting forms prior to the patient's arrival at the health care facility

**Preoperative Checklist** • A checklist used by the health unit coordinator to ensure that the patient's chart is ready for surgery

**Preoperative Nursing Checklist** • A checklist used to ensure the chart and the patient are properly prepared for surgery

**Preoperative Orders** • Orders written by the doctor before surgery to prepare the patient for the surgical procedure

**Registration** • The process of entering personal information into the hospital information system to enroll a person as a hospital patient and create a patient record; patients may be registered as inpatients, outpatients, or observation patients

**Routine Admission** • A patient admission planned in advance; it may be routine urgent or routine elective

**Surgery Consent** • A patient's written permission for an operation or invasive procedure

**Surgery Schedule** • A list of all the surgeries to be performed on a particular day; the schedule is delivered to the unit 1 day in advance

**Valuables Envelope** • A container for storing the patient's jewelry or money; it is placed in the hospital safe for safekeeping

## ABBREVIATIONS

| Abbreviation | Meaning | Example of Usage on a Doctors' Order Sheet |
| --- | --- | --- |
| Dx | diagnosis | Dx: anemia |
| H&P | history and physical | H&P by surgical resident |
| Hx | history | Resident will do Hx |
| MSSU | medical short stay unit | Admit to: MSSU |
| NKA | no known allergies | Allergies: NKA |
| postop | after surgery | Resume all medications postop |
| preop | before surgery | Dr. Smith will write preop orders |
| OBS | observation | Pt in for obs |
| OPS | outpatient surgery (ambulatory surgery) | Send pt to OPS |

## ADMISSION OF THE PATIENT

As a health unit coordinator, your role in the admission procedure is a very important one. You are the first person the new patient encounters on the nursing unit, which will be his or her "home" for several days or longer. You have an opportunity at this time to demonstrate the caring nature of the hospital by greeting the patient warmly and making him or her feel welcome.

Your ability to perform tasks in an efficient manner enables the health care team to provide, as soon as possible, the care and treatment ordered for the patient.

### Types of Admissions

A person may become a hospital patient in a variety of ways. The way in which a person enters the hospital determines the admission type. There are three main types of admissions: entry, patient, and service.

## Entry Type

**Routine Admissions.** Routine admissions are planned in advance. Patients enter the hospital through the admitting department or front door. Routine admissions can further be classified as urgent, scheduled, or elective. When a physician sees a patient in the office and decides that person should be admitted to the hospital, the physician will call the hospital and arrange a **routine urgent** admission. The admission is routine because the hospital receives some advance notice, but it is urgent because the patient will be admitted that day as soon as a hospital bed becomes available. When a physician sees a patient and determines a procedure or surgery is necessary, the physician will call the hospital and arrange a **routine scheduled** or **routine elective** admission. The admission is routine because it is planned in advance, but is scheduled in accordance with the physician's and patient's preference.

**Emergency Admissions.** Emergency admissions are unplanned and are the result of an accident or sudden illness. Patients enter the hospital through the emergency department. These patients are processed through the emergency department and are referred to as an emergency admissions. An emergency department record (Fig. 19–1) is prepared by the emergency department personnel.

Should the patient's condition warrant that he or she remain in the hospital, the patient will be admitted to a nursing unit. The emergency department record is sent to the nursing unit with the patient and placed in the patient's medical record. The health unit coordinator reviews this record to see if all requested tests have been completed. For example, the emergency room physician may have ordered a urinalysis, but the patient may not have voided yet. If the tests have not been completed, the health unit coordinator processes those that remain to be done.

**Direct Admissions.** Direct admissions bypass the admitting office and the emergency room and go directly to the nursing unit or patient care area. Direct admissions may be routine or emergency. Examples of direct admissions would be a pregnant woman going directly to labor and delivery or a patient being transported by ambulance or helicopter from another health care facility such as an extended care facility.

> **HIGHLIGHT**
> The three entry types of admissions are routine, emergency, and direct.

## Patient Type

Admission types are categorized according to a patient's type of entry to the hospital. Patient types may also be categorized. Patient type may be categorized according to purpose and length of hospitalization. The three patient types are **inpatient**, **observation patient**, and **outpatient**.

**Inpatient.** An **inpatient** is a patient who has been admitted to the hospital and assigned to a bed on the nursing unit. A health unit coordinator will prepare a chart and process orders for the patient.

**Observation Patient.** An **observation patient** is a patient who is assigned to a bed on a nursing unit to receive care for a period of less than 24 hours. An observation patient may also be referred to as a medical short-stay or ambulatory patient. Some hospitals may have a specific unit such as a **medical short stay unit (MSSU)** or **ambulatory care unit** to provide short-term care. If the patient requires further hospital care beyond 24 hours, the physician must write an order for hospital admission. The criteria for observation patients varies from facility to facility. A health unit coordinator will prepare a chart and process orders for the observation patient.

**Outpatient.** An **outpatient** is a patient receiving care in a hospital, but not admitted or staying overnight. An outpatient is usually scheduled to receive treatments, therapies, or tests. The department providing care for the outpatient will process the outpatient's orders. Assembly of a chart is not required.

## Service Type

Service type refers to the type of nursing unit (See Chapter 2, "Hospital Nursing Units").

# Admission Arrangement

In all types of admissions, the physician authorizes or arranges the admission. The attending physician, the physician's staff, or the staff of a health maintenance organization arranges for the admission of patients. The physician gives the admitting diagnosis or medical reason for admission.

> **HIGHLIGHT**
> Whatever the patient's route to the hospital may be, it is the physician who authorizes the admission.

# Bed Assignment

Most hospitals are open for admissions 24 hours a day. The admitting department or registration staff performs many tasks in relation to the admission of the patient to the hospital. Most hospitals will have a computerized **census** in the hospital information system that provides an accurate, up-to-date list of occupied and unoccupied hospital beds. For **routine urgent, emergency**, and **direct admissions**, bed assignments will be made when the patient arrives at the hospital and is ready for a room. For **routine scheduled** or **routine elective** admissions a list of expected patients is sent to each nursing unit. The bed as-

**EMERGENCY ROOM**

| MEDICAL RECORD NO. | | MED SERVICE | FINANCIAL CL | DATE | | SOC. SEC. NO./MEDICARE NO. | |
|---|---|---|---|---|---|---|---|
| 567-435 | | Orth | | 5/23/XX | | 527-48-XXXX | |

PATIENT NAME  LAST Lowrey  FIRST Holly  MIDDLE Elinor   HOSPITALIZATION INSURANCE - 1 Sunstate   POLICY/GROUP NO 100-0000

PATIENT'S PERMANENT ADDRESS 10001 North Mountain, CITY Sky, STATE AZ ZIP 85000   TEL 942-XXXX  ADDRESS 2222 N. Tower Pl. Sky, AZ

PATIENT'S TEMPORARY ADDRESS   CITY   STATE   ZIP   TEL   HOSPITALIZATION INSURANCE 2   POLICY/GROUP NO

BIRTHDATE 5/3/XX   AGE 22   HAS PATIENT EVER BEEN TREATED IN THIS HOSPITAL ☐ INPATIENT ☐ OUTPATIENT   WHEN _____ UNDER WHAT NAME _____   ADDRESS

EFFECTIVE DATE - 1 1/06/XX   EFFECTIVE DATE - 2

SEX ☐ MALE ☒ FEMALE   MARITAL STATUS ☐ SINGLE ☒ MARRIED ☐ SEPARATED ☐ DIVORCED ☐ WIDOWED   RACE ☐ WHITE ☒ BLACK ☐ INDIAN ☐ ORIENTAL ☐ OTHER   RELIGION ☐ CATHOLIC ☐ JEWISH ☐ PROTESTANT ☒ OTHER   INDUSTRIAL - PATIENT'S EMPLOYER ☐ YES ☒ NO

RESPONSIBLE PARTY NAME SELF   RELATIONSHIP   TEL   ADDRESS   TEL

ADDRESS STREET P.O. BOX APT NO CITY   STATE   ZIP   RELATIVE NOTIFIED

SPOUSE OR NEAREST RELATIVE (NEXT OF KIN) Iris Lowrey   RELATIONSHIP Mother   TEL 943-XXXX   TIME 1800   BY WHOM M. Loor

ADDRESS STREET P.O. BOX APT NO CITY 211 E. Sun Dr. Sky, AZ   STATE   ZIP 85000   POLICE NOTIFIED   TIME 1730   BY WHOM M. Loor

E R PHYSICIAN Thomas V. Riggs   ATTENDING PHYSICIAN B. Urself

EVENTS AND CARE GIVEN PRIOR TO ARRIVAL

CHIEF COMPLAINT *Pt. states she was involved in an auto accident 10am to-day - no loss of consciousness. Complaint of pain Right shoulder - right knee - 3 inch lac. to left cheek area - abrasion Ⓡ hand*

VITAL SIGNS TEMP 98⁴ ORAL/RECTAL P 88 R 24 BP 130/80

ALLERGIES Codeine

| | ADMIT | EXAM | CALLED | CALLED | CALLED | CONTACTED | ARRIVED | | LAB | X-RAY | DISCHG | | HOME | ADMIT TO ROOM |
|---|---|---|---|---|---|---|---|---|---|---|---|---|---|---|
| INITIAL | | | | | | | | CALLED | | 5³⁰p | | DR OFF | | |
| TIME | 5pm | | | | | | | SPEC TAKEN | | | | OTHER | | |
| PHYSICIANS NAME | B. Urself | | 5⁴⁵p | 5⁵⁵p | | 6¹⁰p | 7pm | RESULTS OBY | | | | WORK | | |

LAST TETANUS July 1971

BROUGHT IN BY (NAME OF PERSON OR AMBULANCE) Associated ambulance   MEDICAL EXAMINER   DISPOSITION OF VALUABLES to husband   NURSES SIGNATURE Mable Jones RN

| ORDERS | HISTORY: PHYSICAL FINDINGS & TREATMENT |
|---|---|
| | S. ↓ ROM ✓R SHOULDER |
| 1. CERVICAL - X-TABLE 1ST | 2° TO PAIN |
| 2. SKULL | Obj 1. VS - STABLE |
| 3 R SHOULDER | 2. HEAD Ⓛ PERLA, EOM's, disc NORMAL |
| R KNEE | ② EAR'S - NO BLOOD |
| R HAND | ③ Ū CRANIAL NERVE SENSATION L=R |
| 4. 1% LIDOCAINE | 4. 3" lac FACE |
| 4.0. - NYLON WHITE | 3. NECK - SUPPLE |
| 6-0 NYLON - BLACK | 4 CHEST - GOOD EXPANSION |
| abrasion, laceration | LUNGS CLEAR P |
| cleansed c̄ betadine soln | 5. ABD - GOOD BS, NO HS MEGLY, NO |
| dressed c̄ neosporin, dry, | TENDERNESS, REBND OR REFERRED |
| dressing. | PAIN. |
| | 6 EXT - R SHOULDER - ECHYMOSIS, ↓ROM |
| | · R KNEE - CONTUSION + ABRASION |
| | R - HAND - ABRASION |
| | 7 XRAYS - SKULL, CERVICAL, R SHOULDER - NEG |
| | Dx A/A, LACERATION ABRASION + CONTUSION |
| | PLAN / HEAD SHEET STITCHES OUT - 4 DAYS |
| | ICE ↓ |

FINAL DIAGNOSIS   CODE

FINAL DISPOSITION - DESCRIBE

SIGNATURE OF E R PHYSICIAN Thomas V. Riggs MD   SIGNATURE OF ATTENDING PHYSICIAN

00-2912 1-77

**MEDICAL RECORDS**

**F I G U R E  19–1** • Emergency department record.

signment may be determined at the beginning of the shift of the patient's expected arrival.

The admitting diagnosis usually determines the type of nursing unit that is suitable and the nursing staff usually determines the specific bed. In many hospitals, bed assignment is decided by the staff on the nursing unit. The nursing personnel is familiar with staffing and roommate issues and can best decide which bed is appropriate for the new patient. After receiving patient information such as name, diagnosis, and sex, the HUC or nurse may assign the bed number.

## Escort to the Nursing Unit

Once the bed assignment has been made, the patient will be escorted to the assigned unit by a volunteer, a member of the hospital transportation department, or admitting personnel. If the patient has already been registered, the admitting papers are delivered to the receiving unit.

## Patient Registration

**Registration** is the process of entering personal information into the hospital information system to enroll a person as a hospital patient and create a patient record. The patient must be registered before any orders can be processed for the patient. The patient registration responsibilities may be performed by an admitting clerk, admission representative, or patient representative in the admitting department. A trend has developed for the HUC to register the patient on the nursing unit.

> **HIGHLIGHT**
>
> Performing the patient registration tasks is becoming the responsibility of the health unit coordinator in many health care facilities.

## Patient Registration Tasks

Patient registration tasks include:

- Interview patient or family to obtain personal information.
- Prepare forms (admission agreement and facesheet) and obtain signatures. Include any test results or prewritten orders or consents.
- Prepare patient's identification bracelet.
- Prepare patient's imprinter card or identification labels.
- Secure patient valuables.
- Supply and explain required information.

> **HIGHLIGHT**
>
> The patient registration tasks must be completed before orders can be processed for the patient.

## Interview

When admissions are arranged in advance, such as for planned or elective surgery, preadmission information may be obtained by mail or by phone by the registration staff. This information, such as the patient's name, address, and telephone number; employer's name and address; insurance carrier; doctor's name, and diagnosis, is placed on a record called the **information sheet** (Fig. 19–2). If the patient information was not obtained previously, it is done at the time of admission.

### INTERVIEW TECHNIQUES

When interviewing a patient to obtain personal information, it is imperative to utilize the interpersonal skills discussed in Chapter 5. Being admitted to the health care facility is a stressful situation and many patients will also be experiencing physical discomfort. The following guidelines should be observed when interviewing patients.

- Protect confidentiality.
  - Ensure privacy when asking for personal information.
- Be proficient and professional.
  - Do not ask repetitive questions.
  - Asking if the patient was previously hospitalized or obtaining the patient's insurance card can hasten the registration process.
  - Treat each patient as an individual.
- Listen carefully.
- Project a friendly, courteous attitude.

## Forms

The **admission agreement** or **treatment consent** lists the general services that the hospital will provide. It is an agreement between the patient and the hospital (Fig. 19–3). This consent may specify financial responsibility also. The patient is to sign the form upon admission. Patients who are unable to sign the form may have a representative sign for them. A copy of the admission agreement/treatment consent is given to the patient after it is signed, and another copy will become part of the patient's medical record.

The **facesheet** or **summary sheet** is the form that is generated after the hospital information from the information sheet is entered into the hospital information system. It is usually filed as the first page of the patient's medical record.

Routine admissions may have had tests performed prior to their admission. Test results are forwarded to the hospital and sent to the nursing unit with the other chart forms. Physicians may write orders or obtain consents in advance. Physician orders and consents are also for-

| PATIENT HOSP.NO.(M.R.#) | INFO STATUS | | | | | ACCOUNT NO. (BUS. OFF.) |
|---|---|---|---|---|---|---|
| 1  987-654 | | | | | | 123-456 |

| PATIENT NAME   LAST | FIRST | MIDDLE | ADM. DATE MO./DAY/YR. | ADM. TIME | HOW BROUGHT TO HOSPITAL |
|---|---|---|---|---|---|
| 2  Andrews | Iver | S. | 8/7/XX | 1345 | Amb. |

| PATIENT'S CURRENT ADDRESS   STREET, P.O. BOX, APT. NO. | CITY | STATE | ZIP CODE | TELEPHONE NO. |
|---|---|---|---|---|
| 3  701 East Danish Lane | Carpenterville, AZ | | 85013 | 246-XXXX |

| PATIENT'S PERMANENT ADDRESS   STREET, P.O. BOX, APT. NO. | CITY | STATE | ZIP CODE | TELEPHONE NO. |
|---|---|---|---|---|
| 4  Same | | | | |

| SEX  1. MALE  2. FEMALE | MARITAL STATUS  1. SINGLE  2. MARRIED  3. SEPARATED  4. DIVORCED  5. WIDOWED | RACE  1. WHITE  2. BLACK  3. INDIAN  4. ORIENTAL  5. OTHER | RELIGION  1. CATHOLIC  2. JEWISH  3. PROTESTANT  4. OTHER  5. LDS | AREA OF RESIDENCE |
|---|---|---|---|---|
| 5  [1] | [5] | [1] | [3] | |

| BIRTHDATE | AGE | PLACE OF BIRTH | MAIDEN NAME | SOC. SEC. NO./MEDICARE NO. |
|---|---|---|---|---|
| 6  10/6/XX | 69 | N.J. | | 151-18-XXXX |

| PATIENT'S OCCUPATION | UNION & LOCAL NO. | PATIENT'S EMPLOYER | ADDRESS | TELEPHONE NO. |
|---|---|---|---|---|
| 7  Retired | | | | |

| PREVIOUSLY TREATED HERE? | NAME USED | PREV. ADM. DATE MO. DA. YR. | PREV. ADMISSION  1. INPATIENT  2. OUTPATIENT | IF NEWBORN, MOTHER'S HOSP. NO. |
|---|---|---|---|---|
| 8  [X] YES  [ ] NO | Same | 2/3/XX | [1] | |

| UNIT | ROOM NO. | ACCOM. CODES  1. PRI  2. SEMI  3. NURSERY  4. PREMIE  5. ICU  6. RCU  7. CCU  8. VIP | ROOM RATE | PAY STATUS | CLASS OF ADMISSION  1. EMERGENCY  2. ELECTIVE  3. URGENT  4. OTHER |
|---|---|---|---|---|---|
| 9  A5 | | [2] | | | [3] |

10  ADMITTING DIAGNOSIS

Cerebrovascular accident

| PHYSICIAN NAME | PHYSICIAN NO. | ADM. SERVICE | INFORMATION OBTAINED FROM: |
|---|---|---|---|
| 11  I.M. Human | 432 | Med. | daughter |

| SPOUSE OR NEAREST RELATIVE (NEXT OF KIN) | RELATIONSHIP | ADDRESS | TELEPHONE NO. |
|---|---|---|---|
| 12  Kay Ellis | daugh | 301 West Restful Dr. Phoenix | 258-XXXX |

| SECOND RELATIVE OR FRIEND | RELATIONSHIP | ADDRESS | TELEPHONE NO. |
|---|---|---|---|
| 13  Marie Darrow | sister | 12 Center St. Danstown, CA | 837-XXXX |

| RESPONSIBLE PARTY NAME | RELATIONSHIP | SOC. SEC. NO. |
|---|---|---|
| 14  Self | | |

| RESP. PARTY ADDRESS   STREET   P.O. BOX   APT. NO. | CITY | STATE | ZIP CODE | TELEPHONE NO. |
|---|---|---|---|---|
| 15 | | | | |

| RESP. PARTY OCCUPATION | NO. YRS. IN THIS EMPLOY | RESP. PARTY EMPLOYER | ADDRESS | TELEPHONE NO. |
|---|---|---|---|---|
| 16 | | | | |

| LENGTH OF TIME IN ARIZ. | 1. OWN HOME  2. RENT HOME | TYPE OF HOME | BANK NAME & BRANCH | 1. SAVINGS  2. CHECKING |
|---|---|---|---|---|
| 17  10 yrs. | [1] | Single | Desert National - Camelhead | [1] |

| CREDIT REFERENCES  1. NAME | ADDRESS | TELEPHONE NO. |
|---|---|---|
| 18  Deep River S&L | 9832 N. LasVegas Pl.   Phoenix | 943-XXXX |
| 19  2. NAME  Yucca Federal | ADDRESS  1903 W. Bottletree Ave. Phoenix | 246-XXXX |

| INDUSTRIAL INJURY  DATE:  MO. DA. YR. | CLAIM NO. | EMPLOYER'S NAME AND ADDRESS AT TIME OF INJURY |
|---|---|---|
| 20 | | |

| BLUE CROSS  NAME OF PLAN | GROUP NO. | IDENTIFICATION | EFFECTIVE DATE MO. DA. YR. | CITY | STATE |
|---|---|---|---|---|---|
| 21 | | | | | |

| CHAMPUS DATA  PATIENT'S ID NO. | CARD EFFECTIVE MO. DA. YR. | CARD EXPIRES ON MO. DA. YR. | PATIENT OR SPONSORS BRANCH OF SERVICE | SERVICE CARD NO. |
|---|---|---|---|---|
| 22 | | | | |

| SPONSORS NAME | RANK-SERVICE NO. | DUTY STATION |
|---|---|---|
| 23 | | |

| OTHER INSURANCE (INC. BLOOD BANK & BLUE SHIELD)  INS. CO. NO. | COMPANY NAME | POLICY HOLDER NAME | POLICY NO. | DATE ISSUED MO. DA. YR. | CITY | STATE |
|---|---|---|---|---|---|---|
| 24  1000 | Desert State | Iver Andrews | A657483 | 2/17/XX | | AZ |
| 25  INS. CO. NO. | COMPANY NAME | POLICY HOLDER NAME | POLICY NO. | DATE ISSUED MO. DA. YR. | CITY | STATE |

| NAME OF HEALTH FACILITY DISCHARGED FROM WITHIN LAST 60 DAYS | ADDRESS |
|---|---|
| 26  None | |

| OTHER INFO.  V. A. [ ] | COORDINATION OF BENEFITS [ ] | INTERVIEWED BY  G. Talker | TYPED BY  W.K.S. |
|---|---|---|---|
| 27 | | | |

28  REMARKS:

FIGURE 19–2 • Information sheet.

warded to the hospital and sent to the nursing unit upon admission.

At the time of admission each patient is assigned a **health records number**. This number identifies the patient and all chart forms. It also serves to identify all charges for equipment, supplies, and procedures. The health re-cords number is used by the business office for billing purposes. Patients who have had previous hospitalizations in the same hospital may be assigned their previous health records number. Some hospitals assign the patient a new number for each hospitalization and give all the old records the updated number.

**CONSENT FOR TREATMENT and**
**AUTHORIZATION TO RELEASE INFORMATION**

1. I, the undersigned, being a patient in _____ Hospital, do hereby consent to the administration and performance of such medical treatment, diagnostic and patient care procedures, including necessary patient safety measures that may be deemed advisable during the course of my hospitalization by my attending physician or his/her designee(s).

2. I am aware that the practice of medicine is not an exact science and I acknowledge that no guarantees have been made to me as to the results of treatments or procedures in this hospital.

3. I understand that the Hospital is a teaching institution, providing clinical education opportunities for medical, nursing, and allied health care professionals in training. These training programs are provided by the Hospital solely and/or in cooperation with other institutions. I understand that the treatment and care provided me at _____ Hospital may involve one or more healthcare professionals in training (from the Hospital's clinical educational programs) functioning under the direct supervision of my physician(s) and/or duly authorized designee(s) or the professional nurses and therapists assigned to my care.

4. I hereby authorize _____ Hospital to furnish my insurance company(ies) and authorized external review agency(ies) with such pertinent information, relative to my hospitalization or treatment deemed necessary to process insurance claims and conduct utilization review procedures of third party payor.

5. I hereby authorize _____ Hospital to furnish my medical records covering this hospitalization (surgery or treatment) to educational or scientific institutions, physicians, physician representatives or authorized healthcare professionals in training, to internal hospital quality improvement, risk/claims management, hospital counsel/insurer when it is judged that medical research, quality improvement, education of science will be benefited.

6. Any tissues or parts surgically removed may be disposed of by the hospital in accordance with accustomed practice.

7. I consent to the taking and use of clinical photographs in the course of this operation or procedure for the purpose of advancing medical education. Use of information and pictures is approved provided my identity is disguised.

8. If I am a Medicare beneficiary, I acknowledge that I have received a copy of **An Important Message From Medicare** in accordance with federal regulations. PPS _____ PPS Exempt _____

9. I acknowledge receipt of the _____ brochures entitled, **Resuscitation, Making the Choice and Advance Directives, Your Right to Choose**, as well as a copy of the IDPH publication entitled: **Statement of Illinois Law on Advance Directives.**

10. Do you have a **Living Will?** ____ Yes ____ No

11. Do you have a **Durable Power of Attorney for Health Care with Agent named?** ____ Yes ____ No

    **Name of Agent** _____

    **Address** _____ **Phone #** _____

    **Signed** _____

    **Witnessed** _____ **Relationship** _____
    (If signed by other than patient, state reason)

    _____ 19 ___ AM
    (Date/Time)                ___ PM

    **Consent For Treatment and Authorization to Release Information**

    **White—Medical Record    Yellow—Patient**

F I G U R E  19–3 • Admission agreement/treatment consent. (From Rockford Memorial Hospital, Rockford, IL, with permission.)

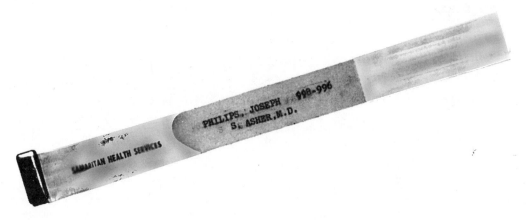

F I G U R E  19–4 • ID bracelet.

### Identification Bracelet

An **identification bracelet** or **band** (Fig. 19–4) is prepared by the registration staff upon admission of the patient to the hospital. The bracelet is a plastic band with a thin cardboard insert on which identification is printed. The identifying information consists of: (1) the patient's name, (2) the attending physician's name, and (3) the health records number. The bracelet is worn throughout the patient's hospitalization. All personnel performing services for the patient must read the identification bracelet to ensure correct patient identification.

### Imprinter Card or Labels

The **imprinter card** is a plastic charge card with the patient name, physician name, health records number, and room number (see Chapter 8). Some hospitals may generate self-adhesive labels in place of the imprinter card. The imprinter card or labels are used to identify forms, requisitions, specimens, etc. The imprinter card and labels are prepared by the registration staff.

---

**H I G H L I G H T**

The facesheet, ID bracelet, and imprinter card are prepared upon admission.

---

### Valuables

Patients who have large amounts of money or expensive jewelry with them at the time of admission are requested to place these items in the hospital safe. The items are placed in a numbered valuables envelope (Fig. 19–5) and the patient is given a duplicate numbered claim check. This number may also be written on the patient's chart. This serves as a reminder that there are valuables in the hospital safe. A clothing and valuables form may also be prepared, signed, and witnessed (Fig. 19–6).

### Information

The registration staff will explain the registration process and hospital rules for the patient. Due to various state laws, the hospital may be required to inform the patient of specific information. Upon admission the patient may be supplied with written information regarding patient rights, Medicare and Medicaid, anesthesia, resuscitation, and advance directives (Fig. 19–3).

## Advance Directives

There is an increasing awareness in the general public concerning one's rights to self-determination in the issues of death and disability. Because of this awareness more patients upon admission are requesting information about advance directives.

**Advance directives** are instructions given by the patient in advance regarding his or her preferences about future medical treatment.

The patient has several options for advance directives:

1. To give instructions by using
   a. the living will declaration form (Fig. 19–8) or
   b. writing in the patient's own words patient's personal beliefs and preferences.
2. To appoint an agent (proxy) to make health care decisions using the power of attorney for health care, should the patient become incapable of making these decisions (19–8).
3. To appoint an agent (proxy) using the power of attorney for health care *and* give some instructions, combining a part of (1) with (2).

An advance directive or living will **ONLY** become effective when the patient no longer can make decisions for himself or herself. The patient may change or destroy any directive or living will at any time.

A **living will** is a declaration made by the patient to family, medical staff, and all concerned with the patient's

## PATIENT'S VALUABLE ENVELOPE

### 01903
ENVELOPE NUMBER

IMPRINT AREA OR PATIENT'S NAME AND HOSPITAL NO

HOSPITAL TAKES ALL POSSIBLE PRECAUTIONS TO SAFEGUARD YOUR PROPERTY BUT DISCLAIMS RESPONSIBILITY FOR VALUABLES SURRENDERED TO WRONGFUL HOLDER OF IDENTIFICATION SLIP AND WILL NOT BE RESPONSIBLE FOR ANY CLAIM FOR LOSS

| CONTENTS OF ENVELOPE | ARTICLES RETAINED BY |
| DEPOSITED WITH HOSPITAL | PATIENT OR RESPONSIBLE PARTY |

CONTENTS OF ENVELOPE — DEPOSITED WITH HOSPITAL

[X] CASH  $100 ___  $20 5  $5 1  LOOSE CHANGE
       $50 ___  $10 ___  $1 2  .

[ ] CHECKS (LIST SEPARATELY) _____

[X] CREDIT CARDS (LIST SEPARATELY) VISA _____

[ ] WATCH _____

[ ] RINGS _____

[X] WALLET _____

[ ] OTHER EXPLAIN _____

[ ] OTHER EXPLAIN _____

ARTICLES RETAINED BY — PATIENT OR RESPONSIBLE PARTY

[X] CASH  $3.00

[ ] WATCH _____

[ ] RINGS _____

[ ] WALLET _____

[ ] RAZOR _____

[X] DENTURES PARTIAL  LOWER

[X] GLASSES _____

[ ] OTHER EXPLAIN _____

00-1346 REV 5-77

I HAVE CHECKED THE ABOVE AND ACKNOWLEDGE THE LISTS TO BE CORRECT I, THE PATIENT, OR RESPONSIBLE PARTY ASSUME FULL RESPONSIBILITY FOR THOSE ITEMS RETAINED IN MY POSSESSION DURING MY HOSPITALIZATION OR BROUGHT TO PATIENT AFTER SIGNATURES HAVE BEEN OBTAINED

| TIME 1400 | DATE 11/2/xx | PATIENT'S SIGNATURE OR RESPONSIBLE PARTY X Wendy Leigh | WITNESSED BY Kay Iver, R.N. |
| VALUABLE ENVELOPE CHART COPY RECEIVED BY Kay Iver, R.N. | | | HOSPITAL EMPLOYEE |
| CASHIER'S USE ▶ | DATE 11/2/XX | RECEIVED AND CERTIFIED Mark Palmer | |
| EMERGENCY ROOM USE ▶ | DATE | PROPERTY COLLECTED BY | WITNESSED BY |

### WITHDRAWALS

| DATE | DESCRIPTION | CASHIER INITIALS | PATIENT SIGNATURE |
| --- | --- | --- | --- |
|  |  |  |  |
|  |  |  |  |

NOT RESPONSIBLE FOR ARTICLES AFTER 30 DAYS FROM DISCHARGE

### LOST RECEIPT DOCUMENTATION
CLAIMANT MUST PROVIDE SOME INDEPENDENT EVIDENCE OF HIS IDENTITY FOR RELEASE OF THE ENVELOPE CONTENTS PLEASE DESCRIBE THIS IDENTIFICATION

FIGURE 19–5 • Valuables envelope.

care stating what is to be done in the event of a terminal illness. It directs the withholding or withdrawing of life-sustaining procedures. The patient may also define what she or he means by *meaningful quality of life*.

**Power of attorney for health care** allows the patient to appoint another person or persons (called a proxy or agent) to make health care decisions for the patient should the patient become incapable of making decisions. The proxy (agent) has a duty to act consistently with the patient's wishes. If the proxy does not know the patient's wishes, the proxy has the duty to act in the patient's best interests.

Advance directives vary according to state regulations.

> **TO THE STUDENT**
>
> To practice preparing the newly admitted patient's chart and Kardex forms, complete **Activity 19–1** in the Skills Practice Manual.

**PATIENT VALUABLES**

**VALUABLES**

| QUANTITY | DESCRIPTION |
|---|---|
| | |
| | |
| | |
| | |
| | |
| | |
| | |

☐ I have been informed that a safe is available in the Patient Accounts Department for the safekeeping of my valuables.

☐ I understand that the Hospital will assume responsibility for eyeglasses, bridgework, dentures and clothing (up to $50) lost or damaged due to negligence of Hospital personnel.

☐ I agree to assume full responsibility for any valuables not turned over to the Hospital for safekeeping in the Hospital safe by myself or my personal representative. I will hold the Hospital responsible for only those valuables listed above.

Signed: _____  Date _____ 19 _____
            (Patient or Representative)

Witnessed by: _____
                    (Admission Representative)

Received by: _____  Deposit Envelope No. _____
                 (Cashier or Nursing Office Representative)

Verified by: _ _____
                 (Admissions Representative or Other Employee)

Safe Deposit Envelope No. _____ Date of Deposit _____ 19 _____

Comments: _____

_____

Patient Valuables

F I G U R E  19-6 • Clothing and valuables list. (From Rockford Memorial Hospital, Rockford, IL, with permission.)

## Admission Notes

967 896
MART TED
DR Y STOCKS
M 40 MED INS

| Date: 10/22/XX | Time of arrival: 1300 | Admitted to: 711/1 |
|---|---|---|

From: *home*          How arrived: *car*

Accompanied by: *Mother*          Relationship:

Orientation to physical environment: *yes*

Height: *5'7"*     Weight: *140#*     T. *37*   P. *86*   R. *20*   B/P *140/80*

Valuables brought to floor: *None*          Disposition:

Allergies and Reaction: *all mycins*

Admitted by:

ADMISSION ASSESSMENT: *S. Mirth, N.A.*

Reason for admission: *Broken Left radius*   Previous adm's: *None*

MEDS — Medications used at home and why:
*none*

Anticoagulant Therapy *No* When & Why          Cortisone Therapy _____ When & Why

Disposition: Sent home _____ Retained _____ If retained - identify Rx No. and am't in Nurses Notes

EENT/SENSORY — Patient's vision, hearing, prosthesis (glasses, contacts, hearing aids).
*Pt. denies wearing glasses or hearing aid*

NEUROLOGICAL — Level of consciousness, alertness and orientation, if indicated.
*Alert and oriented to person, place and time. Speech clear. Answers questions appropriately.*

CARDIOVASCULAR — B/P, pulse (rate, quality) color, A/R and peripheral pulses as indicated.
*No Hx of cardiovascular problems. Skin warm and dry. Pt. able to wiggle L fingers. C/o numbness in L thumb*

RESPIRATORY — Rate, quality, breath sounds as indicated. Sputum production, cough, dyspnea —
influence of activity, smoking *Smokes pack of cigarettes a week. Denies constant cough or SOB. Breath sounds clear bilaterally. No Hx of asthma or bronchitis.*

00-6002  Rev. 3-80

**ADMISSION NOTES**

FIGURE 19-7 • Admission nurse's notes.

## ADMISSION PROCEDURE

| Task | Notes |
| --- | --- |
| Greet the patient upon arrival at the nurse's station. | Introduce yourself and give your status. *Example*: "I'm Ted Mart, the health unit coordinator for this unit." |
| Inform the patient that you will notify the nurse of his or her arrival. | Notify the nurse caring for the patient of the patient's arrival. |
| Record the patient's admission in the unit admission, discharge, and transfer book and/or the census sheet. | In hospitals with computers, the patient's information is placed on the unit census screen. |
| Check the patient's signature on the admission agreement form. | Compare the spelling of the patient's name on the information sheet and the imprinter card with the signature on the admission agreement form. Also check to see that the physician's name is correct. |
| Complete the procedure for the preparation of the chart.<br>　a. Imprint all the chart forms.<br>　b. Fill in all the needed headings.<br>　c. Place all the forms in the chart behind the proper dividers. | |
| Label the outside of the chart. | Identify the chart with the patient's and the doctor's names and the health records number. |
| Prepare any other labels or identification cards used by your facility. | |
| Place the imprinter card in the correct place in the imprinter card holder. | |
| Fill in all the necessary information on the patient's Kardex forms or on the computer Kardex. Place the Kardex forms in the proper place in the Kardex folder. | The information is obtained from the information sheet prepared by the admitting department. |
| Record the data from the admission nurse's notes (Fig. 19–7) on the graphic sheet. | |
| Place the allergy information in all the designated areas or write NKA. | Allergy information (the information obtained from the patient about any sensitivity to medication, food, or other substance) is usually placed on the front of the patient's chart, Kardex form, and medication record. The allergy information is obtained from the admission nurse's notes. Writing NKA indicates to the staff that the allergy information has been checked. |
| Notify the attending physician and/or hospital resident of the patient's admission, and obtain orders. | |
| Add the patient's name to the required unit forms. | |
| Transcribe the admission orders according to your hospital's policy. | For example, diet sheet, TPR sheet, unit assignment sheet. |

## ADMISSION ORDERS

### Introduction

**Admission orders** are written directions by the doctor for the care and treatment of the patient upon entry into the hospital. Most orders are written on the unit or received by telephone immediately after the patient's arrival. However, there are times when the admission orders arrive before the patient. Physicians who use typewritten order sets may leave them on the nursing unit when they make morning rounds. Some physicians may also write admission orders before the arrival of the patient on the nursing unit. The health unit coordinator must be sure these orders are identified. The patient's name should be written on the order sheet in pen or pencil. The orders are stamped later when the imprinter card arrives on the nursing unit.

### Admission Order Components

The common components of admission orders are:

■ The admitting diagnosis.
■ Diet.
■ Activity.
■ Diagnostic orders.
■ Medications. Usually medications are needed for the patient's disease condition, for sleeping, and/or for pain.
■ Treatment orders.
■ Request for old records.
■ Patient care category or code status. The patient care category or code status may be indicated on the patient's admission orders. The patient care category or code status refers to the patient's wishes regarding resuscitation. Code status may be written as full code, modified support, or do not resuscitate.

# LIVING WILL DECLARATION

To my family, doctors, and all those concerned with my care:

I, _____, being of sound mind, make this statement as a directive to be followed if for any reason I become unable to participate in decisions regarding my medical care.

I direct that life-sustaining procedures should be withheld or withdrawn if I have an illness, disease or injury, or experience extreme mental deterioration, such that there is no reasonable expectation of recovering or regaining a meaningful quality of life. For me, life would not have a meaningful quality when _____

_____

I have circled and initialed those procedures that may be withheld or withdrawn. Other procedures may also be withheld or withdrawn except any listed under personal instructions.

    1. Surgery          2. Antibiotics          3. Dialysis

    4. Respiratory       5. Artificially Administered    6. Cardiac
       Support            Feeding and Fluids       Resuscitation

I further direct that treatment be limited to comfort measures only, even if they shorten my life. Other personal instructions:

These directions express my legal right to refuse treatment. Therefore, I expect my family, doctors, and all those concerned with my care to regard themselves as legally and morally bound to act in accordance with my wishes, and in so doing, to be free from any liability for having followed my directions.

Signed _____Date_____

Witness _____Witness _____

# PROXY DESIGNATION CLAUSE

*If you wish, you may use this section to designate someone to make treatment decisions if you are unable to do so. Your Living Will Declaration will be in effect even if you have not designated a proxy.*

I authorize the following person to implement my Living Will Declaration by accepting, refusing and/or making decisions about treatment and hospitalization:

Name_____
Address_____

If the person I have named above is unable to act on my behalf, I authorize the following person to do so:
Name_____
Address_____

I have discussed my wishes with these persons and trust their judgment on my behalf.

Signed _____Date_____

Witness _____Witness _____

F I G U R E  19–8 • Form for living will declaration and power of attorney for health care.

## PHYSICIAN'S ORDER SHEET

| Date | Time | Orders |
|------|------|--------|
| 5-4-00 | 1315 | Diagnosis: acute pulmonary edema |
| | | -P.T. to help c̄ ambulation at least BID |
| | | -1800 cal ADA NAS diet |
| | | -Chest X-ray today and in am |
| | | -EKG today and in am |
| | | -CBC, lytes, ABGs, cardiac isoenzymes stat |
| | | -chem 12, TSH in am |
| | | -Schedule lung scan |
| | | -Vasotec 15 mg po BID |
| | | -Bumex 2 mg po now and qd |
| | | -Cordarone 400 mg po qd |
| | | -Dalmane 30 mg po hs prn sleep |
| | | -VS q 2h for 8h, then q 4h |
| | | -Daily wts |
| | | -I/O |
| | | -O$_2$ at 2l/nc |
| | | -Old record to unit |
| | | -Pt is a full code status |

FIGURE 19–9 • Admission orders.

Figure 19–9 is an example of a set of admission orders.

TO THE STUDENT

To practice transcribing a set of admission orders for a medical patient, complete **Activity 19–2** in the Skills Practice Manual.

## THE SURGERY PATIENT

### Information

The procedure for the routine admission of a medical or surgical patient is the same except that the diagnostic tests are performed on surgery patients as soon as possible following their arrival at the hospital. This allows the time needed to perform the diagnostic studies and to have the test results on the patient's chart prior to surgery. A blood count that is too low or a chest x-ray that is abnormal may require that the surgery be postponed until further investigation is made.

Historically, surgeries were scheduled for the day after the patient's admission. Some surgeries, such as open heart surgery or kidney transplant surgery, may require additional patient preparation and careful explanation of the procedure to the patient and the family. It may also be arranged for patients to tour the intensive care unit, so that they will be aware of their surroundings and the activities that will take place following surgery. Also, other diagnostic studies may need to be carried out before extensive surgery may be performed.

Currently, the trend is to admit the patient the day of surgery.

### Admission Day Surgery and Preoperative Care Unit

The purpose of the **admission day surgery** area is to admit patients the *day of* their scheduled surgery. All preoperative tests have been completed before admission. The patient then is admitted to a surgical unit once the surgery and recovery room care have been completed. Since cost is a major factor in health care today, this type of area is promoted by health insurance companies. Other terms for this practice include same-day surgery and AM admission

(AMAD). The preadmission assessment and testing area may coordinate the advance preparation for admission day surgical patients.

Days before surgery the patient:

■ Visits the doctor.
■ Provides the patient registration staff with personal information either by phone, in person, or written form.
■ Has had blood tests and any other required or doctor-requested tests, such as a chest x-ray or EKG. In many facilities an EKG is automatically done on persons over 40 years of age.
■ Visits with anesthesiologist. This visit may also include patient and family education of the procedure.

On the day of the surgery, the patient reports to the admission area several hours before surgery. The patient is taken to the admission day surgery unit with:

■ Identification band
■ Doctor's orders
■ Laboratory reports (if ordered)
■ EKG (if ordered)
■ X-ray report (if ordered)
■ Addressograph plate (imprinter card) or computer labels
■ Admission forms including any consent forms or physicians' orders

The health unit coordinator performs the routine admission tasks as well as checking to see that all ordered laboratory and other diagnostic tests were completed.

After surgery and the recovery room (postanesthesia care unit), the patient is assigned a bed and is transported to an inpatient surgical unit.

## The Preoperative Orders

The physician who is to perform surgery on a patient writes orders relative to the surgery before the surgery is performed. For example, the surgeon who is performing an abdominal hysterectomy may wish the patient to receive a medicated vaginal irrigation the morning of the surgery. He or she may also order a urinary catheter to be inserted before the patient leaves the nursing unit for surgery.

The surgeon may also designate the anesthesiologist who will write the preoperative preparation orders. The name of the surgery for the preparation of the operative permit also is written on the physicians' order sheet. Any discrepancy between the procedure named on the operative permit and information on the patient's chart should be checked by calling the physician's office. For example, the operative permit as written on the physicians' order sheet may state that the patient is to have an "open reduction of the *left* femur," whereas the patient's diagnosis and physical examination indicate that the patient has a fracture of the *right* femur; obviously such a discrepancy

must be corrected before any orders are carried out. All charting rules must be followed when preparing consent forms. Consents must be written in ink and be legible. Abbreviations are not allowed on surgical consents.

The anesthesiologist also writes orders on the physicians' order sheet the day before the surgery. His or her orders concern the time the food and fluids are to be discontinued and the preoperative medication to be given to help relieve anxiety and aid in the induction of the anesthesia.

### Preoperative Order Components

Orders related directly to the surgery have certain common components.

#### SURGEON'S ORDERS

**Name of Surgery for Operative Permit.** The permit must be signed before the patient receives any "mind-clouding" drugs. In the case of surgery that may result in sterility or in loss of a limb (amputation), two permits may be required.

**Enemas.** The order for an enema depends upon the type of surgery. For surgeries within the abdominal cavity, all wastes must be removed from the intestines. This allows the surgeon more room for exploration.

**Shaves and Scrubs.** The site of the surgical incision must be prepared. This order requires the removal of body hair by shaving. The procedure is referred to as a "surgical prep." The surgeon may also require a special scrub at the surgical site. In some facilities, shaves and scrubs may be done by the operating room staff.

**Name of Anesthesiologist.** It is necessary to know this physician's name in the event that preoperative medication orders are not received. The health unit coordinator may then call the anesthesiologist or person responsible for writing the preoperative orders. (In hospitals where nurse anesthetists administer the anesthesia, the surgeon may write the preoperative orders.)

**Miscellaneous Orders.** Other orders may be for additional diagnostic studies, blood components to be given during surgery, or intravenous preparations to be started before surgery. Treatments and additional medications may also be ordered.

#### ANESTHESIOLOGIST'S ORDERS

**Diet.** When surgery is to be performed during the morning hours, the patient is usually NPO at midnight. A patient having late afternoon surgery may be NPO after 6:00 AM, liquid breakfast. Food and/or fluids by mouth are not allowed for 6 to 8 hours before surgery in which an anesthetic is used that renders the patient unconscious. The NPO rule is maintained to lessen the possibility of the patient aspirating vomitus while under anesthesia.

**Preoperative Medications.** The patient is usually given a hypnotic to ensure that he or she rests well the night before surgery. Approximately 1 hour before the surgery, the patient receives a preoperative intramuscular injection as ordered by the anesthesiologist. (Figure 19–10 is an example of preoperative orders.)

## PREOPERATIVE PROCEDURE

| Step | Task | Notes |
|---|---|---|
| 1. | Imprint the surgery forms and requisitions with the patient's imprinter card and place them within the patient's chart holder. | The surgery forms may include such things as the nurse's preoperative checklist, operating room record, the anesthesiologist's record, and the operating room record (Fig. 19–16). Other forms may be included depending on hospital policy. |
| 2. | Check the patient's chart for the history and physical report. | If the history and physical report is not found on the chart, call the health records department to check if it has been dictated. Call the attending physician if the report is not located. |
| 3. | Check the patient's chart for the following signed consent forms:<br>    a. Informed surgical consent.<br>    b. Blood consent.<br>    c. Admission agreement/treatment consent. | Check the consent forms for the patient's and witness's signature and the correct spelling of the surgical procedure. |
| 4. | Check the patient's chart for any previously ordered studies such as labs and x-rays. | If the diagnostic test results are not on the patient's chart, call the laboratory or diagnostic testing area to confirm that the tests have been done. If they have not been done, notify the patient's nurse. |
| 5 | Chart the patient's latest vital signs. | |
| 6 | File the current medication administration record in the patient's chart. | |
| 7. | Place the imprinter card or printed labels with the chart. | The imprinter card may be taped to the chart. |
| 8. | Notify the appropriate nursing personnel when surgery calls for the patient. | |

## PHYSICIANS' ORDER SHEET

| DATE | TIME | SYMBOL | ORDERS |
|---|---|---|---|
| 5/13/xx | 1530 | | Full liquid diet tonight.<br>T + C 2 U packed cells and hold for surgery.<br>CBC, U A and chest x-ray.<br>ECG this p.m.<br>Consent: Partial Gastrectomy, Vagotomy and pyloroplasty.<br>Rx surg. skin prep.<br>H + P by surgical resident.<br>Preops by Dr. A. Sleep<br>Start 1000 cc 5% D/W 1 hour before surgery.<br>                    Dr. G. Astro |
| 5/13/xx | 1700 | | NPO midnight<br>Nembutal 100 mg. hs tonight MR X 1<br>Demerol 75 mg.  ⟩ IM @ 0700<br>Atropine 0.4 mg. ⟩<br>                    Dr. A. Sleep |

FIGURE 19–10 • Example of a set of preoperative orders.

# PATIENT'S REQUEST FOR SURGERY OR OTHER INVASIVE PROCEDURE, TREATMENT OR THERAPY, AND INFORMED CONSENT

**I ACKNOWLEDGE MY INFORMED CONSENT FOR** and request the described surgical or other invasive procedure(s), treatment or therapy as scheduled by my physician and _____ Hospital. I also understand that I may revoke this consent prior to the performance of the procedure(s), treatment, or therapy.

| SURGICAL OR OTHER INVASIVE PROCEDURE(S), TREATMENT OR THERAPY TO BE PROVIDED: |

**(Please designate in both <u>scientific and plain English terminology</u>.)** _____

_____

_____

_____

**SURGICAL SITE/SIDE (if applicable):** _____

As part of this request, I state that I am satisfied that I have made an informed consent for such surgical or other invasive procedure(s), treatment or therapy which my physician and I have discussed. Specifically, my physician has informed me about:

1. My medical condition, problem or diagnosis;

2. The nature and purpose of the proposed procedure, treatment, or therapy;

3. The significant risks and consequences of the proposed procedure, treatment or therapy;

4. The probability of success of the proposed procedure, treatment, or therapy;

5. Appropriate alternatives to the proposed procedure, treatment, or therapy;

6. The probable prognosis if the proposed procedure, treatment, or therapy is **NOT PROVIDED**; and

7. The fact that some aspects of my care may be provided by my physician's duly authorized designee(s) in the event that he/she is ill or absent.

**I FULLY UNDERSTAND** what my physician and I have discussed, and all my questions have been answered.

_____  AM
Date/Time                        ___PM        _____
                                              Patient's Signature

_____              _____
Witness                                       Relationship (if signed by other than patient, state reason)

I have secured an informed consent to such invasive procedures, treatment, or therapy from the patient.

_____              _____ AM
Physician's Signature                         Date/Time                        ___PM

As part of this request, I state that I have received a copy of the _____ Hospital brochure entitled, *Anesthesia, Your Options,* and have been offered additional information and opportunity to talk with an anesthesiologist. I have had the opportunity to have my questions concerning anesthesia answered and have made an informed consent for anesthesia services.

_____  AM
Date/Time                        ___PM        _____
                                              Patient's Signature

_____              _____
Witness                                       Relationship (if signed by other than patient, state reason)

**Other Participants In Consent Process**

Name: _____ Relationship        Name: _____ Relationship

_____              _____

_____              _____

White – Medical Record;  Yellow – Patient;  Pink – Physician        Informed Consent

F I G U R E  19–11 • Surgical consent. (From Rockford Memorial Hospital, Rockford, IL, with permission.)

**BLOOD TRANSFUSION CONSENT**

I hereby consent to the transfusion of blood or blood components derived from whole blood as my attending physician, or his/her physician designee, may decide is necessary or advisable in the course of my treatment.

My attending physician_____ or his/her physician designee, has explained to me why I need a blood transfusion. I understand that although every unit of blood is tested for evidence of infectious diseases and for quality of the blood cells, there is no set of tests that guarantees the absolute safety of every blood transfusion.

No guarantees have been made to me about the outcome of transfusion or the fitness or quality of the blood to be used.

The physician has answered my questions concerning this transfusion, and I understand the need for the transfusion and the risks involved.

                              Signature_____

                              Date_____19____Hour_____

Signature Witnessed

By_____          Relationship_____
                            if signed by other than patient,
                            state reason:_____
By_____          _____


- - - - - - - - - - - - - - - - - - - - - - - - - - - - - - - - - - - - - - - - -
**REFUSAL OF BLOOD TRANSFUSION**

After discussing the risks and benefits of this treatment with my physician I exercise my right to refuse this blood transfusion because:

Religious_____

Other_____
_____

                              Signature_____

                              Date_____19___Hour_____

Signature Witnessed

By_____

By_____

                              Blood Transfusion Consent/Refusal

F I G U R E  19–12 • Blood consent. (From Rockford Memorial Hospital, Rockford, IL, with permission.)

## Preoperative Routine

The overall responsibility of the health unit coordinator for the surgery chart is to see that it is properly prepared to be sent to surgery with the patient. Although many clerical duties are involved in preparing the patient's chart, the most important task is to have the following records on the chart. It is often hospital policy that surgery cannot begin if any of the required reports is missing.

■ The current history and physical record (H&P)—essential in most health care facilities.
■ Consents.
  • Surgery consent—an informed consent must be obtained prior to surgery (Fig. 19–11).
  • Blood consent—a consent must be signed to accept or refuse blood products (Fig. 19–12).
  • Admission agreement or treatment consent—check to see if signed upon admission.
■ Nursing preoperative checklist—should be checked and signed by nursing personnel.
■ MAR—current medication administration record should be placed in chart prior to transport to surgery.
■ Test results—preoperative test requirements will vary due to patient age, patient condition, type of surgery, and type of anesthetic. It will be necessary to check hospital policy regarding test requirements.
  • Laboratory test results—CBC, U/A, chem screen.
  • Chest x-ray report.
  • Other diagnostic studies—EKG, pulmonary functions screen.

To ensure that the patient's chart is ready for surgery, a preoperative checklist may be used (Fig. 19–13). This checklist should not be confused with the nursing preoperative checklist (Fig. 19–14), which is checked and signed by the patient's nurse to ensure proper patient preparation for surgery. The nursing preoperative checklist is a legal chart form in some facilities.

Each unit receives a surgery schedule (Fig. 19–15), which lists all the surgeries to be performed on the following day. To maintain confidentiality it is common practice that the patient's name not appear on the schedule. In place of the name there might be a room number or medical records number. The health unit coordinator may underline in red ink the patients scheduled for surgery from his or her unit. All the underlined patients should be placed on the checklist. As the required records are placed on the chart, they are checked off. Any reports or records that are missing must be located by calling the particular department or person responsible for the records.

Health unit coordinator tasks performed to prepare the patient's chart for surgery are listed at the top of p. 358.

## Postoperative Routine

Immediately after surgery, most patients spend 1 to 2 hours in the recovery room or postanesthesia care unit. A record of their progress is kept on the recovery room record. The postoperative orders (written by the surgeon immediately following surgery) are often initiated here. For example, the doctor's order for antiembolism hose to be placed on the patient's legs may be carried out by the recovery room staff. The recovery room personnel indicate on the physicians' order sheet those orders that have already been executed. (Note order No. 7 on Fig. 19–17.)

Health unit coordinator tasks performed during the postoperative procedure are listed at top of p. 368.

HEALTH UNIT COORDINATOR PREOPERATIVE CHECKLIST

| PATIENT'S NAME | CHEST X-RAY | UA | CBC | H&P | OR PERMIT | VITAL SIGNS | OR PACKET | IMPRINTER CARD | OTHER |
|---|---|---|---|---|---|---|---|---|---|
| 305 HEALTH, PAT | ✓ | ✓ | ✓ | | ✓ | | ✓ | | ECG ✓ |
| 311 Juniper, June | ✓ | ✓ | ✓ | ✓ | ✓ | | | | ECG ✓ |
| 325 Palooza, LoLA | ✓ | | ✓ | ✓ | ✓ | | | | |

FIGURE 19–13 • A preoperative checklist for the health unit coordinator.

| NURSING UNIT CHECK LIST | YES | NO |
|---|---|---|
| 1. Pre-op bath/Oral hygiene given | ✓ | |
| 2. Make-up/Nail polish removed | | ✓ |
| 3. Bobby Pins, Combs, Hair Pieces Removed<br>Disposition: | ✓ | |
| 4. Sanitary Belt removed | — | — |
| 5. Jewelry, Rings, Religious Medals, or other items removed<br>(May be worn during cardiac catheterization) when<br>removed disposition is: | ✓ | |
| 6. Voided/Retention catheter | ✓ | |
| 7. Preoperative medicine given as ordered | ✓ | |
| 8. Addressograph with chart | ✓ | |
| 9. Pre-anesthetic patient questionnaire completed | ✓ | |

10. Where family can be located during and immediately
after surgery *Surgery Waiting room*

### NURSING UNIT AND OPERATING ROOM NURSES CHECK LIST

| | UNIT NURSE YES | UNIT NURSE NO | O.R. NURSE YES | O.R. NURSE NO |
|---|---|---|---|---|
| 11. Surgical consent for: Rt. (Lt.)<br>*Inguinal herniorrhaphy* | ✓ | | | |
|     as obtained from Doctor's Order sheet | ✓ | | | |
| 12. Consultation<br>Special Consents | | | | |
| 13. History and Physical Dictated On Chart | ✓ | | | |
| 14. Allergies Noted | ✓ | | | |
| 15. Hematology | ✓ | | | |
| 16. Urinalysis | ✓ | | | |
| 17. Surgical/Cardiac cath prep done | ✓ | | | |
| 18. Type and Cross Match */* Units *P.C.* | ✓ | | | |
| 19. Culture site: Results: | | | | |
| 20. Admission Chest X-Ray Report | ✓ | | | |
| 21. EKG Report if over 40 years | ✓ | | | |

| 22. Prosthetic Teeth<br>May be worn during cardiac catheterization | REMOVED YES | NO | REMOVED YES | NO |
|---|---|---|---|---|
| Permanent cap or caps | | | | |
| Permanent bridge | | | | |
| Removable bridge | | | | |
| Removable plate or plates | | | | |
| Loose teeth | | | | |
| 23. Prosthesis and Disposition: | | | | |
| Artificial eye in out | | | | |
| Contact lens in out | | | | |
| Pacemaker | | | | |
| Other | | | | |

R.N. Signature         O.R. Nurse Signature

00-6015 Rev. 12-79

### PATIENT IDENTIFICATION ON UNIT

A. Person from surgery calling for patient

1. Ask for patient by name
2. Check patient's chart
3. Check patient's chart with call slip (not necessary with cardiac catheterization)

B. Person from unit must accompany

1. Ask patient his/her name
 Ask patient his/her doctor's name
2. Check chart face sheet for patient's name and hospital number with patient identiband
3. Check call slip with identiband (not necessary for cardiac catheterization)

*Winifred Marshall, R.N.*
Signature Nursing Unit Personnel

*Bill Standard, Ord.*
Signature Surgery Personnel

### SPECIAL COMMENTS TO OPERATING ROOM AND RECOVERY ROOM NURSES FROM NURSING UNIT: (PLEASE SIGN YOUR COMMENT)

B.P.:H.S. *130/70* a Pre-op *140/82* p Pre-op *136/80*

Pre-op TPR _____ NPO p *Mm* WT. *136*

Pertinent Drug Therapy:

*Demerol 75 mg* ⎫ *IM.*
*Atropine 0.4 mg* ⎭ *8:30 am*

*none*

*none*

PREOPERATIVE CHECK LIST

FIGURE 19–14 • Nurse's preoperative checklist.

SURGERY SCHEDULE FRIDAY JUNE 10, 19XX

| Time | Surgeon | Procedure | Patient's Bed Number |
|------|---------|-----------|----------------------|
| **Operating Room 1** | | | |
| 0730 | Dr. Singsong | Anterior Colporrhaphy; left Bartholin's cystectomy | 412A |
| 0930 | Dr. Prossert | Dilatation & curettage; FS, possible vag. hysterectomy, bil. salpingo-oophorectomy | 321 |
| 1130 | Dr. Broad | Laparoscopy | 621B |
| 1330 | Dr. Street | Rt. breast biopsy, FS, Poss. rt. radical mastectomy | 416 |
| **Operating Room 2** | | | |
| 0730 | Dr. Patellar | Arthrotomy lt. knee, open reduction, internal fixation with plateau medial meniscectomy | 502B |
| 0930 | Dr. Home | Arthroplasty rt. elbow, insertion of prosthesis; reconstruction rheumatoid rt. hand | 511 |
| 1330 | Dr. Bowl | Bone graft lt. radius | 516A |
| **Operating Room 3** | | | |
| 0730 | Dr. Branch | Cystoscopy, TURP | 212 |
| 0930 | Dr. Signe | Cystoscopy, manipulation ureteral stone | 222A |
| 1130 | Dr. Blake | Circumcision | 316B |
| **Operating Room 4** | | | |
| 0730 | Dr. Throat | Tonsillectomy | 304A |
| 0930 | Dr. Ober | Hemorrhoidectomy | 601 |
| **Operating Room 5** | | | |
| 0730 | Dr. Love | Cholecystectomy, biopsy rib cage | 617B |
| 0930 | Dr. Solano | Repair of lt. inguinal hernia | 600 |

F I G U R E  19–15 • A surgery schedule.

## Postoperative Order Components

The postoperative orders that relate to the patient's treatment following surgery usually contain the following components:

**Diet.** The patient may remain NPO or be given sips of water or ice chips (sips and chips). The diet is then increased as tolerated.

**Intake and Output.** The patient's intake and output is closely watched for 24 to 48 hours (Fig. 19–18).

**Intravenous Fluids.** Most surgery patients have at least one bottle of intravenous fluids ordered following surgery. A record of the intake of intravenous fluids is maintained on a parenteral fluid sheet (see Fig. 8–24).

**Vital Signs.** The patient's vital signs are monitored carefully after surgery—usually every 4 hours for 24 to 48 hours.

**Catheters, Tubes, and Drains.** Postoperative patients often have a retention or indwelling urinary catheter. Other orders may pertain to the catheterization of the patient, as necessary. Some patients may require a suction machine when nasogastric or other tubes are in place.

**Activity.** The activity following surgery may be only bedrest, and will be increased as the patient continues to recuperate.

**Positioning.** Some surgeons require the patient's position to be changed frequently. The elevation of the bed may also be very important.

**Observation of the Operative Site.** It is imperative that the site of the operation or the bandages be observed closely for bleeding, excessive drainage, redness, and swelling.

**Medications.** Orders for medications to relieve pain (narcotics) and nausea and vomiting (antinauseants), and to help the patient to sleep or rest (hypnotics) are issued for a period after surgery. Other medications are ordered as needed. (Fig. 19–17 is an example of postoperative orders.)

## HIGHLIGHT

Surgery orders cancel all previous orders.

## TO THE STUDENT

To practice transcribing a set of postoperative orders, complete **Activity 19–4** in the Skills Practice Manual.

```
967 801
CHAIR MORRIS
DR C SCOPE
M 68 SURG INS
```

## OPERATING ROOM NURSES NOTES

Date: _11 / 06 / XX_
        Mo.   Day   Yr.

Operating Room # _4_

Anesthesia Method:   ☒ General       ☐ Caudal
                     ☐ Local Infiltrate   ☐ Regional Blk.
                     ☐ Spinal        ☐ Epidural

Begin Anesthesia _0740_
Begin Surgery _0810_
End Surgery _0910_
Leave Room _0925_

Administered By: _Gerald Sleep, M.D._

Surgeon: _Robert Cutt, M.D._          Assistant: _Rufus String, M.D._

Perfusionist: _____     Observers: _____

Scrub Nurse: _L. Smythe O.R.T._        Circulating Nurse: _P. Bridge, R.N._

Relief: _____ @ _____       Relief: _____ @ _____

Pre-Operative Diagnosis: _Left Rotator Cuff Tendonitis_

Post-Operative Diagnosis: _Same_

Operation: _Exploratory arthrotomy left shoulder, Bristow procedure_

| Radiopaque Sponges 4x4 | | Laparotomy Sponges | No Sponge Count Taken ☐ | | |
|---|---|---|---|---|---|
| | | 5 5 | | Yes | No |
| | | | Sponge Count Correct | | |
| | | | Before Incision Made | ☑ | ☐ |
| | | | Cavity Closure | ☐ | ☐ |
| | | | Skin Closure | ☑ | ☐ |
| Rondic | Laminectomy | Cottoniods | Wound Classificaiton | A | ☑ |
| | | | | B | ☐ |
| | | | | C | ☐ |
| Dissect. | | | | D | ☐ |
| | | | | E | ☐ |

Tissue: _____      To Path Lab By: _____
Culture: _____      To Bacteriology By: _____
Implants:  Manufacturer: _Zimmer_       Serial # _____ Size: _1 inch_
           Type: _Bone screw_

| Date | Time | Comments/Complications |
|---|---|---|
| | | T + C  3 PC. |
| | | Adhesive for closure caused skin reaction near incision |

RN Signature: _Phoebe Bridge, R.N._

A         OPERATING ROOM NURSE'S NOTES

FIGURE 19–16 • Surgery forms. (A) Operating room nurse's notes. *Illustration continued on opposite page*

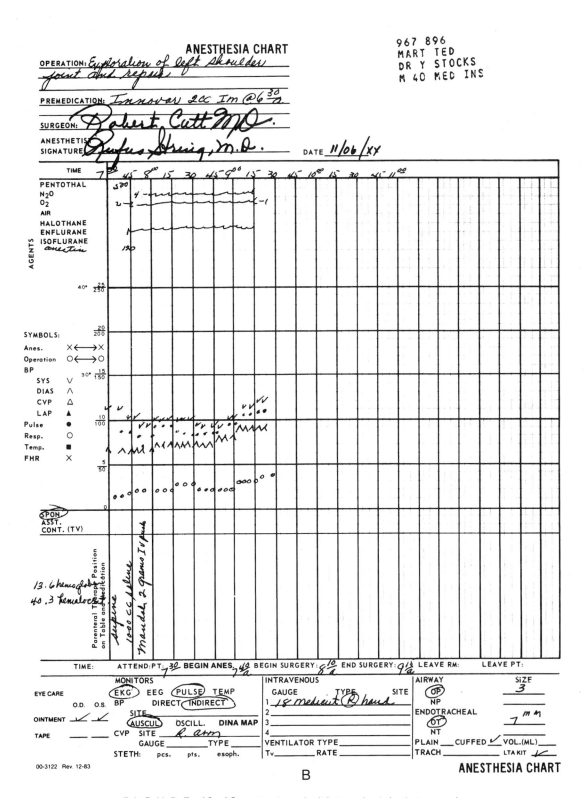

F I G U R E 19–16 • *Continued* (*B*) Anesthesiologist's record.

**PHYSICIAN'S ORDER SHEET**

| Date Ordered | Physician's Orders |
| --- | --- |
| 6/7/xx | Post op |
| | 1. NPO |
| | 2. NG tube to low Gomco |
| | 3. Follow present IV c̄ 5% D/LR @ 125 cc/h |
| | 4. Demerol 75 mg IM q4h prn pain |
| | 5. Compazine 10 mg IM q4h prn N/V |
| | 6. Encourage to TCDB |
| | 7. Knee length elastic hose ⌐above RR @ 1050 |
| | 8. May dangle this evening |
| | Dr. G. Astro |

F I G U R E   **19–17** • Example of a set of postoperative orders.

**24 - Hour Intake & Output**

Name *Rose Philips*
Room *316' West*
Date *5/13/XX*

| Shift | Fluid Intake | | | Fluid Output | | Other | Stools |
|---|---|---|---|---|---|---|---|
| | Oral | I.V. | Piggy Back | Urine | Emesis | Suction ☐ | |
| 0700-1500 | NPO | Credit *150cc* <br> Add *1000cc* <br> Add ____ | *50cc* | *100 cc* <br> *200 cc* <br> *200 cc* | *50 cc* | | |
| 8 Hr. | | *1150* | *50cc* | *500cc* | *50cc* | | |
| 1500-2300 | *50cc* <br> *50cc* <br> *100cc* <br> *50cc* <br> *100 cc* <br> *100 cc* <br> *50 cc* | Credit ____ <br> Add ____ <br> Add ____ | *50cc* | *225cc* <br> *200cc* | | | |
| 8 Hr. | *500cc* | | *50cc* | *450cc* | | | |
| 2300-0700 | | Credit ____ <br> Add ____ <br> Add ____ | | | | | |
| 8 Hr. | | | | | | | |
| 24 Hr. | | | | | | | |

Iced Tea - 6 oz. (180 cc)
Water Glass - 6 oz. (180 cc)
Milk (carton) - 8 oz. (240 cc)
Fruit Juice - 4 oz. (120 cc)
Soup - 4 oz. (120 cc)
Ice Cream - 3 oz. (90 cc)
Jello - 3½ oz. (105 cc)

Cup of Coffee or Tea - 7 oz. (210 cc)
Styrofoam Cup - 150 cc
Paper Cup - 150 cc
Coffee Creamer - ½ oz. (15 cc)
Cereal Creamer - 2 oz. (60 cc)
Coca Cola and Sprite - 12 oz. (360 cc)
$H_2O$ Pitcher - 30 oz. (900 cc)

F I G U R E   19–18 • Intake and output record.

## POSTOPERATIVE PROCEDURE

| Step | Task | Notes |
|---|---|---|
| 1. | Inform the patient's nurse of the patient's arrival in the PACU. | PACU personnel will notify the unit when the patient arrives from the operating room. The nurse caring for the patient may be informed verbally, or the message may be written on a communications board.<br>*Example*: 10:15 AM Joan Stein PACU OK. |
| 2. | Inform the patient's nurse of the expected arrival of the patient from the recovery room. | The recovery room personnel will notify the nursing unit prior to returning the patient to his or her room. |
| 3. | Remove the patient's imprinter card from the chart and place it in the imprinter card holder. | |
| 4. | Place all operating records behind the proper divider, if they have not already been placed there. | |
| 5. | Write the date of surgery and the surgical procedure in the designated place on the patient's Kardex form or on the computer. | |
| 6. | Fill in the date of the surgery on the patient's graphic sheet. | |
| 7. | Transcribe the physicians' postoperative orders. Notify the nurse caring for the patient of stat physicians' orders. | **All preoperative orders are automatically discontinued postoperatively**. The health unit coordinator will erase or cancel all preoperative orders from the patient's Kardex forms and destroy all medicine cards. However, the doctor may write "Continue all preoperative orders." To transcribe this order, only the dates on the preoperative orders should be erased and the operative date substituted. Check the entire set of orders carefully before erasing the patient's Kardex forms. |

## SUMMARY

For most patients, admission to the hospital is a frightening experience. The health unit coordinator can do much in the field of public relations for the hospital at this time. The health unit coordinator is usually the first person with whom the new patient has contact on the nursing unit. A warm welcome and a pleasant smile may help to relieve some anxiety. The expediency with which the patient's chart is prepared and the new orders transcribed allows the health care team to initiate care and treatment sooner.

The health unit coordinator needs to recognize the common components in the admission, preoperative, and postoperative order sets. As in all orders, the quick yet accurate and thorough transcription of orders is a must.

**REVIEW QUESTIONS**

1. Place the letter of the correct answer in the second column in the space provided in the first column.

_____ admission orders

a. admission necessitated by an accident or a medical emergency

_____ admission agreement

b. entry into hospital planned in advance

_____ emergency admission

c. directions for care and treatment written by doctor on patient's entry into hospital

_____ routine admission

d. contains general services the hospital will provide

2. Define the following:

a. health records number _____

_____

_____

_____

b. identification bracelet _____

_____

_____

c. nursing preoperative checklist _____

_____

_____

d. surgery schedule _____

_____

_____

e. valuables envelope _____

_____

_____

f. preoperative orders _____

_____

_____

g. postoperative orders _____

_____

_____

h. allergy information _____

_____

_____

i. information sheet _____

_____

_____

j. health unit coordinator preoperative checklist _____

_____

_____

k. elective surgery _____

_____

_____

l. allergy identification bracelet _____

_____

_____

m. preadmit _____

_____

_____

n. registration _____

_____

_____

o. informed consent _____

_____

_____

3. Eight common components of a set of admission orders are:

a. _____     e. _____

b. _____     f. _____

c. _____     g. _____

d. _____     h. _____

4. Three items prepared by the registration staff that are sent to the unit as part of the admission procedure are:

a. _____

b. _____

c. _____

5. List health unit coordinator tasks regarding the patient's admission.

a. _____     h. _____

b. _____     i. _____

c. _____     j. _____

d. _____     k. _____

e. _____     l. _____

f. _____     m. _____

g. _____     n. _____

6. Explain the health unit coordinator's responsibilities regarding the preoperative patient's chart.

_____

_____

_____

_____

_____

_____

7. Five records or reports that might be on the patient's chart prior to surgery are:

a. _____    d. _____

b. _____    e. _____

c. _____

8. List six components that may be part of preoperative orders.

a. _____    d. _____

b. _____    e. _____

c. _____    f. _____

9. List nine components that may be part of a set of postoperative orders.

a. _____    f. _____

b. _____    g. _____

c. _____    h. _____

d. _____    i. _____

e. _____

10. List three tasks the health unit coordinator may perform concerning the postoperative patient's chart and Kardex.

a. _____

b. _____

c. _____

11. Write the meaning of each of the following abbreviations.

a. H&P       _____

b. preop     _____

c. postop    _____

d. Dx        _____

e. Hx        _____

f. NKA       _____

12. Define advance directives.

_____

_____

_____

13. List six patient registration tasks.

    a. _____    d. _____

    b. _____    e. _____

    c. _____    f. _____

14. List three types of entry admissions.

    a. _____

    b. _____

    c. _____

15. What is the difference between a living will and power of attorney for health care?

    _____

    _____

    _____

16. When does an advance directive or living will become effective?

    _____

    _____

    _____

# References

Barber, L. G.: *Being a Medical Admissions Clerk*. Englewood Cliffs, NJ, Prentice-Hall Career & Technology, Prentice-Hall, Inc., 1994.

Cox, Kay, Hospital Research and Education Trust: *Being a Health Unit Coordinator*. Englewood Cliffs, NJ, Prentice-Hall, 1991.

Lewis, Marcia A. and Warden, Carol D.: *Law and Ethics in the Medical Office*. Philadelphia, F. A. Davis Co., 1983.

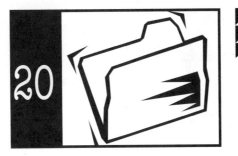

CHAPTER **20**

# DISCHARGE, TRANSFER, AND POSTMORTEM PROCEDURES

## CHAPTER OBJECTIVES

*Upon completion of this chapter, you will be able to:*

1. Define the terms in the vocabulary list.

2. Write the meaning of each abbreviation in the abbreviations list.

3. List 14 tasks that may be required to complete a routine discharge.

4. List the additional tasks that may be required when a patient is discharged to a nursing home.

5. Describe the tasks necessary to prepare the discharged patient's chart for the health records department.

6. List seven clerical tasks performed upon the death of a patient.

7. List 12 tasks that are performed in the transfer of a patient from one unit to another.

8. Describe the duties of the health unit coordinator in the transfer of a patient from one room to another room on the same unit.

9. List nine clerical tasks performed when a transferred patient is received on the unit.

## VOCABULARY

**Autopsy** • An examination of a body after death; it may be performed to determine the cause of death or for medical research

**Coroner's Case** • A death that occurs due to sudden, violent, or unexplained circumstances

**Custodial Care** • Care and services of a nonmedical nature, which consist of feeding, bathing, watching, and protecting the patient

**Expiration** • A death

**Extended Care Facility** • A medical facility caring for patients requiring expert nursing care or custodial care       *long term care*

**Organ Donation** • Donating or giving one's organs and/or tissues after death; one may designate specific organs (i.e., only cornea) or any needed organs

**Organ Procurement** • The process of removing donated organs; it may be referred to as harvesting

**Postmortem** • After death (a postmortem examination is the same as an autopsy)

**Shroud** • A covering placed around a dead body

**Release of Remains** • A signed consent that authorizes a specific funeral home or agency to remove the deceased from a health care facility

**Terminal Illness** • An illness ending in death

## ABBREVIATIONS

| Abbreviation | Meaning |
| --- | --- |
| AMA | against medical advice |
| ECF | extended care facility |

# DISCHARGE OF A PATIENT

Once it is written by the physician, the order for the discharge of a patient from the hospital requires the prompt attention of the health unit coordinator. Most patients wish to leave the hospital as soon as possible after the discharge order is written. Environmental Services (or housekeeping) must also prepare the vacated room and bed for the admission of a new patient. Your instructor will indicate which of the following tasks are performed by the health unit coordinator in your hospital. There are five types of discharges:

- Discharged home
- Discharged to another facility
- Discharged home with assistance
- Discharged against medical advice (AMA)
- Expiration

All discharges, with the exception of expiration and AMA, require a physician's order.

## Routine Discharge Procedure

Most discharges from the hospital are routine in nature; that is, the patient is discharged alive to go home in the company of a family member or a friend.

The following tasks are related to the discharge of a patient.

## Discharge to Another Facility

Hospitals that accept Medicare patients and are accredited by the Joint Commission on the Accreditation of Healthcare Organizations are required to maintain a utilization review committee. The committee's purpose is to review the condition of all patients remaining in the hospital longer than a stated period. When the patient no longer needs expert nursing care but still requires **custodial care**—care and services of a nonmedical nature, which consist of feeding, bathing, watching, and protecting the patient—the doctor is requested to transfer the patient from the hospital to a nursing home.

Other patients who are discharged may also be sent to a nursing home or an extended care facility. Frequently, arrangements for nursing home care are arranged by the hospital social service department.

The discharge to another facility is not unlike a routine discharge, with additional steps.

Many patients need care or assistance at home as part of their recovery process. Additional steps are required when a patient needs home health care.

## Discharge against Medical Advice

A client may feel that he or she is not receiving the care that is needed. Or perhaps the patient believes that there is no improvement of the condition for which he or she is hospitalized. Whatever the reason, the patient may decide to leave the hospital without the doctor approving the discharge.

The client may appear at the nurse's station and announce that he or she is leaving the hospital. The health unit coordinator should ask the patient to be seated until the nurse manager, charge nurse, or team leader is notified. A resident may be called to speak with the patient. The attending physician is notified. Everything possible is done to encourage the patient to remain in the hospital until the treatment is completed. However, the patient cannot be restrained from leaving.

In the event that the patient is not convinced to stay, a release form (Fig. 20–8) is prepared. The form is signed by the patient or his or her representative, and witnessed by an appropriate member of the hospital staff. The patient is then permitted to leave the hospital, and the discharge procedure is the same as for a routine discharge.

*pastoral care may be called*

## Discharge of the Deceased Patient

### Patient Deaths

Not all clients who enter the hospital for care and treatment are discharged alive. Some patients who enter the hospital are well advanced in age. Other clients, in any age group, may have a terminal illness—one that results in death—and make many visits to the hospital, knowing that each admission may be their last. Sometimes, death is unexpected, as in the case of complications from surgery. Frequently, the patient's death is slow, and there is an opportunity to offer support to family members as time permits.

You may be requested to call a religious counselor to speak with the patient. In the event that the patient is a member of a particular religious group, it is necessary for you to notify the religious leader in the community to perform any rites required in the event of impending death. A notation should be made on the patient's Kardex form of any final rites that have been performed.

### Certification of Death

In cases where a death is expected, the nurse or family members may be with the patient at the time of expiration (death). At other times, the patient may die unexpectedly. In either instance, the physician must be notified in order to pronounce the patient dead. The patient is examined for any signs of life. If none can be determined, the patient is pronounced dead and the official time is recorded on the doctors' progress notes. A death certificate must also

## DISCHARGE PROCEDURE

| Step Task | Notes |
|---|---|
| 1. Transcribe the discharge order. | The order may be written on the physicians' order sheet the day before or the day of the expected discharge. |
| 2. Notify the nurse caring for the patient of the discharge order. | |
| 3. Notify the admitting or discharge desk of the patient's discharge. | Notification may be by telephone, a written discharge requisition, or by computer (Fig. 20–1) |
| | The business office or the admitting department notifies the nursing unit if the patient is financially cleared for dismissal. |
| | Some patients may be required to stop at the business office before leaving the hospital. If the patient does not plan to leave during the regular dismissal hours, inform the admitting department of the expected time of departure. |
| 4. Explain the procedure for discharge to the patient and/or the patient's relatives. | The explanation may also be given by the nurse; however, many patients come to the health unit coordinator in the nurse's station for the explanation. |
| 5. Notify other departments that may be giving the patient daily treatments. | Departments such as physical therapy and respiratory care may need to be notified. This may be communicated by telephone, by written communication, or by computer. |
| 6. Communicate the patient's discharge to the dietary department on the diet sheet or by computer. | If the patient is not planning to leave the hospital during the regular discharge hours (usually before lunch), indicate on the diet sheet the expected departure time. |
| 7. Arrange for clinic appointment if doctor requests it. | Write out the appointment date and the time on a piece of paper and give it to the patient. |
| | A discharge instruction sheet is prepared by the nurse and is given to the patient (Fig. 20–2). |
| 8. Arrange transportation if needed. | The patient who does not have family or friends available to provide transportation may need to have a call made for a taxi. |
| 9. Prepare credit slips for medications returned to the pharmacy or equipment and supplies from CSD. | Supplies specifically ordered for the patient from CSD and not used by the patient must be returned to CSD with a credit slip (Fig. 20–3). |
| 10. Notify nursing personnel or transportation service to transport patient to the discharge area. | Patients should never be allowed to go to the discharge area without an escort from the hospital staff. Also, the patient should be transported via a wheelchair. |
| 11. Write the patient's name in the unit admission, discharge, and transfer book, and on the census sheet, or enter in the computer. | |
| 12. Delete the patient's name from the unit TPR sheet. | Draw a line through the patient's name. |
| 13. Notify environmental services to clean the discharged patient's room. | Notification may be by telephone; computer; checking the admission, discharge, and transfer book; or by telling the environmental services personnel on the unit. See Figure 20–4. |

*Hill burton act in case of no insurance bill is paid for* [handwritten note]

*(Continued)*

be completed by the physician, and a report of the death filed with the bureau of vital statistics.

### Release of Remains

The patient's family or guardian must indicate the funeral home to which the body will be released. Usually, a form must be signed by the family before the patient can be released to the funeral home. The nursing office staff may notify the funeral home of the expiration. The funeral home personnel may pick up the patient from the unit or the hospital morgue. A hospital security officer may need to accompany the funeral home personnel.

## DISCHARGE PROCEDURE (Continued)

| Step | Task | Notes |
|---|---|---|
| 14. | Prepare the chart for the health records department:<br>a. Check the summary/DRG worksheet for the physician's summation and the patient's final diagnosis. It is important to have this information upon patient discharge so that coding of diagnosis-related groups may be placed on the chart by the health records department.<br>b. Check for the correct name on the chart form.<br>c. Check for the presence of a final discharge note by a nursing staff member (Fig. 20–6).<br>d. Check for "old records" or "split chart." Place the split chart forms in the chart in the proper sequence.<br>e. Rearrange the chart forms in discharge sequence for your hospital.<br>f. Send the chart of the discharged patient to the health records department along with any old records of the patient. This task is usually performed at the end a shift so that all the charts of the discharged patients on the unit can be sent at the same time. Charts should be enclosed in a folder or manila envelope to preserve the confidentiality of the chart. | Many hospitals use a discharge checklist (Fig. 20–5) to prepare the chart for the health records department. |

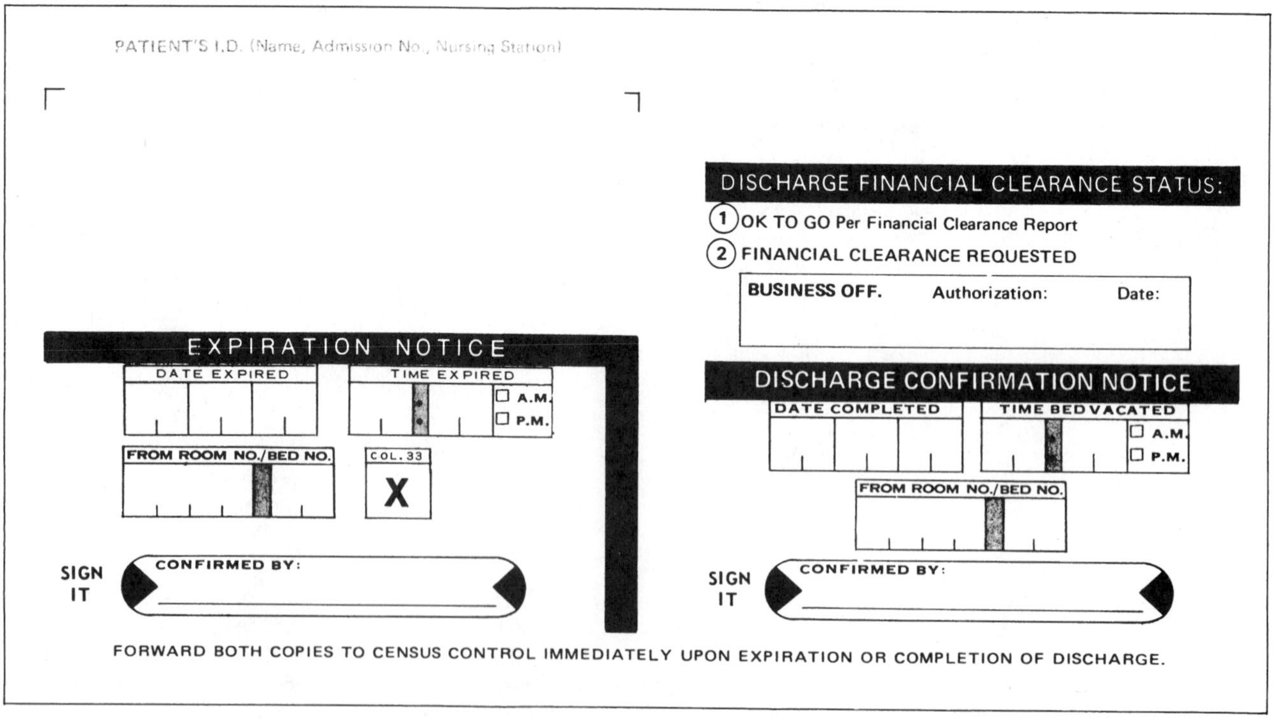
PATIENT'S I.D. (Name, Admission No., Nursing Station)

DISCHARGE FINANCIAL CLEARANCE STATUS:

(1) OK TO GO Per Financial Clearance Report

(2) FINANCIAL CLEARANCE REQUESTED

BUSINESS OFF. Authorization: Date:

EXPIRATION NOTICE

DATE EXPIRED

TIME EXPIRED ☐ A.M. ☐ P.M.

FROM ROOM NO./BED NO.

COL. 33

X

SIGN IT

CONFIRMED BY:

DISCHARGE CONFIRMATION NOTICE

DATE COMPLETED

TIME BED VACATED ☐ A.M. ☐ P.M.

FROM ROOM NO./BED NO.

SIGN IT

CONFIRMED BY:

FORWARD BOTH COPIES TO CENSUS CONTROL IMMEDIATELY UPON EXPIRATION OR COMPLETION OF DISCHARGE.

FIGURE 20–1 • Discharge slip.

# DISCHARGE INSTRUCTIONS

DIAGNOSIS: _____

_____

SURGERY/PROCEDURE: _____

| 1. **ACTIVITY** | NO LIMIT | LIMIT |
|---|---|---|
| Bathing | | |
| Driving | | |
| Sexual | | |
| Work | | |
| Exercise | | |
| Ambulation | | |

2. **MEDICATION:**

____ Patient/family knows what medications are for.

____ Prescriptions sent with patient or family.

| **NAME OF MEDICATION** | **DOSAGE** | **FREQUENCY/TIMES** |
|---|---|---|

3. **DIET:**

Your diet will be _____

Please call dietition at _____ if you have any questions.

4. **SPECIAL INFORMATION:** (include wound care, further treatments, referrals, equipment, etc.)

5. **RETURN VISIT TO PHYSICIAN:** Please call Dr. _____ Phone: _____

to make an appointment in _____ days. Please call the doctor if you cannot take your medicine

or to answer any questions.

6. **INSTRUCTION SHEETS GIVEN:** (Please list pamphlets, written instructions or other standardized information.)

_____

Signature of R.N.

The above was discussed with me and
I understand all of the information.

_____

Date

_____

Signature of Patient/Guardian

Patient ( original)   Medical Records (yellow)   Other (pink)      DISCHARGE INSTRUCTIONS

F I G U R E   20–2 • Discharge instruction sheet. (From Rockford Memorial Hospital, Rockford, IL, with permission.)

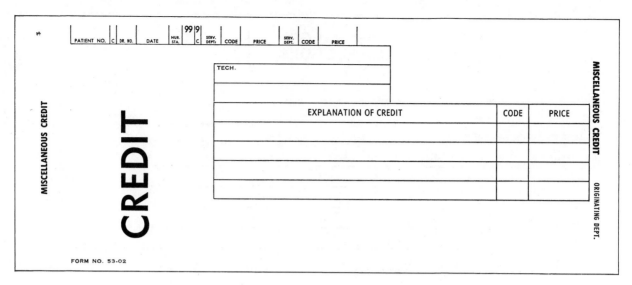

FIGURE 20-3 • Credit requisition.

DISMISSAL-TRANSFER LOG *

NURSING STATION: _____                                                              DATE: _____

| #1 Room Number | #2 Patient Name | #3 Physician | #4 Time Order Written and Called | #7 Time Room Vacated | #8 Time Room Released by E.S. Specialist | #9 E.S. Specialist Initials |
|---|---|---|---|---|---|---|
| **DISCHARGES** | | | | | | |
|  |  |  |  |  |  |  |
|  |  |  |  |  |  |  |
|  |  |  |  |  |  |  |
|  |  |  |  |  |  |  |
|  |  |  |  |  |  |  |
|  |  |  |  |  |  |  |
|  |  |  |  |  |  |  |
|  |  |  |  |  |  |  |
|  |  |  |  |  |  |  |
|  |  |  |  |  |  |  |
|  |  |  |  |  |  |  |
|  |  |  |  |  |  |  |

| #1 Room Number | #2 Patient Name | #3 Physician | #4 Time Order Written and Called | #5 Specific Unit and Type Room Requested | #6 Patient Transferred To What Unit and Room No. | #7 Time Room Vacated | #8 Time Room Released by E.S. Specialist | #9 E.S. Specialist Initials |
|---|---|---|---|---|---|---|---|---|
| **TRANSFERS** | | | | | | | | |
|  |  |  |  |  |  |  |  |  |
|  |  |  |  |  |  |  |  |  |
|  |  |  |  |  |  |  |  |  |
|  |  |  |  |  |  |  |  |  |

FIGURE 20-4 • Housekeeping log. (From Rockford Memorial Hospital, Rockford, IL, with permission.)

---

## DISCHARGE CHECKLIST

*(To be completed and sent with chart to the Medical Records Department by end of shift on which the patient is discharged. Check Yes or No box.)*

Date of Admission __12/4/XX__

*Check List*

*HISTORY & PHYSICAL*

Yes   No

☒   ☐   *1. History and Physical on chart within 48 hours. Due* __12/6/XX__
         *(IF NO, ANSWER NUMBER TWO.)*

☐   ☐   *2. History and Physical Notification Form # 00-0531 sent to Medical Records. Date sent* _____

*Health Unit Coordinator Signature* __Ima Clerke__

*Check List*

*FINAL DISPOSITION OF CHART*

Yes   No

☐   ☐   *1. All sheets embossed with correct patient master card and legible, and all reports are for this patient.*

☐   ☐   *2. Portions of chart which have been removed are replaced in proper order, with chart dividers removed.*

☐   ☐   *3. Reports are correctly inserted or attached.*

         *4. FRONT SHEET:*

☐   ☐       *a. Discharge diagnosis written on Front Sheet by Doctor. If No, answer 4b.*

☐   ☐       *b. Final diagnosis noted on Telephone Tentative or Final Discharge Diagnosis Form #00-0523 attached to chart and send to Medical Records with check list. If unable to complete, state reason on form.*

☐   ☐   *5. Previous Medical Records return to Medical Record Department.*

☐   ☐   *6. Accordion folders used for sending records to Medical Record Department.*

☐   ☐   *7. Discharge entered in Unit Transit Book.*

*Date of Discharge* _____

*Health Unit Coordinator Signature* _____

☐   ☐   *8. Nurses notes are complete.*

*R.N. or L.P.N. Signature:* _____

F I G U R E  20–5 • Discharge checklist.

NURSES NOTES

| DATE TIME | |
|---|---|
| | |
| | |
| | |
| | **10**$^{00}$ **AM** DISCHARGE NURSES NOTES |
| | TIME: PM MODE: WC ✔ STRETCHER AMB. |
| | EXIT: DISCHARGE AREA ✔ EMERGENCY ENTRANCE |
| | ACCOMPANIED BY: EMPLOYEE TITLE *L.P.N.* FAMILY *Husband* |
| | HEALTH STATUS: *Good – Normal post surgery recovery.* |
| | |
| | INSTRUCTIONS GIVEN: *Instruction sheet given to patient.* |
| | |
| | RN SIGNATURE: *Candace M.E. Sutton* |

FIGURE 20–6 • Nursing discharge note.

## ADDITIONAL STEPS FOR DISCHARGE TO ANOTHER FACILITY

| Step | Task | Note |
|---|---|---|
| 1. | Notify social service of the physicians' orders to discharge to another facility. | |
| 2. | Arrange for transportation. | The patient who is confined to bed may require an ambulance when requested. |
| 3. | Complete the continuing care form or transfer form. | The continuing care form requires some information that the health unit coordinator may fill in from the facesheet. The nurse and MD complete their sections of the form (Fig. 20–7). |
| 4. | Photocopy forms as necessary. | Requirement of forms will vary from facility to facility. It is also necessary to check hospital policy to determine who is responsible for making copies—the HUC or the health records department. Once the copies are made, it is important to place the originals back in the chart in proper sequence. |
| 5. | Distribute continuing care form and copies as required. | The photocopies and a copy of the continuing care form are placed in a sealed envelope to be given to the ambulance driver or a family member. This person delivers the envelope to the nurse at the nursing care facility. |
| 6. | Perform routine discharge steps. | |

*(Use Typewriter or Ballpoint Pen – Press Firmly)*                                                    *(See Instructions on back of Page 3)*

## CONTINUING CARE TRANSFER INFORMATION

**TO BE COMPLETED AND SIGNED BY NURSING SERVICE (Please attach a copy of the Nursing Care Plan)**

| PATIENT'S NAME   Last   First   MI | DATE OF BIRTH | SEX | RELIGION | HEALTH INSURANCE CLAIM NUMBER |
|---|---|---|---|---|

PATIENT'S ADDRESS (Street number, City, State and Zip Code)    ATTENDING PHYSICIAN    Name    Address

RELATIVE OR GUARDIAN    Name    Address    Phone Number

Name and Address of Facility Transferring FROM    Dates of Stay at Facility Transferring FROM    Facility Name and Address Transferring TO

Admission    Discharge

PAYMENT SOURCE FOR CHARGES TO PATIENT:

☐ Self or Family    ☐ Private Insurance ID Number _____    ☐ Blue Cross/Blue Shield ID Number _____    ☐ Employer or Union

☐ Public Agency _____    ☐ Other (specify) _____

**PATIENT EVALUATION:**

SPEECH: ☐ Normal    ☐ Impaired    ☐ Unable to speak

HEARING: ☐ Normal    ☐ Impaired    ☐ Deaf

SIGHT: ☐ Normal    ☐ Impaired    ☐ Blind

MENTAL STATUS: ☐ Always Alert    ☐ Occasionally Confused    ☐ Always Confused

FEEDING: ☐ Independent    ☐ Help with Feeding    ☐ Cannot Feed Self

DRESSING: ☐ Independent    ☐ Help with Dressing    ☐ Cannot Dress Self

ELIMINATION: ☐ Independent    ☐ Help to Bathroom    ☐ Bedpan or Urinal    ☐ Incontinent

BATHING: ☐ Independent    ☐ Bathing with Help    ☐ Bed Bath with Help    ☐ Bed Bath

AMBULATORY STATUS: ☐ Independent    ☐ Walks with Help    ☐ Help from Bed to Chair    ☐ Bed Bound

NURSING ASSESSMENT AND RECOMMENDATIONS:

TREATMENTS:

Last Medication: _____ / Dose: _____

Date: _____ Time: _____

APPLIANCES OR SUPPORTS:    or check none ☐

Signature    Title    Date

**TO BE COMPLETED AND SIGNED BY THE ATTENDING PHYSICIAN**

ECF Admitting Diagnosis:

Please send a copy of the following records with patient:

☐ Summary Sheet (face sheet)
☐ Discharge Summary
☐ Physical Examination and History
☐ Consultation
☐ Other (specify) _____

Patient knows diagnosis: ☐ Yes    ☐ No

Surgical Procedures: (current admission)

Transfer by: ☐ Ambulance    ☐ Car    ☐ Other (specify) _____

Allergies: ☐ No    ☐ Yes (specify) _____

VDRL: ☐ Positive    ☐ Negative

Anticoagulant: ☐ Taking now    ☐ Previously

Orders:   Diet, medication and special therapy   *(To be renewed in 48 hours)*

Chest X-Ray Diagnosis: _____

I will care for this patient after admission to new facility: ☐ Yes    ☐ No

Medication Regimen is stabilized: ☐ Yes    ☐ No

Anticipated length of stay for extended care _____ days

Physician's Signature    Date

*If necessary, attach order sheet – The above constitutes valid temporary orders only if signed by a physician.*

Address    Telephone Number

F I G U R E   20–7 • Continuing care transfer form.

## ADDITIONAL STEPS FOR DISCHARGE HOME WITH ASSISTANCE

| Step | Task | Notes |
|---|---|---|
| 1. | Notify social service, discharge planning, or home health care department. | The responsible department will vary from facility to facility. |
| 2. | Prepare the continuing care form. | HUC to complete personal information section. |
| 3. | Obtain a release of information from patient for home health care agency. | |
| 4. | Photocopy forms as necessary. | |
| 5. | Distribute continuing care form and copies as required. | |
| 6. | Perform routine discharge steps. | |

## POSTMORTEM PROCEDURE

| Step | Task | Notes |
|---|---|---|
| 1. | Contact the attending physician, staff physician, or resident to verify the patient's death. | |
| 2. | Prepare any forms that may be needed. | These forms may consist of a release of remains form, a request for autopsy or donation of body organs. Some hospitals use a postmortem checklist to ascertain that all postmortem tasks have been completed (Figs. 20–9, 20–10, and 20–11). |
| 3. | Notify the mortuary that has been requested by the family. | If the family is not familiar with mortuaries in the area, a list of mortuaries is usually available from the hospital telephone switchboard operator. The nursing office personnel may notify the funeral home. |
| 4. | Obtain a shroud pack, if needed. | Not all hospitals require the patient's body to be placed in a **shroud** (a covering placed around the dead body). A shroud pack may be kept in the unit CSD stock supply cupboard or may be obtained from CSD. |
| 5. | The nurse or health unit coordinator may gather the deceased's clothing and place it in a paper sack; label it with the patient's name, the room number, and the date. | The clothing is given to the family or to the mortician. |
| 6. | Obtain the mortuary book from the nursing office or have a mortuary form prepared when the mortician arrives. | The mortician claiming the body must complete forms to show that he or she has claimed the body, the clothing, or any valuables (Fig. 20–12). |

LEAVING HOSPITAL AGAINST ADVICE

Date_____

This is to certify that_____,
a patient in The Above Named Hospital, is leaving the hospital against the advice
of the attending physician and the hospital administration. I acknowledge that I
have been informed of the risk involved and hereby release the attending physician,
and the hospital, from all responsibility and any ill effects which may result from
this action.

_____
PATIENT

_____
OTHER PERSON RESPONSIBLE

_____
RELATIONSHIP

Witness_____

Witness_____

00-0434                                         **LEAVING HOSPITAL AGAINST ADVICE**

F I G U R E  20–8 • Form for discharge against medical advice.

## AUTHORIZATION FOR REMOVAL OF REMAINS/ AUTOPSY/ORGAN AND TISSUE DONATION

**★Area requiring signature of Family/Responsible Party**

**Implanted Devices** _____ **Type** _____
_(i.e., Epidural or Venous access, implanted pump, etc.)_

### AUTHORIZATION FOR REMOVAL OF REMAINS

The undersigned hereby authorizes and directs _____ and/or its
_(Funeral Home)_

agents to remove and take possesion of the remains of _____.
I (We) hereby represent that I am (we are) the next of kin and/or are legally authorized with this responsibility.

_____ 19 _____
**★(Signature)**                    _(Relationship)_        _(Witness)_                    _(Date)_

Please ask that dentures remain with the deceased.
The Funeral Director would appreciate a phone number where the family can be reached:

**Name:** _____  **Phone** _____
☐ Infection Control Precautions should be followed if an "Infection Hazard" tag is attached.

### AUTHORIZATION FOR AUTOPSY

**Autopsy Requested  ☐ NO  ☐ YES  If Yes, by** _____
I (We) request and authorize the physicians and surgeons in attendance at _____ . Hospital to perform a complete

autopsy on the remains of _____,
and I (we) authorize removal and retention or use for diagnostic, scientific or therapeutic purposes, of such organs, tissues and
parts, at this hospital, and at such other institutions as such physicians and surgeons deem appropriate. This authority is granted

subject to the following restrictions: _____

_____
_(If no restrictions, write "None")_

I (We) hereby represent that I am (we are) the next of kin and/or legally authorized by law to control the disposition of the remains.

_____ 19 _____
**★(Signature)**                    _(Relationship)_        _(Witness)_                    _(Date)_

_____ 19 _____
**★(Signature)**                    _(Relationship)_        _(Witness)_                    _(Date)_

When consent is given by telephone, two auditing witnesses must sign.
Name of person obtaining authorization:

                                                                                    AM
_____ Date _____ 19 ___ Time _____ PM
Autopsy performed _____ by _____ M.D.

### ORGAN/TISSUE DONATION REQUEST

1. Please complete the Organ/Tissue Donation Screening Record        One copy is for the
   patient's medical record and one copy for       Administration.

2. In addition to completing the Authorization for the Removal of the Remains
   please complete the       Consent Record

3.       donor manual available for reference.

### Nursing Office notified           ### Coroner notified _____
                                                            _(Name)_              _(Date/Time)_
                                       Coroner to Autopsy ☐ Yes  ☐ No _____
_____
_(Name)_                    _(Date/Time)_

### Primary physician notified        ### Possessions and belongings released to

_____      _____
_(Name)_                    _(Date/Time)_   **★(Signature)**                    _(Date/Time)_

Authorization for Removal of Remains/Autopsy/Organ and Tissue Donation
Original – Med. Records      Copy – Patient

F I G U R E  20–9 • Expiration form, release of remains, authorization for autopsy, and organ donation request. (From Rockford Memorial Hospital, Rockford, IL, with permission.)

AUTHORIZATION FOR DISPOSITION
OF BODY OR PARTS THEREOF

NAME OF PATIENT:_____ DATE:_____

STATUS OF SIGNER:  Patient ☐          Surviving Spouse ☐      Parent ☐      Child ☐      Brother ☐

Sister ☐          Other person entitled by law to control disposition of remains ☐  **Specify:**

_____

ORGAN OR TISSUE DONATED  (Should be specified unless whole body is donated):_____

_____

DONEE:  (a) University of Arizona ☐          (b) Arizona Eye Bank, Inc. ☐          (c) to be determined by hospital or any

available physician ☐      (d) specify if other ☐ _____

The Undersigned hereby donates the body of the above-named patient, or the parts thereof above specified, to the donee above specified for such humanitarian, research, educational, or transplant purposes or other disposition or use as the donee may in its discretion determine.  If the entire body is donated, it is to be delivered unembalmed and without autopsy other than such as may be required by law.

_____                                        _____
          WITNESS                                                              SIGNATURE


_____
          WITNESS


**IF SIGNER IS THE PATIENT THIS FORM MUST BE SIGNED BY A NOTARY PUBLIC.**

STATE OF ARIZONA          )
                         )  ss.
County of Maricopa        )


This instrument was acknowledged before me this_____day of_____, 19_____.



                                                        _____
                                                              NOTARY PUBLIC

My Commission Expires:

_____

                                                        AUTHORIZATION FOR DISPOSITION
                                                        OF BODY OR PARTS THEREOF

F I G U R E  20–10 • Consent form for donation of body organs.

CHECK LIST
Post-Mortem Care

1) Telephone Notification
☐ Family
☐ ALL physicians involved in patient care
☐ Whether or not an autopsy is to be done
☐ Switch Board (name, room number, time, mortuary)
☐ Police in event of Coroner's Case (check to see if physician called)
☐ Mortuary if known - and if mortician is to come to the unit.

2) Forms
Mortuary Form
When mortician comes to unit
☐ white copy to chart
☐ yellow to mortician
☐ pink to Business office with discharge requisition
☐ Patient Information Form remains on the unit
When patient goes to morgue
☐ entire completed form goes with patient
☐ Patient Information Form attached to mortuary form
Autopsy
☐ single copy remains on chart - send to Medical Records as soon as possible

3) Preparation of Body
When patient goes to Morgue
☐ Shroud and tag properly
☐ Mark on the shroud tag if patient is in isolation and causative organism, if known
☐ Complete #1 and 2
If a Coroner's Case
☐ Do not remove drains, IV's, etc., until police come. They may take the body with them.
☐ Notify mortuary of this
When patient goes to mortuary from the unit
☐ Do not shroud unless isolated
☐ Mark on tag causative organism

4) Transport Patient
☐ Patient elevator on E Wing 7:00 a.m. to 3:30 p.m., Mon. thru Fri.
☐ A, B, and C to 5th floor and cross to elevator #8 to 1st floor of S Building, S-4
☐ If body goes to refrigerator, mark 3 x 5 card on door
☐ Two people go with patient and their names are charted

5) Chart
☐ Complete all of Check List for Medical Records
☐ All of items noted in ''Telephone Notification''
☐ Who takes body to morgue
☐ Name of mortuary
☐ Follow Discharge Procedure

6) Please refer to Procedure Book for clarification of any and all of the above points, especially in reference to Coroner's Case, fetal death and autopsy.

_____ R.N.
Signature

00-0585

F I G U R E   20–11 • Example of a postmortem check list.

**MORTUARY FORM**

Name _____

Address _____

Doctor _____ Religion _____
☐ Date Admitted _____

**Religious Rites Performed** ☐ **desired** ☐ Date of Death _____ Time _____ Home Phone_____

---

**I. Clothing and Valuables from Room:**

Listed by_____
Registered Nurse

**II. Jewelry and/or Valuables sent to safe.**

Valuables Envelope Number_____

Witness_____
Registered Nurse

**III. Items on body:**

**IV. Number_____
Valuables envelope on admission (in safe).**

---

Disposition of possessions

To Family:

Items:

Received by_____

Relationship_____

Witness_____
Registered Nurse

To Mortuary:

Items:

Received by_____

Mortuary_____

Witness_____
Hospital Representative Title

---

I accept the body and valuables (as listed above) of the patient named above.  The identity has been verified by:

_____          _____
Mortuary                                                      Mortuary Representative

Telephone number of nearest
relative or responsible party _____

Miscellaneous:

Witness_____

Title _____

Autopsy:   Yes _____   No _____          Time _____   Date _____

DISPOSITION:  1. When body goes to the Morgue, send all 3 copies with the body.
2. When the Mortician comes to the unit, distribute copies as follows:

00-0308          WHITE – To Patient's Chart  ●  YELLOW – To Mortician  ●  PINK – To Business Office

FIGURE 20–12 ● Mortuary form.

## Organ Donation

Many patients indicate their wishes for organ donation before their death. A patient may designate specific organs (i.e., only cornea) or any needed organs or tissues. Due to state laws, the nursing staff may be required to ask the family about organ donation. It will be necessary to check the hospital's policies regarding organ donation. Additional consent forms will be necessary in the event of organ procurement.

## Autopsy or Postmortem Examination

An **autopsy**, or **postmortem examination**, of the body is performed to determine the cause of death or for medical research. The family may ask that an autopsy be done, or the doctor may request it. Before an autopsy can be performed, however, permission must be granted by the family. A consent for autopsy form (Fig. 20–9) must be signed by the next of kin.

## Coroner's Cases

A **coroner's case** is one in which the patient's death is due to sudden, violent, or unexplained circumstances, such as an accident, a poisoning, or a gunshot wound. Deaths that occur less than 24 hours after hospitalization may also be termed coroner's cases. State, county, and local governments have regulations defining a coroner's case in their particular locality. The law gives the coroner permission to study the body by dissection to determine if there is evidence of foul play.

### PROCEDURE FOR TRANSFER FROM ONE UNIT TO ANOTHER

| Step | Task | Notes |
|---|---|---|
| 1. | Transcribe order for a transfer. | Notify admitting department of transfer order to get a new room assignment. |
| 2. | Notify the nurse caring for the patient of the transfer order. | |
| 3. | Communicate to the nurse caring for the patient the receiving unit and room number as given by the admitting department. | |
| 4. | Notify the receiving unit of the transfer. | In some hospitals, the admitting department notifies the receiving unit. |
| 5. | Record the transfer in the unit admission, discharge, transfer book and/or the census sheet, and/or computer. | |
| 6. | Just before the transfer of the patient, remove the chart forms from the chart holder and the Kardex forms from the Kardex holders and obtain any medication administration records not filed in the chart. | It is easier for the health unit coordinator if the dividers of the chart are left in. A set of dividers may be given in exchange. |
| 7. | Put medications in a bag and place them with the chart. | |
| 8. | Remove the patient's imprinter card from the imprinter card holder and place with the chart forms. | If your hospital has the room number on the imprinter card, return the imprinter card to the admitting department for imprinting of new room number. Indicate the change to be made on a piece of paper and attach the paper to the imprinter card with a paper clip before forwarding it. |
| 9. | Notify all departments that perform regularly scheduled treatments on the patient. | |
| 10. | Indicate the transfer on the diet sheet or in the computer and on the TPR sheet. | |
| 11. | Notify environmental services to clean the room. | Environmental services may be notified by telephone, computer, or by checking the admission, discharge, and transfer book. |
| 12. | Notify the attending physician, the switchboard, the information desk, the flower desk, and the mail room of the transfer. | The admitting department may prepare an admission, discharge, and transfer list to be circulated to the switchboard, the information desk, the flower desk, and the mail room. |

## TRANSFER PROCEDURE TO ANOTHER ROOM ON THE SAME UNIT

| Step | Task | Notes |
|------|------|-------|
| 1. | Transcribe the order for the transfer. | |
| 2. | Notify the nurse caring for the patient when request for transfer is granted. | |
| 3. | Remove patient's chart from chart holder and place it in chart holder labeled with the new room number. | |
| 4. | Place all Kardex forms in their new places in the Kardex form holders. | |
| 5. | Indicate change on the diet sheet or in the computer and on the TPR sheet. | |
| 6. | Record the transfer in the unit admission, discharge, and transfer book, and on the census sheet and/or the computer. | |
| 7. | Notify environmental services to clean the room. | Environmental services may be notified by telephone or by checking the admission, discharge, or transfer book. |
| 8. | Notify the switchboard and the information center of the change. | The admitting department in some hospitals notifies the switchboard and the information center of all transfers. |

## PROCEDURE FOR RECEIVING A TRANSFERRED PATIENT

| Step | Task | Notes |
|------|------|-------|
| 1. | Notify the nurse caring for the patient of the expected arrival of a transferred patient. | If your facility does not assign each patient to a room but transfers to the unit only, the nurse manager or charge nurse will tell you where to place the patient. |
| 2. | Introduce yourself to the transferred patient upon his or her arrival on the unit. | |
| 3. | Notify the nurse caring for the patient of the transferred patient's arrival. | |
| 4. | Place the patient's chart in the correct chart holder.<br>a. Label the chart with the patient's name, the doctor's name, and the health records number.<br>b. Place allergy label on front of chart. | If the chart dividers have been removed before transfer, place chart forms behind the proper dividers. |
| 5. | Place all Kardex forms in the proper places. | |
| 6. | Note the receiving of a transfer patient in the unit admission, discharge, and transfer book and on the census sheet. | |
| 7. | Place the patient's name on the diet sheet or in the computer and on the TPR sheet. | |
| 8. | Place the imprinter card in the imprinter card holder. | |
| 9. | Transcribe any new doctors' orders. | When a patient is transferred from an intensive care unit to a regular unit the doctor must write new orders. The intensive care unit orders are to be discontinued. |

The box on p. 382 lists tasks related to the death of a patient which may be performed by the health unit coordinator.

Upon completion of the preceding tasks, the regular discharge procedure is carried out.

---

### HIGHLIGHT

Five Types of Discharges
- Home
- To another facility
- Home with assistance
- Against medical advice
- Expiration

AMA and expiration do not require a doctor's order.

---

## TRANSFER OF A PATIENT

A variety of circumstances may necessitate a patient transfer. A patient condition may change; a patient improves and is transferred out of intensive care. A patient may need a private room for infection control or isolation. A patient may be transferred if their original room request becomes available; the patient wanted a semiprivate room that is now available. A patient may be transferred due to roommate incompatibilities.

In Chapter 18, you had the opportunity to transcribe orders related to the transfer of patients within the hospital. The clerical duties performed in a series of tasks allow for an orderly transfer of the patient from one area to another.

Transfer may be from one unit of the hospital to another, or it may be from one room to another on the same nursing unit.

The tasks that may be performed for the transfer of a patient from one hospital unit to another are listed in the box on p. 388.

## SUMMARY

The health unit coordinator's duties for discharge and transfer procedures are many. If you learn these procedures in a particular order and do not deviate from it, you can be sure that you will always perform the tasks thoroughly and completely.

---

### REVIEW QUESTIONS

1. List 14 tasks performed in a routine discharge of a patient from the hospital.
   a. _transcribe discharge order_
   b. _notify the patient being discharged's nurse_
   c. _notify admitting or discharge desk_
   d. _explain discharge procedure to patient or patient relatives_
   e. _notify other dept giving treatment to the patient of the discharge_
   f. _notify the dietary dept_
   g. _arrange clinical appointment at Drs request_
   h. _arrange transportation if needed_
   i. _prepare credit slips for unused return of equipment supplies, med_
   j. _notify nursing personel or transportation service to transport_
   k. _write the patients name in unit admission discharge + transfer b_
   l. _Delete name from patient TRR sheet_
   m. _notify environmental to clean the discharged patients room_
   n. _Prepare the chart to send to health records department_

2. AMA is the abbreviation for __against medical advice__

3. ECF is the abbreviation for __extended care facility__

4. Describe the duties of the health unit coordinator in the preparation of the discharged patient's chart for the health records department.

check the summary sheet for physicians summation of patient. Note that all forms are imprinted with the same imprinter card

5. List the additional tasks performed when a patient is discharged to a nursing home.

arange transportation
Initiate continuing care forms
Photo copy portions of the chart requested by doctor
place forms in sealed envelope for transportation to nursing home

6. List the additional tasks when a patient is discharged home with assistance.

7. Define the following:
   a. shroud  a covering for a dead body

   b. terminal illness  illness ending in death

   c. expiration  to die

   d. postmortem  after a death

   e. custodial care  care & services that consist of bathing, feeding, watching and protecting the patient

   f. autopsy  examination internally and externally of a dead body

   g. organ donation  donating organs or tissue after death for reharvesting

   h. release of remains  a consent authorized to remove a body from the healthcare facility to the funeral home

i. coroner's case ___a death due to sudden, violent or unexplained circumstances___

j. extended care facility ___medical facility caring for patients requiring expert nursing care or custodial care___

8. List six tasks performed upon the death of a patient.

a. ___contact patients physician for verification of patients death___

b. ___prepare any forms that may be needed___

c. ___notify mortuary requested by family___

d. ___obtain shroud pack if needed___

e. ___gather deceased clothing bag it and label it___

f. ___obtain mortuary book or fill out mortuary form for the mortician on his arrival___

9. Describe the duties performed in the transfer of a patient from one room to another room on the same unit.

_____

_____

_____

_____

_____

_____

_____

_____

_____

10. List 12 tasks that are performed in the transfer of a patient from one unit to another unit.

a. _____

_____

b. _____

_____

c. _____

_____

d. _____

_____

e. _____

f. _____

g. _____

h. _____

i. _____

j. _____

k. _____

l. _____

11. List nine tasks performed when a transferred patient is received on the unit.

a. _____

b. _____

c. _____

d. _____

e. _____

f. _____

g. _____

h. _____

i. _____

## References

Cox, K. L.: *The Hospital Research and Educational Trust: Being a Health Unit Coordinator*, rev. ed. Englewood Cliffs, NJ, Prentice-Hall, Inc., 1991.

Miller, Benjamin F. and Keane, Claire Brackman: *Encyclopedia and Dictionary of Medicine and Nursing*, 3rd ed. Philadelphia, W. B. Saunders Co., 1983.

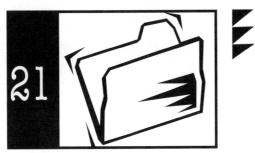
# RECORDING VITAL SIGNS, ORDERING DIETS, SUPPLIES, DAILY LABORATORY TESTS, AND FILING

*Upon completion of this chapter, you will be able to:*

1. Define the terms in the vocabulary list.
2. Write the meaning of each abbreviation in the abbreviations list.
3. Describe the health unit coordinator's responsibilities for recording the vital signs and other information on the patient's graphic sheet.
4. Explain the correct procedure for correcting three kinds of errors on the graphic sheet.
5. Convert Fahrenheit scale to Celsius scale, and Celsius scale to Fahrenheit scale.
6. Describe the health unit coordinator's responsibilities for ordering the mealtime diets.
7. List two reasons for efficient, accurate filing of the records on the patient's chart.
8. List four guidelines for filing the records on the patient's chart.
9. Compare the health unit coordinator's responsibilities in ordering the daily laboratory tests to those involved in ordering the other laboratory tests.
10. Name five hospital departments that may provide supplies to the nursing unit, and write the type of supplies that may be obtained from each department.
11. Briefly explain two systems for restocking the supplies on the nursing unit.

**Bowel Movement** • The passage of stool

**Celsius** • A scale used to measure temperature in which the freezing point of water is 0° and the boiling point is 100° (formerly called centigrade)

**Daily TPRs** • Taking each client's temperature, pulse, and respiration at a certain time(s) each day

**Diet Change Sheet** • A form used by the nursing unit to order the patient's meals three times a day from the dietary department

**Fahrenheit** • A scale used to measure temperature in which 32° is the freezing point of water and 212° is the boiling point

**Pulse Deficit** • The difference between the radial pulse and the apical heartbeat

**Stool** • The body wastes from the digestive tract that are discharged from the body through the anus

*8 Am*
*4 Pm*

## A B B R E V I A T I O N S

| Abbreviation | Meaning |
| --- | --- |
| BM | bowel movement |
| C | Celsius |
| Days aft. Ad. | days after admission |
| Days aft. Op. | days after operation |
| F | Fahrenheit |
| PO Day | postoperative day |
| PP | postpartum |
| TPR(s) | temperature, pulse, and respiration |

## RECORDING THE VITAL SIGNS AND OTHER DATA ON THE GRAPHIC SHEET

In Chapter 10 we discussed what vital signs are, different methods for obtaining them, and doctors' orders relating to vital signs.

Review the terms and abbreviations relating to vital signs presented in the vocabulary and abbreviations lists (Chapter 10), and the doctors' orders relating to vital signs written under the heading "Doctors' Orders for Nursing Observation" (Chapter 10).

It is hospital routine to take each patient's temperature, pulse, respiration (TPR), and blood pressure (BP) once (8:00 AM) or twice (8:00 AM and 4:00 PM) each day (according to hospital policy), to monitor the patient's condition. This process is often referred to as routine vital signs. If the doctor wishes the vital signs to be observed more often than the routine set forth by the hospital, he or she writes the order for such.

The normal vital signs vary from one person to another; however, the following values are considered normal: temperature 98.6°F or 37°C (Table 21–1); pulse: 60–80; respiration: 16–20; and blood pressure: 120/80.

It is routine to check each client for bowel movements daily and to record this information along with the daily vital signs. If the doctor has ordered the patient to be weighed daily, this is also done routinely with the morning vital signs.

The usual practice in most health care facilities is for the nurse caring for the patient to both take the vital signs and record them directly onto the graphic record form. In some instances, the nurse records the vital signs and other information in a unit vital signs book or on a sheet (Fig. 21–1). It is then the health unit coordinator's task to record the data from the vital signs sheet onto each patient's graphic record form. The process is often referred to as recording the vital signs, or recording vital signs.

The health unit coordinator should record the vital signs and other data as soon as it is recorded on the vital signs sheet so that the information is readily available to the doctors when they make their hospital rounds. *Accuracy in the transfer of the vital signs is a must*, as the doctor may use this information to prescribe treatment for the patient.

### TABLE 21–1   CELSIUS/FAHRENHEIT TEMPERATURE EQUIVALENTS

| °C | °F | °C | °F | °C | °F | °C | °F |
| --- | --- | --- | --- | --- | --- | --- | --- |
| 34.0 | 93.2 | 35.8 | 96.4 | 37.6 | 99.7 | 39.4 | 102.9 |
| 34.1 | 93.4 | 35.9 | 96.6 | 37.7 | 99.9 | 39.5 | 103.1 |
| 34.2 | 93.6 | 36.0 | 96.8 | 37.8 | 100.0 | 39.6 | 103.3 |
| 34.3 | 93.7 | 36.1 | 97.0 | 37.9 | 100.2 | 39.7 | 103.5 |
| 34.4 | 93.9 | 36.2 | 97.2 | 38.0 | 100.4 | 39.8 | 103.6 |
| 34.5 | 94.1 | 36.3 | 97.3 | 38.1 | 100.6 | 39.9 | 103.8 |
| 34.6 | 94.3 | 36.4 | 97.5 | 38.2 | 100.8 | 40.0 | 104.0 |
| 34.7 | 94.5 | 36.5 | 97.7 | 38.3 | 100.9 | 40.1 | 104.2 |
| 34.8 | 94.6 | 36.6 | 97.9 | 38.4 | 101.1 | 40.2 | 104.4 |
| 34.9 | 94.8 | 36.7 | 98.1 | 38.5 | 101.3 | 40.3 | 104.5 |
| 35.0 | 95.0 | 36.8 | 98.2 | 38.6 | 101.5 | 40.4 | 104.7 |
| 35.1 | 95.2 | 36.9 | 98.4 | 38.7 | 101.7 | 40.5 | 104.9 |
| 35.2 | 95.4 | 37.0 | 98.6 | 38.8 | 101.8 | 40.6 | 105.1 |
| 35.3 | 95.5 | 37.1 | 98.8 | 38.9 | 102.0 | 40.7 | 105.3 |
| 35.4 | 95.7 | 37.2 | 99.0 | 39.0 | 102.2 | 40.8 | 105.4 |
| 35.5 | 95.9 | 37.3 | 99.1 | 39.1 | 102.4 | 40.9 | 105.6 |
| 35.6 | 96.1 | 37.4 | 99.3 | 39.2 | 102.6 | 41.0 | 105.8 |
| 35.7 | 96.3 | 37.5 | 99.5 | 39.3 | 102.7 | | |

Most often the temperature is taken and recorded using the Fahrenheit scale, but is sometimes taken and recorded on the Celsius scale, also known as the centigrade scale. There may be times when the health unit coordinator will have to convert the temperature from one scale to another. The following conversion formula is used to convert Fahrenheit to Celsius and Celsius to Fahrenheit. Using this formula, a temperature of 98.6° Fahrenheit converts to 37.0° on the Celsius scale.

**Conversion of F to C**

Subtract 32
Multiply by 5
Divide by 9

**Conversion of C to F**

Multiply by 9
Divide by 5
Add 32

## Method for Correcting Errors on the Graphic Sheet

Minor graphic errors may be corrected on the original graphic sheet. However, correction of major errors may require that the original graphic sheet be recopied. The following procedure for correcting errors should be followed.

1. To correct a *minor error on the graphic portion* of the graphic sheet, write "mistaken entry" in ink on the incorrect connecting line, record your first initial, your last name and status about the error, then graph the correct value (see Fig. 21–2).
2. To correct a *numbered entry*, such as the respiration value, draw a line through the entry in ink and write in ink "mistaken entry," your first initial, your last name, and status near it. As close as possible, insert the correct numbers (see Fig. 21–2).

| Rm. No. | NAME | BM | WT | 8:00 A.M. | | | | 12:00 Noon | | | | 4:00 P.M. | | | | 8:00 P.M. | | | |
|---|---|---|---|---|---|---|---|---|---|---|---|---|---|---|---|---|---|---|---|
| | | | | T | P | R | BP | T | P | R | BP | T | P | R | BP | T | P | R | BP |
| 301 | Breach Les | ÷ | | 37 | 80 | 18 | 144/80 | 37 | 82 | 18 | | | | | | | | | |
| 302 | Katt Kitty | ÷o | 120 | 36.6 | 96 | 24 | | | | | | | | | | | | | |
| 303 | Pickens Slim | ÷ii | | 36.8 | 70 | 18 | | | | | | | | | | | | | |
| 304 | Bee Mae | ÷o | | 37 | 82 | 16 | | | | | | | | | | | | | |
| 305 | Honey Mai | ÷o | | 37.2 | 96 | 22 | 122/68 | 37.1 | 96 | 18 | | | | | | | | | |
| 306 | Net Clair | ÷ | | 35.9 | 72 | 18 | | | | | | | | | | | | | |
| 307 | Ibaul Iris | ÷ | | 39 | 102 | 18 | | 37.4 | 80 | 18 | | | | | | | | | |
| 308 | Christmas Mary | ÷iii | | 36.9 | 88 | 20 | | | | | | | | | | | | | |
| 309 | Nerve Lotta | ÷ | | 39.1 | 90 | 24 | | 38.4 | 88 | 20 | | | | | | | | | |
| 310-1 | Sofortche Anne | ÷ | | 38.8 | 92 | 18 | 140/88 | | | | | | | | | | | | |
| 310-2 | Soo Ah | ÷o | 144 | 35.7 | 80 | 20 | | | | | | | | | | | | | |
| 311-1 | Buggy June | ÷ii | | 38.6 | 100 | 18 | | 38.9 | 80 | 20 | | | | | | | | | |
| 311-2 | Kynde Bee | ÷ | | 37.4 | 94 | 16 | | 37 | 80 | 20 | | | | | | | | | |
| 312-1 | Cider Ida | ÷ | | 36.4 | 80 | 18 | 120/80 | | | | | | | | | | | | |
| 312-2 | Saynt Joanne | ÷ | 200 | 36 | 74 | 20 | | | | | | | | | | | | | |

FIGURE 21–1 • A TPR sheet with the 8:00 AM and 12:00 noon data recorded on it. The straight line drawn through the values indicates that the information has been recorded (Celsius temperature scale).

3. To correct a *series of errors* on the graphic sheet, the entire sheet needs to be recopied showing the correct data (see Fig. 21–3).

   a. Imprint a new sheet with the patient's imprinter card (Fig. 21–3B).

   b. Transfer in ink *all* the information onto the new graphic sheet, including the correction of errors (Fig. 21–3B).

   c. Draw a diagonal line through the old graphic sheet in ink and record in ink "mistaken entry" on the line (Fig. 21–3A).

   d. Write that the graphic sheet was recopied, and write in ink your name, your status, and the date on the old graphic sheet (Fig. 21–3A).

   e. Place the old sheet in the back of the chart holder; it remains a permanent part of the chart.

   f. Write "recopied" followed by your name, status, and the date in ink on the new graphic sheet (Fig.

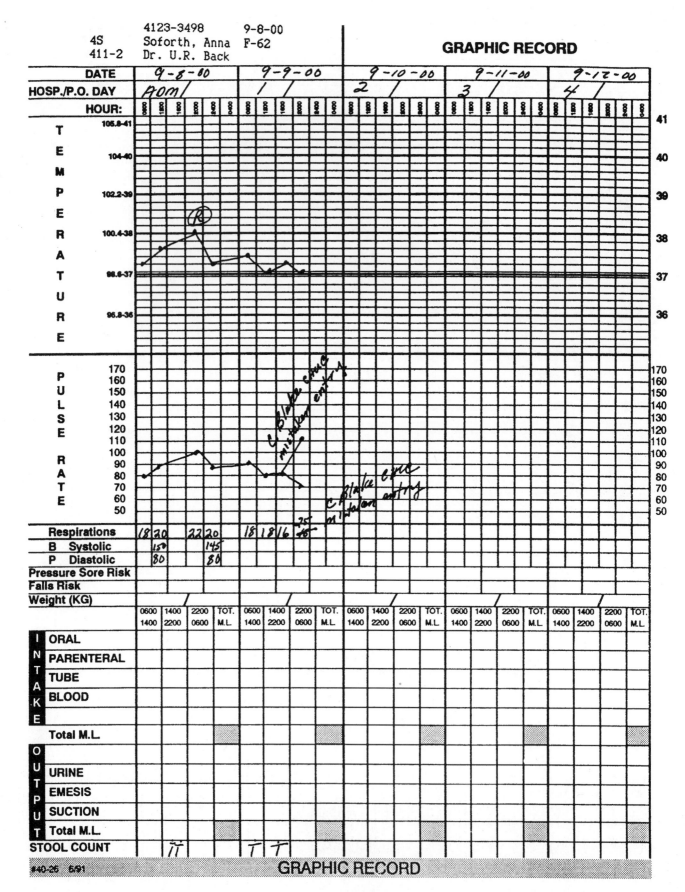

FIGURE 21–2 • An example for the correction of minor errors on the graphic sheet.

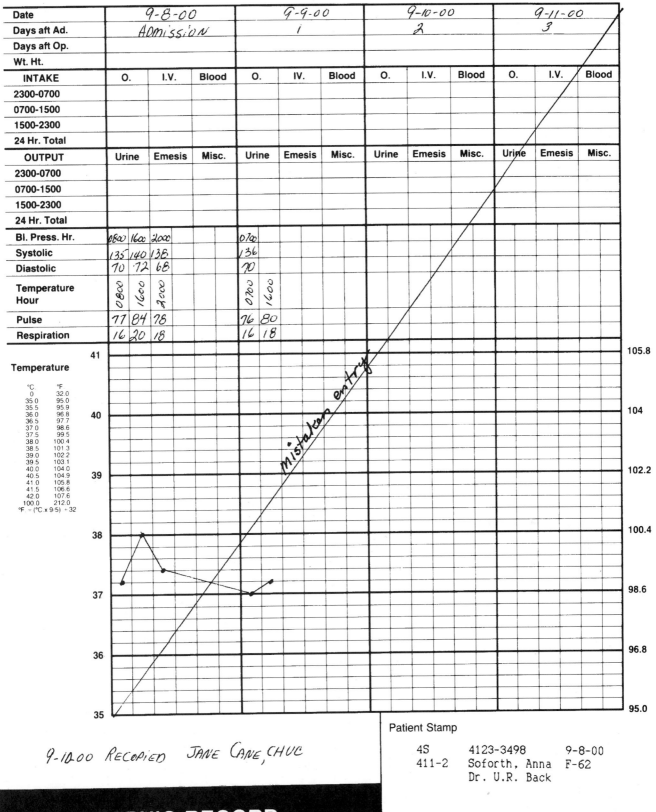

| Date | 9-8-00 | | | 9-9-00 | | | 9-10-00 | | | 9-11-00 | | |
|---|---|---|---|---|---|---|---|---|---|---|---|---|
| Days aft Ad. | ADMISSION | | | 1 | | | 2 | | | 3 | | |
| Days aft Op. | | | | | | | | | | | | |
| Wt. Ht. | | | | | | | | | | | | |
| INTAKE | O. | I.V. | Blood | O. | IV. | Blood | O. | I.V. | Blood | O. | I.V. | Blood |
| 2300-0700 | | | | | | | | | | | | |
| 0700-1500 | | | | | | | | | | | | |
| 1500-2300 | | | | | | | | | | | | |
| 24 Hr. Total | | | | | | | | | | | | |
| OUTPUT | Urine | Emesis | Misc. | Urine | Emesis | Misc. | Urine | Emesis | Misc. | Urine | Emesis | Misc. |
| 2300-0700 | | | | | | | | | | | | |
| 0700-1500 | | | | | | | | | | | | |
| 1500-2300 | | | | | | | | | | | | |
| 24 Hr. Total | | | | | | | | | | | | |
| Bl. Press. Hr. | 0800 | 1600 | 2000 | 0700 | | | | | | | | |
| Systolic | 135 | 140 | 138 | 136 | | | | | | | | |
| Diastolic | 70 | 72 | 68 | 70 | | | | | | | | |
| Temperature Hour | 0800 | 1600 | 2000 | 0700 | 1600 | | | | | | | |
| Pulse | 77 | 84 | 78 | 76 | 80 | | | | | | | |
| Respiration | 16 | 20 | 18 | 16 | 18 | | | | | | | |

Temperature

| °C. | °F |
|---|---|
| 0 | 32.0 |
| 35.0 | 95.0 |
| 35.5 | 95.9 |
| 36.0 | 96.8 |
| 36.5 | 97.7 |
| 37.0 | 98.6 |
| 37.5 | 99.5 |
| 38.0 | 100.4 |
| 38.5 | 101.3 |
| 39.0 | 102.2 |
| 39.5 | 103.1 |
| 40.0 | 104.0 |
| 40.5 | 104.9 |
| 41.0 | 105.8 |
| 41.5 | 106.6 |
| 42.0 | 107.6 |
| 100.0 | 212.0 |

°F = (°C. x 9·5) ÷ 32

*mistaken entry*

9-10-00 RECOPIED    JANE CANE, CHUC

Patient Stamp

4S         4123-3498        9-8-00
411-2      Soforth, Anna    F-62
           Dr. U.R. Back

**GRAPHIC RECORD**

A

FIGURE 21-3 • An example of a recopied graphic sheet used to correct a series of errors. (A) The original graphic sheet. *Illustration continued on following page*

| Date | 9-8-00 | | | 9-9-00 | | | 9-10-00 | | | 9-11-00 | | |
|---|---|---|---|---|---|---|---|---|---|---|---|---|
| Days aft Ad. | ADmission | | | 1 | | | 2 | | | 3 | | |
| Days aft Op. | | | | | | | | | | | | |
| Wt. Ht. | | | | | | | | | | | | |
| **INTAKE** | O. | I.V. | Blood | O. | IV. | Blood | O. | I.V. | Blood | O. | I.V. | Blood |
| 2300-0700 | | | | | | | | | | | | |
| 0700-1500 | | | | | | | | | | | | |
| 1500-2300 | | | | | | | | | | | | |
| 24 Hr. Total | | | | | | | | | | | | |
| **OUTPUT** | Urine | Emesis | Misc. | Urine | Emesis | Misc. | Urine | Emesis | Misc. | Urine | Emesis | Misc. |
| 2300-0700 | | | | | | | | | | | | |
| 0700-1500 | | | | | | | | | | | | |
| 1500-2300 | | | | | | | | | | | | |
| 24 Hr. Total | | | | | | | | | | | | |
| Bl. Press. Hr. | 0800 1600 2000 | | | 0700 | | | | | | | | |
| Systolic | 135  140  160 | | | 125 | | | | | | | | |
| Diastolic | 70  72  88 | | | 90 | | | | | | | | |
| Temperature Hour | | | | 0700  0900 | | | | | | | | |
| Pulse | | | | 80  60 | | | | | | | | |
| Respiration | | | | 20  22 | | | | | | | | |

**Temperature**

| °C | °F. |
|---|---|
| 0 | 32.0 |
| 35.0 | 95.0 |
| 35.5 | 95.9 |
| 36.0 | 96.8 |
| 36.5 | 97.7 |
| 37.0 | 98.6 |
| 37.5 | 99.5 |
| 38.0 | 100.4 |
| 38.5 | 101.3 |
| 39.0 | 102.2 |
| 39.5 | 103.1 |
| 40.0 | 104.0 |
| 40.5 | 104.9 |
| 41.0 | 105.8 |
| 41.5 | 106.6 |
| 42.0 | 107.6 |
| 100.0 | 212.0 |

°F. = (°C x 9/5) + 32

9-10-00   RECOPIED   JANE CRANE, CHUC

## GRAPHIC RECORD

B

FIGURE 21-3 • *Continued*   (*B*) A copied graphic sheet.

21–3B), and place it behind the correct divider in the patient's chart.

## ORDERING DIETS FOR MEALTIME

Many hospitals require that daily diets be ordered approximately 2 hours prior to each mealtime.

To order the mealtime diets, the health unit coordinator checks each diet ordered for the client on the **diet change sheet**, under the heading diet order (Fig. 21–4) with the current diet order on the patient's Kardex form. The diet change sheet is usually initiated during the 11 PM to 7:30 AM shift; therefore checking with the Kardex form reflects any new diet changes. Diet changes from the previous mealtime are recorded in the appropriate column (breakfast, lunch, or dinner) on the diet change sheet. Patient admission, discharge, and transfer, and patients who are NPO for diagnostic studies or surgery are also considered diet changes and must be recorded on the diet change sheet. The appropriate copy of the diet change sheet (breakfast, lunch, or dinner) is then forwarded to the dietary department for use in preparing each patient's tray. For computerized nursing units, diet changes are sent directly to the diet department (via the computer) as each individual patient's order is transcribed.

Order mealtime diets at the same time each day. For example, at 9:30 AM leave other tasks and complete the diet change sheet and forward it to the dietary department. This gives the dietary department sufficient time to prepare the patient's trays for mealtime. Also, ordering diets at the same time each day prevents you from forgetting to perform the task and having to catch up later, which would interfere with both your own work schedule and that of the dietary department.

Guest trays may be requistioned from the dietary department for guests who want to eat in the room with the hospitalized patient. A requisition form (Fig. 21–5) is used to order the tray and for charging purposes.

On pediatric units the nursing mother may receive a meal tray. Because dietary cost is included in the room rate, the nursing mother's tray is ordered in the patient's name. Unlike a guest tray, this tray is not billed separately.

## FILING RECORDS ON THE PATIENT'S CHART

Each day the nursing unit receives many written records, such as diagnostic results and history and physical reports to be filed on the patient's chart. Efficient, accurate filing on the patient's chart is necessary for two reasons. First, during the patient's hospital stay, the filed written records are readily available for use by the attending physician and other hospital personnel. Second, upon the patient's discharge, the health records department personnel have the legal responsibility of assembling and storing *all* records produced during the patient's hospital stay. Correct filing methods used during the patient's hospitalization assist the health records personnel to complete this task.

Below are listed guidelines for filing records on the patient's chart on the nursing unit.

### Guidelines for Filing Records on the Patient's Chart

■ *File at the same time each day.* Filing near the end of the shift allows you to file all the records received during the shift at one time. It is important for the nurse in charge to see all laboratory results as soon as they arrive on the nursing unit.

■ *Separate the records according to the patient's name.* This prepares you to file all the records for a given patient at one time, so that you need obtain and open the chart holder only once.

■ *Always check the patient's name on the chart back with the name on the record before filing it.* Never select the chart by the room number recorded on the record, since the room number on the record is incorrect if the patient has been transferred to another bed on the nursing unit after the records were initiated. Often a doctor prescribes treatment according to test results.

---

**H I G H L I G H T**

Be especially alert when there are two patients on the unit with the same name. When this happens, both patient's charts are flagged with a "name alert" sticker. File all medical record's by their medical records number. Many times you will have patients with the same or very similar names on your nursing unit. The medical records number will never be duplicated.

---

■ *Place the record behind the correct chart holder.* Use consistent sequencing in filing the reports on the patient's charts, to make it easier for the doctor and other health personnel to locate them. Reports are filed either to read like a book, or the reverse—that is, the latest report is filed in front, right behind the divider.

■ *Initial all records you file.* Follow the policy in your health care facility about *where* on the form you should place your initials.

**DIET CHANGE SHEET**

DAY  _Sunday_          DATE  _6-4-00_          UNIT  _3E_

| Room | Name | Diet Order | Breakfast | Lunch | Dinner |
|------|------|-----------|-----------|-------|--------|
| 301 | ~~Robett Harry~~ ~~Breach Les~~ | Reg | Transferred from | 400-1 ✓ | Reg home |
| 302 | Katt Kitty | High Potassium | ✓ | ✓ | ✓ |
| 303 | Pickens Slim | Clear liq | ✓ | Full liq | ✓ |
| 304 | Bee Mae | NPO surg | ✓ | ✓ | ✓ |
| 305 | Honey Mai | Soft | NPO diagnostic test | resume Soft | ✓ |
| 306 | ~~Stone John~~ ~~Flot Clair~~ | Reg | | ✓ | ✓ | admission diet home |
| 307 | Ibaul Iris | Mechanical soft | ✓ | ✓ | ✓ |
| 308 | Christmas Mary | 1000 cal | ✓ | ✓ | ✓ |
| 309 | Nerve Lotta | 2500mg Na | ✓ | ✓ | ✓ |
| 310-1 | Soforche Anne | Reg | NPO diagnostic test | Reg resume | ✓ |
| 310-2 | Soo Ah | Reg force fluids | ✓ | ✓ | ✓ |
| 311-1 | Bugg June | NPO surg | ✓ | ✓ | cl liq |
| 311-2 | Kynde Bee | Full liq | ✓ | soft | ✓ |
| 312-1 | Cider Ida | Bland | ✓ | ✓ | ✓ |
| 312-2 | Saynt Joanne | Modified fiber | ✓ | ✓ | ✓ |

| FS-100 |
|--------|
| **DINNER** |

| FS-100 |
|--------|
| **BREAKFAST** |

| FS-100 |
|--------|
| **LUNCH** |

| FS-100 |
|--------|
| **NURSING** |

F I G U R E  21-4 • A diet change sheet, which has been used to order the patient's breakfast, lunch, and dinner for one day.

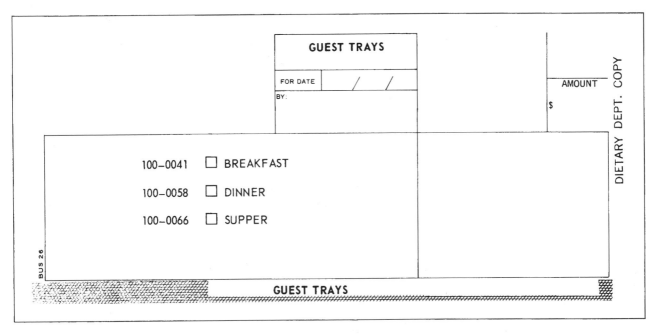

FIGURE 21–5 • A guest tray requisition.

Unfiled records for patients who have been discharged should be forwarded to the health records department. Unfiled records for patients who have been transferred within the hospital should be forwarded to the receiving unit. *Never discard any patient's record.* If in doubt, check with the nurse in charge or with the health records department.

┌──────────────────────────────┐
│     T O   T H E   S T U D E N T     │
└──────────────────────────────┘

To practice filing records on the patient's charts, complete **Activity 21–4** in the Skills Practice Manual.

## ORDERING DAILY LABORATORY TESTS

In Chapter 14, "Laboratory Orders," you practiced transcription of many different types of laboratory orders, including doctors' orders for daily laboratory tests. As you recall, daily laboratory tests are repeated each day until they are discontinued by the doctor, as compared with other laboratory tests, which are ordered one time only. It is the health unit coordinator's task to continue to order the daily laboratory tests each day until the order is cancelled by the doctor.

To order daily laboratory tests, check each patient's Kardex form (Fig. 21–6) and enter the test in the computer or fill out the appropriate laboratory requisition form every day. Some computer systems allow you to enter daily tests one time, thereby saving the health unit coordinator a daily entry. Note on the Kardex that the daily laboratory

test has been ordered for the following day. Each unit has a method of indicating that daily laboratory orders have been ordered.

Ordering the daily laboratory tests may be the task of either the day or the evening shift health unit coordinator. The ordering should be done at a certain time each day to avoid omission; if done on the day shift, it should be scheduled toward the end of the day, to allow for possible cancellation of the order by the doctor.

┌──────────────────────────────┐
│     T O   T H E   S T U D E N T     │
└──────────────────────────────┘

To practice ordering daily laboratory tests, complete **Activity 21–5** in the Skills Practice Manual.

## ORDERING SUPPLIES FOR THE NURSING UNIT

As you can imagine, a busy nursing unit stocks a variety of supplies to keep the unit functioning smoothly. Nursing unit supplies are obtained from the purchasing department, the central service department, the dietary department, the pharmacy, and the laundry department.

Two systems for restocking the supplies are used. One system is for the health unit coordinator to determine the supplies needed and order them from the supplying department; the other is for the supplying department to make rounds throughout the hospital and restock the supply as needed (similar to restocking shelves in a grocery store).

An aspect to be considered regarding supplies is who pays for them. Some items, such as catheter trays and

| DATE ORD. | TREATMENTS | DATE ORD. | DIAGNOSTIC STUDIES | TO BE DONE |
|---|---|---|---|---|
| 6-1 | K-pad to left shoulder | 6-1 | CBC  UA  Chest xray | |
| | | 6-2 | T3 uptake | |
| | | | | |
| | | | | |
| | | | | |
| | | 6-1 | * Daily Hg + Hct | |

| DATE | | DIAGNOSTIC RESULTS | |
|---|---|---|---|

860 - 25

**F I G U R E   21–6** • Kardex form with a daily laboratory order recorded on it.

medications, are usually paid for by the client, whereas other items, such as requisition forms, hand soap, paper clips, and so forth, are paid for from the nursing unit budget. Requisition forms are often used for items charged to the patient for billing and restocking purposes. Failure to complete the requisition form on items normally charged to the patient usually results in the cost being deducted from the nursing unit's budget. Carelessness in this area may play havoc with the overall management of money for the nursing unit supplies.

## Purchasing Department Supplies

Purchasing department supplies consist of nonnursing items, such as chart and requisition forms, pencils, staples, flashlights, and numerous other items. See Figure 21–7 for an example of a purchasing department order form. Items received from the purchasing department are usually paid for from the nursing unit budget. A cost control center number for the nursing unit is placed on all requisitions issued from the unit. Restocking of purchasing department supplies is done weekly or bimonthly and is the most demanding of all the supply areas.

## Central Service Department Supplies

Central service department supplies consist of items used for nursing procedures that are either charged to the patient or charged to the nursing unit's budget. Items charged to the patient, such as catheter trays and irrigation trays, usually have a requisition form with them. (See Fig. 11–2 for examples of CSD requisitions.) Smaller items,

such as Band-Aids, tongue blades, alcohol, and sponges, are a part of the nursing unit's budget.

A recent trend is for many frequently used disposable nursing items (such as catheter trays and enema bags), usually supplied by the central service department, to be obtained directly from the purchasing department. As you know, the purchasing department originally buys all hospital supplies; therefore, this method of bypassing the central service department is both efficient and economical.

## Pharmacy Supplies

The pharmacy supplies include all medications administered to the patients. Medications are kept on the nursing unit in three classifications: (1) the controlled substances, which are locked in the narcotics cupboard or in a computerized dispensing cart; (2) the other daily and prn medications currently being administered to the patients according to the doctors' orders; and (3) a unit stock supply of frequently used medications, such as aspirin. Restocking of daily medications is usually performed on a daily basis and the stock supply is replenished as needed. The patient is charged for medications that he or she has received, and therefore pharmacy supplies are not a part of the nursing unit's budget. The charges, which cover the cost of administration supplies, such as needles and syringes, are usually determined from the patient's medication record sheet.

## Dietary Department Supplies

Dietary department supplies include food items such as milk, orange juice, and ginger ale that are stored in the

STANDARD REGISTER
STOCKLESS FORMS REQUISITION

NO. 01132

| NAME OF REQUESTOR | TELEPHONE NO. | AUTHORIZED SIGNATURE | DATE ORDERED |
|---|---|---|---|
| DEPARTMENT NAME | BUILDING/LOCATION | FLOOR | COST CENTER |

.460

**Column group 1**

| QTY | UNIT OF MEASURE | FORM NUMBER | DESCRIPTION |
|---|---|---|---|
| | 500/BX | 2044 | ENV BLUE #9 SPEC WINDOW |
| | 500/BX | 2045 | ENV INTER OFFICE BLUE #10 |
| | 1/EA | 2046 | ENV INTER OFFICE MAN/10x13 |
| | 500/BX | 2051 | ENV MANILLA PAYROLL WIND |
| | 500/BX | 2061 | ENV WHITE ST JOSEPH #10 |
| | 1000/ROLL | 2093 | LABEL WHT 2-7/8 x 1-7/16 |
| | 500/PK | 2177 | ST JOSEPH LETTERHEAD |
| | 500/BX | 2881 | ENV WHITE #9 OUTGOING |
| | 1000/CTN | 3224 | PURCH 5 PT PAPER COLOR |
| | 500/BX | 3387 | ENV WT WINDOW #10 PAT ACT |
| | 2000/PK | 3481 | LABEL-ADDRESSOGRAPH-PACK |
| | 25/PK | 3623 | HIV CONSENT FORM |
| | 3000/CTN | 61911G | WARD REPORT |
| | 25/PD | ADM-1-4 | CLASS ATTENDANCE SHEET |
| | 1000/CTN | ADM-1104 | ST JOE OCCURRENCE RPT |
| | 10/PK | ADM-1196 | ESP GRAM |
| | 25/PK | ADM-1426 | EMPL EXP REINBURSE |
| | 50/PK | ADM-1775 | PATIENT COMPLAINT SHEET |
| | 100/PD | ADM-3-140 | WHILE YOU WERE OUT PAD |
| | 100/PD | ADM-503-127 | REQ SPEC FOOD SERV |
| | 100/PK | ADM-505 | SPEED MEMO |
| | 1930/CTN | ADMIT 1271 | PATIENT INFO |
| | 1000/CTN | ADMIT-1637 | 4 PT REQ INFO |
| | 100/PK | ADM-1-222 | OCCUPATIONAL THPY CHG |
| | 100/PK | BUS-10 | GENERAL X-RAY |
| | 200/PK | BUS-1000 | RADIOLOGY CONSULT |
| | 100/PK | BUS-1001 | SP PROC X-RAY |
| | 100/PK | BUS-1002 | DPT RAD CARDIO NUC MED |
| | 250/PK | BUS-1007 | GEN SERG DIAG CHGS |
| | 100/PK | BUS-1008 | CDV DIAG LAB |
| | 50/PK | BUS-1016 | EEG CHARGE SLIP |
| | 100/PK | BUS-15 | CONTROLLED DRUGS ORAL A |
| | 10/PK | BUS-1040 | CONTROLLED DRUGS II |
| | 10/PK | BUS-1045 | CONTROLLED DRUGS-INJECT |
| | 10/PK | BUS-1055 | MEDICARE AS 2nd PAYOR |
| | 100/PD | BUS-1057 | MEDICARE ADDENDUM A |
| | 1450/CTN | BUS-1057A | OP/PT CHRG-PROCEDURE |
| | 200/PK | BUS-1280 | BLOOD GAS LAB |
| | 250/PK | BUS-1476 | EEG CHARGE SLIP |
| | 100/PK | BUS-1597 | PERINATAL AMNI BLOOD TEST |
| | 100/PD | BUS-16-134 | PHYS MED CHGE SLIP |
| | 100/PD | BUS-178 | CONDITIONS FOR TREATMENT |
| | 2500/CTN | BUS-18 | PHARMACY CHARGE SLIP |
| | 100/PD | BUS-29-2 | MISC CHARGE SLIP |

**Column group 2**

| QTY | UNIT OF MEASURE | FORM NUMBER | DESCRIPTION |
|---|---|---|---|
| | 5700/CTN | BUS-30-135 | CREDIT SLIP |
| | 1300/CTN | BUS-33 | SPEECH OTOLOGY CHARGE |
| | 3000/CTN | BUS-35-295 | MEMO PADS |
| | 100/PD | BUS-35-295A | FULL SIZE MEMO PAD |
| | 4950/CTN | BUS-42 | BLOOD BANK CONTINUOUS |
| | 100/PK | BUS-42B | OUTPT LAB REQUISITION |
| | 100/PD | BUS-447 | NEW INV CODING SHEET |
| | 100/PD | BUS-448 | PREPAID A/C CODE |
| | 100/PK | BUS-50B | MICRO URNE FLDS LAB REQ |
| | 100/PD | BUS-510-143 | REQ FOR CK OR CASH |
| | 200/PK | BUS-53B | CHEM, HEMA, SEROLO LAB REQ |
| | 50/PK | BUS-60A | CYTOLOGY |
| | 100/PK | BUS-61 | TISSUES FORM |
| | 100/PK | BUS-63 | GENERAL SURGERY CHARGES |
| | 250/PK | BUS-641 | SPD CHARGE CARD |
| | 100/PK | BUS-674 | ER MEDICATION CHARGES |
| | 100/PK | BUS-677 | DELIVERY ROOM CHARGES |
| | 100/PD | BUS-817 | OCCUP THERAPY CHG SLIP |
| | 100/PK | CRS-1421 | GENERAL DIAGNOSTIC-CRS |
| | 950/CTN | CRS-1483 | CRS MTST PAPER |
| | 100/PK | CS-3-291 | NURSING CARE PLAN |
| | 100/PK | DORM-508 | DORM VISITATION SLIP |
| | 250/PK | DORM-510 | PRENATAL REC 2A MT ST |
| | 250/PK | DP-2-163 | BATCH HEADER/TRAILER |
| | 250/PK | DP-2-163C | BATCH HEADER/TRAILER BLUE |
| | 100/PD | DP-960 | CREDIT/DEBIT RECORD |
| | 100/PD | DP-962 | BALANCE TRANSFER |
| | 100/PD | DP-963 | CREDIT/DEBIT SHEET |
| | 250/PK | DP2-163B | BATCH HEADER/TRAILER PBS |
| | 100/PD | EEG-609 | PHYSICIAN TRANSCRIPTION |
| | 100/PD | ENG-445 | PLANT SERV SERVICE CALL |
| | 100/PD | ER-508-172 | PHONE REPORT OF LAB |
| | 500/PK | ER-514 | ER C/SERV ITEMS CHG SLIP |
| | 5000/CTN | FS-1427 | MENU LABEL |
| | 100/PD | HB-17-96 | WORK ORDERS |
| | 1450/CTN | HB-1720 | A/P BLUE |
| | 200/PK | HB-54 | RECEIPTS-PEGBOARD |
| | 250/PK | HB-55 | JOURNAL-PEGBOARD |
| | 100/PK | HRS-2027 | OPERATING ROOM PATH CONST |
| | 2500/CTN | LAB-1684 | 1 PART LAB REPORT |
| | 5000/CTN | LAB-1352 | LAB LABEL-GREEN, MULTI-CUT |
| | 5000/CTN | LAB-1353 | LAB LABEL-WHT, SINGLE CUT |
| | 2500/CTN | LAB-1354 | LAB LABEL-RED |
| | 1600/CTN | LAB-1428 | 12 PART CANARY-CONTINUOUS |

**Column group 3**

| QTY | UNIT OF MEASURE | FORM NUMBER | DESCRIPTION |
|---|---|---|---|
| | 50/PD | LAB-1557 | HEMO-CONTINUOUS |
| | 100/PD | LAB-1621 | 3 PART LAB REPORT |
| | 100/PD | LAB-1979 | PATHOLOGY REPORT-LASER |
| | 100/PD | LAB-501-79 | PATHOLOGY CONSULTATION |
| | 2500/CTN | LABEL-2-7/16 x 4 | WHITE LABEL 2-7/16 x 4 |
| | 100/PK | MD-17 | ADULT MCC ENCOUNTER |
| | 100/PK | MD-300-01 | MD PED HEME CHARGE |
| | 100/PK | MR-1-302 | SUMMARY SHEETS |
| | 100/PD | MR-10-303 | CONSENT TO OPERATION |
| | 100/PD | MR-1012 | ICU MEDICATION RECORD |
| | 200/PK | MR-1016 | MEDICATION REC UNIT DOSE |
| | 100/PK | MR-1017 | RESP THERAPY MOUNT SHEET |
| | 100/PD | MR-1019-232 | 24-HR NWBRN NURSERY OBS |
| | 100/PD | MR-1025-248 | NB DEFICENCY SLIP |
| | 100/PD | MR-1030-270 | OB DEFICENCY SLIP |
| | 100/PD | MR-11-41 | GEN/BNI ANESTHESIA RECORD |
| | 100/PK | MR-1117 | MEDICATION ADMIN RECORD |
| | 1350/CTN | MR-1134 | MED ADMINISTRATION REC |
| | 100/PK | MR-1142 | MATERNITY PT CARE PLAN |
| | 100/PK | MR-1156 | PHYSICIAN IN CHARGE |
| | 100/PK | MR-116 | PED ADMISSION ASSESSMENT |
| | 100/PK | MR-1262 | MATERNITY PT CARE SUP |
| | 100/PD | MR-1490 | NURSES CARE PLAN |
| | 250/PK | MR-1542 | DISCHG CARE PLAN WORKSHEET |
| | 100/PD | MR-18-304 | NURSES RECORD |
| | 100/PD | MR-19-305 | PROGRESS REPORT |
| | 50/PK | MR-1904 | BLANK FORM CARRIER |
| | 25/PK | MR-1904A | ATRIAL LABEL |
| | 25/PK | MR-1904ART | ARTERIAL LABEL |
| | 25/PK | MR-1904CVP | CVP LABEL |
| | 25/PK | MR-1904GP | GENERAL PURPOSE LABEL |
| | 25/PK | MR-1904ICP | ICP LABEL |
| | 50/PK | MR-1904IV | IV LABEL |
| | 10/PK | MR-1904PA | PA LABEL |
| | 250/PK | MR-20B-306 | BLUE MD ORDERS |
| | 200/PK | MR-20W-507 | WHITE MD ORDERS |
| | 100/PK | MR-210 | ADMISS STATUS REC DORM |
| | 100/PD | MR-245 | PRE ADMIT PHYS ORDERS |
| | 200/PK | MR-27 | FOLLOW UP INSTRUCTIONS |
| | 100/PK | MR-275 | LABOR-DELIVERY FORM |
| | 100/PD | MR-283 | HEMODYNAMIC FLOWSHEET |
| | 100/PK | MR-32 | ER CLINICAL RECORD |
| | 100/PK | MR-34-309 | RECOVERY RM RECORD |
| | 100/PK | MR-34A-318 | RECOVERY RM REC CONT |

**Column group 4**

| QTY | UNIT OF MEASURE | FORM NUMBER | DESCRIPTION |
|---|---|---|---|
| | 100/PK | MR-41-282 | CONSENT PHOTOG-PUBLS |
| | 100/PD | MR-417 | REQ FOR PRIOR ORDERS |
| | 100/PK | MR-43-216 | MEDICATION RECORD |
| | 100/PD | MR-46-158 | DIABETIC CHART |
| | 2850/CTN | MR-47 | DISCHARGE FINAL REPORT |
| | 2850/CTN | MR-48 | WEEKLY LAB SUMMARY |
| | 100/PK | MR-480 | PHYS PARENTERAL NUT ORDER |
| | 200/PK | MR-5 | LAB REPORT |
| | 100/PK | MR-509-98 | ADMISSION ASSESSMENT |
| | 500/CTN | MR-522 | 6-PLY MTST PAPER/CBNLESS |
| | 650/CTN | MR-522 | MTST 5-PT PAPER CBN |
| | 50/PD | MR-533 | MEDICAL RECORD OUT CARD |
| | 100/PK | MR-571 | VENTILATOR RESP THERAPY |
| | 100/PK | MR-581 | PATIENT RECORD |
| | 100/PD | MR-583 | CDV ICU FLOW SHEET |
| | 100/PD | MR-593 | DEFICIENCY RECORD |
| | 100/PD | MR-595-179 | PROBLEM SHEET |
| | 100/PK | MR-600-643 | PREOP CHECK LIST |
| | 1100/CTN | MR-616 | PULMONARY LAB REPORT |
| | 2500/CTN | MR-616A | PULMONARY LAB REPORT 1-PT |
| | 100/PD | MR-650 | VITAL SIGNS |
| | 100/PK | MR-671-730 | PRE-ANESTHESIA QUES |
| | 100/PD | MR-675 | NEONATAL RECORD I |
| | 100/PK | MR-676 | NEONATAL II |
| | 100/PK | MR-677 | OB SUMMARY |
| | 100/PK | MR-684 | CONDITIONS OF ADMISSION |
| | 100/PK | MR-685-755 | NURSING DISCHARGE ASSESS |
| | 100/PD | MR-692-783 | X-RAY CASSETTES |
| | 100/PK | MR-717 | PERIOPERATIVE RECORD |
| | 100/PD | MR-803 | DIET SERVICE PROG NOTE |
| | 100/PK | MR-895 | CRITICAL CARE FLOWSHEET |
| | 100/PK | MRS-1157 | BACKING SHEET |
| | 50/PK | NS-12-240 | NOURISHMENT ORDER FORM |
| | 50/PK | NS-507-114W | WEEKLY SCHEDULES |
| | 100/PD | NS-510-215 | REV TEAM ASSIGNMENT |
| | 50/PK | NS-518-14 | RN CLINICAL REPORT |
| | 50/PK | NS-529-478 | TREAT AND TEST PLAN |
| | 100/PD | NS-530-115 | FLUID FORMS |
| | 100/PD | NS-7-100 | TPR RECORD |
| | 100/PD | NS-9-21 | INTAKE/OUTPUT SHEETS |
| | 1/EA | NSY-325 | INFO ABOUT YOUR BABY |
| | 50/PK | NSY-761 | NURSERY ICU KARDEX |
| | 200/PK | OPD-19 | CLINICAL PRESCRIPTIONS |
| | 100/PK | OPD-60-253 | PED-PROGRESS NOTES |

**Column group 5**

| QTY | UNIT OF MEASURE | FORM NUMBER | DESCRIPTION |
|---|---|---|---|
| | 100/PK | PER-1-196 | EMPLOYMENT APPLICATION |
| | 25/PD | PER-13-37 | ACCIDENT EXPOSURE RC |
| | 50/PK | PER-663-793 | EMP/POS CHG REQUEST |
| | 100/PD | PH-1-299 | PRESCRIPTION BLANKS |
| | 100/PD | PH-2-637 | PHONE ORDER FOR MEDS |
| | 4900/CTN | PRD-1923 | NOTICE OF DEPOSIT |
| | 100/PD | PULF-526 | PULF TELEPHONE REPORTS |
| | 100/PK | PUR-1 | PURCHASE ORDERS |
| | 25/PK | PUR-1622 | OFFICE SUPPLY REQ |
| | 25/PK | PUR-203 | REQUISITION TO PURCHASE |
| | 100/PD | PUR-4-53 | GEN REQUISITION SM |
| | 100/PK | PUR-IV | PURCHASE ORDER TOP COPY |
| | 25/PK | PUR-9 | FORMS REQUISITION |
| | 2500/CTN | QA-1247 | RSQUM WORKSHEET |
| | 10/PK | QA-842 | MONITORING SYSTEMS |
| | 1/EA | RO-11-214 | RADIATION ONCOLOGY BROCH |
| | 25/PD | RAD-18 | CAT HISTORY FORM |
| | 100/PK | RAD-511-667 | RADIOLOGY PRELIM REPT |
| | 250/PK | RAD-516 | DAYLIGHT FLASHER CARD |
| | 250/PK | RAD-516A | BLANK DAYLIGHT FLASHER |
| | 200/PK | RTD-504 | RESP THERAPY CHG |
| | 400/CTN | RTD-507 | RESP THERAPY SCHEDULE |
| | 100/PD | SSD-104-283 | MED RECORD |
| | 100/PD | TRAN-363 | TUBE ROOM ROUTE SLIP |
| | 100/PD | TRAN-564 | TRAN CALL SLIP |

### PROCEDURE FOR COMPLETING FORM

1. FILL IN QUANTITY OF FORMS DESIRED, COMPLETE ALL BLANKS AT TOP OF FORM.
2. FOR ITEMS NOT APPEARING ON THIS REQUISITION, CONSULT FORMS CATALOG AND WRITE IN BELOW. (FOR NON-CATALOG FORMS, SPECIAL ORDERS OR NEW FORMS, CONTACT PURCHASING).
3. KEEP "REQUESTOR'S COPY" FOR YOUR RECORDS.
4. SEND ALL REMAINING COPIES TO PURCHASING.
5. FOR ASSISTANCE, CALL EXT. 3443.

| QTY | UNIT OF MEASURE | FORM NUMBER | DESCRIPTION |
|---|---|---|---|
| | | | |
| | | | |
| | | | |
| | | | |
| | | | |
| | | | |

FIGURE 21-7 • A purchasing department order form.

nursing unit kitchen and issued to the patients as needed. These supplies are restocked daily and are usually charged to the nursing unit's budget. See Figure 21–8 for an example of a dietary department stock supply order form.

## Laundry Department Supplies

The laundry department supplies all linen, including towels, washcloths, and bathmats, for the nursing unit. A common practice is for the laundry department to deliver large carts of supplies to the nursing unit each morning. If supplies run low during the day, the health unit coordinator may need to call the laundry department for more items. The cost for laundry department supplies is usually absorbed in the cost of the patient's room.

## PREPARING FORMS

As a health unit coordinator, it may be your task to prepare forms for use by the nurse manager or team leaders, such as the patient assignment sheet (see Fig. 2–2) and work schedules. Since preparing these forms usually involves recording data pertinent to your nursing unit, we will not discuss it further. Find out what your responsibilities are regarding filling out forms. If filling out forms is a daily health unit coordinator task on your unit, plan to fill them out at the same time each day.

## SUMMARY

All the tasks included in this chapter, except for ordering the nursing unit supplies, are performed daily; therefore, you will soon become skilled at performing them.

Accuracy and efficiency are extremely important in charting the vital signs, filing reports on the patients' charts, ordering daily laboratory tests, and ordering the mealtime diets. Performing these tasks at the same time each day is necessary for efficient management of your time, as we shall see in a later chapter.

| NOURISHMENT ORDER FROM FOOD SERVICE | |
|---|---|
| UNIT_____ ORDERED BY_____ | |
| DATE_____ | |
| | |
| DESCRIPTION | ORDER |
| Homogenized Milk | |
| Skim Milk | |
| Chocolate Milk | |
| Orange Juice (unsw) (qts) | |
| Apple Juice | |
| Cranberry Juice | |
| Prune Juice | |
| Tomato Juice | |
| Nectar | |
| Decaffeinated Coffee (pkg of 20) | |
| Tea Bags (pkg of 30) | |
| Graham Crackers (pkg of 12) | |
| Saltines (pkg of 20) | |
| Powdered non-dairy Creamers (50 per box) | |
| Sugar (per 100 ind.) | |
| Ice Cream | |
| Sherbet | |
| Jello | |
| Custard | |
| Oleo (ind.) | |
| Bread (pkg of 10 ind.) | |
| Bouillon -Beef or Chicken (pkg/12) | |
| 7-Up (6 pk) | |
| Cola (6 pk) | |

NOTE: BETWEEN MEAL FEEDINGS, TUBE FEEDINGS OR LIQUID SUPPLEMENTS ARE TO BE ORDERED ON THE "DIET CHANGE SHEET" AND ON THE "SPECIAL DIET" CARD.

NS-12-240    Received by_____

FIGURE 21–8 • A dietary department stock supply order form.

**REVIEW QUESTIONS**

1. If it is the health unit coordinator's task to transfer information from the vital sign sheet onto each patient's graphic sheet, at what time should you perform this task? Why?

   as soon as possible so that when the doctors make their rounds the TPR sheet is available

2. Why is accuracy important in the recording of vital signs?

   the doctor may use vital signs to prescribe treatment

3. You have recorded an incorrect temperature on the graphic sheet. How would you correct this error?

   recopy or write mistaken entry on wrong line and graph correctly

4. You are recording a set of vital signs and you notice that an error was made in the recording of a set of vital signs 2 days previously, which resulted in the following day's entries being incorrect. To correct this series of errors, you need to ___ recopy correct data ___

   The original copy is placed ___ back of the chart folder ___

5. Convert the following Fahrenheit temperatures to Celsius.

   a. 98.6° _____   b. 101.4° _____   c. 99.8° _____   d. 96.7° _____

6. Convert the following Celsius temperatures to Fahrenheit.

   a. 38.2° _____   b. 39.5° _____   c. 36.4° _____   d. 37.8° _____

7. Why is it considered "good planning" to order mealtime diets at approximately the same time each day?

   to avoid forgetting to do it

8. Diet changes may be ordered by the doctor or may be the result of:

   a. admission          c. discharge
   b. transfer           d. NPO for diagnostic studies

9. List two reasons for the need for efficient, accurate filing of records on the patient's chart.

   a. to have the records available for attending physician and other hospital personel
   b. to assist health records in assembling all the patients records for storage

10. List four guidelines for filing records on the patient's chart.

a. Select the seachard time every day

b. Separate the records according to patients names

c. check the name on the chart + match with record befor filing

d. place the record behind the correct divider

11. How does the health unit coordinator's responsibility differ when handling a doctor's order for a daily laboratory test as compared with an order for other laboratory tests?

you have to requisition for these lab tests every day until the doctor dis continues the order. other Lab tests are only ordered one time

12. Name five hospital departments that may provide the nursing unit supplies, and list the type of supplies that may be obtained from each department.

a. Purchasing Dept non nursing Items pencils

b. Central Service — Items used in nursing

c. pharmacy — medications

d. dietary Dept - Food Items

e. laundry Dept Linens

13. Describe two systems for restocking nursing unit supplies.

a. order supplys

b. the supplying dept aut omatically restocks

14. Define the following terms:

a. pulse deficit: the difference between radial and Apical pulse heart beat

b. Celsius scale: scale used to measure temp

c. stool: body waste discharged through the anus

d. diet change sheet: a form to order patients meals 3 times a day from the dietary dept

15. Write the meaning of each of the following abbreviations:

a. BM Bowel Movement

b. TPR Temperature pulse Respiration

c. C Celsius

d. F Farenheit

e. Days aft. Ad. days after admission

f.  PO day _____ *Post Operative Day* _____

g.  PP _____ *post partum* _____

## References

Blackburn, Elsa: *Health Unit Coordinator.* Englewood Cliffs, NJ, Prentice-Hall, Brady Division, 1991.

Sorrentino, Shelia A.: *Textbook for Nursing Assistants*, 3rd ed. St. Louis, The C.V. Mosby Co., 1992.

Taylor, Carol, Lillis, Carol, and LeMone, Priscilla: *Fundamentals of Nursing*, 2nd ed. Philadelphia, J.B. Lippincott Co., 1993.

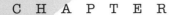

CHAPTER 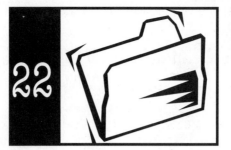 22

# REPORTS, INFECTION CONTROL, EMERGENCIES AND SPECIAL SERVICES

## CHAPTER OBJECTIVES

*Upon completion of this chapter, you will be able to:*

1. Define the terms in the vocabulary list.
2. Write the meaning for each abbreviation in the abbreviations list.
3. List three conditions that may cause a patient to become immunocompromised.
4. List four general isolation categories.
5. List four categories of incidents that require a written report.
6. Explain the importance of incident reports.
7. Name three methods by which bacteria may be spread.
8. Name three pathogenic microorganisms that are frequently responsible for hospital-acquired infections.
9. Explain how AIDS is spread.
10. List nine tasks that the health unit coordinator may perform in a medical emergency.
11. Explain the duties carried out during a fire or fire drill.
12. Describe how to handle mail and flowers delivered to the unit.

## VOCABULARY

**Cardiac Arrest** • The patient's heart contractions are absent or insufficient to produce a pulse or blood pressure (may also be referred to as *code arrest*) ~fire Alarm~ ~code blue~

**Census** • A daily listing of all patient activity (admissions, discharges, transfers, and deaths) within the hospital ~when nurse ask no of people on unit~

**Centers for Disease Control** • Division of the U.S. ~CDC~ Public Health Service that investigates and controls diseases that have epidemic potential

**Communicable Disease** • A disease that may be transmitted from one person to another

**Disaster Procedure** • A planned procedure that is carried out by hospital personnel when a large number of persons have been injured

**Epidemiology** • The study of the occurrence, distribution, and causes of health and disease in humans; the specialist is called an *epidemiologist*

**Incident** • An episode that does not normally occur within the regular hospital routine

**Isolation** • The placement of a patient apart from other patients insofar as movement and social contact are concerned, for the purpose of preventing the spread of infection

**Medical Emergency** • An emergency that is life-threatening ~white code~

**Nosocomial Infection** • Infections that are acquired from within the health care facility

**Pathogenic Microorganisms** • Disease-carrying organisms too small to be seen with the naked eye

**Protective Care** • Another term for isolation

**Respiratory Arrest** • When the patient ceases to breathe or when respirations are so depressed that the blood cannot receive sufficient oxygen and therefore the body cells die (may also be referred to as *code arrest*)

**Reverse Isolation** • A precautionary measure taken to prevent a patient with low resistance to disease from becoming infected   *you dress to protect them*

**Universal Precautions** • The creation of a barrier between the health care worker and the patient's blood and body fluids

## A B B R E V I A T I O N S

| Abbreviation | Meaning |
|---|---|
| AIDS | acquired immunodeficiency syndrome |
| ARC | AIDS-related complex |
| CDC | Centers for Disease Control |
| HBV | hepatitis B virus |
| HBC | hepatitis C virus |

## CENSUS RECORDING

Each hospital keeps a daily **census** record of patient activity for daily operational purposes, such as assigning the nursing staff, and for statistical purposes. The gathering of this information begins with record keeping on each nursing unit, and it is usually the health unit coordinator's responsibility.

Because the method of collecting census data varies among hospitals, it is impossible to present an exact procedure. However, most hospitals require that each nursing unit record on the census sheet the name of each patient hospitalized on the unit, including new admissions, transfers, and discharges (including deceased patients), and the level of nursing care that the patients on that unit need. The census data is collected for a 24-hour period, usually ending at midnight, and is then given to the department (often the admitting department) that compiles the information for the entire hospital. Figure 22–1 is an example of a 24-hour census sheet for a nursing unit. Census information may also be placed on a computer.

It is important that the data recorded on this census sheet be accurate and complete. The health unit coordinator should develop the habit of recording information as it becomes census data. For example, as a new client arrives on the nursing unit, the data should be immediately recorded on the census sheet. Failure to record the information immediately may result in a waste of time later on, when locating the data may be difficult or may result in an omission of the data.

## INCIDENT REPORTS

An **incident** is an episode that does not normally occur within the regular health care facility routine. The incident may be an accident, such as a patient falling while on the way to the bathroom. It also may be a situation, such as spilled liquids in a hospital corridor, that causes someone to slip and sustain an injury.

Incidents may occur to patients, visitors, or health care facility personnel and students. Events other than accidents that occur within the hospital or on hospital property are also reportable. Examples of incidents that require written reports are:

- Accidents
- Thefts from persons on hospital property
- Errors of omission of patient treatment or errors of administration of patient treatment
- Exposure to blood and body fluids such as caused by a needlestick

Many incidents occur in the patient's room and are not viewed by the health unit coordinator. In such cases, the health unit coordinator prepares the incident report form for the nurse by imprinting the patient's name on the report. The nurse and any witnesses complete the report. However, anything that is seen or that you have knowledge of regarding an incident should be written up immediately so that all details can be communicated as they occurred.

An **incident report form** (Fig. 22–2) should be written for all incidents occurring to anyone, no matter how insignificant they may seem. Documentation of all incidents is important in the case of a lawsuit arising from them. The incident is also studied by risk management in order to prevent similar incidents from happening in the future.

Employee hospital incidents must be documented and the employee seen by the employee health nurse or physician in order for him or her to be eligible for coverage by the state workman's compensation commission. Hospital employees who fail to put into writing something which may appear trivial, such as a finger puncture with a thumb tack, have no evidence to present should an infection follow the injury.

Incidents occurring to patients are reported to the patient's physician. After the patient is examined by the physician, the report is signed and forwarded to the proper hospital authority. The incident report never becomes part of the patient's permanent record.

The health unit coordinator is also responsible for maintaining a supply of incident report forms for the nursing unit.

## INFECTION CONTROL

### Isolation

In order to control infections or **communicable diseases** (those diseases that may be transmitted from one person to another), a patient may be placed in **isolation**. To isolate, in the strictest sense, requires that a patient be placed

| CU | PEDS | P-ICU | 2-ICU | 2-CCU | 2-W | 3-E | 3-W | 3-BNI | 3-ICU | 4-E | 4-W | 4-ICU | 5-E | 5-W | 5-BNI | 5-ICU | 6-BNI | 7-BNI | 7-ICA | 7-ICU | |

# CENSUS ACTIVITY WORK SHEET

DATE:

### ADMISSIONS

ACCOMMODATION/CARE TYPE      TEACHING PATIENT

| | LAST NAME | M/F | ADMISSION NO. | ROOM/BED | A/G/E | HOSP. SERV. | TIME ARRIVED ON UNIT | ✓ | DIAGNOSIS/DOCTOR | |
|---|---|---|---|---|---|---|---|---|---|---|
| 1 | Sel Patricia | | 064 501 | 516 / 1 | 27 | M | 3:45ᵖ | ✓ | Salpingo-oophoritis / Dr Twyla | |
| 2 | Brown Helene | | 064509 | 516 2 | 51 | M | 4:00ᵖ | | Sinus Infection / Dr Sammy | |
| 3 | Anderson Richard | | 064506 | 518 / 1 | 22 | M | 3:20ᵖ | | Slipped Disc / Dr Blew | |
| 4 | Jenkins Gary | | 064 518 | 579 / 1 | 28 | M | 2:00ᵖ | | Gastritis / Dr Aaron | |
| 5 | Smith Jerry | | 064 524 | 522 2 | 30 | M | 1:00ᵖ | | Fx Femur / Dr Michaels | |
| 6 | Henry Joan | | 064-221 | 514 / 1 | 34 | M | 1:30ᵖ | | Pharyngitis / Dr Holly | |
| 7 | | | | | | | | | | |
| 8 | | | | | | | | | | |
| 9 | | | | | | | | | | |
| 10 | | | | | | | | | | |
| 11 | | | | | | | | | | |
| 12 | | | | | | | | | | |
| 13 | | | | | | | | | | |
| 14 | | | | | | | | | | |

### TRANSFERS /CHANGES OF CLASSIFICATIONS

ACCOMMODATION/CARE TYPE      CONFIRMATION NOTICE SENT      TEACHING PATIENT

| | LAST NAME | M/F | ADMISSION NO. | TIME COMPL. | FROM ROOM/BED | TO ROOM/BED | HOSPITAL SERVICE | ✓ | TIME | AGE | ✓ | DIAGNOSIS/DOCTOR | |
|---|---|---|---|---|---|---|---|---|---|---|---|---|---|
| 1 | ENDER GEORGE | | 064 488 | | 518 / 1 | 316 / 1 | M | | 3:00 | 36 | | Fx Humerus / Dr Mark | |
| 2 | Arthur Bryce | | 064-460 | | 59 / 1 | 34 / 1 | M | | 12ⁿ | 36 | | Laceration Head / Dr Paul | |
| 3 | FAYD LESLIE | | 064-440 | | 514 / 1 | 20 / 1 | S | | 9ᵃ | 14 | | T&A   Dr Douce | |
| 4 | | | | | | | | | | | | | |
| 5 | | | | | | | | | | | | | |
| 6 | | | | | | | | | | | | | |
| 7 | | | | | | | | | | | | | |
| 8 | | | | | | | | | | | | | |
| 9 | | | | | | | | | | | | | |
| 10 | | | | | | | | | | | | | |
| 11 | | | | | | | | | | | | | |
| 12 | | | | | | | | | | | | | |

### DISCHARGES

1 OK TO GO   2 F/C REQUESTED      NOTIFIED      CONFIRMATION NOTICE SENT (TIME)

| | LAST NAME | M/F | ADMISSION NO | TIME VACATED | ROOM/BED | FIN. CLEAR STAT. | FAMILY | ADMIT'G | ✓ | EXPIRED TIME | REMARKS: | Rxs |
|---|---|---|---|---|---|---|---|---|---|---|---|---|
| 1 | Russ Barbara | | 064 391 | 10ᵃ | 514 / 1 | 1 | 9:35ᵃ | 9:30ᵃ | ✓ | | Home c̄ Rx | |
| 2 | BELL LINDA | | 064 399 | 11ᵃ | 516 / 1 | 1 | 8:30ᵃ | 8:30ᵃ | ✓ | | | |
| 3 | Roper Lucille | | 064 310 | 12:30ᵃ | 216 | 2 | 1 | 9:00ᵃ | 9:00ᵃ ✓ | | | |
| 4 | | | | | | | | | | | | |
| 5 | | | | | | | | | | | | |
| 6 | | | | | | | | | | | | |
| 7 | | | | | | | | | | | | |
| 8 | | | | | | | | | | | | |
| 9 | | | | | | | | | | | | |
| 10 | | | | | | | | | | | | |
| 11 | | | | | | | | | | | | |
| 12 | | | | | | | | | | | | |
| 13 | | | | | | | | | | | | |
| 14 | | | | | | | | | | | | |

NS-400

VERIFIED BY: _____
SIGNATURE

FIGURE 22–1 • A census sheet.

**Confidential Information**
## INCIDENT REPORT
(Patient or Visitor)
Not a Part of Patient's Permanent Chart

1. Date of Admission

2. Diagnosis

3. Date of Incident      Time    M   | Room No., Name, Age, Sex, Hospital Number, Attending Physician

4. Were Bed Rails up?     5. Hi Lo Bed Position
        (YES OR NO)                         (UP OR DOWN)

6. Was Safety Belt or Restraints in use?
                                  DESIGNATE SPECIFICALLY

7. Activity (Complete Bed Rest, Bathroom Privileges, Etc.)

8. Sedatives      Dose      Time    M  ⎱ Given

9. Narcotics      Dose      Time    M  ⎰ within 12 hours

10. Tranquilizers      Dose      Time    M  ⎰ previous to incident

11. Nurse's Account of Incident (State incident, where discovered, condition of patient, etc.)

12. History of Incident as related by Patient

13. List Witnesses or Persons Familiar with Details of Incident (Include roommate's name and hospital number.)

    Name                           Address

    Name                           Address

    Name                           Address

14. Time Doctor was called    AM     PM     15. Time Doctor Responded    AM     PM

16. Time Supervisor called    AM     PM

17. Date of Report

18. _____
            SIGNATURE OF PERSON REPORTING

19. _____
            SIGNATURE OF DEPARTMENT SUPERVISOR

20. _____
            SIGNATURE OF DEPARTMENT HEAD

A      Complete **IMMEDIATELY** for **EVERY** incident and send to Administrator via Department Head.

F I G U R E 22–2 • An incident report. (*A*) General information. *Illustration continued on following page*

---

PHYSICIAN'S STATEMENT

21. State injuries or other result, if any, from this incident _____

_____

_____

22. How, if at all, did the results of this incident affect the patient's original condition? _____

_____

_____

23. What treatment was given? _____

_____

24. Were X-rays or other tests ordered (specify) _____

_____

_____

25. Results of X-ray or other tests _____

_____

_____

26. Patient Examined:  Date _____ Hour_____ AM _____ PM

27. Signed _____ M.D. (House Physician)

B                                28. Signed _____ M.D. (Attending Physician)

---

FIGURE 22-2 • *Continued*  (*B*) Physician's statement.

completely apart from other patients insofar as movement and social contact are concerned. Not all patients with disease conditions that may be transferred to others are in total or strict isolation. Many conditions require only precautions, such as good handwashing technique and careful disposal of the patient's surgical dressings. While the term **isolation** is used by most health care facilities, some hospitals, because of the somewhat negative implications of the term, call the procedure **protective care**.

Another type of isolation is referred to as **reverse isolation**. This, again, is a precautionary measure that is practiced in order to prevent a patient with impaired or low resistance to disease from becoming infected. For example, a burn patient is very susceptible to infection and must be protected from as many **pathogenic microorganisms** (disease-causing organisms too small to be seen by the naked eye) as possible.

Some patients enter the hospital with an infectious disease, such as meningitis, and are placed immediately in an isolation unit. Other patients may develop infections while in the hospital (**nosocomial infections**) that require them to be placed in isolation. Three pathogenic microorganisms that are frequently responsible for hospital-acquired infections are *Streptococcus*, *Staphylococcus*, and *Pseudomonas*.

For statistical purposes, records must be kept of infectious diseases. A report should be submitted to the proper hospital authority (Fig. 22-3). Most hospitals employ an epidemiologist or infection-control officer who maintains all infection records as well as investigating all hospital acquired infections.

The Centers for Disease Control, a division of the U.S. Department of Health and Human Services, has designed a card system to assist hospitals to carry out the proper procedure for each type of isolation (Fig. 22-4). These cards are placed on the isolation patient's door and indicate what precautions are to be taken. The extent of the precautions to be taken depends upon the method by which the disease is spread. Disease may be spread by the following means:

Report # _____

**REPORT OF INFECTION**

COMPLETE ALL BLANKS IN TOP SECTION          UNIT _____

1. Diagnosis is: _____

_____

_____

2. Date of admission: _____

3. Evidence of Infection on admission?
   Yes ☐  No ☐

4. Date of last previous admission here:

   _____

5. Hospitalized at another hospital?
   Yes ☐  No ☐

   If yes, name hospital?

   _____

Date:_____

6. Date of surgery/delivery _____

7. Procedure done: _____

   _____

8. Culture sent?  Yes ☐  No ☐
   (If yes, what was cultured?)
   _____ Blood
   _____ Urine
   _____ Sputum
   _____ Drainage from _____
   _____ Other(specify)_____

   _____

9. *Fever?    Yes ☐    No ☐
   NOTE: *Fever = temp. greater than
   100.4°F (38°C) Oral
   101°F (38.4°C) Rectal

10. Pt. Isolated?  Yes ☐    No ☐

    If yes, enter date next to type initiated

    _____ a. Limited
    _____ b. Respiratory
    _____ c. Wound & Skin
    _____ d. Enteric
    _____ e. Strict
    _____ f. Protective

11. Date of Discharge: _____

CHECK ALL THAT APPLY:

DIARRHEA:

_____ Over 3 stools/24 hrs. for more than 2 days s̄ laxatives, enemas, x-rays preps, cardiac drugs or antibiotics

PHLEBITIS: Location _____

Non-Suppurative:
_____ Mechanical Intracath
_____ Drug
_____ Possible focal site of infection
_____ Observed by Nurse
_____ Diagnosis by Physician

Suppurative:
_____ Purulent drainage

POST PARTUM:

_____ *Fever(exclude 1st PP day)
_____ Purulent vaginal discharge
_____ Diagnosis by Physician

POST-OP:
_____ Continuous *Fever for 2 consecutive days
_____ Abscess(usually documented at time of surgery)

RESPIRATORY TRACT:
Upper
_____ Coryza(profuse nasal drainage)
_____ Pharyngitis
_____ Diagnosis by Physician

Lower:
_____ Sudden on set of cough
_____ Purulent sputum
_____ Suppuration of trachea
_____ X-ray Dx - Pneumonia
_____ Diagnosis by Physician

SKIN:
_____ Abscess
_____ Boil
_____ Cellulitis
_____ Purulent decubiti
_____ Suppuration

BLOOD:
_____ HAA Pos.
_____ HAA Neg.
_____ Positive Culture

URINARY TRACT:
Asymptomatic:
_____ No clinical symptoms
_____ Positive bacteriology X 100,000/ml
_____ Positive bacteriology X 10,000/ml c̄ previous urine culture negative
_____ Pyuria X 10 WBC

Symptomatic:
_____ Frequency
_____ Burning
_____ Urgency
_____ CVT(costo-vertebral tenderness)

WOUND:
_____ Abscess(usually documented at surgery time)
_____ Continuous *Fever for 2 consecutive days
_____ Stitch abscess
_____ Suppuration of wound
_____ Diagnosis by Physican

_____ Other _____

Report completed by: _____          Date:_____

COMMENTS: _____

_____

_____

(DO NOT WRITE IN THIS SECTION. FOR USE BY INFECTION CONTROL OFFICER ONLY)

F I G U R E   22–3 • An infection report.

Front of Card

**Drainage/Secretion Precautions***
**Visitors—Report to Nurses Station Before Entering Room**

1. Masks are not indicated.
2. Gowns are indicated if soiling is likely.
3. Gloves are indicated for touching infective material.
4. HANDS MUST BE WASHED AFTER THE PATIENT OR POTENTIALLY CONTAMINATED ARTICLES AND BEFORE TAKING CARE OF ANOTHER PATIENT.
5. Articles contaminated with infective material should be discarded or bagged and labeled before being sent for decontamination and reprocessing.

Back of Card

Infectious diseases included in this category are those that result in production of purulent material, drainage, or secretions, unless the disease is included in another isolation category that requires more rigorous precautions. (If you have questions about a specific disease, see the listing of infectious diseases in Guideline for Isolation Precautions in Hospitals, Table A, Disease-Specific Isolation Precautions).

The following infections are examples of those included in this category provided they are not a) caused by multiply-resistant microorganisms, b) major (draining and not covered by a dressing or dressing does not adequately contain the drainage) skin wound, or burn infections, including those caused by Staphylococcus aureus or group A Streptococcus, or c) gonococcal eye infections in newborns. See Contact Isolation if the infection is one of these three.

Abscess, minor or limited

Burn infection, minor or limited

Conjunctivitis

Decubitus ulcer, infected, minor or limited

Skin infection, minor or limited

Wound infection, minor or limited

*A private room is usually not indicated for Drainage/Secretion Precautions

**F I G U R E  22–4** • An example of the CDC card system for an isolation category.

- Air—through breathing
- Personal contact
- Body excretions, such as stool, urine, nose, and throat secretions, or drainage from an infected wound

### General Isolation Categories

The general isolation categories are:

- *Strict isolation*—To prevent transmission of highly contagious or virulent infections that are spread by air, direct contact, or indirect contact
- *Reverse isolation*—To protect patients with a decreased immune system function by reducing their risks of exposure to potentially infectious organisms. Reverse isolation is also known as immunocompromised isolation. An example of patients who are immunocompromised are organ transplant recipients, burn victims, or patients receiving chemotherapy.
- *AFB isolation (tuberculosis)*—To prevent transmission of active pulmonary tuberculosis. A positive PPD (Mantoux) does not necessarily mean active tuberculosis. Infants and children with pulmonary tuberculosis do not require isolation.
- *Respiratory isolation*—To prevent transmission of infectious diseases that spread mainly through the air by large droplets traveling over short distances (<3 ft)

and landing in the nose or mouth of a susceptible person.

## Universal Precautions

In 1987 the CDC developed and presented a concept to protect health care providers from blood-borne pathogens such as human immunodeficiency virus (HIV), hepatitis B virus, and hepatitis C virus. During that time there was a quiet panic among health care providers. They were not sure of how HIV was spread or how they could protect themselves. The CDC called this new concept "universal precautions" (for blood and body fluids). Nationwide, hospitals and other health care facilities accepted and taught this new concept to their employees.

**Universal precautions** are the creation of a barrier between the practitioner (health care worker) and the patient's body fluids. Body fluids considered potentially infectious include blood, semen, vaginal secretions, peritoneal fluid, pleural fluid, pericardial fluid, synovial fluid, cerebrospinal fluid, amniotic fluid, urine, feces, sputum, saliva, wound drainage, and vomitus.

The *barrier* in universal precautions is created by wearing or using such items as gloves, gown, mask, goggles or glasses, pocket masks with one-way valves, moisture-resistant laundry bags, and moisture-resistant gowns. Many hospital rooms are equipped with some or all of these barriers.

Universal precautions should be practiced with *every single patient* by *every health care employee*.

## AIDS

AIDS stands for **acquired immunodeficiency syndrome**. It is caused by a virus called HIV, also called HTLV-III or the AIDS virus. The AIDS virus attacks the immune system and thereby reduces the body's ability to defend itself against infection and disease. Persons who have AIDS become open to many opportunistic infections that are not usually a threat to persons with a normal functioning immune system. These infections are called *opportunistic* because the organisms take advantage of the patient's weakened immune system. As the immune system becomes weaker, these opportunistic illnesses may overwhelm the AIDS patient and cause death.

AIDS is spread by blood, vaginal fluids, and semen. There are four main ways AIDS is spread. The first is by sexual intercourse, both homosexual and heterosexual. The second is by injecting drugs intravenously using needles previously injected into someone carrying the AIDS virus. The third way is from an infected mother to her infant during pregnancy or birth. The fourth is transmission of the virus through blood transfusions; this mode is especially common if the patient received the transfusion before blood was routinely tested for the virus. Surgical patients, hemophiliac patients, and mothers who received transfusions during or after birth have contracted the HIV virus this way. In rare instances, it has been reported that

AIDS was spread through the blood of an infected person entering another person's bloodstream either through a cut, open sore, or blood being splashed into the mouth or eye.

An *AIDS virus carrier* is a person who carries the AIDS virus in his or her blood, but who may stay healthy for a long time. Some may never get sick. The only indication of AIDS infection in the carrier is usually a positive blood test for antibodies to the AIDS virus. Once a person has been infected with the AIDS virus, he or she remains infected for life.

**ARC** stands for **AIDS-related complex**. Months or years after the initial infection, some people carrying the virus develop symptoms that may include tiredness, fevers, night sweats, swollen lymph glands, or mental deterioration resembling Alzheimer's disease. Often the symptoms are recurrent and disable the person. This person is said to have ARC or AIDS-related complex.

AIDS is the most severe form of the infection. A full-blown case may not appear until months or years after the initial infection. ARC symptoms may or may not have appeared. The two most frequent opportunistic illnesses that may overtake the AIDS patient are (1) *Pneumocystis carinii* pneumonia (PCP), a pneumonia caused by *Pneumocystis carinii*; and (2) Kaposi's sarcoma (KS), an otherwise rare skin cancer.

## Hepatitis B Virus

Hepatitis B is an inflammation of the liver caused by the **hepatitis B virus (HBV)**. It was formerly called "serum hepatitis." Like AIDS, hepatitis B is spread by body fluids but it is even more contagious than AIDS. Health care providers are at risk for exposure. Strict universal blood and body fluid precautions must be practiced.

A vaccine to prevent hepatitis B is available.

## Health Unit Coordinator Tasks to Control Infection

The health unit coordinator tasks for infection control and isolation vary from institution to institution. It is necessary in any health care facility for the health unit coordinator to have a basic understanding of infection-control policies and isolation categories. *Accurate* information must be given to inquiring visitors. If you are unable to answer a question or are unsure of what to say, get a nurse to speak with the visitor. If there is an infectious or communicable disease on the unit and the nurse has not informed infection control, the health unit coordinator should get in touch with infection control. Infection control works best with good communication among the different groups in the health care setting. The health unit coordinator should wear gloves when handling or transporting specimens. Some health care facilities put the specimen jar in plastic baggies and then gloves are not necessary. The health unit coordinator should practice good handwashing techniques throughout the working day. The health unit coordinator transcribes laboratory orders pertaining to infection control. The following is an example of a set of orders and the subdepartment of the laboratory to which they are sent:

- CSF for
  - cell count—hematology
  - protein—chemistry
  - glucose—chemistry
- LDH—chemistry
- KOH and fungus culture—microbiology
- AFB and TB—microbiology
- Lyme titer—chemistry

Another area in which the health unit coordinator must be fully aware of institution policy is in disclosure of information such as in cases of AIDS. Laws regarding AIDS and confidentiality vary from state to state, as do laws regarding disclosure of HIV-positive persons. When in doubt, *do not disclose information.* In many health care facilities, guidelines have been established to assist the health care worker. Examples of some of these guidelines include:

- *Not* putting diagnosis of AIDS or rule out AIDS on the computer; the primary diagnosis is the infection, symptoms, or cancer. AIDS becomes the secondary diagnosis and appears on the medical record but not in the computer.
- All orders for the laboratory, x-ray, PT, OT, RT, and so on should be marked "blood precautions," but only those people who perform invasive procedures on the patient are told of the AIDS diagnosis.
- Family, friends, and other persons may not know about the AIDS diagnosis and must not be told by any health care employee unless so advised by the physician. Confidentiality and knowledge of the health care facility's policies and guidelines is essential information for the health unit coordinator to complete tasks and offer quality patient care in the area of infection control.

## EMERGENCIES

### Medical Emergencies

Two **medical emergencies**—that is, life-threatening situations—that require remaining calm, swift action, and good communication by the health unit coordinator are **cardiac arrest** and **respiratory arrest.** (It is common hospital terminology to refer to these as *code arrests*). In a cardiac arrest the patient's heart contractions are absent or grossly insufficient, and there is no pulse and no blood pressure. In respiratory arrest, the patient may cease to breathe or the respirations become so depressed that the blood cannot receive oxygen and the body cells die. Both conditions require quick action by hospital personnel and the use of emergency equipment. Treatment must be in-

stituted within 3 to 4 minutes, since the brain cells deteriorate rapidly from lack of oxygen.

Each hospital nursing unit and department maintains an emergency cart. This is taken to the code arrest patient's room immediately. Fully equipped code arrest carts are also stationed in designated areas of the hospital and are wheeled to the patient's room when a code arrest occurs. These carts contain medications and more equipment than the unit emergency carts. It is important for the health unit coordinator to know the location of the emergency cart and any other emergency equipment so that it can be brought quickly to their nursing unit when needed.

Hospitals have designated hospital personnel who report to each code arrest. They are members of the code arrest team. They may be employed in various hospital departments, such as intensive or coronary care, other nursing units, the respiratory care department, pulmonary function department, surgery, and so forth.

As a member of the health care team, the health unit coordinator may be asked to perform the following tasks (see p. 419). (see p. 419)

### Fire Procedures

During the employment orientation period, the health unit coordinator tours the hospital and the unit to which he or she will be assigned. Particular note should be made of the placement of fire alarms and such fire apparatus as extinguishers and hoses. The proper procedure to use in case of fire should be learned. The term *fire* is not used, as it may trigger responses that could be fatal to a patient or create panic among patients. A code number, such as Code 1000, or a name such as "Code Red," is usually used when a fire or fire drill takes place.

The health unit coordinator may be expected to assist with the evacuation of patients who are endangered by the fire. If the fire is not on the unit, the health unit coordinator may help the nursing personnel to close the doors to the patient rooms. Each hospital unit or section of the hospital is separated by fire doors. These specially constructed doors serve to help contain the fire in one area. They must also be closed during a fire.

Fires may be of several types:

- Those occurring in combustible materials, such as rags, paper, mattresses, and so forth
- Electrical
- Burning liquids

Each type requires a specific kind of extinguisher to put out the fire. Demonstration of the use and type of extinguisher to be used in specific fires are given periodically by the local fire department.

Each fire, no matter how small, is reported to the hospital fire marshal.

### Disaster Procedure

A **disaster procedure** is a planned procedure that is carried out by hospital personnel when a large number of

## TASKS RELATED TO MEDICAL EMERGENCIES

| Step | Task | Notes |
|------|------|-------|
| 1. | Notify the switchboard operator to alert the code arrest team. | Notification may be made by dialing a special number on the telephone, stating code arrest, and giving the location. Some health care facilities use the expression "Code Blue" to designate a cardiac or respiratory arrest. |
| 2. | Direct the code arrest team to the patient's room. | |
| 3. | Remove the patient information sheet from the patient's *vital signs sheet* chart and take or send the chart to the patient's room. | |
| 4. | Notify all physicians connected with the patient's case (attending physician, consultants, and residents). | |
| 5. | Notify the patient's family of the situation. | The telephone call may be made by a member of the nursing staff, such as the clinical manager. |
| | | If the health unit coordinator does communicate with the family, the conversation should be carried on in as controlled a manner as possible, so as to not cause panic. The dialogue might be, "Mr. Whetstone, your brother's condition has changed, and the doctor feels you would like to know. The doctors are with him now. Will you be coming to the hospital?" *Not Likely* |
| 6. | Call the departments for treatments and supplies as needed. | Usually respiratory care, pulmonary function, and CSD are the departments involved. |
| 7. | Alert the admissions department for possibility of transfer to ICU. | If the code procedure is successful, the patient is transferred to ICU or possibly CCU, where he or she can be closely monitored. |
| 8. | Prepare any requisitions or charge slips that may be needed. | Many medications, equipment from CSD, and cardiac equipment such as EKG and monitoring equipment are used during the code procedure. |
| 9. | For a successful code, follow the procedure for a transfer to another unit. | See Chapter 20. |
| 10. | For an unsuccessful code procedure, follow the procedure for postmortem care. | See Chapter 20. |

persons have been injured. The disaster may occur during a flood, a fire, a bombing, or an accident, such as a train derailment, or plane crash. Each hospital maintains a disaster plan book. Disaster drills are held once or twice a year to keep the hospital personnel informed and in practice. The disaster procedure is activated by announcing a code such as "Code 5000" on the hospital public address system.

The role you may play during this procedure will be explained by your instructor, as it differs from hospital to hospital. In the case of a disaster, all off-duty hospital personnel must return to the hospital. Their assistance is needed to care for the hospital patients and disaster victims.

## SPECIAL SERVICES

### Flowers

When a health care facility is large enough to have a specific area to which all flowers are delivered, the task of conveying the flowers to clients may be an assignment for the volunteer. In that case, the health unit coordinator may need only to direct the volunteer to the correct room.

In hospitals where the representative from the florist delivers the flowers directly to the unit, the health unit co-ordinator should ascertain that the patient is still on the unit or within the hospital before dismissing the representative. After signing the delivery slip, the health unit coordinator may deliver the flowers to the patient's room.

### Mail

Mail is delivered to the nursing unit daily. The mail is checked and the patient's room and bed numbers are written on each envelope. In the event that the patient has been discharged, you write "discharged" in pencil on the envelope and return it to the mail room. The mail may be distributed to the patients as time allows or the task may be designated to a hospital volunteer.

## SUMMARY

While there are many things the new health unit coordinator needs to learn upon employment, it is important to know the routines and be able to perform the tasks related to medical emergencies, fires, and disasters. When emergencies occur there is no time to look in a book for directions about what you must do.

The other tasks discussed in this chapter may not be part of your regular routine, and therefore it is necessary for you to review the procedures in your hospital as time permits.

**REVIEW QUESTIONS**

1. Write the meaning of each abbreviation listed below in the space provided.
   a. AIDS _Acquired Immunodificiency Syndrome_
   b. ARC _Aids Related complex_
   c. CDC _Center for disease control and prevention_
   d. HBV _Hepatitis B Virus_

2. List four categories of incidents that require a report to administration.
   a. _Accidents_
   b. _thefts of personal property or hospital property_
   c. _errors of admission of patient treatment, errors of omission_
   d. _exposure to blood & body fluids_

3. Describe the duties of a health unit coordinator during a fire drill.
   _may assist with evacuation, may help close_
   _doors to patients room, close fire doors_

4. Name three pathogenic microorganims that are frequently responsible for hospital-acquired infections.
   a. _Streptococcus_
   b. _staphylococcus_
   c. _Psuedomonos_

5. Define the following:
   a. Centers for Disease Control _division of the US Public Health_
   _service that investigates and controls diseases of epidemic Potencial_
   b. verbal orders _orders given orally by a doctor for a nurse_
   _or HUC_
   c. reverse isolation _precautionary measure taken to prevent patients_
   _with low resistence to disease from becoming infected_
   d. respiratory arrest _when a person stops breathing and respirations_
   _become so depressed that the blood cannot recieve oxygen._
   e. protective care _another form for isolation_
   f. pathogenic microorganisms _disease carrying organisms too small_
   _to be seen by the naked eye_
   g. medical emergency _life threatening emergency_
   h. isolation _to place a patient apart from other_
   _patients to prevent spread of disease_

i. incident __something that happens thats out of the regular routine of the hospital__

j. communicable disease __a disease that can be transmitted from one person to another__

k. census __a daily listing of all patient activity admissions, transfers, discharges, deaths__

l. cardiac arrest __absence or insufficient heart contractions so no, pulse or blood pressure is found__

m. disaster procedure __preplanned procedure carried out by a hospital when a large no of people are injured__

n. nosocomial infections __infections acquired by patient while in the hospital__

o. universal precautions __creation of a barrier between a health care worker and patients blood & body fluids__

6. List nine tasks that the health unit coordinator may perform during a medical emergency.

a. _____

_____

b. _____

_____

c. _____

_____

d. _____

_____

e. _____

_____

f. _____

_____

g. _____

_____

h. _____

_____

i. _____

_____

7. What should the health unit coordinator do when handling or transporting specimens?

__wear rubber gloves unless the specimen is double bagged.__

8. Why is reporting in writing of each hospital incident important?

_____documentation_____

_____

9. Three methods by which bacteria may be spread are:

a. _____airborne_____

b. _____personal contact_____

c. _____body excreations_____

10. Describe how to handle:

a. patient mail _____

_____

_____

b. patient flowers _____

_____

_____

11. List the four general isolation categories and their purpose.

a. _____strict isolation — to prevent transmission of highly contagios disease - air, director, indirect contact_____

b. _____reverse isolation - to protect patients with lowered immun system_____

c. _____AFB - prevent transmission of active TB_____

_____

d. _____respiratory to prevent infectious disease spread mainly through the air_____

12. Name three conditions that may cause a patient to become immunocompromised.

a. _____burn victims_____

b. _____chemo therapy_____

c. _____organ transplant_____

13. List four barriers used in universal precautions.

a. _____gloves_____

b. _____masks_____

c. _____gown_____

d. _____goggles or glasses_____

14. In AIDS, what is meant by an "opportunistic infection"?

_____It takes advantage of a weakened immune system_____

*PCP Pneumonia*

*KS Karposis sarcoma*

15. Name the two opportunistic diseases related to AIDS.

a. _____

b. _____

## References

Beaufoy, A.: HIV Infection employee education and infection control measures. *Canadian Journal of Public Health* 80 (Suppl.1):31–33, 1989.

Blackburn, E.: *Health Unit Coordinator*. Englewood Cliffs, NJ, Prentice-Hall, Brady Division, 1991.

Collier, Idolia Cox: *Medical Surgical Nursing*, 3rd ed. St. Louis, The C.V. Mosby Co., 1992.

Good Samaritan Hospital: *Unit Secretary Manual*, rev. ed. Phoeniz, AZ, Good Samaritan Hospital, 1995.

O'Toole Marie: *Miller-Keane Encyclopedia and Dictionary of Medicine Nursing and Allied Health*, 6th ed. Philadelphia, W.B. Saunders Co., 1997.

Taylor, C., LeMone, P., and Lillis, C.: *Fundamentals Of Nursing*, 2nd ed. Philadelphia, J.B. Lippincott Co., 1993.

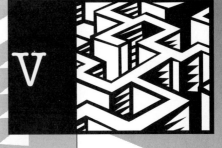

# SECTION V

# INTRODUCTION TO ANATOMIC STRUCTURES, MEDICAL TERMS, AND ILLNESS

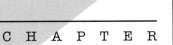 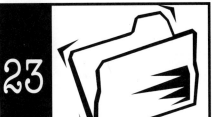

# MEDICAL TERMINOLOGY, BASIC HUMAN STRUCTURE, DISEASES, AND DISORDERS

# UNIT I

# Medical Terminology: Word Elements, Analyzing, and Word Building

## OBJECTIVES

*Upon completion of this unit, you will be able to:*

1. Name and define the four word elements that are commonly used in building medical terms.
2. Define *analysis of medical terms* and *word building*.
3. Given a list of medical terms and a list of word elements, divide the medical terms into their component elements—that is, word roots, prefixes, suffixes, and combining vowel—and identify the kinds of word elements present in each term by name.
4. Given a description of the medical condition and a list of word endings—that is, words root, prefixes, suffixes, and combining vowel—write out the medical term that represents a stated medical condition.

## INTRODUCTION TO MEDICAL TERMS

Most medical terms are made up of Greek and Latin words; however, some have been adapted from modern languages. Although a background of Greek or Latin is not necessary to learn the meaning of medical terms, it is necessary to learn the English translation of the Greek or Latin word parts. In this course of study the parts of the word are memorized rather than the whole word. By learning word parts you will be able to build words according to a given definition and break down words into word parts to determine their meaning.

For example, in the medical term

nephr/ectomy

nephr is the word part that means "kidney" and ectomy is the word part meaning "surgical removal." Thus the word nephrectomy means "surgical removal of the kidney."

Once you have memorized the meanings of the word parts (nephr and ectomy), you will know their meanings when they appear in other medical terms.

In the preceding example, you can define the term by literally translating it. However, a few medical terms have an *implied meaning*.

For example, the word

an/emia

literally translated means without (an) blood (emia). However, the correct interpretation of anemia—an implied meaning—is a *deficiency* of red blood cells.

Knowledge of the meanings of the word parts for a medical term with an implied meaning takes you almost, but not quite, to the exact meaning of the term.

Medical terms are used instead of English words because one word says what it would take many English words to say. For example, *nephrectomy* means "surgical removal of the kidney." Medical terms are efficient, factual, save space, and often describe a situation or procedure more exactly.

Pronunciation of medical terms varies. What is acceptable pronunciation in one part of the country may not be used in another part of the country; therefore, flexibility is necessary in the pronunciation of medical terms.

As you begin working with medical terminology, you will feel overwhelmed at the task of learning this new language. However, repeated use of the word parts will assist you in building your vocabulary, and you will soon be using medical terms fluently in your everyday speech.

This unit deals with the word elements and how they are used together to form medical terms. *Remember*: it is important for you to master Unit I before proceeding to Unit II, and so forth, because each unit is a continuation of the previously studied units.

## WORD ELEMENTS

In this course of study the development of a medical vocabulary is based upon memorizing parts of words rather than the whole word. **Word element** is the term we will use to describe the components of words. To build or analyze (divide into parts) medical terms, you must first learn the following four word elements:

1. The word *root*
2. The *prefix*
3. The *suffix*
4. The *combining vowel*

### The Word Root

The **word root** is the basic part of the word; it expresses the principal meaning of the word. For example, in the medical term gastr/ic

gastr (which means stomach) is the word root.

## The Prefix

The **prefix** is the part of the word placed *before* the word root to alter its meaning. For example, in the medical term

intra/gastr/ic

intra (which means within) is the prefix.

## The Suffix

The **suffix** is the part of the word added *after* the word root to alter its meaning. For example, in the medical term

gastr/ic

ic (which means pertaining to) is the suffix.

## The Combining Vowel

The **combining vowel** is usually an *o* used between two word roots or between a word root and a suffix to ease pronunciation. When connecting a *word root* to a *suffix*, a combining vowel is usually *not used* if the suffix begins with a *vowel*. For example, in the word

gastr/ectomy

ectomy (surgical removal) begins with the word *e*; thus the combining vowel *o* is not used.

When connecting *two word roots*, the combing vowel is usually *used* even though the second root begins with a vowel. For example, in the word

gastr/o/enter/itis

the second word root enter (intestinal) begins with the vowel *e*, but the combining vowel *o* is still used.

*Note*: A combining form is simply the word root and the combining vowel. For example, gastr/o is a combining form.

Throughout this chapter the word roots are listed in combining forms.

## ANALYZING MEDICAL TERMS

To **analyze medical terms** means to divide the term into word elements and identify each word element. Divide the word into word elements by use of vertical slashes and identify the word element by labeling it as follows: P—prefix; WR—word root; S—suffix; CV—combining vowel.

| Word Roots | Meaning |
|---|---|
| electr | electricity |
| gastr | stomach |
| hepat | liver |
| cyt | cell |
| cardi | heart |
| nephr | kidney |

| Prefixes | Meaning |
|---|---|
| intra | within |
| sub | under |
| trans | across |

| Suffixes | Meaning |
|---|---|
| itis | inflammation |
| ectomy | surgical removal (excision) |
| gram | a record |
| ic | pertaining to |
| ology | the study of |

## EXERCISE 1

### ANALYZING MEDICAL TERMS

Analyze the following medical terms by dividing each into word elements and writing P, WR, S, or CV above the appropriate part, as in the following examples. Use the following list to help you identify word elements.

WR CV WR S      P  WR S
gastr/ o /enter/itis   intra/gastr/ic

*Examples*:

1. cytology      3. subhepatic      5. cardiology

2. gastrectomy   4. electrocardiogram   6. transhepatic

## WORD BUILDING

**Word building** is the process of creating a medical term using word elements. In building medical terms from a given definition, keep in mind that the *beginning* of the definition usually indicates the *suffix* that is needed to build the term.

## EXERCISE 2

### WORD BUILDING

Build medical terms from the following definitions. Use the above list to assist you.

*Example*: study of the stomach _____gastrology_____

1. the study of the heart _____

2. the study of cells _____

3. surgical removal of the stomach _____

4. inflammation of the stomach _____

5. pertaining to the stomach _____

6. pertaining to within the stomach _____

7. surgical removal of the kidney _____

## REVIEW QUESTIONS

1. List the four word elements. Define and give an example of each.

a. _____

_____

b. _____

_____

c. _____

_____

d. _____

_____

2. Define:

a. analysis of medical terms

_____

_____

b. word building

_____

_____

## UNIT II

# Body Structure and Skin

### OBJECTIVES

*Upon mastery of basic human structure for this unit, you will be able to:*

1. Define cell, tissue, organs, and system.
2. Name four kinds of tissue.
3. List five body cavities and name a body organ contained in each.
4. Define the directional terms outlined in this unit.
5. Describe the function and structure of skin.
6. Briefly describe the structure of the living cell.
7. Describe cancer, abscess, laceration, burns, gangrene, and infection.

## BODY STRUCTURE

### Body Cells

The **cell** is the basic unit of all life. The human body is made up of trillions of cells. Cells perform specific functions, and their size and shape vary according to function. Bones, muscles, skin, and blood are each made up of different kinds of cells. The cell was discovered by Robert Hooke over 300 years ago. Body cells are microscopic; approximately 2000 are needed to make an inch. Cells are constantly growing and reproducing. Such growth is responsible for the development of an embryo into a child and a child into an adult. This growth is also responsible for the replacement of cells that have a relative short life span and cells that are injured, diseased, or worn out.

To visualize the structure of a cell we can compare the three main parts of the cell with the three parts of an egg: the egg shell, the egg white, and the egg yolk.

- *Cell Membrane*
  The **cell membrane** (egg shell) (Fig. 23–1) is porous, flexible, and elastic, which allows for a solution to move in and out. The cell membrane keeps the cell intact. The cell dies if the cell membrane can no longer carry out this function.
- *Cytoplasm*
  **Cytoplasm** (egg white) is the main body of the cell. Cell activities take place here. For example, in the muscle cell the contracting is done by the cytoplasm.
- *Nucleus*
  The **nucleus** (egg yolk) is small and is located near the center of the cell. It is the control center of the cell and plays an important role in reproduction. Chromosomes located in the nucleus contain the genes that determine hereditary characteristics. All cells do not contain a nucleus, such as the mature red blood cell (Fig. 23–2). Some other cells contain several nuclei, an example is the skeletal muscles.

### Body Tissues

A **tissue** is made up of a group of similar cells that work together to perform particular functions.

Four types of tissues are:

- *Epithelial Tissue*
  **Epithelial tissue** forms protective coverings (skin), lines body openings (respiratory tract), and forms glands.
- *Connective Tissue*
  The main function of the **connective tissue** is to connect tissues to one another, as implied in its name. Connective tissue forms bones, fat, and cartilage and provides immunity.
- *Muscle Tissue*
  **Muscle tissue** forms the muscles of the body, which contract and relax to produce movement.
- *Nerve Tissue*
  **Nerve tissue** forms parts of the nervous system, which conducts impulses and helps to coordinate body activities.

### Body Organs

An **organ** is made up of several kinds of tissues. The stomach is an organ. It is made up of muscle, nerve, connective, and epithelial tissue.

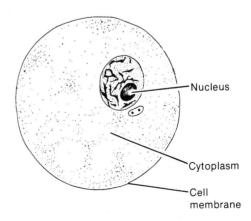

**FIGURE 23–1 •** A body cell. (From Mayes, M. E.: *Nurses' Aide Study Manual*, 3rd ed. Philadelphia, W.B. Saunders Co., 1976, with permission.)

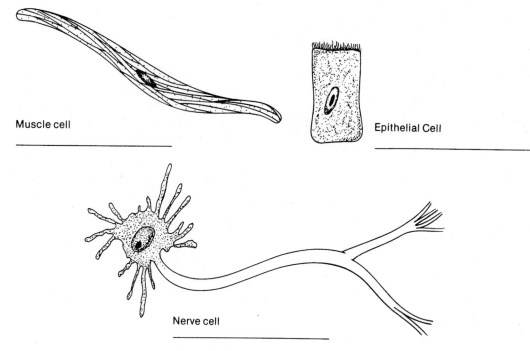

Muscle cell

Epithelial Cell

Nerve cell

F I G U R E  23–2 • Types of cells.

## Body Systems

A **system** is a group of organs that work together to perform complex body functions (Fig. 23–3). For example, the urinary system is made up of the following organs: kidneys, ureters, urinary bladder, and urethra. Its function is to remove wastes from the blood and eliminate them from the body. Other body systems are digestive, musculoskeletal, nervous, reproductive, endocrine, circulatory, and respiratory. Some organs are a part of more than one system. The pharynx, for example, is part of both the digestive and respiratory systems. In the digestive system the pharynx allows for the passage of food; in the respiratory system it allows for the passage of air.

## Body Cavities

Large spaces within the body that contain internal organs are called **body cavities** (Fig. 24–4). The body cavities are:

- *Cranial*
  Contains the brain.
- *Thoracic*
  Contains the heart, lungs, and esophagus.
- *Abdominal*
  Contains the stomach, intestines, kidneys, liver, pancreas, gallbladder, and spleen. The abdominal cavity is separated from the thoracic cavity by a muscle called the **diaphragm**.
- *Pelvic*
  Contains the bladder, urethra, ureters, and reproductive organs.
- *Spinal*
  Contains the spinal cord.

## Body Directional Terms

Directional terms are used to describe a location on or within the body.

- *Superior (cranial)*
  Pertaining to *above*. (The eye is located *superior* to the mouth.)
- *Inferior (caudal)*
  Pertaining to *below*. (The mouth is located *inferior* to the nose.)
- *Anterior (ventral)*
  Pertaining to *in front of*. (The ribs are located *anterior* to the shoulder blade.)
- *Posterior (dorsal)*
  Pertaining to *in back of*. (The shoulder blade is located *posterior* to the ribs.)
- *Lateral*
  Pertaining to the *side*. (The little toe is *lateral* to the big toe.)
- *Medial*
  Pertaining to the *middle*. (The big toe is *medial* to the little toe.)
- *Abduction*
  Pertaining to *away* from.
- *Adduction*
  Pertaining to *towards*.

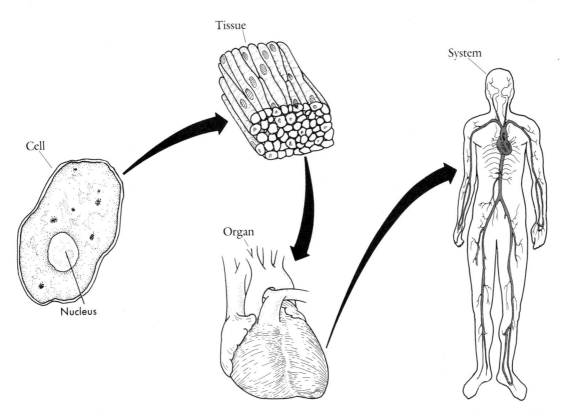

**F I G U R E  23–3 •** Organization of the body. (From LaFleur, M., and Starr, W.: *Exploring Medical Language*. St. Louis, The C.V. Mosby Co., 1985, with permission.)

## SKIN

The **skin** is the largest organ of the body (Fig. 23–5). The skin of an adult may weigh 20 lb or more.

The skin has many functions. The main one is to protect underlying tissues from pathogenic (disease-causing) microorganisms and other environmental hazards. The skin also assists in the regulation of body temperature and is a sensory organ that passes messages of pain, cold, and touch to the brain.

The outer layer of skin is called the **epidermis** and is made of epithelial tissue. The cells of the innermost layer produce themselves. As they move toward the surface, the outermost cells are shed. Millions of cells are produced and shed each day. The epidermis contains no blood vessels.

The layer directly below the epidermis is called the **dermis**, or true skin. It is made up of connective tissue and contains blood vessels, nerve endings, and sweat and oil glands.

The **subcutaneous tissue** is thick, fat-containing tissue located below the dermis and is a means of connecting the skin proper to surface muscles.

The **hair follicle** is a pouch-like depression in the skin from which the hair grows to extend above the skin surface. **Oil glands** (sebaceous glands) connect to the hair follicle by tiny ducts. Each sebaceous gland produces oil (sebum), which lubricates the hair and skin.

The **sweat glands** are coiled, tube-like structures located mainly in the dermis. Each extends to the surface in the form of a tiny opening called a **pore**. There are approximately 3000 pores in the palm of a hand and approximately 2,000,000 on the body surface. Sweat is produced by the sweat glands. As sweat evaporates on the body surface, it cools the body. Skin color is determined by the amount of melanin in the skin. Skin color varies from pale yellow to black.

## DISEASES AND CONDITIONS OF THE SKIN AND BODY CELLS

### Cancer

**Cancer** (CA) is a disease in which unregulated new growth of abnormal cell occurs. It is normal for worn-out body cells to be replaced by new cell growth and also for

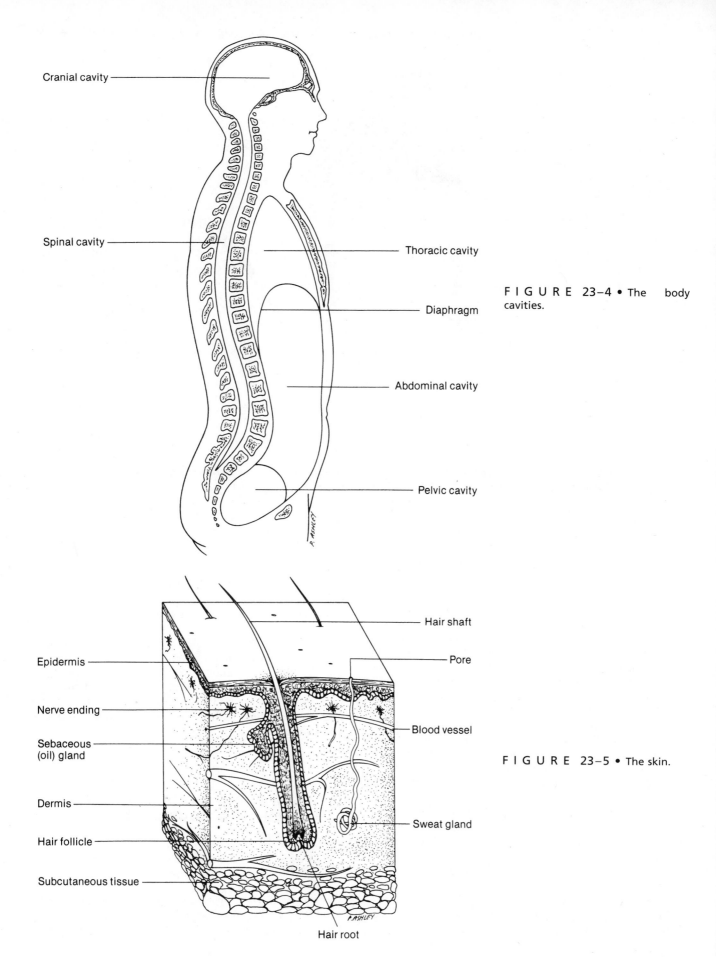

Cranial cavity

Spinal cavity

Thoracic cavity

Diaphragm

Abdominal cavity

Pelvic cavity

FIGURE 23-4 • The body cavities.

Hair shaft

Pore

Epidermis

Nerve ending

Sebaceous (oil) gland

Dermis

Hair follicle

Subcutaneous tissue

Blood vessel

Sweat gland

Hair root

FIGURE 23-5 • The skin.

new cells to form to repair tissue damage. Normal cell growth is regulated; in cancer the growth is unregulated, and it continues to reproduce until a mass known as a **tumor**, or **neoplasm**, forms.

Cancerous tumors are malignant, which means they become progressively worse, whereas noncancerous tumors are benign or nonrecurrent. Malignant tumors grow in a disorganized fashion, interrupting body function and interfering with the food and blood supply to normal cells. Malignant cells may **metastasize** (spread) from one organ to another through the bloodstream or lymphatic system.

Cancer is many different diseases, and one cause cannot be pinpointed. Cigarette smoking, exposure to carcinogenic substances, and ultraviolet rays are believed to cause 80% of cancers.

Treatments of cancer include surgery, chemotherapy, and radiation therapy.

### Cancer's Seven Warning Signals

■ Change in bowel or bladder habits
■ Unusual bleeding or discharge
■ Thickening or lump in the breast or elsewhere
■ Change in a wart or mole
■ Nagging cough or hoarseness
■ A sore that does not heal
■ Indigestion or difficulty in swallowing

## Burns

All burns are dangerous if not treated properly because infection can occur and because shock is possible in more serious burns. Burns are classified according to degrees of severity (Fig. 23–6).

1. First-degree burns damage the epidermis.
2. Second-degree burns damage the epidermis and the dermis.
3. Third-degree burns damage the epidermis, dermis, and subcutaneous tissue.

## Abscesses

An **abscess** is a cavity containing pus. Abscesses are usually caused by pathogenic microorganisms that invade the tissue through a break in the skin. As the microorganisms destroy the tissue an increased blood supply is rushed to the area, causing inflammation in the surrounding tissue. Abscesses are formed by the body to wall off the pathogenic microorganisms and keep them from spreading throughout the body.

## Lacerations

A **laceration** is a wound produced by tearing body tissue. Cleaning the laceration is important because of the danger of infection. Suturing may be required to repair lacerations.

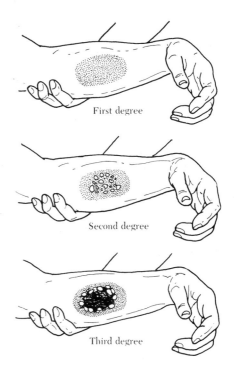

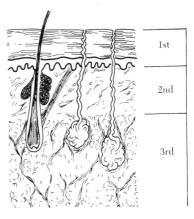

**FIGURE 23–6** • First-degree burns damage the epidermis; second-degree burns damage the epidermis and the dermis; third-degree burns damage the epidermis, dermis, and the subcutaneous tissue. (From Miller, B. F. and Keane, C. B.: *Encyclopedia and Dictionary of Medicine, Nursing, and Allied Health*, 4th ed. Philadelphia, W.B. Saunders Co., 1987, with permission.)

## Gangrene

**Gangrene** is the death of body tissue caused by lack of blood supply to an area of the body; often it is the result of infection or injury. Symptoms include fever, pain, darkening of the skin, and an unpleasant odor. Treatment includes surgical debridement (removal with a sharp instrument) of the necrotic tissue, which must occur before healing can begin.

## Infection

**Infection** is the invasion of the body by pathogenic microorganisms that reproduce and multiply, causing disease. Infections may be caused by streptococcal, staphylococcal, or *Pseudomonas* bacteria; by viruses; or by other organisms.

Bacterial infections are treated with antibiotic therapy.

---

**REVIEW QUESTIONS**

1. Define:

   a. cell _____

   b. tissue _____

   c. organ _____

   d. system _____

2. Name four kinds of tissues:

   a. _____     c. _____

   b. _____     d. _____

3. List five body cavities and name one internal organ contained in each:

   a. _____     d. _____

   _____     _____

   b. _____     e. _____

   _____     _____

   c. _____

   _____

4. Match the following directional terms in Column I with the correct meaning in Column II.

   | Column I | Column II |
   | --- | --- |
   | a. superior | _____ in front of |
   | b. inferior | _____ pertaining to the middle |
   | c. lateral | _____ pertaining to away from |
   | d. medial | _____ pertaining to the side |
   | e. anterior | _____ above |
   | f. posterior | _____ below |
   | g. adduction | _____ pertaining to towards |
   | h. abduction | _____ in back of |

5. List three functions of the skin:

   a. _____

   b. _____

   c. _____

6. The outermost layer of the skin is called the _____ . The layer of

   skin directly below this layer is called the _____ . The next thick

   layer of fat-containing tissue is called the _____ tissue.

7. Skin color is determined by the amount of _____ in the skin.

8. _____ glands produce oil that lubricates the skin and hair.

9. _____ open to the surface of the skin in tiny openings called
   pores.

10. Describe the structure of a living cell.

    _____

    _____

    _____

11. Match the terms in Column I with the phrases in Column II.

|  | **Column I** | **Column II** |
|---|---|---|
| a. | burns | _____ cavity containing pus |
| b. | abscess | _____ classified according to degree |
| c. | laceration | _____ invasion of the body by pathogenic microorganisms |
| d. | gangrene | _____ new growth of abnormal cells |
| e. | infection | _____ death of body tissue |
| f. | cancer | _____ wound produced by tearing |
| g. | dermatitis | |

## MEDICAL TERMINOLOGY RELATING TO BODY STRUCTURE AND SKIN

### OBJECTIVES

*Upon mastery of medical terminology for this unit, you will be able to:*

1. Define, spell, and pronounce the medical terms listed in this unit.

2. Analyze the medical terms that are built from word elements.

3. Given a meaning of a medical condition, build the corresponding medical terms, using word elements.

Listed below are the word elements you will be working with in this unit. You will need to memorize each one because you will continue to use them in this chapter and in your work environment. The exercises following the lists will assist you in this task. Practice pronouncing each word element aloud.

To review, a word root is the basic part of the word; a combining form is the word root plus a combining vowel

(*o*); and a suffix is the part added on to the end of a word root.

| Word Roots/Combining Forms | Meaning |
|---|---|
| carcin/o (kar'-sĭn-ō) | cancer |
| cyt/o (sī'-tō) | cell |
| derm/o (der'-mō) | skin |
| dermat/o (der'-mah-tō) | skin |
| epitheli/o (ĕp-ĭ-thē'-lē-ō) | epithelium |
| hist/o (hĭs'-tō) | tissue |
| lip/o (lĭp'-ō) | fat |
| path/o (păth'-ō) | disease |
| sarc/o (sar'-cō) | connective tissue |
| trich/o (trĭk'-ō) | hair |
| viscer/o (vš'-er-ō) | internal organs |

Many of the suffixes presented in this course of study are made up of word roots and suffixes. For example, the suffix <u>ology</u> is built from <u>log</u> (word root for "study") plus <u>y</u> (suffix). For learning purposes, these will be studied as suffixes and be analyzed as one word element.

| Suffixes | Meaning |
|---|---|
| al | pertaining to |
| genic (jĕn′-ĭk) | producing |
| itis (i′-tĭs) | inflammation |
| oid (oyd) | resembling |
| ologist (ŏl′-ō-jĭst) | one who studies and practices (specialist) |
| ology (ŏl′-ō-jē) | study of |
| oma (ō′-mah) | tumor |

| Prefix | Meaning |
|---|---|
| trans (trăns) | through, across, beyond |

### EXERCISE 1

Define each combining form listed below.

1. viscer/o _____

2. dermat/o _____

3. cyt/o _____

4. hist/o _____

5. derm/o _____

6. trich/o _____

7. path/o _____

8. carcin/o _____

9. sarc/o _____

10. epitheli/o _____

11. lip/o _____

### EXERCISE 2

Define each suffix and prefix listed below.

1. al _____

2. ology _____

3. ologist _____

4. oid _____

5. itis _____

6. oma _____

7. genic _____

8. trans _____

### EXERCISE 3

Write the word element for each definition below. Indicate which word elements are suffixes by writing S in the space provided, indicate which word elements are word roots or combining forms by writing WR in the space provided, and indicate which word elements are prefixes by writing P in the space provided.

| | Meaning | Word Element | Type of Word Element |
|---|---|---|---|
| Example | inflammation | itis | S |
| 1. | cell | _____ | _____ |
| 2. | skin | _____ | _____ |
| 3. | specialist | _____ | _____ |
| 4. | resembling | _____ | _____ |
| 5. | internal organs | _____ | _____ |
| 6. | tissues | _____ | _____ |
| 7. | pertaining to | _____ | _____ |
| 8. | study of | _____ | _____ |
| 9. | through | _____ | _____ |
| 10. | cancer | _____ | _____ |

## MEDICAL TERMS RELATING TO BODY STRUCTURE AND SKIN

Listed below are the medical terms you need to know for this unit. Practice pronouncing these words aloud. Following the list are exercises that will assist you in learning these terms.

| General Terms | Meaning |
|---|---|
| carcinogenic (kar'-sĭn-ō-jĕn'-ik) | cancer producing |
| cytoid (sī-toyd) | resembling a cell |
| cytology (sī-tŏl'-ō-jē) | study of cells |
| dermal (dĕr'-mal) | pertaining to the skin |
| dermatoid (dĕr'-măh-toyd) | resembling skin |
| dermatologist (dĕr-măh-tŏl'-ō-jĭst) | a doctor who specializes in dermatology |
| dermatology (dĕr-măh-tŏl'-ō-jē) | the branch of medicine that deals with diagnosis and treatment of skin disease |
| epithelial (ĕp-ĭ-thē'-lē-al) | pertaining to epithelium |
| histology (hĭs-tŏl-ō-jē) | study of tissues |
| pathogenic (păth-ō-jĕn'-ĭk) | disease producing |
| pathologist (pĥ-thŏl'-ō-jĭst) | a doctor who specializes in pathology (body changes caused by disease) |
| pathology (păh-thŏl'-ō-jē) | the study of body changes caused by disease |
| trichoid (trĭk'-oyd) | resembling hair |
| visceral (vĭs'-er-al) | pertaining to internal organs |
| transdermal (trăns-dĕr'-mal) transcutaneous | pertaining to through (entering) the skin |

| Diagnostic Terms | Meaning |
|---|---|
| carcinoma (kăr-sĭ-nō'-mah) | cancerous tumor (malignant) |
| dermatitis (dĕr-mah-tī'-tĭs) | inflammation of the skin |
| epithelioma (ĕp-ĭ-thē-lē-ō'-ah) | a tumor composed of epithelial cells |
| lipoma (lī-pō'-mah) | a tumor containing fat |
| sarcoma (sar-kō'-mah) | a tumor composed of connective tissue |

## EXERCISE 4

Analyze and define each term listed below.

*Example:*                    a doctor who specializes in pathology
WR/  S
path/ologist

*Analyzing note*: If the *o*, as in the word path/ology, is studied as a part of the suffix, it is not considered a combining vowel in this course of study and remains as part of the suffix.

**Analyze**                                                    **Define**

1. cytology  _____

2. trichoid  _____

3. pathology  _____

4. pathogenic  _____

5. dermal  _____

6. cytoid  _____

7. visceral  _____

8. histology  _____

9. dermatologist _____

10. dermatitis _____

11. carcinogenic _____

12. epithelial _____

13. carcinoma _____

14. epithelioma _____

15. sarcoma _____

16. lipoma _____

17. pathologist _____

18. dermatoid _____

19. dermatology _____

20. transdermal _____

## E X E R C I S E  5

Build the medical terms that correspond with the definitions listed below. Remember that the *beginning* of the definition usually indicates the *suffix* that is needed to build the term.

1. resembling a cell _____

2. resembling hair _____

3. resembling skin _____

4. a doctor who specializes in pathology _____

5. a doctor who specializes in the treatment of skin diseases _____

6. pertaining to the skin _____

7. pertaining to the internal organs _____

8. the study of tissues _____

9. the study of body changes caused by disease _____

10. the branch of medicine that deals with skin disease _____

11. disease producing _____

12. study of cells _____

13. inflammation of the skin _____

14. a tumor containing fat _____

15. a tumor composed of epithelial cells _____

16. pertaining to epithelium _____

17. cancer producing _____

18. a tumor composed of connective tissue _____

19. cancerous tumor _____

20. pertaining to through the skin _____

## E X E R C I S E 6

Build each medical term studied in this unit by having someone dictate the terms to you.

1. _____
2. _____
3. _____
4. _____
5. _____
6. _____
7. _____
8. _____
9. _____
10. _____

11. _____
12. _____
13. _____
14. _____
15. _____
16. _____
17. _____
18. _____
19. _____
20. _____

# U N I T III

# The Musculoskeletal System

## O B J E C T I V E S

*Upon mastery of basic human structures for this unit, you will be able to:*

1. Describe five functions of bones.
2. Describe bone structure.
3. Name and spell correctly the bones of the body.
4. Define joint, ligament, and tendon.
5. Describe three types of muscles.
6. Describe arthritis, herniated disk, Paget's disease, osteoporosis, types of fractures, and hip replacement.

## THE SKELETAL SYSTEM

### Organs of the Skeletal System

Bones (206 in an adult skeleton).

### Functions of the Skeletal System

- To protect the internal organs
- To provide a framework for the body
- To act with the muscles to produce body movement
- To produce blood cells
- To store calcium

### Bone Structure

- Bones have their own system of blood vessels and nerves.
- Bones contain **red bone marrow** (which manufactures blood cells) and **yellow bone marrow** (which is mostly fat).
- Bones are covered with a thin membrane called **periosteum**, which is necessary for growth and repair.

### The Bone Framework of the Head
(Fig. 23–7)

#### Cranium (8 Bones)

- **Frontal bone (1)**: Framework of the forehead and roof of the eye socket.
- **Parietal bones (2)**: Form the upper sides of the cranium.
- **Temporal bones (2)**: Form the lower sides of the cranium and contain parts of the ear.

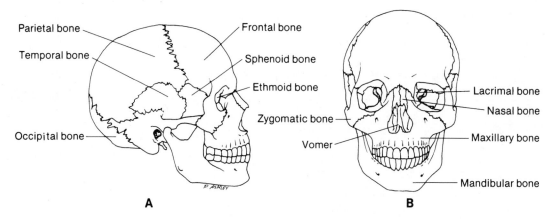

FIGURE 23–7 • The bones of the skull. (A) Cranial bones. (B) Facial bones.

- **Ethmoid bone (1)**: Forms part of the cranial floor and part of the nasal cavity.
- **Sphenoid bone (1)**: A bat-shaped bone that extends behind the eyes and forms part of the base of the skull.
- **Occipital bone (1)**: A bone composing the back and most of the base of the skull. It connects with the parietal and temporal bones.

### Facial Bones (10 Bones)

- **Maxillary bones (2)**: Upper jaw bones.
- **Mandible (1)**: Lower jaw bone. The mandible is the only movable bone in the skull.
- **Nasal bones (2)**: Support the bridge of the nose.
- **Lacrimal bones (2)**: Corner of the eye sockets.
- **Zygomatic bones (2)**: Cheek bones.
- **Vomer (1)**: Lower portion of the nasal septum.

## Vertebral Column (Fig. 23–8)

- **Cervical (7)**: The first seven vertebrae, which form the neck.
- **Thoracic (12)**: The following 12 vertebrae, which form the outward curve of the spine, and join with 12 pairs of ribs.
- **Lumbar (5)**: The next five vertebrae, which are the largest and strongest, and form the inward curvature of the spine.
- **Sacrum (5)**: The next five vertebrae; these are fused together in the adult.
- **Coccyx (3–5)**: The last three to five vertebrae; in the adult, these fuse together to form one coccyx.

The vertebrae form the spinal column. Openings in the vertebrae provide a continuous space through which the spinal cord travels. The vertebrae are separated by disks (plates of cartilage). The central portion of the disk is filled with a pulpy elastic substance called *nucleus pulposus*. The disks allow for flexibility and absorb shock. The lamina is located on the posterior arch of the vertebra.

## Rib Cage

- All 24 ribs are attached posteriorly to the thoracic vertebrae.
- The first seven pairs of ribs (**true ribs**) attach anteriorly to the sternum; the next three pairs converge and join the seventh rib anteriorly; and the last two pairs remain free at the anterior ends. The last five pairs of ribs are called **false ribs**. The last two pairs are often referred to as **free** or **floating ribs**.

### Sternum (1 Bone)

The sternum is the breast bone.

## Upper Extremities

- **Clavicle (2)**: Collar bone.
- **Scapula (2)**: Shoulder blade.

### Arm and Hand Bones (Fig. 23–9)

- **Humerus (2)**: Upper arm bone.
- **Ulna (2)**: Smaller lower arm bone, finger side.
- **Radius (2)**: Larger lower arm bone, thumb side.
- **Carpals (16)**: Wrist bones.
- **Metacarpals (10)**: Bones of the hand.
- **Phalanges (28)**: Three bones in each finger and two bones in each thumb.

## Lower Extremities

The **pelvic bones** are composed of three pairs of bones fused together. These are:

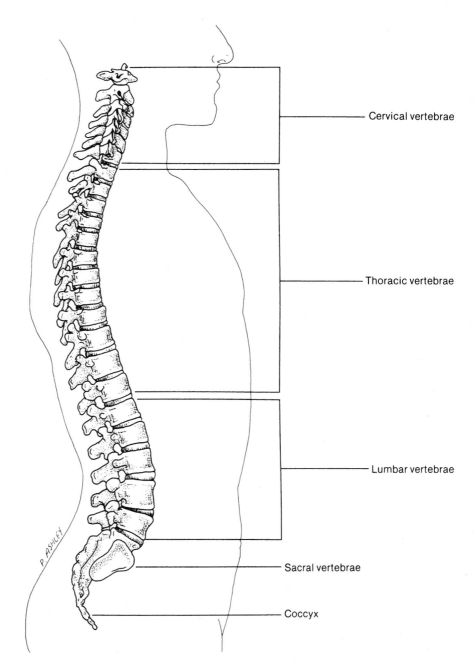

FIGURE 23–8 • The vertebral column.

Cervical vertebrae

Thoracic vertebrae

Lumbar vertebrae

Sacral vertebrae

Coccyx

- **Ilium (2)**: Uppermost, largest portion of the pelvis.
- **Ischium (2)**: Lower, posterior portion of the pelvis.
- **Pubis (2)**: Anterior portion of the pelvis.

## Leg and Foot Bones

- **Femur (2)**: Thigh bone, larges bone in the body.
- **Patella (2)**: Kneecap.
- **Tibia (2)**: Largest, inner lower leg bone (shin bone).
- **Fibula (2)**: Smaller, outer lower leg bone.
- **Tarsals (4)**: Ankle bones.
- **Metatarsals (10)**: Bones of the foot.
- **Phalanges (28)**: Three bones in each toe, except for two in each big toe.

## Joints

A **joint** is that place on the skeleton where two or more bones meet. Joints allow for movement and hold bones together. **Ligaments** are tough bands of tissue that connect one bone with another bone at a joint.

## THE MUSCULAR SYSTEM

## Organs of the Muscular System

Muscles.

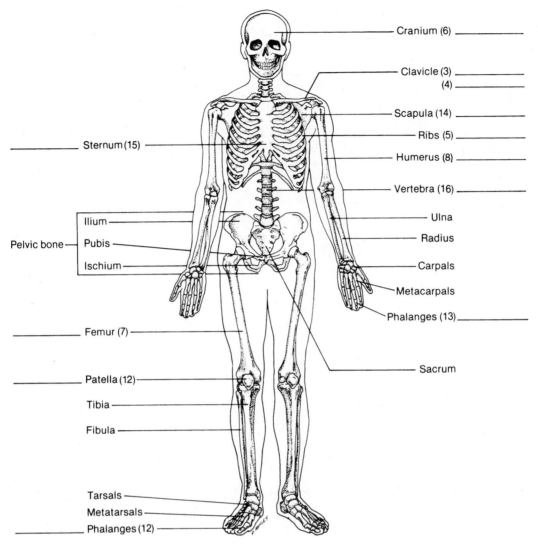

Cranium (6) _____

Clavicle (3) _____
(4) _____

Scapula (14) _____

Ribs (5) _____

Humerus (8) _____

Vertebra (16) _____

Ulna

Radius

Carpals

Metacarpals

Phalanges (13) _____

_____ Sternum (15)

Ilium

Pelvic bone — Pubis

Ischium

_____ Femur (7)

_____ Patella (12)

Tibia

Fibula

Tarsals

Metatarsals

_____ Phalanges (12)

Sacrum

F I G U R E  23–9 • The skeleton.

## Muscular Function

Muscles produce movement of body parts. Oxygen and nerve supply to the muscle are necessary for muscle function.

## Types of Muscles

- **Voluntary Muscle:** The voluntary muscles are controlled by the conscious portion of the brain. There are over 600 voluntary muscles (skeletal muscles) that enable the body to move. The muscles are attached to the bones by **tendons**. Muscle action is produced by a pulling motion, and muscles work in pairs.
- **Involuntary Muscle:** The involuntary muscles are not under the control of the conscious part of the brain but respond to impulses from the autonomic nerves. Involuntary muscles are located in the walls of the blood vessels and in internal organs (such as the stomach).

- **Cardiac Muscle:** The cardiac muscle is found in the heart and is also an involuntary muscle.

## DISEASES AND CONDITIONS OF THE MUSCULOSKELETAL SYSTEM

## Arthritis

Over 100 types of joint diseases exist; the two most common types are rheumatoid arthritis and osteoarthritis. Much is still unknown about the cause of arthritis; however, it has been observed that emotional upset can aggravate the disease.

### Rheumatoid Arthritis

**Rheumatoid Arthritis** usually occurs between the ages of 20 and 40 years, more commonly in women. The onset of symptoms, which include malaise, fever, weight loss, and stiffness of the joints, is gradual. The symptoms come and go. If the disease becomes chronic, degeneration of the joints, with permanent damage, occurs. Treatment consists of heat and drugs, such as aspirin and cortisone, to reduce inflammation and pain.

### Osteoarthritis

**Osteoarthritis** usually occurs in the large, weight-bearing joints, such as the hips. It is the chronic inflammation of the bone and joints caused by degenerative changes in the cartilage covering the surface of the joints. It occurs mostly in older individuals. Treatment consists of drugs to reduce the pain and inflammation and physical therapy to loosen the impaired joints.

## Ruptured Disk

A *ruptured disk* may also be referred to as a slipped or herniated disk or as a herniated nucleus pulposus (HNP). It is the abnormal protrusion of the nucleus pulposus of the intervertebral disk into the neural canal that causes pressure on the spinal cord. Such herniation occurs mostly in the lower back. Treatment consists of bedrest, traction, and analgesics. A laminectomy may be performed to remove a portion of the vertebra, creating more room for the protruding portion of the disk, or a diskectomy may be performed, in which the disk is removed and two or more of the vertebrae are fused together (Fig. 23–10).

## Osteoporosis

Osteoporosis is an abnormal decrease in the amount of bone mass and is the leading cause of fractures. It is the most prevalent bone disease in the world. Over 20 million people in the United States have osteoporosis. Postmenopausal estrogen-deficient women are the most likely to be affected. Age-related osteoporosis affects both men and women equally. Osteoporosis is known as the "silent crippler," resulting in a virtually symptomless process. Symptoms occur after the disease has progressed. The most common symptoms are pain, and loss of height due to the bent-over position that the person assumes. The disease can cause up to an 8-inch loss in height. Fractures occur in all parts of the skeletal system.

The disease is diagnosed by radiologic studies to measure the bone density and serum calcium levels. Since the disease is virtually symptom free, the focus is on prevention to minimize bone loss. Prevention measures include calcium supplements, exercise, hormonal replacement therapy, and correct posture.

## Paget's Disease

Paget's disease, a common condition occurring in 3% of the population over age 40, causes bones to become extremely weak. The bone may fracture with a very slight blow. If the vertebrae is involved, it may collapse. Bones are living substances that are in a constant process of dissolving and rebuilding. Osteoblasts are the cells that rebuild bone, and osteoclasts are the cells that dissolve bone. An imbalance of this dissolving and rebuilding process results in weak areas or lesions of the bone.

The symptoms of Paget's disease depend on the bones that are affected. Lesions in long bones cause pain, bowing, and arthritic changes of the extremities. When the disease affects the skull, the patient may have headaches, ringing in the ears, hearing loss, and dizziness. If the skull involvement affects the occipital region, pressure is placed on the cerebellum that may compress the spinal cord.

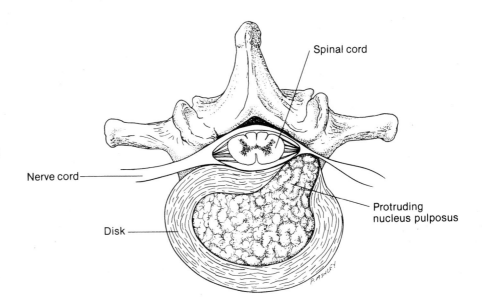

FIGURE 23–10 • A ruptured disk.

Pressure on the spinal cord causes neurologic changes such as muscle weakness, loss of coordination, and ataxia.

Diagnosis is made by radiologic studies of the affected bone. The serum alkaline phosphatase and urinary hydroxyproline levels will be elevated. The treatment for Paget's disease is Didronel, a drug that slows down the dissolving process of the osteoclasts.

## Fractures (FX)

A **fracture** is an injury to a bone in which the bone is broken (Fig. 23–11). A fracture is classified by the bone that is injured, such as "fractured radius." Some types of fractures are:

**Closed**, or **simple**:  a broken bone but no open wound.
**Open**, or **compound**: a broken bone and an open wound in the skin.
**Greenstick**: a bone partially bent and partially broken.
**Comminuted**: the bone is splintered or crushed.
**Spiral**: the bone has been twisted apart.

An **open** or **closed reduction** is used to correct a fracture. A closed reduction is done without an incision, whereas an open reduction is done after an incision is made into the fracture site.

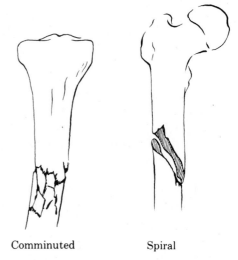

Comminuted          Spiral

**F I G U R E  23–11 •** Types of fractures.

## HIP REPLACEMENT

**Hip replacement** (also called total hip arthroplasty) uses an artificial ball-and-socket joint to replace the patient's hip joint. Hips are replaced in cases of advanced osteoarthritis and improperly healed fractures, or to relieve a chronically painful or stiff hip.

---

**REVIEW QUESTIONS**

1. List five functions of the skeletal system.

   a. _____

   b. _____

   c. _____

   d. _____

   e. _____

2. _____ is a thin membrane that covers bones.

3. Write the names of the bones that make up the cranium and the face. Indicate the number of each.

**Cranium**

| Bone | No. | Bone | No. |
|------|-----|------|-----|
| a. _____ | ____ | d. _____ | ____ |
| b. _____ | ____ | e. _____ | ____ |
| c. _____ | ____ | f. _____ | ____ |

**Face**

| Bone | No. | | Bone | No. |
|------|-----|--|------|-----|
| a. _____ | ____ | d. | _____ | ____ |
| b. _____ | ____ | e. | _____ | ____ |
| c. _____ | ____ | f. | _____ | ____ |

4. List the five regions of the vertebral column.

   a. _____     d. _____

   b. _____     e. _____

   c. _____

5. Write the name of the bone to match the definitions written below.

   a. shoulder blade _____

   b. collar bone _____

   c. upper arm bone _____

   d. lower arm bone, thumb side _____

   e. lower arm bone, finger side _____

   f. wrist bones _____

   g. bones of the hand _____

   h. finger bones _____

6. Write the names of three pairs of bones that are fused together to form the pelvic bones.

   a. _____     c. _____

   b. _____

7. List the bones of the leg and foot.

   a. _____     e. _____

   b. _____     f. _____

   c. _____     g. _____

   d. _____

8. Name the three types of muscles and give an example of each.

   a. _____

   b. _____

   c. _____

9. Define:

   a. joint _____

   b. tendon _____

   c. ligament _____

10. Two types of arthritis are:

   a. _____

   b. _____

11. Two operations that may be performed for a herniated disk are:

   a. _____

   b. _____

12. Define:

   a. closed fracture _____

   b. open fracture _____

   c. spiral fracture _____

   d. comminuted fracture _____

13. Hip replacement is also called _____.

14. Dissolving and rebuilding of bone is called _____ and

   _____.

15. When Paget's disease affects the skull the symptoms are

   a. _____

   b. _____

   c. _____

   d. _____

16. An abnormal decrease in the amount of bone mass is called _____.

17. In osteoporosis, prevention interventions include

   a. _____     c. _____

   b. _____     d. _____

## MEDICAL TERMINOLOGY RELATING TO THE MUSCULOSKELETAL SYSTEM—PREFIXES AND SUFFIXES

### OBJECTIVES

*Upon mastery of the medical terminology for this unit, you will be able to:*

1. Define and spell the word elements and medical terms presented in this unit of study.

2. Analyze the medical terms built from word elements.

3. Given the meaning of a medical condition relating to the musculoskeletal system, build with word elements the corresponding medical term.

4. Given descriptions of hospital situations in which the health unit coordinator may encounter medical terminology, apply the correct medical terms to the situation.

| Skeletal System | Meaning |
|---|---|
| 1. arthr/o (ar'-thrō) | joint |
| 2. chondr/o (kŏn'-drō) | cartilage |
| 3. clavic/o (klăv-ĭ-kō) | clavicle (collar bone) |
| 4. clavicul/o (klah-vĭk'-ū-lō) | clavicle (collar bone) |
| 5. cost/o (kŏs'-tō) | rib |
| 6. crani/o (krā'-nē-ō) | cranium (skull) |
| 7. femor/o (fĕm'-or-ō) | femur (thigh bone) |
| 8. humer/o (hūm'-er-ō) | humerus (upper arm bone) |
| 9. lamin/o (lăm'-ĭ-nō) | lamina (bony arch of the vertebrae) |
| 10. menisc/o (mĕ-nĭs'-kō) | meniscus (cartilage of the knee joint) |
| 11. oste/o (ŏs'-tē-ō) | bone |
| 12. patell/o (pah-tĕl'-ō) | patella (kneecap) |
| 13. phalang/o (fah-lăn'-jō) | phalange (finger or toe bone) |
| 14. scapul/o (skăp'-ū-lō) | scapula (shoulder blade) |
| 15. stern/o (ster'-nō) | sternum (breast bone) |
| 16. vertebr/o (ver'-tĕ-brō) | vertebra(s), vertebrae (pl)—bones of the spine |

| Muscular System | Meaning |
|---|---|
| 17. my/o (mī'-ō) | muscle |

| Other | Meaning |
|---|---|
| 18. electr/o (ē-lĕk'-trō) | electric |

## EXERCISE 1

Write the combining forms for the skeletal system in the spaces provided on the diagram in Figure 23–9. The number preceding the combining form in the list above matches the number of the body parts in the diagram.

## EXERCISE 2

Define each combining form listed below.

1. arthr/o  _____
2. oste/o  _____
3. cost/o  _____
4. crani/o  _____
5. femor/o  _____
6. my/o  _____
7. humer/o  _____
8. patell/o  _____
9. stern/o  _____

10. clavicul/o  _____
11. scapul/o  _____
12. phalang/o  _____
13. vertebr/o  _____
14. clavic/o  _____
15. electr/o  _____
16. lamin/o  _____
17. chondr/o  _____
18. menisc/o  _____

# E X E R C I S E  3

Write the combining forms for each part of the body listed below.

1. finger bone _____
2. joint _____
3. bone _____
4. thigh bone _____
5. kneecap _____
6. shoulder blade _____
7. bones of the spine _____
8. collar bone  a. _____
   b. _____

9. skull _____
10. breast bone _____
11. upper arm bone _____
12. rib _____
13. muscle _____
14. lamina _____
15. cartilage _____
16. meniscus _____

Recall from Units I and II that suffixes are letters that may be added to the end of a word root. Listed below are the suffixes you need to know for this unit. Continue to use these throughout the chapter. The exercises will assist you in learning each suffix.

| Suffix | Meaning |
| --- | --- |
| algia (ăl'-jē-ah) | pain |
| ar | pertaining to |
| centesis (sĕn-tē-sš) | puncture and aspiration of |
| ectomy (ĕk'-tō-mē) | surgical removal or excision |
| gram | record |
| graph | instrument to record |
| graphy | process of recording |
| ic | pertaining to |
| osis (ō'-sĭs) | abnormal condition |
| otomy (ŏt'-ō-mē) | surgical incision |
| plasty (plăs'-tē) | surgical repair or plastic repair |
| scope (skōp) | instrument for visual examination |
| scopy (skōp'-ē) | visual examination |
| trophy (trōf'-ē) (may also be used as a word root) | development |

# E X E R C I S E  4

Write the suffix for each term listed below.

1. surgical repair _____
2. pain _____
3. pertaining to  a. _____
   b. _____
4. surgical incision _____
5. surgical removal _____
6. instrument to record _____

7. process of recording _____
8. record _____
9. development _____
10. abnormal condition _____
11. instrument for visual examination _____
12. visual examination _____
13. puncture and aspiration of _____

E X E R C I S E **5**

Write the definition for each suffix listed below.

1. algia _____     8. plasty _____

2. graph _____     9. ectomy _____

3. gram _____     10. ar _____

4. graphy _____     11. osis _____

5. otomy _____     12. scopy _____

6. trophy _____     13. scope _____

7. ic _____     14. centesis _____

Recall from Unit I that prefixes are letters that may be added to the beginning of a word root. Listed below are six prefixes you need to memorize in this unit.

| Prefix | Meaning |
| --- | --- |
| a, an | without (if used with a word root that begins with a vowel, use _an_; if used with a word root that begins with a consonant, use _a_) |
| dys (dĭs) | bad or painful |
| inter | between |
| intra | within |
| sub | under or below |
| supra | above |

E X E R C I S E **6**

Write the prefix for each term listed below.

1. within _____     5. between _____

2. painful _____     6. above _____

3. under _____

4. without   a. _____

            b. _____

E X E R C I S E **7**

Write the definition for each prefix listed below.

1. intra _____     4. dys _____

2. supra _____     5. a, an _____

3. sub _____     6. inter _____

## MEDICAL TERMS RELATING TO THE MUSCULOSKELETAL SYSTEM

Listed below are the medical terms you need to know for this unit. Most are made up of the word roots, prefixes, and suffixes you have been working with; however, there are some words that relate to the musculoskeletal system that are not made up of the word elements you have studied thus far. These are also included in the list. Following the list are exercises that will assist you in learning the meaning and spelling of each word. Practice pronouncing each word aloud.

| General Terms | Meaning |
| --- | --- |
| atrophy (ăt'-rō-fē) | without development; decrease in the size of a normally developed organ |
| chrondogenic (kŏn-drō-jĕn'-ĭk) | producing cartilage |
| cranial (krā'-nē-al) | pertaining to the cranium |
| dystrophy (dĭs'-trō-fē) | bad or faulty development |
| femoral (fĕm'-ō-ral) | pertaining to the femur or thigh bone |
| humeral (hū'-mĕr-al) | pertaining to the humerus |
| intervertebral (ĭn-tĕr-vĕr'-tĕ-bral) | pertaining to between the vertebrae |
| intracranial (ĭn-trah-krā'-nē-al) | pertaining to within the cranium |
| orthopedics (or-thō-pē'-dĭks) | the diagnosis and treatment of disease or fractures of the musculoskeletal system |
| orthopedist (or-thō-pē'-dist) | a doctor who specializes in orthopedics |
| osteoma (ŏs-tē-ō'-mah) | a tumor composed of bone |
| sternal (stĕr'-nal) | pertaining to the sternum |
| sternoclavicular (stĕr'-nō-klah-vĭk'-ū-lar) | pertaining to the sternum and clavicle |
| sternocostal (stĕr-nō-kŏs'-tal) | pertaining to the sternum and ribs |
| sternoid (stĕr'-noyd) | resembling the sternum |
| subcostal (sŭb-kŏs'-tal) | pertaining to below a rib or ribs |
| subscapular (sŭb-skăp'-ū-lar) | pertaining to below the scapula |
| suprascapular (soo-prah-skăp'-ū-lar) | pertaining to above the scapula |
| vertebrocostal (vĕr'-tĕ-brō-kŏs'-tal) | pertaining to the vertebrae and ribs |

| Surgical Terms | Meaning |
| --- | --- |
| arthroplasty (ar'-thrō-plăs-tē) | plastic repair of a joint |
| arthrotomy (ar-thrŏt'-ō-mē) | surgical incision of a joint |
| chondrectomy (kŏn-drĕk'-tō-mē) | excision of a cartilage |
| clavicotomy (klăv-ĭ-kŏt'-ō-mē) | surgical incision into the clavicle |
| costectomy (kŏs-tĕk'-tō-mē) | excision of a rib |
| cranioplasty (krā'-nē-ō-plăs-tē) | plastic repair to the cranium |
| craniotomy (krā-nē-ŏt'-ō-mē) | surgical incision into the cranium |
| laminectomy (lăm-ĭ-nĕk'-tō-mē) | surgical removal of lamina; often performed to relieve symptoms of a ruptured (slipped) disk |
| meniscectomy (mĕn-ĭ-sĕk'-tō-mē) | excision of the meniscus (of the knee joint) |
| patellectomy (păt-ĕ-lĕk'-tō-mē) | excision of the patella |
| vertebrectomy (vĕr-tĕ-brĕk'-tō-mē) | excision of a vertebra |

| Diagnostic Terms | Meaning |
| --- | --- |
| arthralgia (ar-thrăl'-jē-ah) | pain in a joint |
| arthritis (arthrī'-tĭs) | inflammation of a joint |
| arthrosis (ar-thrŏ'-sĭs) | abnormal condition of a joint |
| chondritis (krŏn-drī'-tĭs) | inflammation of the cartilage |
| meniscitis (mĕn-ĭ-sī'-tĭs) | inflammation of the meniscus (of the knee joint) |
| muscular dystrophy (mŭs'-kū-lar) (dĭs'-trō-fē) | a progressive, crippling disease of the muscles |
| myoma (mī-ō'-mah) | a tumor formed of muscular tissue |

| Terms Relating to Diagnostic Procedures | Meaning |
| --- | --- |
| arthrocentesis (ar-thrō-sĕn-tē'-sĭs) | puncture and aspiration of a joint |
| arthrogram (ar'-thrō-grăm) | a procedure performed to x-ray (record) a joint; contrast medium, dye, or air is used |
| arthroscope (ar'-thrō-scōpe) | instrument used to visualize a joint, usually the knee |
| arthroscopy (ar-thrŏs'-kō-pē) | visual examination of the inside of a joint for diagnosing and identifying problems |
| electromyogram (EMG) (ē-lĕk'-trō-mī'-ō-grăm) | record of electric potential of muscle activity |
| electromyograph (ē-lĕk'-trō-mī'-ō-grăph) | a machine that records the electric potential of muscle activity |

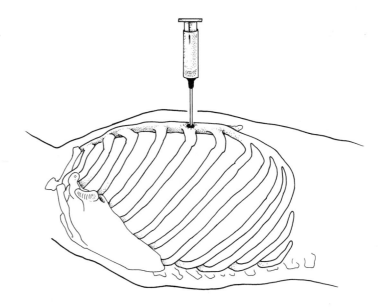

FIGURE 23–12 • Sternal puncture. (From LaFleur, M. and Starr, W.: *Exploring Medical Language*. St. Louis, The C.V. Mosby Co., 1985, with permission.)

| Terms Relating to Diagnostic Procedures | Meaning |
|---|---|
| electromyography (ē-lĕk'-trō-mī'-ōg'-rah-fē) | process of recording the electric potential of muscle activity |
| sternal puncture (stĕr'-nal) (pŭngk'-chŭr) | insertion of a hollow needle into the sternum to obtain a sample of bone marrow to be studied in the laboratory (Fig. 23–12). It is used for diagnosing blood disorders such as anemia and leukemia. |

# E X E R C I S E  8

Analyze and define each medical term listed below.

1. electromyogram  _____

2. myoma  _____

3. sternoclavicular  _____

4. cranial  _____

5. vertebrocostal  _____

6. arthritis  _____

7. intervertebral  _____

8. humeral  _____

9. dystrophy  _____

10. subscapular  _____

11. arthrosis  _____

12. electromyography  _____

13. arthrogram  _____

14. electromyograph  _____

15. sternocostal  _____

16. arthralgia  _____

17. subcostal  _____

18. femoral _____

19. clavicotomy _____

20. arthrotomy _____

21. intracranial _____

22. atrophy _____

23. arthroplasty _____

24. osteoma _____

25. costectomy _____

26. cranioplasty _____

27. patellectomy _____

28. vertebrectomy _____

29. craniotomy _____

30. suprascapular _____

31. sternoid _____

32. chondrogenic _____

33. arthroscopy _____

34. chondritis _____

35. arthroscope _____

36. chondrectomy _____

37. laminectomy _____

38. sternal _____

39. meniscectomy _____

40. arthrocentesis _____

41. meniscitis _____

# E X E R C I S E  9

Using the word roots, prefixes, suffixes, and combining vowels as needed, build medical terms from each definition listed below.

1. pertaining to the cranium _____

2. resembling the sternum _____

3. pertaining to below the scapula _____

4. pertaining to the femur _____

5. surgical incision into a joint _____

6. excision of a cartilage _____

7. pain of a joint _____

8. inflammation of a joint _____

9. abnormal condition of a joint _____

10. pertaining to the humerus _____

11. without development _____

12. pertaining to the vertebrae and ribs _____

13. surgical incision into the cranium _____

14. surgical removal of a rib _____

15. pertaining to below the rib _____

16. x-ray (record) of a joint _____

17. surgical removal of a vertebra _____

18. record of the electric potential of muscle activity _____

19. surgical incision into the clavicle _____

20. process of recording electric potential of muscle activity _____

21. bad or faulty development _____

22. a tumor formed of muscular tissue _____

23. machine to record electric potential of muscle activity _____

24. pertaining to the sternum and clavicle _____

25. pertaining to between the vertebrae _____

26. pertaining to within the cranium _____

27. pertaining to the sternum and rib _____

28. surgical removal of the patella _____

29. plastic repair of the cranium _____

30. a tumor composed of bone _____

31. surgical incision into the clavicle _____

32. producing cartilage _____

33. visual examination of a joint _____

34. instrument to examine a joint visually _____

35. inflammation of cartilage _____

36. excision of cartilage _____

37. surgical removal of the lamina _____

38. pertaining to the sternum _____

39. puncture and aspiration of a joint _____

40. excision of the meniscus _____

41. inflammation of the meniscus _____

E X E R C I S E  **10**

Define each medical term listed below.

1. orthopedics _____

2. orthopedist _____

3. muscular dystrophy _____

4. sternal puncture _____

E X E R C I S E  **11**

Spell each medical term studied in this unit by having someone dictate the terms to you.

1. _____

2. _____

3. _____

4. _____

5. _____

6. _____

7. _____

8. _____

9. _____

10. _____

11. _____

12. _____

13. _____

14. _____

15. _____

16. _____

17. _____

18. _____

19. _____

20. _____

21. _____

22. _____

23. _____

24. _____

25. _____

26. _____

27. _____

28. _____

29. _____

30. _____

31. _____

32. _____

33. _____

34. _____

35. _____

36. _____

37. _____

38. _____

39. _____

40. _____

41. _____

42. _____

43. _____

44. _____

45. _____

# E X E R C I S E  12

Answer the following questions.

1. _____ is the name of the nursing unit in the hospital that cares for the patients with *fractures* or

   *diseases of the bone*. _____ is the name of the doctor who specializes in this area of medicine.

2. A _____ , _____ tray is used by the doctor to obtain a *sample of bone marrow from*

   *the sternum*. The tray is named after the procedure.

3. The doctor ordered a procedure to determine the *electric potential of muscle activity*. The procedure is called

   a(an) _____ .

4. The following is a list of diagnostic phrases. In the space provided tell which bone is fractured.

   *Example*: fractured femur _____ thigh bone _____

   a. fractured tibia            _____

   b. fractured humerus         _____

   c. fractured cervical 6 (C6) _____

   d. fractured ilium           _____

   e. fractured clavicle        _____

   f. fractured radius          _____

5. A surgery schedule is a list of operations to be performed on a given day in the hospital. The following are types of operations recorded on the surgery schedule. Indicate the terms that are incorrectly spelled by rewriting the term correctly in the space provided.

a. castectomy _____

b. craniotomy _____

c. lamonectomy _____

d. clavictamy _____

e. cranioplasty _____

f. patelectomy _____

g. ostoarthrotomy _____

h. meniscectomy _____

6. The doctor ordered a procedure to x-ray a joint that requires the use of contrast medium. The procedure is called a(an) _____ . Puncture and aspiration of a joint is called _____ .

## UNIT IV

# The Nervous System

*Upon mastery of basic human structure for this unit, you will be able to:*

1. Describe the overall function of the nervous system.

2. List and describe the organs of the nervous system covered in this unit.

3. Describe the function of the meninges and locate and name the three layers of tissue that make up the meninges.

4. Describe cerebrovascular accident, Parkinson's disease, transient ischemic attack, Alzheimer's disease, and epilepsy.

## THE NERVOUS SYSTEM

### Organs of the Nervous System

■ Nerves
■ Brain
■ Spinal cord

The nervous system is commonly divided into two parts:

1. The **central nervous system** is called "CNS" and consists of the brain and spinal cord.
2. The **peripheral nervous system** is called "PNS" and consists of the nerves of the body.

### Functions of the Nervous System

All body parts and systems must work together to maintain a healthy body. The nervous system coordinates the functions of body organs and body systems by using nerve impulses to transmit information from one part of the body to another (Fig. 23–13).

### Nerves

A **nerve** is a cord-like structure located outside of the CNS. It contains nerve cells called **neurons**. The nerve transmits nerve impulses from one part of the body to another. Two types of neurons are:

1. **Sensory neurons**, which transmit impulses to the brain and spinal cord.
2. **Motor neurons**, which transmit impulses from the brain and spinal cord to muscles or glands.

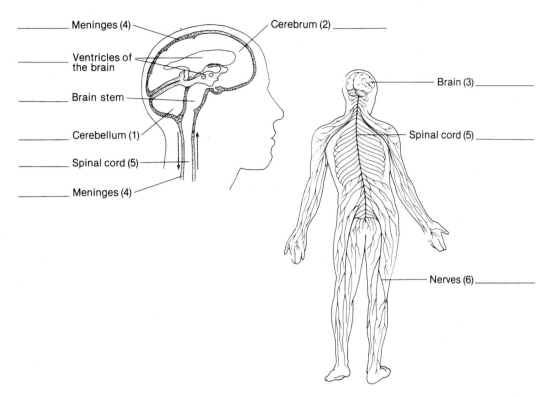

F I G U R E   23–13 • The nervous system.

## The Brain

The **brain** is located in the cranial cavity and is the main center for coordinating body activities. The brain is divided into three parts: the cerebrum, the cerebellum, and the brain stem. Each part of the brain is responsible for controlling certain body functions.

The **cerebrum** is the largest part of the brain. It is located in the upper portion of the cranium. The cerebrum is divided into the right and left hemispheres, which are connected only at the lower middle portion. The cerebrum contains the sensory, motor, sight, and hearing centers. Memory, intellect, judgment, and emotional reactions also take place in the cerebrum.

Spaces within the cerebrum, called **ventricles**, produce a watery fluid known as **cerebrospinal fluid (CSF)**. This fluid surrounds the brain and spinal cord. Its function is to cushion shock that may occur to the spinal cord or brain.

The **cerebellum**, or "hind brain," is situated below the posterior portion of the cerebrum. Its functions are to assist in the coordination of voluntary muscles and to maintain balance.

The **brain stem** is made up of several parts. It contains the nerve fibers that form the connecting links between the different parts of the brain and the centers that control three vital functions: blood pressure, respiration, and heartbeat.

## The Spinal Cord

The **spinal cord** extends from the brain stem and passes through the spinal cavity to between the first and second lumbar vertebrae. The spinal cord is the pathway for conducting **sensory impulses** up to the brain and **motor impulses** down from the brain. Injury to the spinal cord can result in paralysis, the loss of voluntary muscle function.

## Meninges

The **meninges** are made up of three layers of connective tissue that completely surround the spinal cord and brain. The outer tough layer is called the **dura mater**. The middle layer is the **arachnoid mater**, a web-like structure. The inner thin, tender layer is called the **pia mater**. The cerebrospinal fluid flows through a space between the arachnoid and the pia mater called the **subarachnoid space**.

## DISEASES AND CONDITIONS OF THE NERVOUS SYSTEM

### Cerebrovascular Accident

**Cerebrovascular accident (CVA)**, also called stroke, is the interference of blood flow to the brain, which reduces the oxygen supply, causing damage to the brain tissue.

Damage to the brain tissue varies according to the artery affected. Paralysis is a result of the damage, and it may range from slight to complete hemiplegia (paralysis of one side of the body). CVA of the left hemisphere of the brain produces symptoms on the right side of the body, and CVA of the right side of the brain produces symptoms on the left side of the body. The more quickly the circulation returns, the better the chance for recovery.

The major causes of CVA are embolism, thrombosis, and hemorrhage (Fig. 23–14). Strokes affect about 500,000 people each year, causing death in half of them.

## Transient Ischemic Attack

**Transient ischemic attacks (TIA)** are recurrent episodes of decreased neurologic function such as double vision, slurred speech, weakness in the legs, and dizziness lasting from seconds to 24 hours, then clearing. TIAs are considered warning signs for strokes. TIAs are caused by small emboli that temporarily interrupt blood flow to the brain. Treatment includes the administration of aspirin and anticoagulants to minimize thrombosis in the hope of preventing a cerebrovascular accident. Preventive treatment may include a **carotid endarterectomy**, a surgical procedure to remove the thickened inner area of the carotid artery.

## Parkinson's Disease

**Parkinson's disease**, also called shaking palsy, parkinsonism, and paralysis agitans, is one of the most common crippling diseases in the United States.

Parkinson's disease is the result of damage to several small areas of the brain; the cause of the damage is most often unknown, but sometimes it may be the result of viral infection, carbon monoxide poisoning, or cerebral arteriosclerosis. Symptoms include muscle rigidity, tremors, and a shifting gait. Deterioration is progressive. There is no cure; treatment is aimed at relieving symptoms and promoting function as long as possible. Parkinson's disease does not impair intellect.

## Alzheimer's Disease

**Alzheimer's disease** is characterized by confusion, loss of memory, restlessness, hallucinations, and the inability to carry out purposeful movement. The patient may lose bowel and bladder control and refuse to eat. The disease is progressive and usually begins in later midlife. There is no cure, and treatment is mostly routine care plus maintaining nutrition.

## Epilepsy

Epilepsy is a disorder of the CNS as a result of abnormal electrical activity. It is common to hear epilepsy and seizure used synonymously; the difference is that epilepsy is the disease and the seizure is the result of the disease. Epilepsy usually occurs in childhood or after age 50. The disease can be classified as idiopathic (etiology unknown) or acquired. Some of the known causes of acquired epilepsy are, brain tumors, brain injury, and endocrine disorders. Seizures resulting from fever, otitis media, or drug toxicity are usually isolated incidents and do not warrant the diagnosis of epilepsy.

Seizure activity is divided into three stages: during the preictal stage the patient may experience abnormal somatic and psychic sensations and a strange-sounding cry. These sensations and/or cry are called an aura. The second stage is called interictal and includes violent jerking of some parts or total body. The patient may experience incontinence of urine and stool, foaming or frothing from the mouth, changes in skin color, tongue biting, arching of the back, and turning of the head to one side. The period immediately after the seizure is called the postictal stage. During this stage the patient may be confused and lethargic, and reports headache and sore muscles.

Diagnosis is confirmed by observation of the seizure activity, and computed axial tomography scan of the brain that may show a lesion. An electroencephalogram and/or an echoencephalogram may locate the site and possible cause of the disorder.

Treatment requires stabilization on anticonvulsant drugs (see Chapter 13 for a list of these drugs); 95% of the pop-

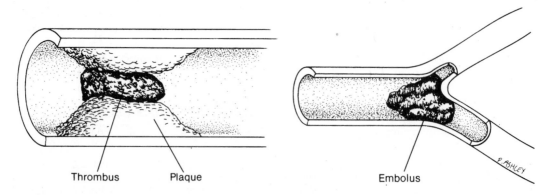

Thrombus  Plaque

Embolus

FIGURE 23–14 • A thrombus (blood clot) or an embolus (a floating mass that blocks a vessel) in a cerebral artery can cause a cerebrovascular accident.

ulation respond to drug therapy. The other 5% is treated surgically to remove the affected brain tissue. Patient education is included in the treatment regimen. Information about seizure triggers and how to avoid those triggers are an important part of the patient education. There is a national association that helps the patient deal with self-esteem issues and the stigma that is still attached to epilepsy. Because of the stigmatization many people who have epilepsy will not wear an identification bracelet, and they will not inform others of their illness.

**HIGHLIGHT**

Patients who are experiencing a seizure need to be protected from injury, especially head injuries. Remove any furniture or other objects that the patient may strike. If possible put a pillow under the patient's head. Call for help. DO NOT TRY TO RESTRAIN THE MOVEMENTS OF THE PATIENT. Protect the patient's privacy. Ask those that are uninvolved with the care of the patients to please leave the area.

**REVIEW QUESTIONS**

1. Name the organs of the nervous system. Write the function of each organ.

   a. _____

   _____

   b. _____

   _____

   c. _____

   _____

2. A nerve cell is called a(an) _____ . The two types of nerve cells

   are _____ and _____ .

3. Name three parts of the brain and describe the functions of each.

   a. _____

   _____

   b. _____

   _____

   c. _____

   _____

4. Describe the location and function of the spinal cord.

   _____

   _____

5. The meninges are made up of three layers of tissue. The outer layer is called the _____

   _____ ; the middle layer is called the _____ ;

   and the inner layer is called the _____ .

6. Match the terms in Column I with the phrases in Column II.

| Column I | Column II |
|---|---|
| a. Parkinson's disease | _____ also called shaking palsy |
| b. Alzheimer's disease | _____ may be idopathic or acquired |
| c. transient ischemic attack | _____ may result in hemiplegia |
| d. cerebrovascular accident | _____ warning sign for strokes |
| e. cerebral palsy | _____ symptoms include hallucinations |
| f. epilepsy | |

7. Name the three stages of a seizure.

a. _____

b. _____

c. _____

## MEDICAL TERMINOLOGY RELATING TO THE NERVOUS SYSTEM AND PSYCHOLOGY

### OBJECTIVES

*Upon mastery of the medical terminology for this unit, you will be able to:*

1. Spell and define the word elements and medical terms that relate to the nervous system.

2. Analyze the medical terms relating to the nervous system that are built from word elements.

3. Given the meaning of a medical condition relating to the nervous system, build with word elements the corresponding medical term.

4. Spell and use in sentence form psychology terminology represented in this unit.

5. Given descriptions of hospital situations in which the health unit coordinator may encounter medical terminology, apply the correct medical terms to the situations.

Listed below are the word elements you need to memorize for the nervous system. The exercises included in this unit will help you with this task. You will continue to use these word elements throughout the course and during employment. Practice pronouncing each word element aloud.

| Word Roots/ Combining Forms | Meaning |
|---|---|
| 1. cerebell/o (sĕr-ĕ-bĕl′-ō) | cerebellum (hind brain) |
| 2. cerebr/o (sĕr′-ē-brō) | cerebrum (main portion of the brain) |
| 3. encephal/o (ĕn-sĕf′-ah-lō) | brain |
| 4. mening/o (mĕ-nĭng′-gō) | meninges (spinal cord covering) |
| 5. myel/o (mī′-ĕl-ō) | spinal cord, also bone marrow |
| 6. neur/o (nū′-rō) | nerve |
| 7. spin/o (spī′-nō) | spine |

| Other Word Roots/ Combining Forms | Meaning |
|---|---|
| 8. pneum/o (nū′-mō) | air |
| 9. poli/o (pō′-lē-ō) | gray matter |

| Suffixes | Meaning |
|---|---|
| 1. cele (sēl) | herniation or pouching out |
| 2. orrhagia (or-ah′-jē-ah) | rapid discharge |
| 3. orrhaphy (or′-ah-fē) | to suture (surgical) |
| 4. orrhea (ō-rē′-ah) | discharge |
| 5. plegia (plē′-jē-ah) | paralysis, stroke |

E X E R C I S E   **1**

Write the combining forms for the nervous system in the spaces provided on the diagram in Figure 23–13. The number preceding the combining form in the list above matches the number of the body part on the diagram.

E X E R C I S E   **2**

Define each combining form listed below.

1. cerebr/o    _____

2. encephal/o    _____

3. neur/o    _____

4. poli/o    _____

5. mening/o    _____

6. spin/o    _____

7. myel/o    _____

8. cerebell/o    _____

9. pneum/o    _____

E X E R C I S E   **3**

Write the combining forms for each term listed below.

1. nerve    _____

2. cerebrum    _____

3. meninges    _____

4. spinal cord    _____

5. cerebellum    _____

6. brain    _____

7. spine    _____

8. air    _____

9. gray matter    _____

E X E R C I S E   **4**

Write the suffix that matches each definition written below. (*Note*: This exercise includes suffixes from this unit and previous units. Refer back as needed.)

1. tumor    _____

2. surgical repair    _____

3. pertaining to    _____

4. to suture    _____

5. discharge    _____

6. inflammation    _____

7. specialist    _____

8. record (x-ray)    _____

9. study of    _____

10. rapid discharge    _____

11. herniation    _____

12. surgical removal    _____

13. incision    _____

14. pain    _____

E X E R C I S E  **5**

Write the definition for each suffix listed below. (*Note*: This exercise includes suffixes from this unit and previous units. Refer back as needed.)

1. gram _____

2. itis _____

3. ology _____

4. orrhea _____

5. orrhagia _____

6. orrhaphy _____

7. cele _____

8. ar _____

9. ectomy _____

10. plasty _____

11. otomy _____

12. algia _____

13. osis _____

## MEDICAL TERMS RELATING TO THE NERVOUS SYSTEM

Listed below are medical terms you will need to know for the nervous system. Exercises following this list will assist you in learning these terms. Practice pronouncing these terms aloud.

| General Terms | Meaning |
| --- | --- |
| aphasia (ah-fā'-zē-ah) | loss of expression or understanding of speech or writing |
| cerebrospinal (ser'-ē-brō-spī'-nal) | pertaining to the brain and spine |
| hemiplegia (hĕm-ĭ-plē-jē-ah) | paralysis of the right or left side of the body, usually caused by a stroke |
| meningorrhea (mĕ-nĭng-gō-rē'-ah) | drainage of blood into the meninges |
| myelorrhagia (mī-ĕ-lō-rā'-jē-ah) | spinal hemorrhage |
| neurologist (nū-rŏl'-ō-jĭst) | a doctor who specializes in neurology |
| neurology (nū-rŏl'-ō-jē) | the branch of medicine that deals with the diagnosis and treatment of disorders or diseases of the nervous system |
| paraplegia (păr-ăh-plē'-jē-ah) | paralysis of the legs and sometimes the lower part of the body, usually caused by an injury to the spinal cord |
| quadriplegia (kwăd-rē-plē'-jē-ah) | paralysis that affects all four limbs |

| Surgical Terms | Meaning |
| --- | --- |
| neuroplasty (nū'-rō-plăs-tē) | plastic surgery of a nerve |
| neurorrhaphy (nū-rŏr'-ah-fē) | suturing of a nerve |

| Diagnostic Terms | Meaning |
| --- | --- |
| cerebral palsy (ser'-ē-bral) (paul'-zē) | partial paralysis and lack of muscle coordination from a defect, injury, or disease of the brain, which is present at birth or shortly thereafter. |
| cerebrovascular accident (CVA) (ser'-ē-brō-văs'-kŭ-lăr) | impaired blood supply to parts of the brain; also called a stroke |
| cerebellitis (ser-ĕ-bĕl-ī'-tĭs) | inflammation of the cerebellum |
| cerebrosis (ser-ĕ-brō'-sĭs) | any brain disease |
| encephalitis (ĕn-sĕf-ah-lī'-tĭs) | inflammation of the brain |
| encephalocele (ĕn-sĕf'-ah-lō-sĕl) | herniation of brain tissue through the skull |
| epilepsy (ĕp'-ĭ-lĕp-sē) | convulsive disorder of the nervous system characterized by recurrent seizures |
| meningitis (mĕn-ĭn-jī'-tĭs) | inflammation of the meninges |
| meningomyelocele (mĕ-nĭng-gō-mī'-ĕ-lō-sĕl) | herniation of the spinal cord and meninges through the vertebral column |
| multiple sclerosis (mŭl'-tĭ-pl) (sklĕ-rō'-sĭs) | a degenerative disease of the nerves controlling muscles, characterized by hardening patches along the brain and spinal cord |

| Diagnostic Terms | Meaning |
| --- | --- |
| neuralgia (nū-răl'-jē-ah) | pain in a nerve |
| neuritis (nū-rī'-tĭs) | inflammation of a nerve |
| neuroma (nū-rō'-mah) | a tumor made up of nerve cells |
| poliomyelitis (pō'-lē-ō-mī-ĕ-lī'-tĭs) | virally caused disease that attacks gray matter of the spinal cord |
| subdural hematoma (sŭb-dū'-ral) (hēm-ah-tō'-mah) | accumulation of blood in the subdural space |

| Terms Relating to Diagnostic Procedures | Meaning |
| --- | --- |
| CAT, or CT scan (computed axial tomography) | use of radiologic imaging that produces images of "slices" of the body |
| echoencephalogram (ĕk'-ō-ĕn-sĕf'-ă-lō-grăm) | a process of recording brain structures by use of sound recorded on a graph |
| electroencephalogram (EEG) (ē-lĕk'-trō-ĕn-sĕf'-ăh-lō-grăm) | the tracing or recording of the electric impulses of the brain |
| magnetic resonance imaging (MRI) | a noninvasive nuclear-medicine procedure for imaging tissues that cannot be seen by other radiologic techniques. |
| myelogram (mī'-ĕ-lō-grăm) | x-ray of the spinal cord; injected dye is used as the contrast medium |
| pneumoencephalogram (nū'-mō-ĕn-sĕf'-ăh-lō-grăm) | x-ray of the ventricles in the brain; air is used as the contrast medium |
| spinal puncture (lumbar puncture) (LP) (spī'-năl) (pŭngk'-chŭr) | the removal of cerebrospinal (CSF) fluid for diagnostic purposes. A hollow needle is inserted into the subarachnoid space between the third and fourth lumbar vertebrae |

# E X E R C I S E  6

Analyze and define each medical term listed below.

1. neurology _____

2. cerebrospinal _____

3. neuralgia _____

4. poliomyelitis _____

5. neuroplasty _____

6. encephalitis _____

7. meningitis _____

8. pneumoencephalogram _____

9. neurorrhaphy _____

10. meningorrhea _____

11. neurologist _____

12. encephalocele _____

13. electroencephalogram _____

14. meningomyelocele _____

15. cerebellitis _____

16. cerebrosis _____

17. neuroma _____

18. myelorrhagia _____

19. myelogram _____

20. neuritis _____

## E X E R C I S E 7

Define each medical term listed below.

1. multiple sclerosis _____

2. epilepsy _____

3. cerebral palsy _____

4. cerebrovascular accident _____

5. echoencephalogram _____

6. hemiplegia _____

7. paraplegia _____

8. quadriplegia _____

9. spinal puncture _____

10. subdural hematoma _____

11. CAT scan _____

12. MRI _____

13. aphasia _____

## E X E R C I S E 8

Using the word elements studied in this unit and previous units, build medical terms from each of the definitions listed below.

1. inflammation of a nerve _____

2. drainage of blood into the meninges _____

3. inflammation of the brain _____

4. inflammation of the meninges _____

5. plastic surgery of a nerve _____

6. a doctor who specializes in neurology _____

7. suture of a nerve _____

8. tumor made of nerve cells _____

9. pain in a nerve _____

10. pertaining to the cerebrum and spine _____

11. herniation of the spinal cord and meninges through the vertebral column _____

_____

12. inflammation of the cerebellum _____

13. herniation of the brain through the skull _____

14. x-ray of the ventricles of the brain with the use of air as contrast medium _____

_____

15. spinal hemorrhage _____

16. tracing or recording of the electrical impulses of the brain _____

17. x-ray of the spinal cord _____

# E X E R C I S E 9

Spell each medical term studied in this unit by having someone dictate the terms to you.

1. _____
2. _____
3. _____
4. _____
5. _____
6. _____
7. _____
8. _____
9. _____
10. _____
11. _____
12. _____
13. _____
14. _____
15. _____
16. _____
17. _____
18. _____
19. _____
20. _____
21. _____
22. _____
23. _____
24. _____
25. _____
26. _____
27. _____
28. _____
29. _____
30. _____
31. _____
32. _____
33. _____

## TERMS RELATING TO PSYCHOLOGY

An extensive knowledge of psychology vocabulary is not necessary for general hospital employment; therefore, we will discuss only those terms that you as a health unit coordinator may encounter in general medical and surgical areas of employment.

*Psych/o* is a combining form meaning "mind." The following words are developed from the word root *psych* and suffixes, most of which you have already studied.

| Psychology Terms | Meaning |
| --- | --- |
| psychiatrist (sī-kī'-ah-trĭst) | a physician who specializes in psychiatry |
| psychiatry (sī-kī'-ah-trē) | a branch of medicine that deals with the study, treatment, and prevention of mental illness |
| psychologist (sī-kŏl'-ō-jĭst) | a person trained to perform psychological analysis, therapy, or research |
| psychology (sī-kŏl'-ō-jē) | study of the mind (behavior) |
| psychosis (sī-kō'-sĭs) | mental disorder |
| psychosomatic (sī'-kō-sō-măt'-ĭk) | pertaining to the mind and body relationship |

*Neur/o* is the combining form that means nerve. However, it may be used to describe certain psychiatric disorders, as in the following terms.

| | |
| --- | --- |
| neurosis (nŭ-rō'-sĭs) | an emotional disorder considered less serious than a psychosis |
| neurotic (nŭ-rŏt'-ĭk) | having a neurosis |

## E X E R C I S E  10

Spell each psychology term studied in this unit by having someone dictate the terms to you.

1. _____     5. _____

2. _____     6. _____

3. _____     7. _____

4. _____     8. _____

## E X E R C I S E  11

Answer the following questions.

1. _____ is the name of the nursing unit in the hospital that cares for patients with disorders of the nervous system. _____ is the name of the doctor who specializes in this area of medicine.

2. The patient is admitted to the hospital with the admitting diagnosis of stroke or _____ . The abbreviation for this term is _____ . The patient is paralyzed on the left side of her body. She has _____ .

3. A child is diagnosed as having an inflammation of the meninges or _____ . The doctor performs a procedure to obtain cerebrospinal fluid for diagnostic study. The procedure is called _____ . To perform this procedure, the doctor uses a special tray named after the procedure. It is called a _____ tray.

4. Name four diagnostic procedures that end in the suffix *-gram* that the doctor may order to gather information about the nervous system organs or about their functions:

a. _____     c. _____

b. _____     d. _____

## UNIT V

# The Eye and the Ear

## O B J E C T I V E S

*Upon mastery of the basic human structure for this unit, you will be able to:*

1. Name and locate the parts of the eye and briefly describe the function of each part.
2. Describe how the eye is protected.
3. Trace the pathway of light from the outside environment to the cerebrum.
4. Name and describe the function of the two types of nerve cells located in the retina.
5. Name and locate the parts of the ear.
6. Trace the travel of sound waves from the outside environment to the brain.
7. Describe cataract, glaucoma, retinal detachment, and tinnitus.

## THE EYE

The eye (Fig. 23–15) is the organ of vision. The eye receives light waves that are focused on the retina and pro-

duces visual nerve impulses that are transmitted to the visual area of the brain by the optic nerve.

The eye is a spherical, delicate structure, protected by the skull bones, eyelashes and eyelids, tears, and the conjunctiva. The **conjunctiva** is a transparent membrane that lines the upper and lower eyelid and the anterior portion of the eye. It helps protect the eye from harmful bacteria.

The **sclera** is the outer protective layer of the eye. We can see the anterior portion of the sclera. It is often referred to as the "white of the eye." The **cornea** is the transparent part of the sclera that lies over the iris of the eye and allows the light rays to enter.

The middle layer of the eye is called the **choroid**. The choroid contains blood vessels that supply nutrients to the eye. The **iris** and the **ciliary muscle** make up the anterior middle portion of the choroid. The iris, the colored portion of the eye, has an opening in the center called the **pupil**. Muscles of the iris regulate the amount of light entering the eye by dilation and contraction of the pupil.

The **lens**, located directly behind the pupil, focuses light rays on the retina. The ciliary muscle regulates the shape of the lens to make this possible.

The inner layer of the eye is called the **retina**. Two different sets of nerve cells, called rods and cones, are responsible for the adaptation to light. The cones are sensi-

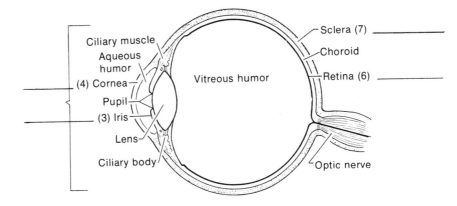

F I G U R E   23–15 • The eye. (From Mayes, M. E.: *Nurses' Aide Study Manual*, 3rd ed. Philadelphia, W.B. Saunders Co., 1976, with permission.)

tive to bright light, and responsible for color vision. The rods adapt to provide vision in dim light. The cones and rods transmit impulses to the optic nerve. The optic nerve carries these impulses to the vision center in the cerebrum, where they are registered as visual sensations.

The spaces inside the eyeball are filled with fluid. The small anterior space in front of the lens is filled with a watery substance called the **aqueous humor**. The large posterior space behind the lens is filled with a jelly-like substance called the **vitreous humor**. The functions of these fluids are to maintain the shape of the eyeball and to assist in bending the light rays to focus on the retina.

### HIGHLIGHT

The pathway of light rays > conjunctiva > cornea > aqueous humor > pupil > lens > vitreous humor > retina > optic nerve (converted to nerve impulses) > cerebrum.

## DISEASES OF THE EYE

### Cataract

**Cataracts** are the gradual development of cloudiness of the lens of the eyes; they usually occur in both eyes. Most cataracts develop after a person is 50 years of age and they are caused by degenerative changes. At first vision is blurred, and if not treated, cataracts eventually lead to loss of eyesight. Treatment is the surgical removal of the lens followed by correction of the visual defects. Two types of surgery used to remove cataracts are the extraction of the entire lens and **phacoemulsification**, which is the use of ultrasonic vibrations to break the lens into pieces, followed by aspiration, or sucking out the pieces.

Correction of visual defects includes a lens implant. Following the removal of the cataract, a synthetic lens is inserted into the eye through a corneal incision. Corrective eyeglasses or contact lens may also be used to correct the visual defect caused by cataract extraction.

### Glaucoma

**Glaucoma** is the abnormal increase of intraocular (within the eye) pressure. It is the most preventable cause of blindness and yet is the cause of 15% of all blindness in the United States. The pressure is caused by overproduction of aqueous humor or obstruction of its outflow, causing damage to the retina resulting in blindness.

Two forms of glaucoma exist, chronic, and acute. Chronic glaucoma affects vision gradually and may not be diagnosed until after some loss of vision has occurred. The acute form causes severe pain and sudden dimming of vision.

Treatment varies, but glaucoma is often treated with drugs that help reduce the intraocular pressure. The patient has to understand that the medication must be taken for the rest of their lives.

### Retinal Detachment

**Retinal detachment** is a separation of the retina from the choroid in the back of the eye, allowing vitreous humor to leak between the choroid and the retina. Retinal detachment may be caused by trauma but is often the result of aging. **Photocoagulation**, **cryosurgery**, and **scleral buckling** are surgical procedures used for treatment.

## THE EAR

Two functions of the ear are hearing and equilibrium (sense of balance). The ear is divided into three main parts: the outer ear, the middle ear, and the inner ear (Fig. 23–16).

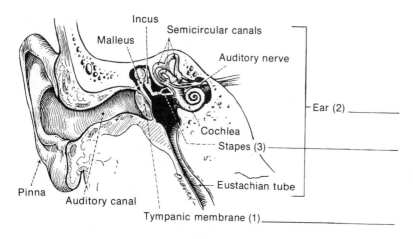

FIGURE 23–16 • The ear. (From Mayes, M. E.: *Nurses' Aide Study Manual*, 3rd ed. Philadelphia, W.B. Saunders Co., 1976, with permission.)

## The Outer Ear

The **outer ear** is made up of two parts, the pinna and the auditory canal. The **pinna** is the appendage we see on each side of the head. The **auditory canal** is a tube that leads from the outer ear to the middle ear.

## The Middle Ear

The **tympanic membrane** (eardrum) separates the outer and middle ear. Located just inside the eardrum are three small bones, or **ossicles**, called the **malleus**, the **incus**, and the **stapes**. These three small bones form a chain across the middle ear from the tympanic membrane (eardrum) to the oval window. The middle ear also contains the **eustachian tube**, which leads from the middle ear to the pharynx (throat). The eustachian tube serves to equalize pressure on both sides of the tympanic membrane. Disease-causing bacteria, especially in children, may travel from the throat to the middle ear through the eustachian tube, resulting in middle-ear infection.

## The Inner Ear

The **oval window** separates the middle ear from the inner ear. The structure next to the oval window in the inner ear is the **cochlea**, which is shaped like a snail. It contains special fluids that carry sound vibrations. The inner ear also contains the **semicircular canals**. The cerebellum interprets the impulses from the semicircular canals to maintain balance and equilibrium.

## Passage of Sound Waves through the Ear

> **HIGHLIGHT**
>
> The pathway of sound waves > pinna > auditory canal > tympanic membrane > ossicles (malleus, incus, stapes) > oval window > cochlea > auditory nerve > (converted to nerve impulses) > cerebrum.

## Tinnitus

Tinnitus is described as ringing, buzzing, or roaring noise in the ears. In some patients this noise can be heard by others (objective tinnitus). Common causes of tinnitus are, chronic infections, head injuries, prolonged exposure to loud environmental noise, hypertension, and cardiovascular disease. Another common cause of tinnitus is taking drugs that are ototoxic. Ringing in the ears is a very common side effect of aspirin.

Persistent and severe noises in the ear can interfere with the person's ability to carry on normal activities including the ability to rest and sleep. Medical treatment begins with trying to determine the underlying cause of the tinnitus. Many cases have been unresponsive to all conventional methods of treatment. One frequent approach to treatment is to try masking the ear noises by providing soft background music. Biofeedback has been marginally effective in cases caused by stress or hysteria.

Because the condition is so prevalent, a national association has been established. One of the primary goals of the association is management and study of the condition.

---

**REVIEW QUESTIONS**

1. Five things that help protect the eye in various ways are

   a. _____    d. _____

   b. _____    e. _____

   c. _____

2. Tell how sound waves (vibrations) travel from the pinna to the cerebrum (brain).

   _____

   _____

   _____

   _____

3. Match the definitions in Column II with the terms in Column I.

**Column I**

a. choroid
b. pupil
c. stapes
d. retina
e. auditory nerve
f. cornea
g. cochlea
h. iris
i. sclera
j. lens
k. optic nerve

**Column II**

_____ anterior transparent part of the sclera

_____ the colored portion of the eye

_____ located directly behind the pupil

_____ outer protective layer of the eye

_____ the opening in the center of the iris

_____ inner layer of the eye

_____ transmits impulses from the retina to the brain

_____ middle layer of the eye

4. List in order, beginning with the conjunctiva, the organs of the eye through which the light rays travel to the retina:

a. _____     d. _____

b. _____     e. _____

c. _____     f. _____

5. Name and describe the function of the two types of nerve cells located in the retina.

**Nerve Cell**                                **Function**

a. _____     _____

b. _____     _____

6. List the parts of:

a. the outer ear _____

_____

b. the middle ear _____

_____

_____

_____

_____

c. the inner ear _____

_____

_____

7. Cataracts are _____

_____

8. Glaucoma is _____

_____

9. List six things that cause tinnitus.

   a. _____

   b. _____

   c. _____

   d. _____

   e. _____

   f. _____

10. List two treatments for tinnitus.

    a. _____

    b. _____

11. Retinal detachment is _____

    _____

12. Three surgical procedures used to treat retinal detachment are

    a. _____

    b. _____

    c. _____

## MEDICAL TERMINOLOGY RELATING TO THE EYE AND THE EAR

### OBJECTIVES

*Upon mastery of the medical terminology for this unit, you will be able to:*

1. Spell and define the word elements and medical terms for the eye and ear.

2. Given the meaning of a medication condition relating to the eye or ear, build with word elements the corresponding medical term.

3. Analyze the medical terms that are built from word elements that relate to the eye and ear.

4. Given a description of hospital situations in which the health unit coordinator may encounter medical terminology, apply the correct medical terms to the situation involved.

Listed below are the combining forms for this unit. Memorize each combining form. Practice pronouncing each word element aloud.

| Word Roots/Combining Forms | Meaning |
| --- | --- |
| *Eye* | |
| 1. blephar/o (blĕf'-ah-rō) | eyelid |
| 2. conjunctiv/o (kŏn-jŭnk'-tĭv-ō) | conjunctiva (membrane covering the eye and lining of the eyelid) |
| 3. irid/o (ī'-rĭd-ō) | iris (colored portion of the eye) |
| 4. kerat/o (kĕt'-ah-tō) | cornea (clear anterior covering of the eye) |
| 5. ophthalm/o (ŏf-thal'-mō) | eye |
| 6. retin/o (rĕt'-ĭn-ō) | retina (inner layer of eye) |
| 7. scler/o (sklĕ'-rō) | sclera (white covering of the eye—also means hard) |
| *Ear* | |
| 1. myring/o (mĭ-rĭng'-gō) | tympanic membrane (eardrum) |
| 2. ot/o (ō'-tō) | ear |
| 3. staped/o (stā-pē'-dō) | stapes |

EXERCISE **1**

a. Write the combining forms for the eye in the spaces provided on the diagram in Figure 23–15. The number preceding the combining form in the list above matches the number of the body part on the diagram.
b. Write the combining forms for the ear in the spaces provided on the diagram in Figure 23–16. The number preceding the combining form in the list above matches the number of the body part on the diagram.

EXERCISE **2**

Define each combining form listed below.

1. retin/o _____
2. kerat/o _____
3. scler/o _____
4. ophthalm/o _____
5. conjunctiv/o _____

6. ot/o _____
7. myring/o _____
8. blephar/o _____
9. irid/o _____
10. staped/o _____

EXERCISE **3**

Write the word roots for each part of the body listed below.

1. eye _____
2. eyelid _____
3. retina _____
4. ear _____
5. eardrum _____

6. sclera _____
7. conjunctiva _____
8. iris _____
9. cornea _____
10. stapes _____

## MEDICAL TERMS RELATING TO THE EYE AND THE EAR

The following list is made up of medical terms you will need to know for the eye and ear. Exercises following this list will assist you in learning these terms. Practice pronouncing these terms aloud.

| General Terms | Meaning |
|---|---|
| ophthalmologist (ŏf′-thal-mŏl′-ō-jĭst) | a physician who specializes in ophthamology |
| ophthalmology (ŏf′-thăl-mŏl′-ō-jē) | the study of the eye and its diseases |
| optometrist (ŏp-tŏm′-ĕ-trĭst) | a professional person trained to examine the eyes and prescribe glasses |
| otorrhea (ō-tō-rē′-ah) | discharge from the ear |

| Surgical Terms | Meaning |
|---|---|
| blepharoplasty (blĕf′-ah-rō-plăs-tē) | plastic repair of the eyelid |
| blepharorrhaphy (blĕf′-ah-rōr′-ah-fē) | suturing of an eyelid |
| cataract extraction (kăt′-ah-răkt) (ĕk-străk′-shŭn) | removal of the clouded lens of the eye |
| corneal (kor′-nē-al) transplant | transplantation of a donor cornea into the eye of the recipient |
| enucleation (ē-nū-klē-ā′-shŭn) | removal of an organ; often used to indicate surgical removal of the eyeball |

| Surgical Terms | Meaning |
|---|---|
| iridectomy (ĭr-ĭ-dĕk'-tō-mē) | excision of a part of the iris |
| iridosclerotomy (ĭr-ĭ-dō-sklĕ-rŏt'-ō-mē) | incision into the sclera and iris |
| keratotomy (kĕr-ah-tot'-ō-mē) | incision into the cornea (radial keratotomy is an operation in which a series of incisions, in spoke-like fashion, are made in the cornea); done to correct myopia (nearsightedness) |
| myringoplasty (mĭ-rĭng'-gō-plăs-tē) | surgical repair of the tympanic membrane |
| myringotomy (mĭ-rĭng-gŏt'-ō-mē) | incision of the tympanic membrane |
| ophthalmectomy (ŏf-thal-mĕk'-tō-mē) | excision of the eye |
| scleroplasty (sklĕ'-rō-plăs-tē) | plastic repair of the sclera |
| sclerotomy (sklĕ-rŏt'-ō-mē) | incision into the sclera |
| stapedectomy (stā-pē-dĕk'-tō-mē) | excision of the stapes |

| Diagnostic Terms | Meaning |
|---|---|
| cataract (kăt'-ah-răkt) | cloudiness of the lens of the eye |
| conjunctivitis (kŏn-jŭnk-tĭ-vī'-tĭs) | inflammation of the conjunctiva (pinkeye) |
| glaucoma (glaw-kō'-mah) | an eye disease caused by increased pressure within the eye |
| keratocele (kĕr'-ah-tō-sĕl) | herniation (protrusion of a layer) of the cornea |
| keratoconjunctivitis (kĕr'-ah-tō-kŏn-jŭnk-tĭ-vī'-tĭs) | inflammation of the cornea and conjunctiva |
| otitis media (ō-tī'-tĭs) (mē'-dē-ah) | inflammation of the middle ear |
| retinal detachment (rĕt'-ĭn-al) (dē-tăch'-mĕnt) | complete or partial separation of the retina from the choroid |
| strabismus (străh-bĭz'-mŭs) | a weakness of the muscle of the eye that causes the eye to look in different directions (medical term for "crossed eyes") |

| Terms Relating to Diagnostic Procedures | Meaning |
|---|---|
| otoscope (ō'-tō-skōp) | an instrument for the visual examination of the ear |
| ophthalmoscope (ŏf-thal'-mō-skōp) | an instrument for the visual examination of the eye |

# E X E R C I S E  4

Analyze and define each medical term listed below.

1. ophthalmoscope _____

2. ophthalmologist _____

3. ophthalmectomy _____

4. otorrhea _____

5. otoscope _____

6. iridosclerotomy _____

7. iridectomy _____

8. blepharoplasty _____

9. blepharorrhaphy _____

10. keratoconjunctivitis _____

11. keratocele _____

12. conjunctivitis _____

13. myringotomy _____

14. myringoplasty _____

15. keratotomy _____

# E X E R C I S E  5

Build medical terms from each definition listed below.

1. inflammation of the middle ear _____

2. instrument to examine the eye visually _____

3. suturing of the eyelid _____

4. discharge from the ear _____

5. incision into the iris and the sclera _____

6. plastic repair of the sclera _____

7. excision of part of the iris _____

8. herniation of the cornea _____

9. instrument to examine the ear _____

10. excision of the eye _____

11. incision of the sclera _____

12. plastic repair of the eyelid _____

13. incision into the tympanic membrane _____

14. plastic repair of the tympanic membrane _____

15. inflammation of the cornea and conjunctiva _____

16. inflammation of the conjunctiva _____

17. incision into the cornea _____

# E X E R C I S E  6

Define each medical term listed below.

1. cataract _____

2. cataract detachment _____

3. retinal detachment _____

4. enucleation of the eye _____

5. stabismus _____

6. glaucoma _____

7. optometrist _____

8. corneal transplant _____

# E X E R C I S E  7

Spell each medical term studied in this unit by having someone dictate the terms to you.

1. _____  5. _____

2. _____  6. _____

3. _____  7. _____

4. _____  8. _____

9. _____    19. _____

10. _____    20. _____

11. _____    21. _____

12. _____    22. _____

13. _____    23. _____

14. _____    24. _____

15. _____    25. _____

16. _____    26. _____

17. _____    27. _____

18. _____    28. _____

## E X E R C I S E  8

Answer the following questions.

1. Instruments used to examine the eye and ear visually are usually part of the equipment stored at the nurses' station in the hospital. The instrument used to examine the eye is called a(an) _____ . The instrument used to examine the ear is called a(an) _____.

2. Children often develop inflammation of the middle ear, called _____ . Children who have had repeated middle-ear infections may have a build-up of fluid in the middle ear. The doctor may surgically treat this condition by making an incision into the eardrum, known as _____ , and inserting tiny tubes.

3. The patient is admitted to the hospital with a diagnosis of cloudiness of the lens of the right eye, or _____ _____ . She is scheduled for surgical removal of the diseased lens. The operation is called _____ .

4. Two medical words are used to describe surgical removal of the eyeball. They are

   a. _____    b. _____

5. _____ is the medical term for "crossed eyes."

# UNIT VI

# The Circulatory System

## THE CIRCULATORY SYSTEM

## Organs of the Circulatory System

- Heart
- Blood vessels
- Blood

## Functions of the Circulatory System

All living cells need nourishment and oxygen for life, and all living cells produce waste. The circulatory system provides the vital transportation service that carries nourishment to the cells of the body and carries the waste away.

The **heart** pumps **blood** to the lungs and the body cells through a network of tubing called **blood vessels**. The blood is the carrying agent for food, oxygen, waste, and other materials needed or produced by cell function.

## THE HEART

The heart is located in the chest cavity between the lungs, situated behind the sternum. It is a four-chambered organ the size of a fist, and it weighs less than a pound. The heart performs the action of pumping the blood through the blood vessels to all parts of the body, circulating it in a one-way movement.

## Structure of the Heart

The heart wall is made up of three layers. The thickest, the muscular middle layer, is called the **myocardium**. The outer double layer, which encloses the heart like a sac, is called the **pericardium**. A small amount of fluid is present between the layers of the pericardium, to prevent friction during the movement of the heartbeat. The **endocardium** is the inner lining of the heart, and it also forms the heart valves.

The heart is divided into four cavities or chambers (Fig. 23–17). The **septum** is a partition dividing the heart into a right and left side. Each side is divided by halves into two upper chambers—the **right atrium** and the **left atrium**—and two lower chambers—the **right ventricle** and the **left ventricle**. The left atrium is separated from the left ventricle by the **bicuspid**, or **mitral**, **valve**. On the right side, the right atrium is separated from the right ventricle by the **tricuspid valve**.

## BLOOD VESSELS

Blood vessels are the tubular structures through which the blood flows to and from the heart to the body parts (Fig. 23–18). There are three major types of blood vessels: arteries, capillaries, and veins.

**Arteries** carry blood away from the heart, except for the pulmonary artery. The pulmonary artery is the only artery in the body that carries blood with low levels of oxygen and a high concentration of carbon dioxide. All other arteries carry blood high in oxygen concentration from the heart to the body cells. Arterial walls are the thickest because they must withstand the pumping force of the heart. Arteries branch into **arterioles**, tiny arteries that connect the arteries to capillaries. The **aorta** is the largest artery of the body, being approximately 1 inch in diameter. It carries blood away from the left ventricle of the heart.

The **veins** are the vessels that carry blood back to the heart. Venous blood carries carbon dioxide and other waste products except for the pulmonary veins. They carry blood high in oxygen concentration from the lungs to the heart. The vein walls are thinner than the arterial walls and contain tiny valves to help prevent the backward flow of blood and to keep it moving in one direction. **Venules** are tiny veins that connect the capillaries with the veins. The **superior vena cava** and the **inferior vena cava** are large veins through which the blood returns from the body to the right atrium.

**Capillaries** are microscopic, thin-walled blood vessels. The exchange of substances takes place between the blood and the body cells while the blood is in the capillaries.

# YOUR HEART AND HOW IT WORKS

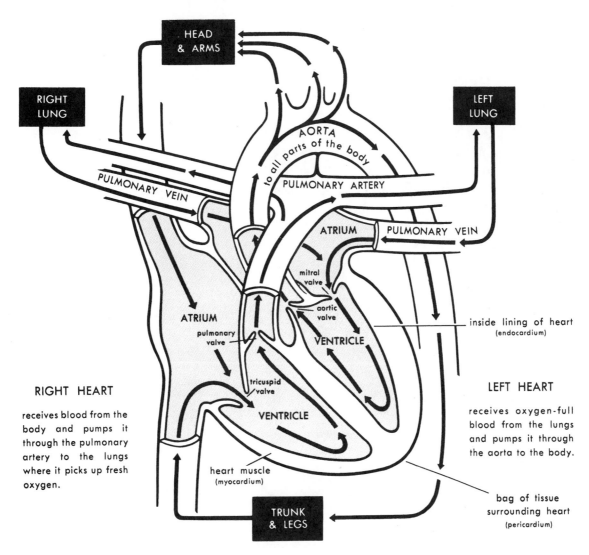

**RIGHT HEART**

receives blood from the body and pumps it through the pulmonary artery to the lungs where it picks up fresh oxygen.

**LEFT HEART**

receives oxygen-full blood from the lungs and pumps it through the aorta to the body.

**F I G U R E   23–17 •** The heart. (Courtesy of The American Heart Association and its affiliates.)

The cells take in nutrients and oxygen from the blood and give off waste and carbon dioxide to the blood. The blood carries the waste to the organ that removes it from the body. The capillaries provide the link between the arteries and veins.

## THE FLOW OF BLOOD THROUGH THE BLOOD VESSELS OF THE BODY

Blood leaves the heart through the aorta. It travels first through the arteries and then through the arterioles to the capillaries, where the exchange of gases, nutrients, and waste takes place. The blood returns from the capillaries by first entering the venules and then flowing through the veins, finally entering the right atrium of the heart through

the superior and inferior venae cavae. The superior vena cava returns blood to the heart from the upper part of the body, and the inferior vena cava returns blood to the heart from the lower part of the body.

### HIGHLIGHT

Pathway: Blood saturated with $CO_2$ returns to the right side of the heart via the inferior and superior vena cava > right atrium > tricuspid valve > right ventricle > pulmonary valve > pulmonary artery > to the lungs > (exchange of $CO_2$ and $O_2$ takes place in the lungs) from the lungs saturated with $O_2$ > pulmonary veins > left atrium > bicuspid valve (mitral valve) > left ventricle > aortic valve > aorta.

■

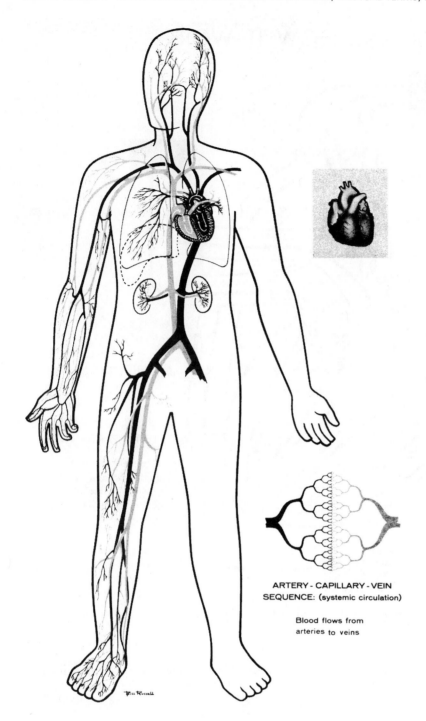

F I G U R E  23–18 • The blood vessels. (Courtesy of The American Heart Association and its affiliates.)

ARTERY - CAPILLARY - VEIN
SEQUENCE: (systemic circulation)

Blood flows from
arteries to veins

## BLOOD

**Blood** is the carrying agent of the transportation system. It is a warm, sticky fluid ranging in color from dark bluish red to bright red, according to the amount of oxygen it is carrying. An adult has approximately 5.7 L (6 qt) of blood.

### Function of Blood

The blood has two main functions: transportation and fighting infection.

### *Transportation*

The blood carries oxygen from the lungs and nutrients from the digestive tract to the body cells. It carries waste products from the cells, carbon dioxide to the lungs, and other waste (urea) to the kidneys. The blood also transports hormones and other chemicals.

### *Fighting Infection*

Certain blood cells help the body fight disease-causing organisms.

## Blood Composition

Blood is made up of plasma and cells.

### Plasma

**Plasma** is the fluid portion of the blood, in which the blood cells are suspended. Plasma is approximately 90% water and contains over 100 other constituents, such as glucose, fibrinogen, and protein. It makes up approximately 50% of the total amount of the blood. Plasma transports nutrients, waste material, hormones, and so forth to and from the body cells. Fibrinogen assists in the blood-clotting process.

### Blood Cells

There are three kinds of **blood cells**, each carrying out certain functions.

**Erythrocytes** (red blood cells) are produced by the red bone marrow. Red bone marrow is found in the flat bones of the body, such as the sternum or the pelvic bones. A **sternal puncture** is a procedure used to obtain bone marrow from the sternum. The bone marrow is then studied to determine its ability to produce red blood cells. The function of the red blood cell is to carry oxygen and carbon dioxide. **Hemoglobin** is the oxygen-carrying pigment of the erythrocyte that gives blood its color. The average red blood cell (RBC) count is 4.5 to 5 million/mm$^3$ of blood. Erythrocytes exist approximately 4 months. It is estimated that each erythrocyte travels approximately 700 miles during its lifetime.

**Leukocytes** (white blood cells) are colorless cells produced by the spleen, bone marrow, and lymph nodes. Their chief function is to fight against pathogenic microorganisms (disease-causing bacteria). The normal white blood cell (WBC) count is 5000 to 9000/mm$^3$ of blood. An elevated blood count may indicate the presence of an infection in the body. Leukocytes last a very short time—approximately 14 hours or less.

**Platelets** are also formed in the red bone marrow. Their prime function is to aid in the clotting of blood. A normal platelet count is about 250,000/mm$^3$ of blood. Platelets exist for a short time in the bloodstream and are replaced approximately every 4 days.

## CIRCULATION OF BLOOD THROUGH THE HEART

Blood carrying the waste product carbon dioxide returns from circulating through the body and enters the right atrium of the heart through the superior vena cava and the inferior vena cava. The blood travels through the tricuspid valve to the right ventricle. The right ventricle pumps the blood through the **pulmonary arteries** to the lungs. (The pulmonary artery is the only artery that transports waste-carrying blood.) The blood, while in the lungs, gets rid of the carbon dioxide and takes on oxygen. This exchange changes the appearance of the blood from a bluish red color to a bright red color. The oxygenated blood returns to the left atrium through the **pulmonary veins**.

**HIGHLIGHT**

Since leukocytes fight incompatible blood cells, it is absolutely essential that patients be typed and cross-matched before receiving blood. Before scientists learned to group blood into types that could be safely given from one person to another, many deaths resulted from incompatible blood transfusions. The blood types are O, A, B, and AB.

(The pulmonary vein is the only vein in the body to carry oxygenated blood.) The blood passes through the bicuspid valve to the left ventricle. The left ventricle pumps the blood through the aorta and out to the body parts. Refer to Figure 23–17; the arrows indicate the passage of blood through the heart.

## THE SPLEEN

The **spleen** is located in the upper left abdomen and is protected by the lower ribs. Two important functions of the spleen are to destroy old red blood cells, bacteria, and germs and to store blood for emergency use. The spleen produces the red blood cells in the fetus.

## DISEASES AND DISORDERS OF THE CIRCULATORY SYSTEM

### Coronary Artery Disease

**Coronary artery disease** (CAD) is usually caused by occlusion, or narrowing of the arteries due to the build-up of plaque on the arterial walls, a condition called **atherosclerosis**. **Angina pectoris** is a condition caused by lack of oxygen to the myocardium as a result of atherosclerosis of the coronary arteries. Atherosclerosis can completely block the artery, creating a condition called **coronary occlusion** (Fig. 23–19); or a **thrombus** can develop on segments of the artery containing plaque, causing a blockage, a condition referred to as **coronary thrombosis**. Both conditions may lead to a **myocardial infarction** (heart attack) because they interfere with the flow of blood to the heart, which denies the myocardium the oxygen and nutrients it needs. A symptom of a myocardial infarction is sudden onset of chest pain, sometimes radiating to the arms. The severity of the heart attack depends on which artery is blocked and to what extent it is blocked.

**Coronary artery bypass surgery** may be performed in coronary artery disease to improve the blood supply to the myocardium. This type of surgery consists of using a vein from the leg grafted to the aorta and the clogged coronary artery to form an alternative route for the flow of blood.

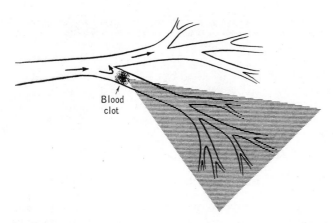

F I G U R E  23–19 • Coronary occlusion. The shaded area represents the infarcted area of the myocardium. (From Keane, C. B.: *Essentials of Medical-Surgical Nursing*. Philadelphia, W.B. Saunders Co., 1979, with permission.)

## Congestive Heart Failure

**Congestive heart failure (CHF)** occurs when the heart is unable to pump the required amount of blood, resulting in the accumulation of blood in the lungs and liver. CHF develops gradually. Symptoms are dyspnea and peripheral edema. Treatment includes rest and the administration of oxygen, digitalis, and diuretics.

## Anemia

**Anemia** is a disorder characterized by a below normal level of hemoglobin in the blood. It may result from decreased red blood cell production, from increased red blood cell destruction, or from blood loss. Treatment varies according to the cause. The anemic person becomes easily fatigued. Pallor may also indicate anemia. Sternal puncture to obtain bone marrow for study and blood tests are used to diagnose anemia.

## Varicose Veins

**Varicose veins** are swollen, distended, and knotted veins usually in the tissue of the leg. Standing or sitting prolonged periods causes weight on the valves from the blood and can result in the valves losing their elasticity. Other causes include pregnancy and obesity. Elevation of the leg and elastic stockings are used for treatment. Surgery, ligation (tying off the vein), and stripping may be required for serious cases.

## Acquired Immunodeficiency Syndrome

**Acquired immunodeficiency syndrome (AIDS)** is manifested by destruction of patients' immune systems, making them very susceptible to infection. AIDS is caused by the human immunodeficiency virus (HIV), which infects certain white blood cells of the body's immune system and gradually destroys the body's ability to fight infection. Many infected persons develop previously rare types of pneumonia (*Pneumocystis carinii* **pneumonia**) and cancer (**Kaposi's sarcoma**).

HIV has been isolated from semen and blood and is transmitted by intimate contact involving the mucous membranes or breaks in the skin, across the placenta from mother to fetus, or before or during birth. The sharing of hypodermic needles among IV drug users, blood transfusions, and needle sticks are other ways of becoming infected. The virus cannot penetrate intact skin. AIDS has become one of the deadliest epidemic diseases of modern times and will remain a major public health concern during the 1990s.

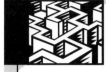

**REVIEW QUESTIONS**

1. a. Label the following diagram of the heart, including the blood vessels through which the blood enters and leaves the heart. Include the following parts:

| | | |
|---|---|---|
| endocardium | pulmonary artery | right atrium |
| myocardium | pulmonary vein | left atrium |
| pericardium | aorta | right ventricle |
| bicuspid valve | superior vena cava | left ventricle |
| tricuspid valve | inferior vena cava | |

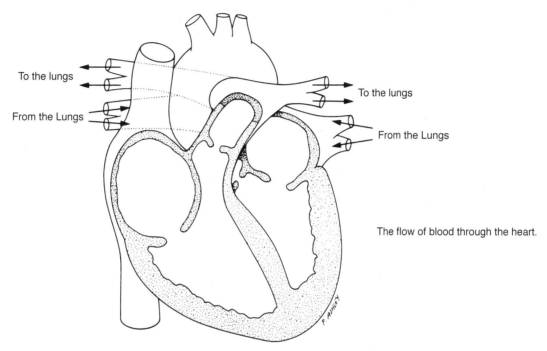

To the lungs

From the Lungs

To the lungs

From the Lungs

The flow of blood through the heart.

   b. Using arrows, trace on the diagram the circulation of blood from the superior and inferior vena cava to the aorta.

2. Blood travels through a network of tubes called blood vessels. Name in sequence the types of blood vessels the blood travels through when leaving the heart to reentry, and write the function of each.

   a. _____

   b. _____

   c. _____

   d. _____

   e. _____

3. The fluid portion of the blood is called the _____ . Its functions are

   a. _____

   b. _____

   c. _____

4. List three types of blood cells and briefly describe the function of each.

   a. _____

   b. _____

   c. _____

5. Name the four blood types.

   a. _____

   b. _____

   c. _____

   d. _____

6. Two functions of the spleen are:

   a. _____

   b. _____

7. Match the terms in Column I with the phrases in Column II.

| Column I | Column II |
|---|---|
| a. anemia | _____ caused by lack of oxygen to the myocardium |
| b. CHF | _____ the heart is unable to pump blood |
| c. CAD | _____ narrowing of arteries |
| d. coronary thrombosis | _____ below normal level of hemoglobin |
| e. myocardial infarction | _____ causes occlusion of an artery |
| f. bypass | _____ surgery for varicose veins |
| g. angina pectoris | _____ damage to the heart muscle |
| h. ligation and stripping | _____ caused by HIV |
| i. AIDS | |

## MEDICAL TERMINOLOGY RELATING TO THE CIRCULATORY SYSTEM

### OBJECTIVES

*Upon mastery of the medical terminology for this unit, you will be able to:*

1. Spell and define the word elements and the medical terms for the circulatory system.

2. Given the meaning of a medical condition relating to the circulatory system, build with word elements the corresponding medical term.

3. Analyze the medical terms that are built from word elements that relate to the circulatory system.

4. Given a list of word elements, identify them as word roots, suffixes, or prefixes.

5. Given descriptions of hospital situations in which the health unit coordinator may encounter medical terminology, apply the correct medical terms to the situation described.

The list below contains the word elements you need to memorize for the circulatory system. The exercises included in this unit will help you with this task. You will continue to use these word elements throughout this course and during your employment. Practice pronouncing each word element aloud.

| Word Roots/Combining Forms | Meaning |
|---|---|
| angi/o (ăn'-jē-ō) | blood vessel |
| aort/o (ā-ōr'-tō) | aorta |
| arteri/o (ar-tē'-rē-ō) | artery |
| cardi/o (kar'-dē-ō) | heart |
| hem/o (hē'-mō); hemat/o (hĕm'-ah-tō) | blood |
| phleb/o (flĕb'-ō); ven/o (vē'-nō) | vein |
| splen/o (splē'-nō) | spleen |
| thromb/o (thrŏm'-bō) | clot |

| Color Word Roots/Combining Forms | Meaning |
|---|---|
| cyan/o (sī'-ah-nō) | blue |
| erythr/o (ĕ-rīth'-rō) | red |
| leuk/o (loo'-kō) | white |

| Suffixes | Meaning |
|---|---|
| emia (ē'-mē-ah) (may also be used as word root) | condition of the blood |
| megaly (mĕg'-ah-lē) | enlargement |
| pexy (pĕk'-sē) | surgical fixation (suspension) |
| sclerosis (sklĕ-rō'-sĭs) (may also be used as word root) | hardening |
| stenosis (stĕ-nō'-sĭs) (may also be used as word root) | narrowing |

| Prefixes | Meaning |
|---|---|
| endo (ĕn'-dō) | inside |
| hyper (hī'-per) | above normal |
| hypo (hī'-pō) | below normal |
| peri (pĕr'-ē) | around |

# EXERCISE 1

Identify each word element listed below by writing P for prefix, S for suffix, or WR for word root in the space provided. Then define each word element in the space provided. Word elements studied in previous units are also included in this exercise.

| Word Element | Type | Meaning |
|---|---|---|
| *Example*: 1. pexy | S | surgical fixation |
| 2. hypo | ____ | _____ |
| 3. a, an | ____ | _____ |
| 4. hem | ____ | _____ |
| 5. splen | ____ | _____ |
| 6. cyt | ____ | _____ |
| 7. stenosis | ____ | _____ |
| 8. endo | ____ | _____ |
| 9. leuk | ____ | _____ |
| 10. erythr | ____ | _____ |
| 11. angi | ____ | _____ |
| 12. cardi | ____ | _____ |
| 13. arteri | ____ | _____ |
| 14. peri | ____ | _____ |

15. inter        _____        _____

16. intra        _____        _____

17. sclerosis    _____        _____

18. emia         _____        _____

19. megaly       _____        _____

20. phleb        _____        _____

21. aort         _____        _____

22. thromb       _____        _____

23. hyper        _____        _____

E X E R C I S E  **2**

Write the word elements for the meanings listed below. Identify each word element you write in the answer column. Use P for prefix, S for suffix, and WR for word root or combining form. For review purposes, word elements from previous units are included in this exercise.

| Meaning | Type | Word Elements |
|---|---|---|
| 1. aorta | _____ | _____ |
| 2. enlargement | _____ | _____ |
| 3. hardening | _____ | _____ |
| 4. between | _____ | _____ |
| 5. artery | _____ | _____ |
| 6. blood vessel | _____ | _____ |
| 7. white | _____ | _____ |
| 8. narrowing | _____ | _____ |
| 9. spleen | _____ | _____ |
| 10. without | _____ | _____ |
| 11. surgical fixation | _____ | _____ |
| 12. inside | _____ | _____ |
| 13. blood | _____ | _____ |
| 14. cell | _____ | _____ |
| 15. below normal | _____ | _____ |
| 16. red | _____ | _____ |
| 17. heart | _____ | _____ |
| 18. around | _____ | _____ |
| 19. blood condition | _____ | _____ |
| 20. vein | _____ | _____ |
| 21. clot | _____ | _____ |

## MEDICAL TERMS RELATING TO THE CIRCULATORY SYSTEM

The following list is made up of medical terms you will need to know for the circulatory system. Exercises following this list will assist you in learning these terms. Practice the pronunciation of these terms out loud.

| General Terms | Meaning |
| --- | --- |
| arrhythmia (ah-rĭth'-mē-ah) | variation from a normal rhythm, especially of the heartbeat |
| aortic (ā-or'-tĭk) | pertaining to the aorta |
| cardiac arrest (kar'-dē-ăk) (ah-rěst') | sudden and often unexpected stoppage of the heartbeat |
| cardiologist (kar-dē-ŏl'-ō-jĭst) | a physician who specializes in cardiology |
| cardiology (kar-dē-ŏl'-ō-jē) | the study of the heart and its functions and diseases |
| cardiomegaly (kar'-dē-ō-měg'-ah-lē) | enlargement of the heart |
| cardiovascular (kar'-dē-ō-văs'-kū-lar) | pertaining to the heart and blood vessels |
| coronary (kŏr'-ō-nā-rē) | a term used to describe blood vessels that supply blood to the heart |
| endocardial (ěn-dō-kar'-dē-al) | pertaining to within the heart |
| erythrocyte (ě-rĭth'-rō-sīt) | red blood cell (RBC) |
| hemorrhage (hěm'-ō-rĭj) | the rapid flow of blood from a blood vessel |
| hypertension (hī-per-těn'-shŭn) | high blood pressure |
| hypotension (hī-pō-těn'-shŭn) | low blood pressure |
| intravenous (ĭn-trah-vē'-nŭs) | within a vein |
| leukocyte (loo'-kō-sīt) | white blood cell (WBC) |
| phlebotomy (flě-bŏt'-ō-mē) | incision into the vein to withdraw blood |
| splenomegaly (splē-nō-měg'-ah-lē) | enlargement of the spleen |
| tachycardia (tăk-ě-kar'-dē-ah) | abnormally rapid heart rate |
| thrombosis (thrŏm-bō'-sīs) | abnormal formation of a blood clot |

| Surgical Terms | Meaning |
| --- | --- |
| angiorrhapy (ăn-jě-ōr'-ah-fě) | suturing of a blood vessel |
| hemorrhoidectomy (hěm-ō-roi-děk'-tō-mē) | excision of hemorrhoids |
| splenectomy (splě-něk'-tō-mē) | excision of the spleen |
| splenopexy (splě'-nō-pěk-sē) | surgical fixation of the spleen |

| Diagnostic Terms | Meaning |
| --- | --- |
| anemia (ah-nē'-mē-ah) | deficiency in the number of erythrocytes (RBC) |
| aneurysm (ăn'-ū-rĭzm) | a dilation of a weak area of the arterial wall |
| arteriosclerosis (ar-tē'-rē-ō-sclě-rō'-sĭs) | hardening of the arteries |
| arteriostenosis (ar-tē'-rē-ō-stě-nō'-sĭs) | constriction (narrowing) of an artery |
| congestive heart failure (CHF) | inability of the heart to pump sufficient amounts of blood to the body parts |
| coronary occlusion (kŏr'-ō-nā-rē) (ō-kloo'-zhŭn) | the closing off of a coronary artery, which usually results in damage to the heart muscle; commonly referred to as a heart attack |
| coronary thrombosis (kŏr'-ō-nā-rē) (thrŏm-bō'-sĭs) | the blocking of a coronary artery by a blood clot; commonly referred to as a heart attack |
| edema (ě-dē'-mah) | an abnormal accumulation of fluid in the intercellular spaces of the body |
| embolism (ěm'-bō-lĭzm) | a floating mass that blocks a vessel |
| endocarditis (ěn-dō-kar-dī'-tĭs) | inflammation of the inner lining of the heart |
| hematology (hē-mah-tŏl'-ō-jē) | study of the blood. Also, a diagnostic division within a hospital laboratory that performs diagnostic tests on blood components |
| hematoma (hē-mah-tō'-mah) | a tumor-like mass formed from blood in the tissues |
| hemophilia (hē-mō-fīl'-ē-ah) | a congenital disorder characterized by excessive bleeding |
| hemorrhoid (hěm'-ōrr-oyd) | enlarged veins in the rectal areas |

| Diagnostic Terms | Meaning |
|---|---|
| leukemia (loo-kē′-mē-ah) | a type of cancer characterized by rapid abnormal production of white blood cells |
| myocardial infarction (MI) (mī-ō-kar′-dē-al) (ĭn-fark′-shŭn) | damage to the heart muscle caused by insufficient blood supply to the area; a condition the lay person refers to as a heart attack |
| pericarditis (pĕr-ĭ-kar-dī′-tĭs) | inflammation around the heart or pericardium |
| thrombophlebitis (thrŏm′-bō-flĕ-bī′-tĭs) | inflammation of a vein as the result of a clot |

| Terms Relating to Diagnostic Procedures | Meaning |
|---|---|
| angiogram (ăn′-jē-ō-grăm) | an x-ray of a blood vessel, with dye used as a contrast medium |
| aortogram (ā-ōr′-tō-grăm) | an x-ray of the aorta, with dye used as a contrast medium |
| arteriogram (ar-tē′-rē-ō-grăm) | an x-ray of an artery, with dye used as a contrast medium |
| cardiac catheterization (kar′-dē-ăk) (kăth′-ĕ-ter-ĭ-zā′-shŭn) | a diagnostic procedure to visualize the heart to determine the presence of heart disease or heart defects. A long catheter is threaded from a blood vessel to the heart cavities. Dye is used as a contrast medium. |
| electrocardiogram (EKG) (ē-lĕk′-trō-kar′-dē-ō-grăm) | a record of the electric impulses of the heart |
| electrocardiograph (ē-lĕk′-trō-kar′-dē-ō-grăf) | the machine used for electrocardiography |
| electrocardiography (ē-lĕk′-trō-kar-dē-ŏg′-rah-fē) | the process of recording the electric impulses of the heart |
| hematocrit (hē′-măt-ō-krĭt) | hematocrit, which means "to separate blood," is a laboratory test that measures the volume percentage of red blood cells in whole blood |
| hemoglobin (hē′-mō-glō′-bĭn) | the oxygen-carrying pigment of the red blood cells |

# E X E R C I S E  3

Analyze and define each medical term listed below.

1. aortic _____

2. splenomegaly _____

3. hemorrhage _____

4. thrombosis _____

5. leukocyte _____

6. erythrocyte _____

7. cardiologist _____

8. cardiomegaly _____

9. phlebotomy _____

10. angiorrhaphy _____

11. splenectomy _____

12. splenopexy _____

13. endocarditis _____

14. arteriosclerosis _____

15. arteriostenosis _____

16. thrombophlebitis _____

17. hematoma _____

18. hematology _____

19. leukemia _____

20. anemia _____

21. electrocardiogram _____

22. electrocardiograph _____

23. electrocardiography _____

24. angiogram _____

25. arteriogram _____

26. aortogram _____

27. pericarditis _____

E X E R C I S E  **4**

Using the word elements you have studied in this unit and previous units, build medical terms from each definition listed below.

1. x-ray of the aorta _____

2. x-ray of an artery _____

3. x-ray of a blood vessel _____

4. a record of the electric impulses of the heart _____

5. inflammation of the inner lining of the heart _____

6. hardening of the arteries _____

7. inflammation of a vein due to a blood clot formation _____

8. study of the blood _____

9. study of the heart _____

10. one who specializes in cardiology _____

11. enlarged heart _____

12. incision into a vein _____

13. excision of the spleen _____

14. surgical fixation of the spleen _____

15. rapid discharge of blood _____

16. white blood cell _____

17. red blood cell _____

18. inflammation around the heart _____

E X E R C I S E  **5**

Define each medical term listed below.

1. hematocrit _____

2. hemoglobin _____

3. cardiac arrest _____

4. cardiovascular _____

5. hemorrhoidectomy _____

6. myocardial infarction _____

7. hemorrhoid _____

8. intravenous _____

9. cardiac catheterization _____

10. aneurysm _____

11. embolism _____

12. hypertension _____

13. hypotension _____

14. congestive heart failure _____

15. coronary _____

16. edema _____

17. arrhythmia _____

18. tachycardia _____

E X E R C I S E  6

Spell each medical term studied in this unit by having someone dictate the terms to you.

1. _____     22. _____

2. _____     23. _____

3. _____     24. _____

4. _____     25. _____

5. _____     26. _____

6. _____     27. _____

7. _____     28. _____

8. _____     29. _____

9. _____     30. _____

10. _____     31. _____

11. _____     32. _____

12. _____     33. _____

13. _____     34. _____

14. _____     35. _____

15. _____     36. _____

16. _____     37. _____

17. _____     38. _____

18. _____     39. _____

19. _____     40. _____

20. _____     41. _____

21. _____     42. _____

43. _____     47. _____

44. _____     48. _____

45. _____     49. _____

46. _____

# E X E R C I S E  **7**

Answer the following questions.

1. _____ is a division within the laboratory that performs diagnostic tests on blood components. _____ and _____ are two tests performed in this laboratory division.

2. The coronary care unit (CCU) in the hospital is an intensive care unit set up to care for patients who have heart attacks. The admitting diagnosis of these patients may be:

   a. _____

   b. _____

   c. _____

3. Below is a list of medical terms. Circle the terms that may be found on the surgical schedule. Underline the part of the word that makes it a surgical procedure.

   |                       |                    |
   | --------------------- | ------------------ |
   | endocarditis          | hypertension       |
   | splenectomy           | hemorrhoidectomy   |
   | electroencephalogram  | cardiology         |

4. A doctor who performs surgery on the heart or blood vessels may be called a _____ surgeon.

5. A patient is having symptoms that indicate a disease or complication involving the circulatory system. The attending doctor is a good practitioner. He wishes the patient to see a heart specialist. He will contact a

   _____.

6. Each hospital has a team of people to call for emergency conditions such as sudden stoppage of the heart or

   _____ . This team may be called the _____ team.

7. The doctor orders a diagnostic procedure to record the electric impulses of the heart. He or she orders a

   _____ . The technician brings a _____ (machine) to the patient's bedside to perform this test.

8. The patient is scheduled for an x-ray of the blood vessels to be visualized by the use of dye as a contrast medium.

   The patient is scheduled for a _____ .

9. The patient is scheduled for a diagnostic test that uses dye as a contrast medium to visualize parts of the heart. A long catheter is threaded from a blood vessel to the heart. _____ is the name of this test.

10. Below are listed three types of blood cells. Look under "Doctors' Orders for Hematology Studies" on p. 257. Write the name of the laboratory test used to study each cell listed below:

    a. leukocyte _____

    b. erythrocyte _____

    c. platelet _____

11. _____ is the clear, fluid portion of the blood that may be ordered by the doctor to be administered intravenously to the patient.

# UNIT VII

## The Digestive System

### OBJECTIVES

*Upon mastery of the basic human structure for this unit, you will be able to:*

1. Define the terms in the vocabulary list.
2. Describe the overall functions of the digestive system.
3. Name the organs of the digestive tract and describe the function of each.
4. Name the digestive enzymes.
5. Trace the passage of food through the digestive tract.
6. Name the four sphincters of the digestive tract.
7. List the accessory organs to the digestive tract and tell how each contributes to the digestive process.
8. Describe peptic ulcer, diverticular disease, gallstones, and pyloric stenosis.

### VOCABULARY

**Absorption** • The transfer of digested food from the small intestine to the bloodstream

**Digestion** • The physical and chemical breakdown of food for use by the body cells

**Elimination** • The removal of solid waste from the body

**Ingestion** • Taking nutrients into the digestive tract through the mouth

**Mastication** • The act of chewing food

**Metabolism** • Utilization of digested food by the body cells

## THE DIGESTIVE SYSTEM

### Organs of the Digestive System

*Digestive Tract*

Mouth
Pharynx
Esophagus
Stomach
Small intestine
Large intestine

### Sphincters of the Digestive System

Sphincters, circular muscles that close or open a natural body opening, regulate the passage of substances. There are four sphincter muscles along the digestive tract. These digestive sphincters are called cardiac, pyloric, ileocecal, and anal sphincters.

**Accessory Organs**

Liver
Gallbladder
Pancreas
Salivary Glands

### Function of the Digestive System

Food passes through a long tubular structure called the **digestive tract** (also called the **alimentary canal** and the **gastrointestinal tract**), which extends from the mouth to the rectum. Along the way food is prepared for absorption by some of the organs of the digestive tract and the accessory organs. The waste material—that material that is not transferred to the bloodstream during absorption—is eliminated from the body. **Ingestion**, **digestion**, **absorption**, and **elimination** are the main functions of the digestive system.

## THE DIGESTIVE TRACT

### The Mouth

In the mouth the chewing of food starts the physical breakdown of food for use by body cells. The salivary glands (Fig. 23–20) produce saliva that contains the enzyme amylase. This enzyme starts the chemical breakdown of food. The three pairs of salivary glands are:

1. **Parotid**, the largest located near the ear.
2. **Submandibular**, located near the lower jaw
3. **Sublingual**, located under the tongue

Each gland has a duct (canal) that opens into the mouth to allow for the flow of saliva.

### The Pharynx

The **pharynx** (throat) allows for the passage of food from the mouth to the esophagus. The pharynx is shared with

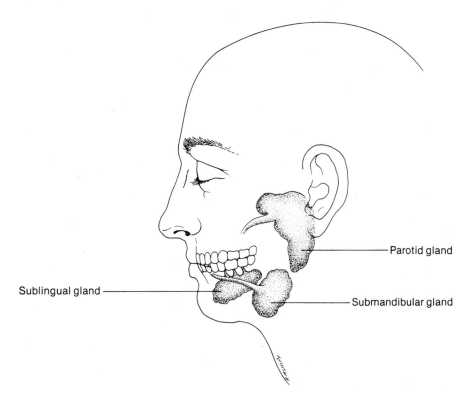

FIGURE 23–20 • The salivary glands.

the respiratory tract, since it is also used for the passage of air.

## The Esophagus

The **esophagus** is a muscular tube that extends from the pharynx to the stomach. It passes through the thoracic cavity, behind the heart, to the abdominal cavity. The esophagus is approximately 9 inches (22.5 cm) long. Its function is simply the passage of food, which is propelled

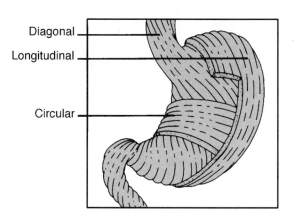

FIGURE 23–21 • The stomach. (Modified from Whitney, E. N. and Hamilton, E. M.: *Understanding Nutrition*, 4th ed. Belmont, CA, Wadsworth Publishing, 1987, with permission.)

along by involuntary wave-like movements; this action is called **peristalsis**. The cardiac sphincter is located between the esophagus and the stomach.

## Stomach

The stomach is located in the upper left portion of the abdomen, below the diaphragm. It is a container for the food during part of the digestive process. Gastric glands located in the mucous membrane lining of the stomach secrete enzymes (lipase and pepsin) and hydrochloric acid. These secretions continue the chemical breakdown of food. The muscles of the stomach are circular, diagonal and longitudinal. This muscle construction of the stomach makes the organ very strong (Fig. 23–21). The function of the stomach is to secrete the enzymes, mix, and churn the food to a liquid consistency. This process of mixing and churning continues the physical breakdown of food. When the food is liquefied it is referred to as chyme.

After about 30 minutes the food begins to leave the stomach at 30-minute intervals. It passes through the pyloric sphincter muscle into the duodenum, which is the first part of the small intestine. It takes 2 to 4 hours for the stomach to empty completely.

## The Small Intestine

The small intestine, so called because it is smaller in diameter than the large intestine, is approximately 20 feet

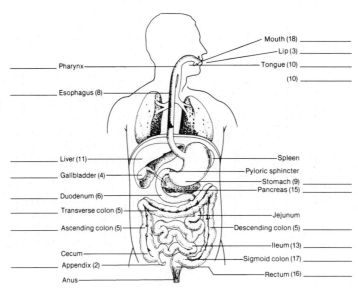

F I G U R E  23–22 • The digestive system. (From Applegate, E. J.: *The Anatomy and Physiology Learning System*. Philadelphia, W. B. Saunders, 1995, with permission.)

long. It extends from the stomach to the large intestine (Fig. 23–22). The first part of the small intestine is called the duodenum. Two accessory organs, the pancreas and the gallbladder secrete into the duodenum through tiny tubes called ducts. The pancreas secretes enzymes. The gallbladder secretes bile that has been produced by the liver and stored in the gallbladder. The jejunum followed by the ileum forms the remainder of the small intestine. (Ilium, part of the pelvic bone studied in the musculoskeletal system, has the same pronunciation as ileum. Correct spelling of the word to communicate the correct meaning is absolutely essential.) The muscosal cells located in the lining of the small intestine secrete enzymes that continue the chemical breakdown of food. Some of these enzymes are sucrase, maltase, lipase, peptidase, and lactase. Digestion is completed in the small intestine and absorption takes place here.

Absorption is the passage of the end products of digestion from the small intestine into the bloodstream. The passage of nutrients from the small intestine to the bloodstream is facilitated through the capillary walls of the villi, which has a surface area of approximately 100 square feet. The villi are tiny finger-like projections that line the walls of the small intestine (Fig. 23–23). The blood carries the nutrients to all body cells, where they are used according to need. The process of cell utilization of nutrients is called metabolism.

The food substance (waste) that is not absorbed continues to move by peristalsis through the ileocecal sphincter into the large intestine.

## The Large Intestine

The **large intestine** is approximately 5 feet long. Peristalsis continues into the large intestine. The large intestine ex-

tends from the ileum to the **anus**, the opening at the end of the rectum to the outside. The large intestine is divided into the following parts, listed in sequence extending from the ileum: the **cecum**; the **colon**, which is divided into four parts—the **ascending colon**, the **transverse colon**, the **descending colon**, and the **sigmoid colon**—and the **rectum**. The function of the large intestine is the absorption of water and the elimination of the solid waste products of digestion from the body.

> ### HIGHLIGHT
>
> **The Pathway**: Food ingestion > mouth > esophagus > cardiac sphincter > stomach > pyloric sphincter > small intestine (duodenum, jejunum, ileum) > **nutrients** absorption by the blood and carried to all cells for metabolism **waste** > ileocecal sphincter > large intestine (cecum, ascending colon, transverse colon, descending colon, sigmoid colon, rectum) > anal sphincter > elimination.

The **appendix** is a small blind tube attached to the cecum. It has no function.

## THE ACCESSORY ORGANS

## The Liver, Gallbladder, and Pancreas

ood does not pass through the accessory organs, but they play a vital role in the digestive process.

The **liver**, the largest gland in the body, is located in the upper right portion of the abdominal cavity. Although it has many important functions, we will discuss only one, the production of bile. The liver secretes bile, which aids

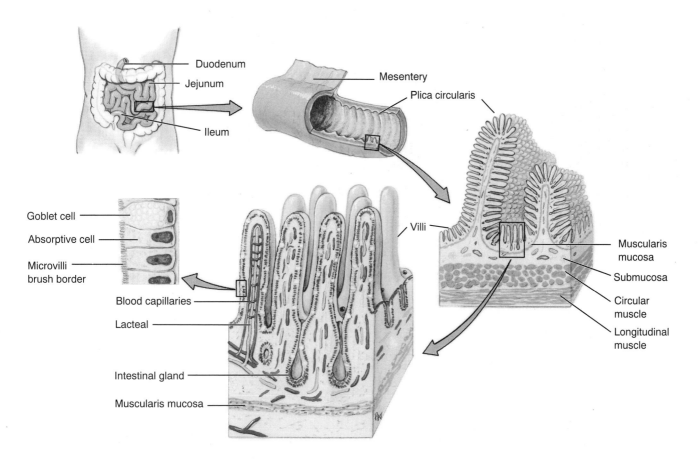

F I G U R E   23–23 • Villi intestine. (From Applegate, E. J.: *The Anatomy and Physiology Learning System*. Philadelphia, W. B. Saunders, 1995, with permission.)

in the digestion of fats. Bile is stored in the **gallbladder**, a small sac located under the liver. The gallbladder concentrates the bile by reabsorbing water. When bile is present in the duodenum the gallbladder is stimulated to contract and release bile into the duodenum.

The **pancreas** is located behind the stomach. Part of its function is to secrete the enzymes lipase, protease, amylase, and bicarbonate into the duodenum. These enzymes continue the digestion process by chemically breaking down the food particles. The **islets of Langerhans** are contained in the pancreas. They produce a hormone called **insulin**, which is released directly into the bloodstream. Insulin is necessary for the metabolism of carbohydrates in the body.

## DISEASES AND CONDITIONS OF THE DIGESTIVE SYSTEM

### Peptic Ulcer

A **peptic ulcer** is a lesion, or sore, of the mucous membrane of the esophagus, stomach (gastric ulcer), or duodenum (duodenal ulcer) (Fig. 23–24). A combination of

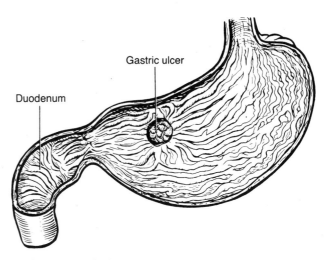

F I G U R E   23–24 • Peptic ulcer. (From Miller, B. F. and Keane, C. B.: *Encyclopedia and Dictionary of Medicine, Nursing and Allied Health*, 4th ed. Philadelphia, W. B. Saunders Co., 1987, with permission.)

factors cause peptic ulcers, including excessive secretion of gastric enzymes, hydrochloric acid, stress, heredity, and taking certain drugs.

Symptoms include pain 1 to 3 hours after eating, which is usually relieved by eating or taking antacids. Also a gnawing sensation in the epigastric region is experienced.

If untreated, bleeding, hemorrhage, or perforation may occur. Perforation allows the contents of the stomach or small intestine to escape into the peritoneal cavity.

The GI series, gastroscopy, and gastric analysis are used for diagnosing peptic ulcers. Since symptoms of peptic ulcer are similar to symptoms of stomach or duodenal cancer, early diagnosis is important.

Early treatment includes diet control and medication. Surgery may be indicated when there is scarring, recurrent bleeding, or perforation.

## Diverticular Disease

**Diverticular disease** is caused by the forming of small pouches, called **diverticula**, on the intestine wall (Fig. 23–25). These are two forms of diverticular disease: diverticulosis and diverticulitis. In **diverticulosis**, diverticula are present but cause no symptoms. In **diverticulitis**, the diverticula are inflamed and may cause obstruction, infection, or hemorrhage.

Symptoms include cramping in the abdomen and muscle spasms. Medical treatment includes using enemas, diet, and drugs for infection. Severe cases may require surgical removal of the involved segment of the intestine and a temporary colostomy (surgical opening between the colon and the body surface).

## Cholelithiasis and Choledocholithiasis

**Cholelithiasis**, or gallstones, is a common condition affecting 20% of the population over 40 years of age (Fig. 23–26). The stones form because of changes in the bile content.

Gallstones can lodge in the common bile duct, which leads to the duodenum. This condition is called **choledocholithiasis**. Pain is caused by pressure building up in the gallbladder.

Symptoms of a typical gallbladder attack include acute abdominal pain after eating a fatty meal. Sometimes the pain is so severe the patient may seek emergency treatment. Other symptoms are digestive disturbances, such as belching.

A cholecystogram is used for diagnosing gallstones. Treatment includes laparoscopy, cholecystectomy, choledocholithotomy, or **extracorporeal shock wave lithotripsy** (**ESWL**), which shatters gallstones using high-energy shock waves for removal without surgery.

## Pyloric Stenosis

Pyloric stenosis is an obstruction caused by narrowing of the pyloric sphincter muscle. The condition may be congenital or acquired. In adults the condition is most often

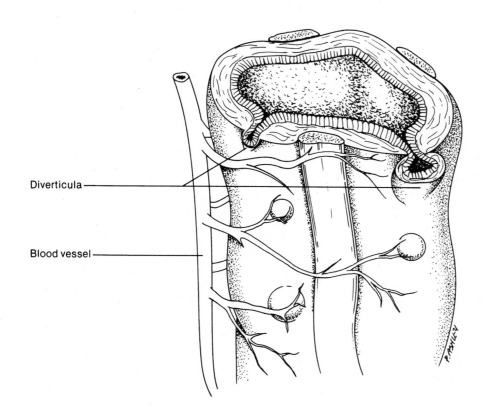

Diverticula ———

Blood vessel ———

F I G U R E  23–25 • Diverticula.

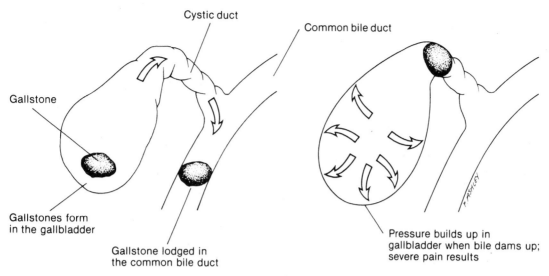

F I G U R E   23–26 • Gallstones.

caused by peptic ulceration or tumors that may be cancerous. Symptoms include vomiting that becomes progressively more frequent and forceful. Infants with pyloric stenosis may at first be diagnosed as failure to thrive. Adults will experience a gradual weight loss.

Diagnosis is confirmed by an upper gastrointestinal examination using barium as a contrast medium. Treatment is usually surgical. In infants a formula that is thickened with cereal may be enough to stretch out the sphincter muscle if the stenosis is not severe.

## REVIEW QUESTIONS

1. Define:

   a. ingestion _____

   b. digestion _____

   c. elimination_____

2. Describe the overall function of the digestive system.

   _____

   _____

3. Beginning with the mouth, list in order the organs that food passes through during ingestion, digestion, and elimination. Include the names of the parts of the small intestine, large intestine, and the sphincter muscles.

   _____

   _____

   _____

   _____

4. List the digestive enzymes, the organs that secrete the digestive enzymes, and the digestive organ in which they perform their functions.

| Name of Digestive Enzyme | Organ of Secretion | Organ of Function |
|---|---|---|
| a. _____ | _____ | _____ |
| b. _____ | _____ | _____ |
| c. _____ | _____ | _____ |
| d. _____ | _____ | _____ |
| e. _____ | _____ | _____ |

5. Name the four accessory organs of digestion.

   a. _____

   b. _____

   c. _____

   d. _____

6. A narrowing of the opening between the stomach and the small intestine is called _____

   _____ .

7. Describe the function of the following organs in the digestive process:

   a. mouth _____

   b. stomach _____

   c. small intestine _____

   d. large intestine _____

   e. gallbladder _____

8. Match the terms in Column I with the phrases in Column II.

| Column I | Column II |
|---|---|
| a. diverticulitis | _____ lesion of the mucous membrane of the stomach |
| b. cholelithiasis | _____ inflamed diverticula |
| c. cholecystectomy | _____ stones in the gallbladder |
| d. diverticulosis | _____ stone in the common bile duct |
| e. peptic ulcer | _____ diverticula with no symptoms |
| f. choledocholithiasis | |

# MEDICAL TERMINOLOGY RELATING TO THE DIGESTIVE SYSTEM

## OBJECTIVES

*Upon mastery of the medical terminology for this unit, you will be able to:*

1. Spell and define the word elements and medical terms for the digestive system.

2. Given the meaning of a medical condition relating to the digestive tract, build with word elements the corresponding medical terms.

3. Given a list of medical terms, identify those that are surgical procedures and those that are diagnostic studies.

4. Compare the three *-tomy* suffixes.

5. Analyze and define medical terms, built from word elements that relate to the digestive system.

6. Given a description of hospital situations in which the health unit coordinator may encounter medical terminology, apply the correct medical terms to the situations described.

The list below contains the word elements you need to memorize for the digestive system. The exercises included in this unit will help you with this task. You will continue to use these word elements throughout this course and during your employment. Practice pronouncing each element aloud.

| Word Roots/Combining Forms | Meaning |
|---|---|
| 1. abdomin/o (ăb-dŏm′-ĭ-nō) | abdomen |
| 2. appendic/o (ăp-ĕn-dĕk′-ō) | appendix |
| 3. cheil/o (kī′-lō) | lip |
| 4. chol/o (kō′-lō) or chol/e (kō′-lē) | bile, gall |
| 5. col/o (kō′-lō) | colon |
| 6. duoden/o (doo-ō-dē′-nō) | duodenum |
| 7. enter/o (ĕn′-ter-ō) | intestines |
| 8. esophag/o (ĕ-sŏf′-ah-gō) | esophagus |
| 9. gastr/o (găs′-trō) | stomach |
| 10. gloss/o (glŏss′-ō); lingu/o (lĭng′-gwō) | tongue |
| 11. hepat/o (hĕp′-a-tō) | liver |
| 12. herni/o (her′-nē-ō) | protrusion of a body part |
| 13. ile/o (ĭl′-ĕ-ō) | ileum |
| 14. lapar/o (lăp′-ah-rō) | abdomen |
| 15. pancreat/o (păn′-krē-ă-tō) | pancreas |
| 16. proct/o (prŏk′-tō) | rectum |
| 17. sigmoid/o (sĭg′-moy-dō) | sigmoid colon (part of the colon) |
| 18. stomat/o (stō′-mah-tō) | mouth |

| Other Word Roots/Combining Forms | Meaning |
|---|---|
| 19. cyst/o (sĭs′-tō) | bladder (urinary unless otherwise used) |
| 20. lith/o (lĭth′-ō) | stone or calculus |

| Suffixes | Meaning |
|---|---|
| 21. iasis (ī′-ah-sĭs) | condition of |
| 22. ostomy (ŏs′-tō-mē) | creation of an artificial opening into |

## *-tomy* Suffixes

You are already familiar with two *-tomy* suffixes that are used to describe surgical procedures. They are *-otomy*, which means incision into a part of the body, and *-ectomy*, which means surgical removal of a part of the body. The third *-tomy* suffix you will study in this unit is *-ostomy*,

which describes a surgical procedure performed to create an artificial opening into a part of the body. For example, in the medical term *colostomy* (*col* is the word root for colon), a portion of the colon is attached to the surface of the abdomen, which creates an artificial opening between the colon and the abdominal surface (Fig. 23–27). This artificial opening is used for the passage of stools.

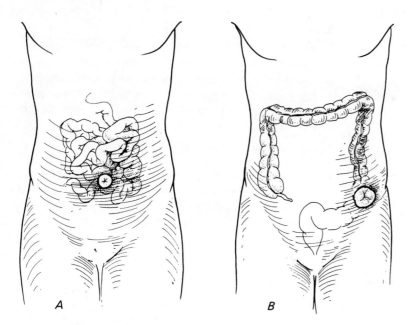

F I G U R E  23–27 • (A) Illeostomy. (B) Colostomy. (From LaFleur, M. and Starr, W.: *Exploring Medical Language*. St. Louis, The C. V. Mosby Co., 1985, with permission.)

## E X E R C I S E  **1**

Write the combining forms for the digestive system in the spaces provided on the diagram in Figure 23–22. The number preceding the combining form in the preceding list matches the number of the body part in the diagram.

## E X E R C I S E  **2**

Define the word elements listed below. Indicate the word elements that are suffixes by writing S after each in the space provided.

| Word Elements | Definition | Suffix |
|---|---|---|
| 1. stomat | | |
| 2. gloss | | |
| 3. gastr | | |
| 4. proct | | |
| 5. pancreat | | |
| 6. enter | | |
| 7. hepat | | |
| 8. cheil | | |
| 9. esophag | | |
| 10. iasis | | |
| 11. chol | | |
| 12. cyst | | |
| 13. duoden | | |
| 14. col | | |
| 15. ile | | |

16. abdomin _____ _____

17. appendic _____ _____

18. lapar _____ _____

19. lith _____ _____

20. ostomy _____ _____

21. herni _____ _____

22. sigmoid _____

## E X E R C I S E  3

Define the three *-tomy* suffixes. Build a medical term using each suffix and write the meaning of each term you have built.

1. otomy _____

_____

2. ectomy _____

_____

3. ostomy _____

## MEDICAL TERMS RELATING TO THE DIGESTIVE SYSTEM

The following is a list made up of medical terms you will need to know for the digestive system. Exercises following this list will assist you in learning these terms. Practice pronouncing each term aloud.

| General Terms | Meaning |
|---|---|
| abdominal (ăb-dŏm'-ĭn-al) | pertaining to the abdomen |
| diarrhea (dī'-ah-rē'-ah) | frequent discharge of watery stool |
| duodenal (doo-ō-dē'-nal) | pertaining to the duodenum |
| dysentery (dĭs'-ĕn-tĕr-ē) | condition of bad or painful intestines accompanied by diarrhea |
| glossoplegia (glŏss-ō-plē'-jē-ah) | paralysis of the tongue |
| hepatoma (hĕp-ah-tō'-mah) | a tumor of the liver |
| hepatomegaly (hĕp'-ah-tō-mĕg'-ah-lē) | enlargement of the liver |
| hernia (her'-nē-ah) | an abnormal protrusion of a body part through the containing structure |
| jaundice (jawn'-dĭs) | yellowness of the skin and eyes; a symptom of hepatitis |
| pancreatic (păn-krē-ăt'-ĭk) | pertaining to the pancreas |
| proctorrhea (prŏk-tō-rē'-ah) | discharge from the rectum |
| stomatogastric (stō'-mah-tō-găs'-trĭk) | pertaining to the stomach and the mouth |
| sublingual (sŭb-lĭng'-gwal) | pertaining to under the tongue |
| ulcer (ŭl'-ser) | a sore of the skin or mucous membrane |

| Surgical Terms | Meaning |
|---|---|
| abdominal herniorrhaphy (ăb-dŏm'-ĭn-al) (her-nē-ōr'-ah-fē) | suturing of a weak spot or opening in the abdominal wall to prevent protrusion of organs |
| appendectomy (ăp-ĕn-dĕk'-tō-mē) | excision of the appendix |

| Surgical Terms | Meaning |
|---|---|
| cheiloplasty (kī'-lō-plăs-tē) | surgical repair of the lip |
| cholecystectomy (kō-lē-sĭs-tĕk'-tō-mē) *Note:* e is used as the combining vowel between the word roots *chol* and *cyst* | excision of the gallbladder |
| colectomy (kō-lĕk'-tō-mē) | excision of the colon |
| colostomy (kō-lŏs'-tō-mē) | an artificial opening into the colon; a portion of the colon is attached to the surface of the abdomen for the passage of stools |
| esophagoenterostomy (ē-sŏf'-ah-gō-ĕn-ter-ŏs'-tō-mē) | creation of an artificial opening between the esophagus and the intestine |
| gastrectomy (găs-trĕk'-tō-mē); pyloroplasty (pī-lōr'-ō-plăs-tē); and vagotomy (vā-gŏt'-ō-mē) | a surgical procedure performed for treatment of ulcers; gastrectomy is the removal of the stomach; pyloroplasty is the plastic repair of the pyloric sphincter, located at the lower end of the stomach; vagotomy is the incision into the vagus nerve, performed to reduce the amount of gastric juices in the stomach |
| gastrostomy (găs-trŏs'-tō-mē) | an artificial opening into the stomach (for feeding purposes) |
| glossorrhaphy (glō-sōr'-ah-fē) | suturing of the tongue |
| herniorrhaphy (her-nē-ōr'-ah-fē) | surgical repair of a hernia (suturing of the containing structure, e.g., the abdominal wall) |
| ileostomy (ĭl-ē-ŏs'-tō-mē) | artificial opening into the ileum; a portion of the ileum is attached to the surface of the abdomen for passage of stools |
| laparotomy (lăp-ah-rŏt'-ō-mē) | incision into the abdominal wall |

| Diagnostic Terms | Meaning |
|---|---|
| appendicitis (ah-pĕn-dĭ-sī'-tĭs) | inflammation of the appendix |
| cholecystitis (kō-lē-sĭs-tī'-tĭs) | inflammation of the gallbladder |
| cholelithiasis (kō-lē-lĭ-thī'-ah-sĭs) *Note:* e is used as the combining vowel between the word roots *chol* and *lith* | a condition of gallstones |
| Crohn's (krōnz) disease | chronic inflammatory disease that can affect any part of the bowel, most often the lower small intestine |
| diverticulitis (dī-ver-tĭk-ū-lī'-tĭs) | inflammation of the diverticula (small pouches in the intestinal wall) |
| duodenal ulcer (dū-ō-dē'-nal) (ŭl'-sĕr) | ulcer (sore open area) in the duodenum |
| gastric ulcer (găs'-trĭk) (ŭl'-ser) | ulcer in the stomach |
| gastritis (găs-trī'-tĭs) | inflammation of the stomach |
| hepatitis (hĕp-ah-tī'-tĭs) | inflammation of the liver |
| ileitis (ĭl-ē-ī'-tĭs) | inflammation of the ileum |
| infectious hepatitis (ĭn-fĕk'-shŭs) (hĕp-ah-tī'-tĭs) | inflammation of the liver (caused by a virus) |
| pancreatitis (păn-krē-ah-tī'-tĭs) | inflammation of the pancreas |
| stomatitis (stō-mah-tī'-tĭs) | inflammation of the mouth |
| ulcerative colitis (ul'-sĕ-rā-tĭv) (kō-lī'-tĭs) | inflammation of the colon with the formation of ulcers |

| Terms Related to Diagnostic Procedures | Meaning |
|---|---|
| abdominocentesis (ăb-dŏm'-ĭ-nō-sĕn-tē'-sĭs) | aspiration of fluid from the abdominal cavity |
| barium enema (BE) (bă'-rē-ŭm) (ĕn'-ē-mah) | x-ray of the colon (fasting x-ray); barium is used as the contrast medium |
| cholangiogram (kō-lăn'-jē-ō-grăm) | x-ray of the bile ducts (fasting x-ray), usually done after a cholecystectomy; dye is the contrast medium |
| cholecystogram (kō-lē-sĭs'-tō-grăm) | x-ray of the gallbladder (fasting x-ray), also known as a GB series; dye is used as the contrast medium |
| colonoscopy (kō-lŏn-ŏs'-kō-pē) | visual examination of the colon |
| colonoscope (kō-lŏn'-ō-skōp) | the instrument used for visual examination of the colon |
| esophagoscope (ē-sŏf'-ah-gō-skōp) | the instrument used for the visual examination of the esophagus |
| esophagoscopy (ē-sŏf'-ah-gŏs'-kō-pē) | visual examination of the esophagus |
| gastroscope (găs'-trō-skōp) | the instrument used for the visual examination of the stomach |
| gastroscopy (găs-trŏs'-kō-pē) | visual examination of the stomach |

| Terms Related to Diagnostic Procedures | Meaning |
| --- | --- |
| proctoscope (prŏk'-tō-skōp) | the instrument used for the visual examination of the rectum |
| proctoscopy (prŏk-tŏs'-kō-pē) | visual examination of the rectum |
| sigmoidoscopy (sĭg-mol-dŏs'-kō-pē) | visual examination of the sigmoid colon |
| upper gastrointestinal (UGI) (găs'-trō-ĭn-tĕs'-tĭ-nal) | x-ray of the esophagus and the stomach (fasting x-ray); barium is used as the contrast medium; UGI with small-bowel follow-through is an x-ray of the stomach and small intestines |

# E X E R C I S E  4

Analyze and define the terms listed below.

1. glossoplegia _____

2. appendectomy _____

3. cholecystectomy _____

4. gastrostomy _____

5. hepatomegaly _____

6. ileostomy _____

7. pyloroplasty _____

8. protorrhea _____

9. cholecystitis _____

10. gastritis _____

11. sublingual _____

12. ileitis _____

13. cholecystogram _____

14. sigmoidoscopy _____

15. gastrectomy _____

16. gastroscopy _____

17. gastroscope _____

18. colitis _____

19. hepatitis _____

20. colostomy _____

21. herniorrhaphy _____

22. colonoscope _____

23. colonoscopy _____

# E X E R C I S E  5

Using the word elements studied in this unit and previous units, build medical terms from the definitions listed below. Also, identify which are surgical procedures by writing S in the space provided, and which are diagnostic studies by writing D in the space provided. Underline the word part that indicates that the word is a surgical procedure or a diagnostic study. (*Note:* Some words in the list will not fall into either of these categories.)

*Examples:*  gastr<u>ectomy</u>  S

gastr<u>oscopy</u>  D

1. inflammation of the mouth  _____  _____

2. inflammation of the gallbladder  _____  _____

3. a condition of gallstones  _____  _____

4. x-ray of the gallbladder  _____  _____

5. excision of the gallbladder  _____  _____

6. inflammation of the pancreas  _____  _____

7. instrument for visual examination of the rectum  _____  _____

8. visual examination of the rectum  _____  _____

9. aspiration of fluid from the abdominal cavity  _____  _____

10. artificial opening into the colon  _____  _____

11. artificial opening into the ileum  _____  _____

12. visual examination of the esophagus  _____  _____

13. instrument to examine the stomach visually  _____  _____

14. creation of an artificial opening between the esophagus and the intestines  _____  _____

15. inflammation of the stomach  _____  _____

16. suturing of the tongue  _____  _____

17. plastic repair of the lip  _____  _____

18. excision of the colon  _____  _____

19. paralysis of the tongue  _____  _____

20. pertaining to the stomach and the mouth  _____  _____

21. pertaining to under the tongue  _____  _____

22. discharge from the rectum  _____  _____

23. enlargement of the liver  _____  _____

24. tumor of the liver  _____  _____

25. pertaining to the pancreas  _____  _____

26. inflammation of the appendix  _____  _____

27. removal of the appendix  _____  _____

28. visual examination of the colon  _____  _____

29. instrument to examine the colon visually  _____  _____

# E X E R C I S E 6

Define the following medical terms:

1. dysentery _____

2. upper gastrointestinal (UGI) _____

3. barium enema _____

4. cholecystogram _____

5. jaundice _____

6. ulcerative colitis _____

7. gastric ulcer _____

8. Crohn's disease _____

# E X E R C I S E 7

Spell each medical term studied in this unit by having someone dictate the terms to you.

1. _____    25. _____

2. _____    26. _____

3. _____    27. _____

4. _____    28. _____

5. _____    29. _____

6. _____    30. _____

7. _____    31. _____

8. _____    32. _____

9. _____    33. _____

10. _____   34. _____

11. _____   35. _____

12. _____   36. _____

13. _____   37. _____

14. _____   38. _____

15. _____   39. _____

16. _____   40. _____

17. _____   41. _____

18. _____   42. _____

19. _____   43. _____

20. _____   44. _____

21. _____   45. _____

22. _____   46. _____

23. _____   47. _____

24. _____   48. _____

49. _____     51. _____

50. _____     52. _____

## E X E R C I S E  8

Answer the following questions.

1. A surgical procedure to make an artificial opening from the small intestine to the abdomen is listed on the surgery schedule. Circle the correct surgical term for this procedure and explain your choice:
   a. iliostomy
   b. ileostomy
   c. ileotomy

   _____

   _____

2. A patient enters the hospital with a diagnosis of gallstones. The admitting diagnosis in medical terms will be

   _____. The doctor orders a diagnostic study to x-ray the gallbladder to determine the

   presence of disease or gallstones. He or she orders a _____. The result of the x-ray

   indicates surgery for the removal of the gallbladder. The medical term for this operation is _____.

3. The doctor orders a medication to be administered under the patient's tongue. _____

   _____ is the word written on the doctors' order sheet to indicate this.

4. List three visual examinations the doctor may order on the digestive tract and name the instrument used for each examination.

   a. _____

   b. _____

   c. _____

5. A patient enters the hospital with an admitting diagnosis of abdominal pain. The doctor orders two x-rays, one of

   the stomach and small intestine, and one of the colon. He or she orders a _____ and a

   _____. Surgery is indicated. The doctor plans to remove the stomach, repair the pyloric

   sphincter, and make an incision into the vagus nerve. The medical terms used to describe the surgery are:

   a. _____

   b. _____

   c. _____

6. The following surgical procedures are listed on the surgical schedule, and you are making out consent forms for them. Indicate, by circling the terms, which terms are spelled incorrectly, and correctly spell the misspelled terms in the space provided.

   a. laportotomy        _____

   b. appendectomy       _____

   c. herniorraphy       _____

   d. collectomy         _____

   e. gastostomy         _____

# UNIT VIII

# The Respiratory System

## OBJECTIVES

*Upon mastery of the basic human structure for this unit, you will be able to:*

1. Describe the overall function of the respiratory system.
2. Name and locate the organs of the respiratory system and tell the function of each.
3. Compare internal respiration with external respiration.
4. Describe the pathway of air from the outside to the capillary blood in the lungs.
5. Describe pneumothorax, hemothorax, pulmonary embolism, and chronic obstructive pulmonary disease (COPD).

## THE RESPIRATORY SYSTEM

## Organs of the Respiratory System

- Nose
- Pharynx
- Larynx
- Trachea
- Bronchus
- Lungs

## Division of the Respiratory System

The upper respiratory system refers to the nose, and pharynx. The lower respiratory system refers to the larynx, trachea, bronchi, and lungs.

## Function of the Respiratory System

The function of the respiratory system is to exchange gases. Oxygen is taken into the body and carbon dioxide is removed. This process is referred to as **respiration**. The respiratory system also helps to regulate the acid-base balance and produce vocal sounds.

## Respiration

**External respiration**, or breathing, is the exchange of gases between the lungs and the external environment. Oxygen is inhaled into the lungs and passes through the capillary wall into the blood to be carried to the blood cells. Carbon dioxide passes out of the capillary blood to the lungs to be exhaled to the outside environment.

The exchange of gases also takes place within the body between the blood in the capillaries and individual body cells. This is called **internal respiration**. The body cells take on the oxygen from the blood and at the same time give off carbon dioxide to the blood to be transported back to the lungs, where it is exhaled from the body.

## The Nose

Air enters the respiratory system through the nose. The nose is divided into a right and left nostril by a partition called the **nasal septum**. The nose prepares the air for the body by (1) warming and moistening the air, (2) removing pathogenic microorganisms, and (3) removing foreign particles, such as dust, from the air. Tiny hair-like growths in the nose called cilia trap and move the foreign particles towards the outside and away from delicate lung tissue. Particles too large to be handled by the cilia produce a sneeze or cough, which forcibly expels the foreign particles.

## The Pharynx

Both air and food travel through the **pharynx** (throat). The food passes from the pharynx to the esophagus, while the air passes from the pharynx into the larynx, which is located anterior to the esophagus.

## The Larynx

The **larynx** (voice box) is a tubular structure located below the pharynx. As mentioned earlier, the pharynx is a passageway for both food and air. A flap of cartilage, called the **epiglottis**, automatically covers the larynx during the act of swallowing to prevent the food from passing from the pharynx into the larynx. The larynx contains the **vocal cords**. As the air is exhaled past the vocal cords, the vibration of the cords produces sounds.

## The Trachea

The **trachea** (windpipe) is a vertical tube extending from the larynx to the bronchi (Fig. 23–28). A series of C-shaped cartilage rings prevents the trachea from collapsing. The function of the trachea is the passage of air.

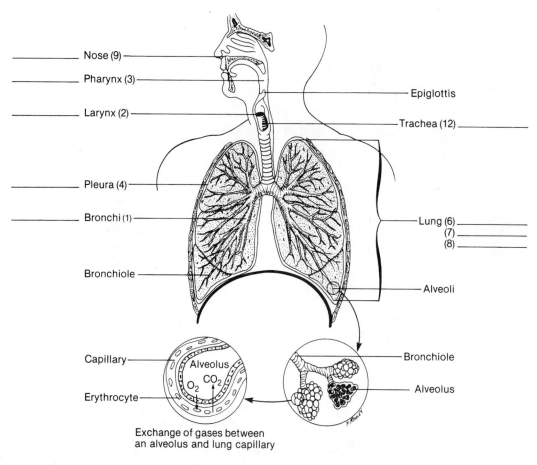

Exchange of gases between
an alveolus and lung capillary

FIGURE 23–28 • The respiratory system.

## Bronchi

Behind the heart, close to the center of the chest, the trachea branches into two tubes: one leading to the right lung and the other leading to the left lung. These tubes are called **bronchi** (singular: *bronchus*). The function of the bronchi is the passage of air.

## The Lungs

The lungs are cone-shaped organs located in the thoracic cavity. The right lung is the larger of the two and is divided into three lobes. The left lung is divided into two lobes. After the bronchus enters the lung, it divides into smaller tubes and continues to subdivide into even smaller tubes called **bronchioles**. At the end of each bronchiole is a grape-like cluster of air sacs called **alveoli** (singular: *alveolus*). The walls of the alveoli are one-celled, which allows for the exchange of gases to take place between the alveoli and the capillaries. The **pleura** is a double sac that surrounds each lung.

### HIGHLIGHT

The Pathway: Air > nose > pharynx > larynx > trachea > bronchi > bronchioles > alveoli where the exchange of $CO_2$ and $O_2$ takes place.

## CONDITIONS OF THE RESPIRATORY SYSTEM

## Pneumothorax and Hemothorax

### Pneumothorax

**Pneumothorax** is the collection of air or gas in the pleural cavity, resulting in a collapsed lung, atelectasis, (Fig. 23–29). It may be caused by a chest wound, or it may be a spontaneous collapse due to lung disease. The pleural cavity is airtight, with negative pressure. As air enters the pleural cavity it creates pressure against the lung, causing it to collapse.

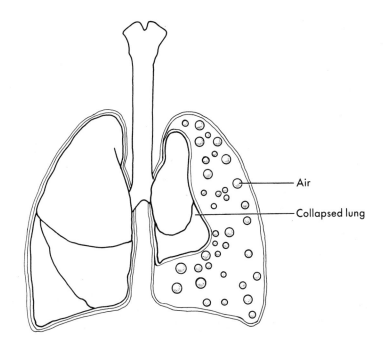

Air

Collapsed lung

F I G U R E 23–29 • Pneumothorax. (From LaFleur, M. and Starr, W.: *Exploring Medical Language*. St. Louis, The C.V. Mosby Co., 1985, with permission.)

Symptoms include sudden sharp chest pain, shortness of breath, cyanosis, and stopping of normal chest movements on the affected side.

Treatment consists of a thoracentesis to remove the air or gas from the cavity and a thoracotomy, with the insertion of chest tubes. The tubes are connected to an underwater drainage system and remain in place until air is no longer expelled from the pleural space.

### Hemothorax

A **hemothorax** is the collection of blood in the pleural cavity; it is usually caused by trauma. Treatment includes stopping the bleeding, evacuating the blood from the pleural space, and reexpanding the lung.

## Pulmonary Embolism

Pulmonary embolism is the most common complication in hospitalized patients. It strikes 6,000,000 adults a year, causing 100,000 deaths.

**Pulmonary embolism** is usually caused by a thrombus that has been dislodged from a leg vein and now blocks a pulmonary artery. Symptoms are dyspnea (difficulty in breathing), chest pain, cyanosis (blue tinge to the skin), and shock. It is difficult to distinguish from pneumonia and myocardial infarction. Chest x-ray, pulmonary angiography, and arterial blood gases are used to diagnose pulmonary embolism. Treatment includes anticoagulant and oxygen therapy.

## Chronic Obstructive Pulmonary Disease (COPD)

COPD is the persistent obstruction of bronchial air flow. This chronic condition of the respiratory system is the second leading cause of hospital admissions in this country. COPD is actually a group of respiratory diseases, of which bronchitis and emphysema are the most common.

COPD is attributed to cigarette smoking, environmental pollution, occupational hazards, and chronic infections. Symptoms include shortness of breath, chronic cough, and fatigability upon even mild exertion. Symptoms are progressive and lung damage is irreversible. There is no known cure. Treatment focuses on maintaining the remaining lung function and relieving symptoms as much as possible.

**REVIEW QUESTIONS**

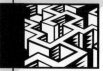

1. In external respiration the blood in the capillaries takes on _____ and gives off _____ to the lungs.

2. In internal respiration the body cells take on _____ from the blood in the capillaries and at the same time give off _____ to the blood in the capillaries.

3. List in sequence the organs through which the air from the outside travels to the blood in the capillaries of the lung.

   a. _____      e. _____

   b. _____      f. _____

   c. _____      g. _____

   d. _____

4. _____ is a passageway for both food and air. _____ is a cartilage flap that prevents food from entering the larynx.

5. List three things that happen to the inhaled air in the nose.

   a. _____

   b. _____

   c. _____

6. The vocal cords are located in the _____

7. Describe the lungs.

   _____

   _____

   _____

   _____

   _____

8. a. Blood in the pleural cavity is called _____

   b. Air in the pleural cavity is called _____

   c. A collapsed lung is known as _____

   d. A thrombus blocking a pulmonary artery is called _____

9. In _____ _____ _____ _____ symptoms are progressive and lung damage is irreversible.

10. List four things that cause COPD.

   a. _____

   b. _____

   c. _____

   d. _____

## MEDICAL TERMINOLOGY RELATING TO THE RESPIRATORY SYSTEM

### O B J E C T I V E S

*Upon mastery of the medical terminology for this unit, you will be able to:*

1. Spell and define the terms related to the respiratory tract.

2. Given the meaning of a medical condition relating to the respiratory system, build with word elements the corresponding medical term.

3. Analyze and define medical terms that are built from word elements that relate to the respiratory system.

4. State the meaning of the abbreviations used in this unit of study.

5. Given a description of a hospital situation in which the health unit coordinator may encounter medical terminology, apply the correct medical term to the situation described.

The list below contains the word elements you need to memorize for the body respiratory system. The exercises included in this unit will help you with this task. You will continue to use these word elements throughout the course and during your employment. Practice pronouncing each word element aloud.

| Combining Forms | Meaning |
| --- | --- |
| 1. bronch/o (brŏn'-kō) | bronchus (s.); bronchi (pl.) |
| 2. laryng/o (lah-rĭng'-gō) | larynx (voice box) |
| 3. pharyng/o (fah-rĭng'-gō) | pharynx (throat) |
| 4. pleur/o (ploo'-rō) | pleura |
| 5. pnea (nē'-ah) | respiration and breathing |
| 6. pneum/o (nū'-mō) | lung (also means air) |
| 7. pneumon/o (nū-mŏn'-ō) | lung |
| 8. pulmon/o (pŭl'-mŏ-nō) | lung |
| 9. rhin/o (rī'-nō) | nose |
| 10. thorac/o (thŏ'-rah-kō) | chest |
| 11. tonsill/o (tŏn'-sĭl-ō) *Note:* the word root for tonsil has a double *l*. | tonsil |
| 12. trache/o (trā'-kē-ō) | trachea (windpipe) |

### E X E R C I S E  1

Write the combining forms for the respiratory system in the spaces provided on the diagram in Figure 23–28. The number preceding the combining form in the list above matches the number of the body part on the diagram.

### E X E R C I S E  2

Write the combining forms for each term listed below.

1. lung _____  _____

   _____

2. pharynx _____

3. larynx _____

4. trachea _____

5. tonsil _____

6. bronchus _____

7. pleura _____

8. nose _____

9. breathing _____

10. chest _____

# MEDICAL TERMS RELATING TO THE RESPIRATORY SYSTEM

The following list is made up of medical terms you will need to know for the respiratory system. Exercises following this list will assist you in learning these terms. Practice the pronunciation of these terms aloud.

| General Terms | Meaning |
| --- | --- |
| adenoids (ăd'-ĕn-oyds) | tissue in the nasopharynx |
| apnea (ăp'-nē-ah) | temporary stoppage of breathing |
| bronchotracheal (brŏn'-kō-trā'-kē-al) | pertaining to the bronchi and trachea |
| dyspnea (dĭsp-nē'-ah) | difficulty in breathing |
| endotracheal (ĕn-dō-trā'-kē-al) | pertaining to within the trachea |
| pharyngocele (fah-rĭng'-gō-sēl) | an abnormal pouch in the pharynx |
| pharyngoplegia (fah-rĭng-gō-plē'-jē-ah) | paralysis of the pharynx |
| pulmonary (pŭl'-mŏ-nĕr-ē) | pertaining to the lungs |
| thoracentesis (thō-rah-sĕn-tē'-sĭs) | surgical puncture and drainage of fluid from the chest cavity for diagnostic or therapeutic purposes |
| thoracic (thō-răs'-ĭk) | pertaining to the chest |
| thoracocentesis (thō'-rah-kō-sĕn-tē'-sĭs) | the same as thoracentesis |
| tracheoesophageal (trā'-kē-ō-ĕ-sŏf-ah-jē'-al) | pertaining to the trachea and esophagus |

| Surgical Terms | Meaning |
| --- | --- |
| adenoidectomy (ăd'-ĕ-noy-dĕk'-tō-mē) | surgical removal of the adenoids |
| laryngectomy (lar-ĭn-jĕk'-tō-mē) | excision of the larynx |
| lobectomy (lō-bĕk'-tō-mē) | excision of a lobe of a lung (may also refer to the brain or liver) |
| pleuropexy (ploo'-rō-pĕk'-sē) | surgical fixation of the pleura |
| pneumonectomy (nū-mŏ-nĕk'-tō-mē) | excision of the lung (may be total or partial removal of a lung) |
| rhinoplasty (rhī-nō-plăs'-tē) | surgical repair of the nose |
| thoracotomy (thō-rah-kŏt'-ō-mē) | incision into the chest cavity |
| tonsillectomy (tŏn-sĭl-lĕk'-tō-mē) | surgical removal of the tonsils |
| tracheostomy (trā-kē-ŏs'-tō-mē) | artificial opening into the trachea (through the neck) |

| Diagnostic Terms | Meaning |
| --- | --- |
| adenoiditis (ăd'-ĕ-noy-dī-tĭs) | inflammation of the adenoids |
| asthma (ăz'-mah) | a chronic disease characterized by periodic attacks of dyspnea, wheezing, and coughing |
| bronchitis (brŏn-kī'-tĭs) | inflammation of the bronchi |
| chronic obstructive pulmonary disease (COPD) | chronic obstruction of the airway that results from emphysema, asthma, or chronic bronchitis |
| emphysema (ĕm-fĭ-sē'-mah) | a degenerative disease characterized by destructive changes in the walls of the alveoli, resulting in loss of elasticity to the lungs |
| laryngitis (lar-ĭn-jī'-tĭs) | inflammation of the larynx |
| pharyngitis (fah-rĕn-jī'-tĭs) | inflammation of the pharynx |
| pleuritis (ploo-rī'-tĭs); pleurisy (ploo'-rĕ-sē) | inflammation of the pleura |
| pneumonia (nū-mōn'-nē-ah) | an inflammation or infection of the lung |
| pneumothorax (noo-mō-thor-ăks) | air in the pleural cavity causes the lung to collapse |
| tuberculosis (too-ber'kū-lō'-sĭs) | a chronic infectious, inflammatory disease that commonly affects the lungs |
| rhinopharyngitis (rī'-nō-făr-ĭn-jī'-tĭs) | inflammation of the nose and throat |
| rhinorrhagia (rī-nō-rā'-jē-ah) | nosebleed, also called epistaxis |
| tonsillitis (tŏn-sī-lī'-tĭs) | inflammation of the tonsils |
| upper respiratory infection (URI) (rĕ-spī'-rah-tō-rē) | infection of pharynx, larynx, or bronchi |

| Terms Related to Diagnostic Procedures | Meaning |
| --- | --- |
| bronchogram (brŏn'-kō-grăm) | an x-ray of the bronchi and lung (with the use of a contrast medium) |
| bronchoscope (brŏn'-kō-skōp) | instrument used to visually examine the bronchi |

| Terms Related to Diagnostic Procedures | Meaning |
|---|---|
| bronchoscopy (brŏn-kŏs'-kō-pē) | the visual examination of the bronchi |
| laryngoscope (lăr-rĭng'-gō-skōp) | instrument for visual examination of the larynx |

*Pulmonary Function:* A diagnostic department within the hospital that is responsible for performing diagnostic tests that relate to respiratory function. Arterial blood gases (ABG) is a test that is frequently performed by this department.

*Respiratory Therapy:* A department within the hospital that is responsible for performing treatment related to respiratory functions.

## E X E R C I S E 3

Analyze and define each medical term listed below.

1. dyspnea _____

2. pharyngocele _____

3. apnea _____

4. bronchotracheal _____

5. tracheoesophageal _____

6. endotracheal _____

7. pharyngoplegia _____

8. rhinopharyngitis _____

9. rhinorrhagia _____

10. bronchoscope _____

11. bronchoscopy _____

## E X E R C I S E 4

Using the word elements studied in this unit and previous units, build medical terms from each definition listed below.

1. inflammation of the bronchi _____

2. inflammation of the larynx _____

3. artificial opening into the trachea _____

4. excision of a lung _____

5. excision of a lobe of the lung _____

6. surgical fixation of the pleura _____

7. plastic repair of the nose _____

8. incision into the chest cavity _____

9. surgical puncture and drainage of the chest cavity _____

10. inflammation of the tonsils _____

11. inflammation of the adenoids _____

# EXERCISE 5

Complete the spelling of each medical term listed below.

| Medical Term | Meaning |
|---|---|
| 1. pn___othor__ | air in the pleural cavity causing the lungs to collapse |
| 2. em___se__ | disease of the alveoli of the lung |
| 3. ___umon__ | an inflammation or infection of the lung |
| 4. pleur____y | surgical fixation of the pleura |
| 5. phar___itis | inflammation of the pharynx |

# EXERCISE 6

Write the meaning of each abbreviation listed below.

1. COPD _____

2. URI _____

# EXERCISE 7

Define each medical term listed below.

1. adenoids _____

2. lobectomy _____

3. emphysema _____

4. pneumonia _____

5. upper respiratory infection _____

6. apnea _____

7. dyspnea _____

8. pharyngocele _____

9. laryngectomy _____

10. pneumothorax _____

11. rhinorrhagia _____

12. bronchogram _____

13. laryngoscope _____

14. asthma _____

15. chronic obstructive pulmonary disease _____

16. tuberculosis _____

# E X E R C I S E 8

Spell each term studied in this unit by having someone dictate the terms to you.

1. _____
2. _____
3. _____
4. _____
5. _____
6. _____
7. _____
8. _____
9. _____
10. _____
11. _____
12. _____
13. _____
14. _____
15. _____
16. _____
17. _____
18. _____
19. _____
20. _____
21. _____

22. _____
23. _____
24. _____
25. _____
26. _____
27. _____
28. _____
29. _____
30. _____
31. _____
32. _____
33. _____
34. _____
35. _____
36. _____
37. _____
38. _____
39. _____
40. _____
41. _____
42. _____

# E X E R C I S E 9

Answer the following questions.

1. The patient was admitted to the hospital with the diagnosis of hemothorax. The doctor is planning to perform a procedure on the patient to remove fluid from the chest cavity by surgical puncture. This procedure is called a

_____.

2. A patient suddenly stops breathing. During this emergency the doctor may perform the following procedure to

assure the opening of the air passageway. The doctor uses a _____ (an instrument for

visual examination of the larynx) to insert a _____ (pertaining to within the trachea) tube. These are two items of equipment that may be used during an emergency. You may be asked to locate these items for the nursing staff or doctor. Upon assignment to a nursing unit, locate and be able to identify this equipment.

3. The patient is having difficulty breathing. The doctor performs a procedure called _____ (artificial opening into the trachea) to facilitate breathing. A tube is inserted into the trachea to prevent it from collapsing. It has the same name as the procedure. It is called a _____ tube. A tray, which has the same name as the procedure, called a _____, is used by the nursing staff to care for the patient. The health unit coordinator orders this tray from the central service department. A throat suction machine is used for the care of the patient. You may also have to order this machine from the central service department. A patient with a tracheostomy may have difficulty talking; therefore, the health unit coordinator should not use the intercom to communicate with this patient.

4. _____ is the hospital department that performs diagnostic tests that relate to respiratory function. _____ is the hospital department that performs treatments related to respiratory function.

5. The patient is scheduled for a visual examination of the bronchus, called a _____. _____ is the instrument the doctor uses to perform the examination.

6. The patient is admitted to the hospital with a _____ (a collapsed lung). The patient is having difficulty breathing; the medical term for this is _____. The doctor treats this condition by making a surgical incision into the chest wall, called a _____, for the purpose of inserting tubes. A tray, which has the same name as the procedure, a _____ tray, is obtained from the central service department for the doctor's use.

7. T & A is the abbreviation for excision of the tonsils, called _____, and excision of the adenoids, called _____. It is a common practice for the doctor to perform these two operations at the same time.

# UNIT IX

# The Urinary System and the Male Reproductive System

## OBJECTIVES

*Upon mastery of the basic human structure for this unit, you will be able to:*

1. Describe the overall functions of the urinary system and the male reproductive system.
2. Name the organs of the urinary system and tell the function of each organ.
3. Name the components of urine.
4. Name the organs of the male reproductive system and describe the function of each organ.
5. Describe the passageway of sperm from the testes to the outside of the body.
6. State the location and describe the function of the seminal vesicle glands and the prostate gland.
7. Describe pyelonephritis, renal calculi, and tumors of the prostate gland.

## THE URINARY SYSTEM

### Organs of the Urinary System

Kidneys
Ureters
Bladder
Urethra

### Function of the Urinary System

The function of the urinary system is to remove some of the waste material from the blood and excrete it from the body. The urinary system may also be referred to as the **excretory system**.

### The Kidneys

The **kidneys** are two fist-sized, bean-shaped organs located in the lumbar region of the spine, posterior to the abdominal cavity. The primary functions of the kidneys are to remove waste from the blood, and balance the fluid in the body by removing and retaining water. Nephrons, the basic unit of the kidney, begin removing waste and water as the blood flows into the kidney through the renal artery. Each kidney contains about 1,000,000 nephrons. The antidiuretic hormone (ADH) released by the posterior

pituitary gland stimulates the production of urine containing soluble waste. When there is a danger of dehydration the posterior pituitary gland will decrease the amount of ADH that is released. The nephrons will continue to remove waste but the fluid portion of urine will decrease. Voided urine is more concentrated and in smaller amounts. This process maintains the fluid balance in the body. After the urine is produced it drains into a space in the kidney called the renal pelvis. From the renal pelvis the urine is transported to the bladder by the ureter.

### Ureters

The **ureters** are tubes that provide the drainage system for urine from the renal pelvis of each kidney to the bladder (Fig. 23–30). They are small in diameter and are approximately 10 to 12 inches (25 to 30 cm) long. They extend from the renal pelvis of the kidney and enter the posterior portion of the bladder.

The ureters have muscular walls that contract to keep the urine moving towards the bladder. A backup of urine into the kidney is prevented by a flap fold of mucous membrane at the entrance of the ureters into the bladder.

### The Urinary Bladder

The **urinary bladder** is a hollow muscular bag located in the pelvic cavity. The bladder is a temporary reservoir for the urine it receives from the ureters. The need to urinate is stimulated by the distention of the bladder as it fills with urine.

### The Urethra

The **urethra** is the tube through which the urine passes from the bladder to the outside of the body. The female urethra is approximately $1\frac{1}{2}$ inches (3.75 cm) long, and the male urethra, which is also a part of the male reproductive system, is approximately 8 inches (20 cm) long.

### Urine

**Urine** is a straw-colored fluid that is approximately 95% water and 5% waste material (urea, uric acid, creatinine, and ammonia). The daily amount of urine produced by the kidneys is about 1500 mL.

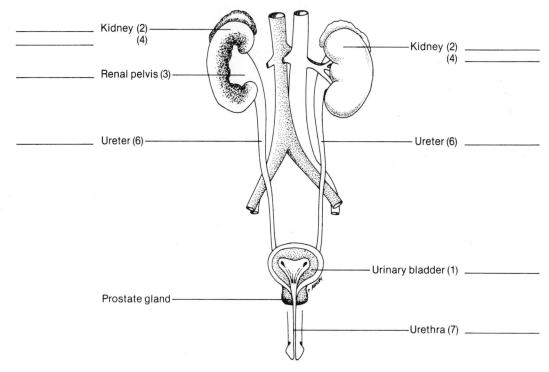

F I G U R E  23–30 • The male urinary system.

## THE MALE REPRODUCTIVE SYSTEM

### Organs of the Male Reproductive System (Fig. 23–31)

Testes
Scrotum
Vas deferens
Urethra
Seminal vesicles
Prostate
Penis

### Functions of the Male Reproductive System

The functions of the male reproductive system are to produce and eject the male reproductive cell (sperm, or spermatozoa), and to secrete the hormone testosterone.

### The Testes

The **testes** (singular: *testis*), or **testicles**, are a pair of egg-shaped organs located outside the body, suspended in a sac called the **scrotum**. They are the main sex glands of the male. The function of the testes is the production of sperm (sex cells) and testosterone (hormone). **Testosterone** is responsible for the development of the male secondary sex characteristics, such as beard and deep voice, and for the function of certain reproductive organs.

### Production of Sperm

Sperm is produced in coiled tubes, located inside the testes, called **seminiferous tubules**. The sperm passes on to a tiny 20-foot tube called the **epididymis**, located in the scrotum. The sperm is stored in the epididymis for a short time, during which it matures and becomes motile (able to move by itself). The sperm then travels through a pair of tubes about 2 feet long called the **vas deferens**. The vas deferens carries the sperm to the **urethra**. The urethra connects with both the bladder and the vas deferens and passes through the penis to the outside. It is a passageway for both semen and urine. The **seminal vesicles** are glands located near the bladder that open into the vas deferens just prior to its joining with the urethra. The seminal vesicles produce a secretion that nourishes the sperm. This secretion makes up much of the volume of **semen** (sperm plus secretions). The junction of the vas deferens and the urethra is surrounded by a gland called the prostate gland.

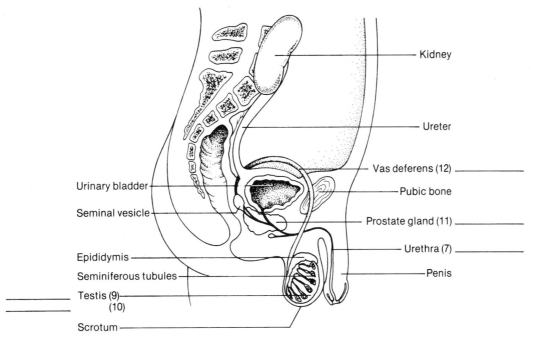

**FIGURE 23–31** • The male reproductive system.

## The Prostate Gland

The **prostate gland** secretes a fluid that aids in the motility of the sperm. The prostate gland also aids in ejaculation (the expulsion of semen from the male urethra). Each ejaculation contains an average of 200 million sperm. Erection (stiffening) of the **penis**, produced by an increased blood supply to the sponge-like tissue of the penis, allows for deposit of the sperm in the female vagina during ejaculation. A fold of skin called the prepuce, or foreskin, covers the tip of the penis; this is often removed shortly after birth by the surgical procedure of **circumcision**.

## DISEASES AND CONDITIONS OF THE URINARY SYSTEM AND THE MALE REPRODUCTIVE SYSTEM

## Pyelonephritis

**Pyelonephritis** is the infection of the renal pelvis and the kidney caused by bacterial invasion of the urinary tract. Typically the infection spreads from the bladder to the urethra to the kidneys. Three stages of the disease process are: pyelitis—inflammation of the renal pelvis; pyelonephritis—inflammation of the renal pelvis and kidney; and pyonephrosis—collection of pus in the renal pelvis. As the disease progresses, the name changes. Symptoms include dysuria (pain during urination), nocturia (excessive urination at night), hematuria (blood in the urine), and burning on urination. Urinalysis and culture and sensitivity of bacterial specimens from the urine are used to diagnose the condition. Treatment includes antibiotic therapy.

## Renal Calculi

**Renal calculi**, or kidney stones, usually form in the renal pelvis, where they may remain, or they may enter the ureter and cause obstruction. Pain, resulting from the obstruction, is usually the key symptom. Kidney, ureter, and bladder x-ray; intravenous pyelogram; and kidney ultrasonography are used in diagnosing renal calculi. Treatment is to promote normal passage of the stone. If it is too large, surgical removal of the stone may be necessary. **Lithotripsy**, the crushing of kidney stones, is replacing the need for surgery. Laser beams are used to crush the stone. If the patient is immersed in a tank of water the procedure is called **hydrolithotripsy**; if done out of water the procedure is referred to as **nephrotripsy**.

## Tumors of the Prostate Gland

Tumors of the prostate gland may be either malignant (cancer of the prostate) or benign (benign prostatic hypertrophy).

Often the growth is not diagnosed until it is large enough to obstruct urinary outflow. Treatment of choice is surgical removal of the tumor. A **radical**, or **perineal, prostatectomy** is the excision of the entire gland and its capsule through an incision in the perineum. **Suprapubic prostatectomy** is removal of the prostate gland through an incision in the abdomen and the bladder. **Retropubic prostatectomy** is the surgical removal of the prostate gland through an incision in the abdomen, but the bladder is not excised. **Transurethral prostatic resection** is the removal of a portion of the prostate gland through the urethra. There is no surgical incision.

## REVIEW QUESTIONS

1. _____ is an organ used by both the urinary system and the male reproductive system.

2. Describe the function of the urinary system.

   _____

   _____

3. The basic unit of the kidney is the _____. Its function is to _____

   _____

   _____

4. Describe the flow of urine from the renal pelvis of the kidney to the outside of the body.

   _____

   _____

5. Urine is made up of 95% _____ and 5% _____.

6. The amount of water removed from the blood is determined by the amount of _____

   that is released by the _____

7. Two functions of the testicles are:

   a. _____

   b. _____

8. Trace the travel of the sperm from the testicles to the outside of the body. Tell what glands add solution to the sperm along the passageway.

   _____

   _____

   _____

   _____

9. Match the terms in Column I with the phrases in Column II.

| Column I | Column II |
|---|---|
| a. nephrotripsy | _____ kidney stone |
| b. pyelonephritis | _____ growth that may obstruct urinary outflow |
| c. renal calculi | |
| d. hydrolithotripsy | _____ infection of the renal pelvis and kidney |
| e. benign prostatic hypertrophy | |
| f. perineal prostatectomy | _____ crushing of a kidney stone |
| g. lithotripsy | |

## MEDICAL TERMINOLOGY RELATING TO THE URINARY SYSTEM AND THE MALE REPRODUCTIVE SYSTEM

### OBJECTIVES

*Upon mastery of the medical terminology for this unit, you will be able to:*

1. Correctly spell and define the terms related to the urinary system and the male reproductive system.

2. Given the meaning of a medical condition relating to the urinary system and the male reproductive system, build with word elements the correct corresponding medical term.

3. Analyze and define medical terms built from word elements that relate to the urinary system and the male reproductive system.

4. Write the meaning of each abbreviation used in this unit of study.

5. Given a description of a hospital situation in which the health unit coordinator may encounter medical terminology, apply the correct medical terms to the situation described.

The list below contains the word elements you need to memorize for the urinary system and the male reproductive system. The exercises included in this unit will help you with this task. You will continue to use these word elements throughout the course and during employment. Practice pronouncing each word element aloud.

## Urinary System

| Word Roots/Combining Forms | Meaning |
|---|---|
| 1. cyst/o (sĭs'-tō) | bladder |
| 2. nephr/o (nĕf'-rō) | kidney |
| 3. pyel/o (pī'-ē-lō) | renal pelvis |
| 4. ren/o (rē'-nō) | kidney |
| 5. ur/o (ū'-rō) | urine |
| 6. ureter/o (ū-rē'-ter-ō) | ureter |
| 7. urethr/o (ū-rē'-thrō) | urethra |
| 8. urin/o (ū'-rĭ-nō) | urine (urinary tract, urination) |

## Male Reproductive System

| Word Roots/Combining Forms | Meaning |
|---|---|
| 9. orchi/o (or'-kē-ō) | testicle, testis |
| 10. orchid/o (or'-kĭ-dō) | testicle, testis |
| 11. prostat/o (prŏs'-tăt-ō) | prostate |
| 12. vas/o (vās'-ō) | vas deferens |

## EXERCISE 1

a. Write the combining forms for the urinary system in the spaces provided on the diagram in Figure 23–30. The number preceding the combining form in the list above matches the number of the body part on the diagram.

b. Write the combining forms for the male reproductive system in the spaces provided on the diagram in Figure 23–31. The number preceding the combining form in the list above matches the number of the body part on the diagram.

### EXERCISE 2

Write the combining forms for each term listed below.

1. urine _____ _____

2. renal pelvis _____

3. kidney _____ _____

4. ureter _____

5. bladder _____

6. testicle _____ _____

7. vas deferens _____

8. urethra _____

9. urinary tract _____

10. prostate _____

## MEDICAL TERMS RELATING TO THE URINARY SYSTEM AND THE MALE REPRODUCTIVE SYSTEM

The following list is made up of medical terms you will need to know for the urinary system and the male reproductive system. Exercises following this list will assist you in learning these terms. Practice pronouncing each term aloud.

| General Terms | Meaning |
| --- | --- |
| hematuria (hēm-ah-tū′-rē-ah) | blood in the urine |
| scrotum (scrō′-tŭm) | the skin-covered sac that contains the testes and their accessory organs |
| urethral (ū-rē′-thral) | pertaining to the urethra |
| urinary (ū′-rĭ-nĕr-ē) | pertaining to the urine |
| urinary catheterization (kăth′-ĕ-ter-ĭ-zā′-shŭn) | insertion of a sterile tube through the urethra into the bladder to remove urine |
| urination (ū-rĭ-nā′-shŭn) | passage of urine from the body, also called micturition |
| urologist (ū-rŏl′-ō-jĭst) | a doctor who specializes in urology |
| urology (ū-rŏl′-ō-jē) | the branch of medicine that deals with the diagnosis and treatment of diseases of the urinary tract and of the male reproductive organs |
| void (voyd) | to pass urine from the bladder to the outside of the body |

| Surgical Terms | Meaning |
| --- | --- |
| circumcision (sur′-kŭm-sĭzh′-ŭn) | surgical removal of the foreskin of the penis |
| nephrectomy (nĕ-frĕk′-tō-mē) | excision of the kidney |
| nephrolithotomy (nĕf′-rō-lĭ-thŏt′-ō-mē) | incision into the kidney to remove a stone |
| nephropexy (nĕf′-rō-pĕk-sē) | surgical fixation of a kidney |
| orchiectomy (ōr-kē-ĕk′-tō-mē) | excision of one or both testes |
| prostatectomy (prŏs-tah-tĕk′-tō-mē) | surgical removal of the prostate gland |
| transurethral resection (TUR) (trăns-ū-rē′-thral) (rē-sĕk′-shŭn) | removal of a portion of the prostate through the urethra |
| ureterolithotomy (ū-rē′-ter-ō-lĭ-thŏt′-ō-mē) | incision into the ureter to remove a stone |
| urethroplasty (ū-rē′-thrō-plăs′-tē) | plastic repair of the urethra |
| urethrorrhaphy (ū-rē-thrōr′-ah-fē) | suturing of a urethral tear |
| vasectomy (vah-sĕk′-tō-mē) | excision of the vas deferens or a portion of the vas deferens (produces sterility in the male) |

| Diagnostic Terms | Meaning |
| --- | --- |
| cystitis (sĭs-tī'-tĭs) | inflammation of the bladder |
| cystocele (sĭs'-tō-sēl) | herniation of the urinary bladder |
| hydrocele (hī'-drō-sēl) | a condition of swelling of the scrotum caused by the collection of fluid |
| nephritis (nĕ-frī'-tĭs) | inflammation of the kidney |
| nephrolithiasis (nĕf'-rō-lĭ-thī'-ah-sĭs) | a kidney stone |
| pyelonephritis (pī'-ĕ-lō-nĕ-frī'-tĭs) | inflammation of the kidney and renal pelvis |
| renal calculus (rē'-nal) (kăl'-cū-lŭs) | a kidney stone |
| uremia (ū-rē'-mē-ah) | urine in the blood caused by inability of the kidneys to filter out waste products from the blood |
| ureteralgia (ū-rē-ter-al'-jē-ah) | pain in the ureter |

| Terms Relating to Diagnostic Procedures | Meaning |
| --- | --- |
| blood urea nitrogen (BUN) | laboratory test performed on a blood sample to determine kidney function |
| cystogram (sĭs'-tō-grăm) | x-ray of the urinary bladder; dye is used as a contrast medium |
| cystoscopy (sĭs-tŏs'-kō-pē) | visual examination of the bladder; usually performed in the operating room so the patient may be anesthetized |
| intravenous pyelogram (IVP) (ĭn-trah-vē'-nŭs) (pī'-ĕ'-lō-grăm) | x-ray of the kidney, especially the renal pelvis and ureters; contrast medium is used |
| kidneys, ureters, and bladder (KUB) | x-ray of the kidneys, ureters, and bladder |
| urinalysis (ū-rī-năl'-ĭ-sĭs) | a laboratory test to analyze urine to assist in the diagnosis of disease |

# E X E R C I S E  3

Analyze and define each medical term listed below.

1. uremia _____

2. urologist _____

3. nephrolithotomy _____

4. prostatectomy _____

5. nephritis _____

6. urology _____

7. orchiectomy _____

8. nephrolithiasis _____

9. cystocele _____

10. cystoscopy _____

11. nephrectomy _____

12. nephropexy _____

13. pyelonephritis _____

14. ureteralgia _____

15. urethral _____

16. ureterolithotomy _____

17. cystitis _____

18. urethroplasty _____

19. urethrorrhaphy _____

E X E R C I S E **4**

Using the word elements studied so far, build medical terms from each definition listed below.

1. instrument to examine the urinary bladder visually _____

2. inflammation of the kidney _____

3. excision of the kidney _____

4. a doctor who specializes in urology _____

5. blood in the urine _____

6. urine in the blood _____

7. suturing of a urethral tear _____

8. excision of the vas deferens or a portion of it _____

9. excision of the prostate gland _____

10. pain in the ureter _____

11. herniation of the bladder _____

12. x-ray of the bladder _____

13. inflammation of the kidney and the renal pelvis _____

14. incision into the kidney to remove a stone _____

15. plastic repair of the urethra _____

16. surgical fixation of a kidney _____

17. branch of medicine that deals with the urinary system and male reproductive system _____

18. excision of the testes _____


E X E R C I S E **5**

Define each medical term listed below.

1. urinalysis _____

2. renal calculus _____

3. hydrocele _____

4. transurethral resection _____

5. circumcision _____

6. urinary _____

7. urination _____


E X E R C I S E **6**

Write the meaning of each abbreviation listed below.

1. IVP _____

2. KUB _____

3. BUN _____

4. TUR _____


# E X E R C I S E  7

Spell each medical term studied in this unit by having someone dictate the terms to you.

1. _____     19. _____

2. _____     20. _____

3. _____     21. _____

4. _____     22. _____

5. _____     23. _____

6. _____     24. _____

7. _____     25. _____

8. _____     26. _____

9. _____     27. _____

10. _____    28. _____

11. _____    29. _____

12. _____    30. _____

13. _____    31. _____

14. _____    32. _____

15. _____    33. _____

16. _____    34. _____

17. _____    35. _____

18. _____    36. _____


# E X E R C I S E  8

Answer the following questions.

1. The patient is unable to void. The doctor writes an order to pass a sterile tube through the urethra into the bladder to remove the urine. This procedure is called a(an) _____. The doctor wants a sample of this urine sent to the lab to be analyzed. He or she writes an order for a _____.

2. The patient is admitted to the hospital with a diagnosis of inflammation of the bladder, or _____ _____.

3. The doctor orders an x-ray of the kidneys, ureters, and urinary bladder. The abbreviation for this x-ray procedure is _____. He or she also ordered a blood test to determine kidney function. He or she may have ordered a _____. The abbreviation for this test is _____.

4. The doctor writes an order on the patient's chart for a consultation with a doctor who specializes in the treatment of diseases of the urinary tract and male reproductive system; this specialist is called a(an) _____

_____

5. The patient is scheduled for the operating room for a procedure to visualize the urinary bladder. The procedure is called _____. The patient may be scheduled for this procedure in the operating room because _____.

# UNIT X
# The Female Reproductive System

## OBJECTIVES

*Upon mastery of the basic human structure for this unit, you will be able to:*

1. Describe the primary functions of the female reproductive system.
2. Name the organs of the female reproductive system and describe the function of each organ.
3. Locate the perineum.
4. Name and describe the functions of two hormones produced by the ovaries.
5. Describe endometriosis, ectopic pregnancy, and pelvic inflammatory disease.

## THE FEMALE REPRODUCTIVE SYSTEM

### Organs of the Female Reproductive System (Fig. 23–32)

Uterus
Ovaries
Fallopian tubes
Vagina

The reproductive organs do not mature and begin performing the reproductive functions until about the age of 11. The maturing of the reproductive organs is called puberty.

### Functions of the Female Reproductive System

The functions of the female reproductive system are to produce the female reproductive cell (ovum), to produce hormones, and to provide for conception and pregnancy.

### The Uterus

The **uterus** is a thick, muscular, pear-shaped organ located in the pelvic cavity between the rectum and the urinary bladder. In pregnancy, the uterus functions to contain and nourish the unborn child. It also plays a role in menstruation and labor. The main body of the uterus is called the **fundus**. The lower narrow end that extends into the vagina is called the **cervix**.

### The Ovaries

The **ovaries** are a pair of small oval-shaped glands located in the pelvic cavity. They are the female sex glands and produce the female reproductive cell called the ovum (plural: *ova*). The female child is born with about 10,000 ova in the ovaries. At puberty the ovaries in response to the follicle-stimulation hormone (FSH) will release a mature ova about every 28 days. This process is called ovulation and it occurs about halfway through the menstrual period.

The ovaries also produce two hormones, estrogen and progesterone. **Estrogen** is responsible for the development of the female reproductive organs and the development of the female secondary sex characteristics, such as breasts and pubic hair.

The hormone **progesterone** plays a part in the menstrual cycle by helping to prepare the uterus for conception, and in pregnancy.

### The Fallopian Tubes

A pair of tubes, each approximately 5 inches (12.5 cm) long, called the **fallopian tubes**, provide a passageway for the ovum from the ovaries to the uterus. The fallopian tubes are not connected to the ovaries; however, after ovu-

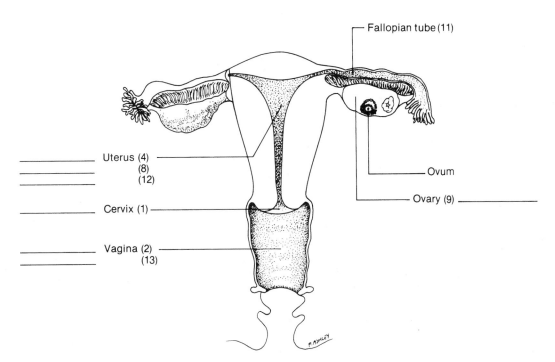

F I G U R E   23–32 • The female reproductive system.

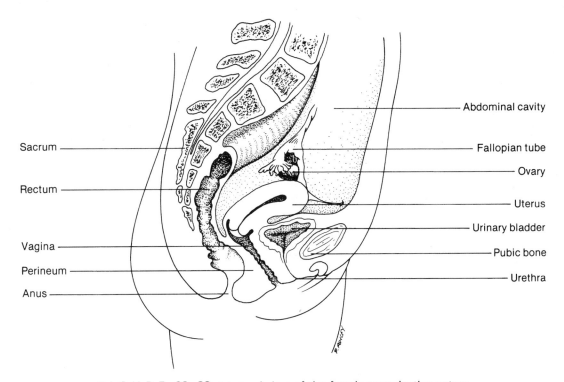

F I G U R E   23–33 • Lateral view of the female reproductive system.

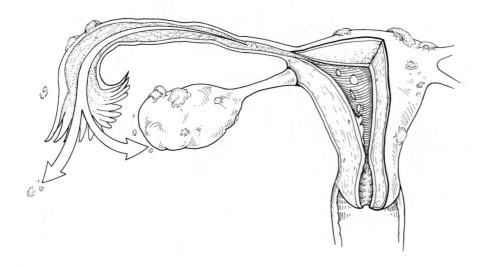

FIGURE 23–34 • Endometriosis. (From LaFleur, M. and Starr, W.: *Exploring Medical Language*. St. Louis, The C.V. Mosby Co., 1985, with permission.)

lation the ovum is swept into one of the fallopian tubes, which are connected to the uterus. Fertilization, the union of the sperm and the ovum, usually takes place in the fallopian tube. It takes approximately 5 days for the ovum to pass through the fallopian tube to the uterus.

## The Vagina

The **vagina** is a muscular tube about 3 in. long that connects the uterus to the outside of the body (Fig. 23–33). The outside opening of the vagina is between the rectum

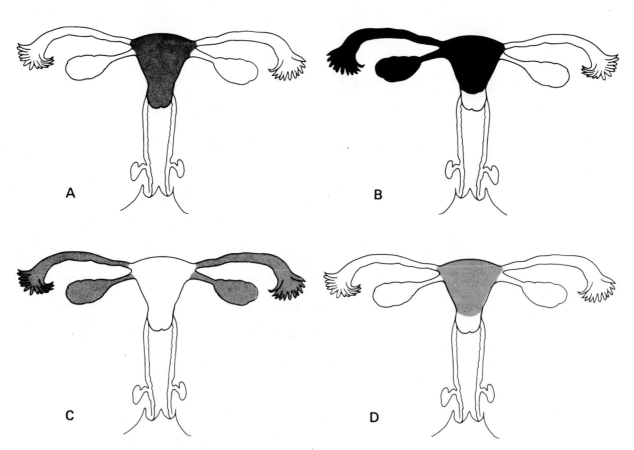

FIGURE 23–35 • (*A*) Total hysterectomy. (*B*) Hysterosalpingo-oophorectomy. (*C*) Bilateral salpingo-oophorectomy. (*D*) Subtotal hysterectomy.

(posterior) and the urethra (anterior) of the pelvic floor. The vagina receives the penis during sexual intercourse and is part of the birth canal through which the newborn baby passes from the uterus to the outside of the body.

## The Perineum

The pelvic floor of both the male and female is called the **perineum**. However, this term is most frequently used to describe the area between the vaginal opening and the anus of the female.

## DISEASES AND CONDITIONS OF THE FEMALE REPRODUCTIVE SYSTEM

### Endometriosis

**Endometriosis** is a condition in which endometrial tissue (lining of the uterus) is found outside of the uterus, especially in the pelvic area, but it can appear anywhere in the body (Fig. 23–34). The misplaced endometrial tissue undergoes changes, including bleeding, during menstruation. Symptoms include dysmenorrhea (painful menstruation), causing constant pain in the vagina and lower abdomen. The cause is unknown.

Treatment varies according to the severity of the disease and according to the age and childbearing desires of the patient. Hormonal treatment may be recommended for milder forms of endometriosis. Conservative surgery may be the removal of cysts or lysis (freeing) of adhesions. For severe cases and for those women not wanting to bear children, a total hysterectomy and bilateral salpingo-oophorectomy is recommended (Fig. 23–35).

### Pelvic Inflammatory Disease

**Pelvic inflammatory disease (PID)** is any infection of the female pelvic organs; it is mostly caused by bacterial infection. Early diagnosis and treatment prevent damage to the reproductive organs. If untreated, PID can lead to infertility and to other severe medical complications. Treatment includes antibiotic therapy.

### Ectopic Pregnancy

In an **ectopic pregnancy** the fertilized ovum is implanted outside of the uterus; over 90% implant in the fallopian tubes. Often the fetus grows large enough to rupture the tube, creating a life-threatening situation. Symptoms of a ruptured fallopian tube include severe abdominal pain on one side and vaginal bleeding. Treatment is surgical removal of the fallopian tube and the fetus.

## REVIEW QUESTIONS

1. _____ and _____ are the names of two hormones produced by the ovaries. _____ is the hormone responsible for the secondary sex characteristics and aids in the development of the female reproductive organs.

2. Fertilization usually takes place in the _____.

3. The _____ is the lower portion of the uterus, which extends into the vagina.

4. Describe the primary functions of the female reproductive system.

   _____

   _____

5. List the organs of the female reproductive system and write a line or two about the function of each organ.

   a. _____

   b. _____

   c. _____

   d. _____

6. An ova begins maturing in response to the _____

   _____   _____.

7. An infection of the female pelvic organs that, if left untreated, can lead to infertility is called

   _____

8. A pregnancy occurring outside the uterus is called a(n) _____.

9. A condition in which endometrial tissue is found outside the uterus is called _____.

## MEDICAL TERMINOLOGY RELATING TO THE FEMALE REPRODUCTIVE SYSTEM

### OBJECTIVES

*Upon mastery of the medical terminology for this unit, you will be able to:*

1. Spell and define the terms related to the female reproductive system.

2. Given the meaning of a medical condition relating to the female reproductive system, build with word elements the correct corresponding medical terms.

3. Analyze and define medical terms that are built from word elements related to the female reproductive system.

4. Define terms related to pregnancy, childbirth, and the newborn.

5. Given a description of a hospital situation in which the health unit coordinator may encounter medical terminology, apply the correct medical term to the situation described.

The list below contains the word elements you need to memorize for the female reproductive system. The exercises included in this unit will help you with this task. You will continue to use these word elements throughout the course and during employment. Practice pronouncing each word element aloud.

| Word Roots/Combining Forms | Meaning |
|---|---|
| 1. cervic/o (ser'-vĭ-ko) | cervix (the neck-like portion of the uterus) |
| 2. colp/o (kŏl'-pō) | vagina |
| 3. gynec/o (gĭ'-nĕ-kō, jĭn'-ĕ-kō) | woman |
| 4. hyster/o (hĭs'-ter-ō) | uterus (womb) |
| 5. mamm/o (măm'-mō) | breast |
| 6. mast/o (măs'-tō) | breast |
| 7. men/o (mĕn'-ō) | menstruation |
| 8. metr/o (mĕ'-trō) | uterus (womb) |
| 9. oophor/o (ō-ŏf'-ō-rō) | ovary |
| 10. perine/o (pĕr-ĭ-nē'-ō) | perineum (the pelvic floor); in the female, the area between the vaginal opening and the anus, and in the male, the region between the scrotum and the anus |
| 11. salping/o (săl-pĭng'-gō) | fallopian or uterine tube |
| 12. uter/o (ū'-tĕr-ō) | uterus (womb) |
| 13. vagin/o (văj'-ĭ-nō) | vagina |

### EXERCISE 1

Write the combining forms for the female reproductive system in the spaces provided on the diagram in Figure 23–32. The number preceding the combining forms in the list above matches the number of the body part on the diagram.

E X E R C I S E **2**

Write the combining form for each of the following.

1. menstruation                                              _____

2. woman                                                     _____

3. vagina                                                    _____          _____

4. perineum                                                  _____

5. fallopian or uterine tube                                 _____

6. ovary                                                     _____

7. uterus                         _____        _____          _____

8. cervix                                                    _____

9. breast                                                    _____          _____

## MEDICAL TERMS RELATING TO THE FEMALE REPRODUCTIVE SYSTEM

The list below contains the medical terms you need to memorize for the female reproductive system. The exercises included in this unit will help you with this task. You will continue to use these medical terms throughout the course and during your employment. Practice pronouncing each term aloud.

| General Terms | Meaning |
| --- | --- |
| gynecologist (gī-nĕ-kŏl′-ō-jĭst, jĭn-ĕ-kŏl′-ō-jĭst) | a doctor who specializes in gynecology |
| gynecology (gī-nĕ-kŏl′-ō-jē, jĭn-ĕ-kŏl′-ō-jē) | the branch of medicine dealing with diseases and disorders of the female reproductive system |
| menopause (mĕn′-ō-pawz) | the period during which the menstrual cycle slows down and eventually stops |
| menstrual (mĕn′-stroo-ăl) | pertaining to menstruation |
| menstruation (mĕn-stroo-ā′-shŭn) | discharge of blood and tissue from the uterus, normally occurring every 28 days |
| ovum (ō′-vŭm) (sing.); ova (ō′-vă) (pl.) | female reproductive cell; may be referred to as the female reproductive egg |
| ureterovaginal (ū-rē′-ter-ō-văj′-ĭ-nal) | pertaining to the ureter and vagina |
| uterine (ū′-ter-ĭn) | pertaining to the uterus |
| vaginal (văj′-ĭ-nal) | pertaining to the vagina |
| vaginoperineal (văj-ĭ-nō-pĕr-ĭ-nē′-al) | pertaining to the vagina and perineum |

| Surgical Terms | Meaning |
| --- | --- |
| cervicectomy (sĕr-vĭ-sĕk′-tō-mē) | excision of the cervix |
| colporrhaphy (kŏl-por′-ah-fē) | suturing of the vagina |
| dilatation and curettage (dĭl-ah-tā′-shŭn) (kū-rĕ-tăhzh′) | surgical procedure to scrape the inner walls of the uterus |
| hysterectomy (hĭs-tĕ-rĕk′-tō-mē) | surgical removal of the uterus |
| hysterosalpingo-oophorectomy (hĭs′-ter-ō-săl-pĭng′-gō-ō-ŏf-ō-rĕk′-tō-mē) | excision of the uterus, ovaries, and fallopian tubes |
| mammoplasty (măm′-ō-plăs-tē) | plastic repair of the breast(s) to enlarge or reduce in size or to reconstruct after surgical removal of a tumor |
| mastectomy (măs-tĕk′-tō-mē) | surgical removal of a breast |
| oophorectomy (ō-ŏf-ō-rĕk′-tō-mē) | excision of an ovary; if both ovaries are removed, it is referred to as a bilateral oophorectomy |

| Surgical Terms | Meaning |
|---|---|
| perineoplasty (pĕr-ĭ-nē′-ō-plăs-tē) | plastic repair of the perineum |
| perineorrhaphy (pĕr′-ĭ-nē-ōr′-ah-fē) | suturing of the perineum |
| salpingo-oophorectomy (săl-pĭng′-gō-ō-ŏf-o-rĕk′-tō-mē) | excision of a fallopian tube and an ovary |
| salpingopexy (săl-pĭng′-gō-pĕk-sē) | surgical fixation of a fallopian tube |

| Diagnostic Terms | Meaning |
|---|---|
| amenorrhea (ā-mĕn-ō-rē′-ah) | without menstrual discharge |
| cervicitis (ser-vĭ-sī′-tĭs) | inflammation of the cervix |
| dysmenorrhea (dĭs-mĕn-ō-rē′-ah) | painful menstruation |
| menometrorrhagia (mĕn-ō-mĕt-rō-rā′-jē-ah) | excessive uterine bleeding during and in between menstrual periods |
| metrorrhagia (mĕ-trō-rā′-jē-ah) | uterine bleeding at irregular intervals |
| metrorrhea (mĕ-trō-rē′-ah) | abnormal uterine discharge |
| oophoritis (ō-ŏf-ō-rī′-tĭs) | inflammation of an ovary |
| salpingitis (săl-pĭn-jī′-tĭs) | inflammation of a fallopian tube |
| salpingocele (săl-pĭng′-gō-sēl) | pouching out or herniation of the fallopian tube |

| Terms Relating to Diagnostic Procedures | Meaning |
|---|---|
| cervical Pap smear | a laboratory test used to detect cancerous cells; commonly performed to detect cancer of the cervix and uterus |
| colposcope (kŏl′-pō-skōp) | an instrument used for visual examination of the vagina and cervix |
| colposcopy (kŏl-pŏs′-kō-pē) | visual examination of the vagina and cervix |
| hysterosalpingogram (hĭs′-ter-ō-săl-pĭng′-gō-grăm) | x-ray of the uterus and fallopian tubes |
| mammogram (măm′-ō-grăm) | x-ray of the breast |
| vaginal speculum (spĕk′-ū-lŭm) | an instrument used for expanding the vagina to allow for visual examination of the vagina and cervix |

# E X E R C I S E  3

Analyze and define the following medical terms:

1. gynecology _____

2. colporrhaphy _____

3. oophorectomy _____

4. oophoritis _____

5. salpingo-oophorectomy _____

6. salpingopexy _____

7. hysterectomy _____

8. dysmenorrhea _____

9. colposcope _____

10. mammoplasty _____

11. amenorrhea _____

12. mammogram _____

13. hysterosalpingogram _____

14. colposcopy _____

# E X E R C I S E  4

Using the word elements you have studied, build medical terms from each definition listed below.

1. excision of the ovary _____

2. the branch of medicine dealing with diseases of the reproductive organs of women _____

_____

3. surgical fixation of a fallopian tube _____

4. inflammation of an ovary _____

5. an instrument used to examine the vagina visually _____

6. abnormal uterine discharge _____

7. excision of the cervix _____

8. excision of the uterus, ovaries, and fallopian tubes _____

9. herniation of a fallopian tube _____

10. pertaining to the ureter and vagina _____

11. inflammation of the cervix _____

12. excision of the uterus _____

13. suture of the vagina _____

14. plastic repair of the perineum _____

15. pertaining to the vagina _____

16. surgical removal of a breast _____

17. excision of a fallopian tube and ovary _____

18. painful menstruation _____

19. x-ray of the uterus and fallopian tubes _____

20. without menstrual discharge _____

21. x-ray of the breast _____

22. plastic repair of the breast _____

23. visual examination of the vagina and cervix _____


# E X E R C I S E  5

1. gynecologist _____

2. uterine _____

3. vaginal speculum _____

4. menometrorrhagia _____

5. dilatation and curettage _____

6. ovum _____

## E X E R C I S E  6

A surgery schedule lists all the operations to be performed in the hospital on a given day. Information on a surgery schedule includes the patient's name, the operation, and the surgeon. In the sample below, identify the terms spelled incorrectly in both the patient's name and operations listed.

Spell the term correctly in the space provided.

| Patient Name | Surgery | Doctor |
|---|---|---|
| Mrs. Utteris _____ | dilation and curettage _____ | Dr. Scrape |
| Mrs. Overy _____ | histero-solpingo-oopherectomy _____ | Dr. Removal |
| Mrs. Peronium _____ | periniplasty _____ | Dr. Repair |
| Mrs. Vagina _____ | colporhaphy _____ | Dr. Suture |
| Mrs. Tube _____ | salpangpexy _____ | Dr. Fixation |

## E X E R C I S E  7

Spell each medical term studied in this unit by having someone dictate the terms to you.

1. _____
2. _____
3. _____
4. _____
5. _____
6. _____
7. _____
8. _____
9. _____
10. _____
11. _____
12. _____
13. _____
14. _____
15. _____
16. _____
17. _____
18. _____
19. _____

20. _____
21. _____
22. _____
23. _____
24. _____
25. _____
26. _____
27. _____
28. _____
29. _____
30. _____
31. _____
32. _____
33. _____
34. _____
35. _____
36. _____
37. _____

## TERMS RELATING TO OBSTETRICS

Below is a list of common terms used in the field of obstetrics and their definitions.

| Obstetric Terms | Meaning |
| --- | --- |
| abortion (ah-bor'-shŭn) | termination of pregnancy before the fetus is capable of survival out of the uterus |
| amniotic fluid (ăm-nē-ŏt'-ĭk) | fluid that surrounds the fetus |
| cesarean section (sē-sǎ'-rē-ăn) | incision into the uterus through the abdominal wall to deliver the fetus |
| congenital (kŏn-jĕn'-ĭ-tal) | a condition that exists at birth |
| ectopic pregnancy (ĕk-tŏp'-ĭk) | the fertilized ovum is implanted outside of the uterus |
| fetus (fē'-tŭs) | the unborn child in the uterus from the third month of development to birth |
| natal (nā'-tal) | pertaining to birth |
| neonatal (nē'-ō-nā'-tal) | pertaining to the first 4 weeks after birth |
| obstetrician (ŏb-stĕ-trĭsh'-ăn) | a doctor who practices obstetrics |
| obstetrics (ŏb-stĕt'-rĭks) | the branch of medicine that deals with pregnancy and childbirth |
| placenta (plah-sén'-tah) (afterbirth) | a spongy structure developed during pregnancy through which the unborn child is nourished |
| postnatal (pōst-nā'-tal) | occurring after birth |
| prenatal (prē-nā'-tal) | occurring before birth |

## E X E R C I S E  8

Match the word in Column I with its meaning in Column II.

**Column I**

_____ congenital

_____ abortion

_____ fetus

_____ postnatal

_____ natal

_____ prenatal

_____ obstetrics

_____ ectopic pregnancy

**Column II**

a. occurring before birth
b. present at birth
c. early termination of pregnancy
d. unborn child
e. a branch of medicine
f. pregnancy outside the uterus
g. occurring after birth
h. birth

## E X E R C I S E  9

Define each term listed below.

1. obstetrician _____

2. placenta _____

3. amniotic fluid _____

4. cesarean section _____

## EXERCISE 10

Answer the following questions.

1. In a large hospital there is usually a nursing unit for patients who are hospitalized for surgery of the female reproductive tract. This unit is called _____. A separate nursing unit is used for delivery and care of the newborn and for care of the mothers. This unit is called _____.

2. The doctor plans to perform a pelvic examination of a female patient. The _____ is the instrument she or he uses to expand the vagina. During the pelvic examination the doctor plans to remove some cells from the cervix to be studied for the presence of cancer. The cells are sent to the laboratory for a _____ test.

---

## UNIT XI

# The Endocrine System

### OBJECTIVES

*Upon mastery of the basic human structure for this unit, you will be able to:*
1. Describe the overall function of the endocrine system.
2. Name the glands of the endocrine system and describe the hormones produced by each gland and the function of each of the hormones.
3. Compare endocrine glands with exocrine glands.
4. Describe diabetes mellitus and Graves' disease.

## THE ENDOCRINE SYSTEM

### Organs of the Endocrine System (Fig. 23–36)

Pituitary
Thyroid gland
Parathyroid gland
Adrenal glands
Islets of Langerhans

### Functions of the Endocrine System

The functions of the endocrine system are much the same as those of the nervous system—communication and control; however, endocrine functions are carried out in a much different manner. The organs of the endocrine system are the endocrine glands, which produce controlling substances called **hormones**. Endocrine, or ductless, glands do not have tubes to carry their secretions to other parts of the body: endocrine secretions go directly into the bloodstream, which carries them to other parts of the body. In contrast to the endocrine glands, the exocrine glands of the body have tubes to carry their secretions from the producing gland to other parts or organs of the body. For example, the saliva produced by the parotid gland (an exocrine gland) flows from the parotid gland through a tube into the mouth.

### The Pituitary Gland

The **pituitary gland** is often referred to as the "master gland" because the hormones it produces stimulate the functions of other endocrine glands. It is a pea-sized gland located in the cranial cavity at the base of the brain. The pituitary gland is divided into two lobes: the anterior and the posterior lobe.

The **anterior lobe** produces the following five hormones:

■ **Adrenocorticotropic hormone (ACTH)**, which stimulates the action of part of the adrenal gland.
■ **Thyroid stimulating hormone (TSH)**, which stimulates the action of the thyroid gland.
■ **Growth hormone (GH)**, which regulates body growth.
■ **Prolactin (PRL)**, which stimulates and sustains milk production following the birth of a child. Prolactin has no known effect in males.

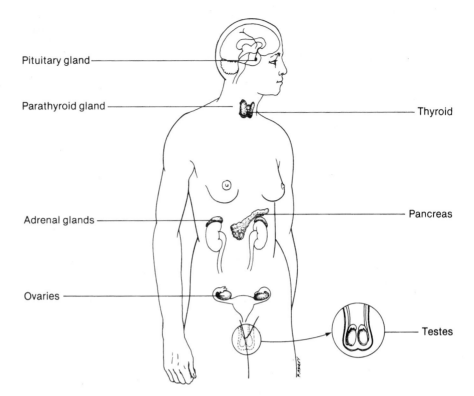

Pituitary gland

Parathyroid gland

Thyroid

Adrenal glands

Pancreas

Ovaries

Testes

F I G U R E  23–36 • The endocrine glands. (From LaFleur, M. and Starr, W.: *Exploring Medical Language*. St. Louis, The C.V. Mosby Co., 1985, with permission.)

■ **Follicle stimulating hormone (FSH)**, which stimulates the production of the male sex cell (spermatogensis).

The pituitary gland also produces hormones that stimulate the growth and hormone production of the ovaries and testes.

The **posterior lobe** produces two hormones:

■ **Antidiuretic hormone (ADH)**, which stimulates reabsorption of water by the kidney.
■ **Oxytocin**, which stimulates contractions of the uterus during childbirth.

## The Thyroid Gland

The **thyroid gland** is located in the neck. It produces the hormone **thyroxine**, which maintains metabolism of the body cells. Iodine is necessary in the body for the production of thyroxin by the thyroid gland.

## The Parathyroid Glands

The **parathyroid glands** are four small bodies located posterior to the thyroid gland. They produce the hormone parathyroid hormone, which regulates the amount of calcium in the blood.

## The Islets of Langerhans

The **islets of Langerhans** are microscopic bunches of cells scattered throughout the pancreas (refer to Unit VII). They produce the hormone **insulin**, which is necessary for the metabolism of carbohydrates in the body.

## The Adrenal Glands

The **adrenal glands**, situated on top of each kidney, are divided into two parts: the adrenal cortex (outer part) and the adrenal medulla (inner part).

The **adrenal cortex** produces three steroid hormones: **mineralocorticoids**, **glucocorticoids**, and **androgens**.

Cortisol and cortisone are two glucocorticoids that influence protein, sugar, and fat metabolism. Cortisone, because of its antiinflammatory effect, is used therapeutically for treatment of various ailments. Extra cortisol is produced by the body during stressful periods to assist the body in responding to stress.

Mineralocorticoids regulate electrolyte balance, which is essential to normal body function and to life itself.

Androgens are hormones that are responsible for the masculinizing effect in males. Testosterone produced by the testes has the same masculinizing effect and is discussed further in Unit IX, "The Urinary System and the Male Reproductive System."

The **adrenal medulla** produces two hormones that help the body to respond to emergency or stressful situations by increasing the function of vital organs (heartbeat and respiration), raising blood pressure, and providing extra nourishment for the voluntary muscles so they can perform an extra amount of work. The names of these two hormones are **epinephrine** (or adrenaline) and **norepinephrine**.

## Sex Glands

The ovaries of the female and the testes of the male are endocrine glands. Ovaries are described in Unit X, "The Female Reproductive System," and the testes are discussed in Unit IX, "The Urinary System and the Male Reproductive System."

# DISEASES OF THE ENDOCRINE SYSTEM

## Diabetes Mellitus

**Diabetes mellitus** results in the inability of the body to store and use carbohydrates in the usual manner. Contributing factors are the inability of the islets of Langerhans to produce enough insulin, increase in the rate that the body uses the insulin, increase in the rate of insulin storage in the body, or drop in the efficiency of the use of insulin.

Symptoms of diabetes mellitus are polyuria, an increase in urine output; polyphagia, an increase in appetite; polydipsia, an increase in thirst; glycosuria, an elevation of sugar in the urine; and hyperglycemia, an elevation of sugar in the blood.

Diagnostic studies include urinalysis, fasting blood sugar, and glucose tolerance test.

Treatment depends on the severity of the disease. Mild diabetes can be controlled by a diet that usually contains limited amounts of sugar and carbohydrates. Moderate to severe diabetes may require insulin therapy.

Too much glucose in the blood may cause a condition called diabetic coma, whereas too much insulin in the blood may cause a condition called insulin shock.

## Graves' Disease

**Graves' disease**, a form of hyperthyroidism, causes overproduction of thyroxine, an increase in the size of the thyroid gland (goiter), and many changes in the other systems. Accompanying symptoms include intolerance to heat, nervousness, loss of weight, and goiter. The cause of Graves' disease is unknown, but it is five times more common in women than in men. It usually occurs between the ages of 20 and 40 years. $T_3$ and $T_4$ uptake tests and a thyroid scan may be used to diagnose Graves' disease.

Treatment includes prescribing antithyroid drugs and performing a subtotal thyroidectomy.

---

**REVIEW QUESTIONS**

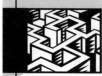

1. _____ is necessary in the body for the production of thyroxine.

2. Indicate the hormones produced by each endrocine gland by writing the number of the hormone listed in **Column II** by the name of the endocrine gland listed in **Column I**. You may want to write more than one number in each space.

   **Column I**

   a. _____ anterior pituitary gland

   b. _____ adrenal cortex gland

   c. _____ thyroid gland

   d. _____ posterior pituitary gland

   e. _____ parathyroid gland

   f. _____ islets of Langerhans

   g. _____ adrenal medulla gland

   **Column II**

   1. parathyroid hormone
   2. GH
   3. TSH
   4. FSH
   5. oxytocin
   6. ACTH
   7. cortisone
   8. epinephrine
   9. insulin
   10. PRL
   11. thyroxine
   12. ADH

3. Explain why the pituitary gland is sometimes referred to as the "master gland."

   _____

   _____

4. What is the overall function of the endocrine system? _____

_____

5. Insulin is secreted by the _____, located throughout the _____.

6. What is the function of insulin in the body? _____

_____

7. Describe the symptoms of diabetes mellitus.

   a. _____

   b. _____

   c. _____

   d. _____

   e. _____

8. Graves' disease is a form of _____.

## MEDICAL TERMINOLOGY RELATING TO THE ENDOCRINE SYSTEM

### OBJECTIVES

*Upon mastery of the medical terminology for this unit, you will be able to:*

1. Spell and define the terms related to the endocrine system.
2. Given the meaning of a medical condition relating to the endocrine system, build with word elements the correct corresponding medical terms.
3. Given a description of a hospital situation in which the health unit coordinator may encounter medical terminology, apply the correct medical terms to the situation described.

The list below contains the word elements you need to memorize for the endocrine system. The exercises included in this unit will help you with this task. You will continue to use these word elements throughout the course and during employment. Practice pronouncing each word element aloud.

| Word Roots/Combining Forms | Meaning |
| --- | --- |
| aden/o (ăd′-ĕ-nō) | gland |
| adren/o (ah-drē′-nō) | adrenal |
| adrenal/o (ah-drē′-nal-ō) | adrenal |
| parathyroid/o (păr-ah-thī′-roy-dō) | parathyroid |
| thyr/o (thī′-rō) | thyroid |
| thyroid/o (thī′-roy-dō) | thyroid |

### EXERCISE 1

Write the combining forms for each medical term listed below.

1. gland _____    3. adrenal _____

2. thyroid _____    _____

   _____    4. parathyroid _____

## MEDICAL TERMS RELATING TO THE ENDOCRINE SYSTEM

The following list is made up of medical terms you will need to know for the endocrine system. Exercises following this list will assist you in learning these terms. Practice pronouncing each term aloud.

| General Terms | Meaning |
|---|---|
| adenitis (ăd-ĕ-nī′-tĭs) | inflammation of a gland |
| adenoid (ăd′-ĕ-noyd) | resembling a gland (adenoids: glandular tissue located in the nasopharynx of children) |
| adenoma (ăd-ĕ-nō′-mah) | a tumor of glandular tissue |
| adenosis (ăd-ĕ-nō′-sĭs) | disease of a gland |
| adrenal (ah-drē′-nal) | near the kidney |
| adrenalitis (ah-drē-năl-ī′-tĭs) | inflammation of the adrenal gland |
| gland | an organ that produces a certain substance |
| secretion (sē-krē′-shŭn) | a substance produced by a gland |

| Surgical Terms | Meaning |
|---|---|
| parathyroidectomy (păr′-ah-thī-roy-dĕk′-tō-mē) | excision of the parathyroid gland |
| thyroidectomy (thī-roy-dĕk′-tō-mē) | surgical removal of the thyroid gland |

| Diagnostic Terms | Meaning |
|---|---|
| Addison's disease (ăd′-i-sŭnz) | a disease caused by lack of production of hormones by the adrenal gland |
| Cushing's disease (koosh′-ĭngz) | a disorder caused by overproduction of certain hormones by the adrenal cortex |
| diabetes insipidus (dī-ah-bē′-tĭs) (ĭn-sĭp′-ĭ-dĭs) | a disease caused by inadequate antidiuretic hormone production by the posterior lobe of the pituitary gland |
| diabetes mellitus (dī-ah-bē′-tĭs) (mĭl-ī′-tĭs) | a disease that results in the inability of the body to store and use carbohydrates in the usual manner. It may be caused by inadequate production of insulin by the islets of Langerhans |
| hyperthyroidism (hī-per-thī′-roy-dĭzm) | excessive production of thyroxin and often an enlarged thyroid gland (goiter); also called Graves' disease or exophthalmic goiter |
| hypothyroidism (hī-pŏ-thī′-roy-dĭzm) | a condition of underproduction of thyroxin by the thyroid gland |

| Terms Relating to Diagnostic Procedures | Meaning |
|---|---|
| blood glucose monitoring | a method of monitoring the patient's glucose level by using a finger stick to obtain blood; performed by nursing staff |
| fasting blood sugar (FBS) | a laboratory test to determine the amount of glucose in the blood; may be used to diagnose and/or monitor diabetes mellitus |
| glucose tolerance test (GTT) | a laboratory test to determine abnormalities in glucose metabolism; may be used to assist the diagnosis of diabetes mellitus |
| protein-bound iodine | a laboratory test performed on a sample of blood to determine thyroid activity |
| $T_3$, $T_4$, and $T_7$ uptake | studies performed on a blood sample that use nuclear substances to determine the function of the thyroid gland |
| thyroid scan | a diagnostic study for thyroid gland function |

# E X E R C I S E  2

Using the word elements studied in this unit and previous units, build medical terms from each definition listed below.

1. inflammation of a gland _____

2. surgical removal of the thyroid gland _____

3. surgical removal of the parathyroid gland _____

4. resembling a gland _____

5. tumor of glandular tissue _____

6. disease of a gland _____

7. inflammation of the adrenal gland _____

## E X E R C I S E 3

The following are conditions caused by over- or undersecretion of endocrine glands. In the space provided write the name of the gland involved with the condition.

1. diabetes mellitus _____

2. hyperthyroidism _____

3. Addison's disease _____

4. hypothyroidism _____

5. Cushing's disease _____

6. diabetes insipidus _____

## E X E R C I S E 4

Complete the following words:

1. dia_t_ _ins_p_d_ _

2. Ad_ _ _on's dis_ _se

3. Cu_ _ing's dis_ _se

4. h_poth_ _oid_ _m

5. sec_ _ti_ns

## E X E R C I S E 5

Spell each term studied in this unit by having someone dictate the terms to you.

1. _____

2. _____

3. _____

4. _____

5. _____

6. _____

7. _____

8. _____

9. _____

10. _____

11. _____

12. _____

13. _____

14. _____

15. _____

16. _____

17. _____

18. _____

19. _____

20. _____

21. _____

22. _____

## E X E R C I S E 6

Answer the following questions.

1. The patient is admitted to the hospital with a possible diagnosis of _____, caused by an inadequate amount of insulin in the body. Insulin is produced by the _____. The doctor may order two laboratory tests, _____ and _____, to assist in diagnosing the patient's condition. He or she also orders _____ to be performed by the nursing staff to determine the patient's glucose level.

2. If the patient is suffering from the lack of a certain hormone in the body, the doctor may order a hormonal medication to be given to the patient to make up for the deficiency. The following is a list of hormonal medications. Indicate which endocrine gland should secrete each hormone.

    a. ACTH _____

    b. cortisone _____

    c. insulin _____

    d. epinephrine _____

    e. Premarin (estrogen) _____

    f. testosterone _____

    g. thyroid preparation _____

3. The patient is admitted to the hospital with a diagnosis of a thyroid condition. List three tests the doctor may order to gather information about the patient's thyroid function.

    a. _____

    b. _____

    c. _____

## References

Hole, John W., Jr.: *Essentials of Human Anatomy Physiology*, 4th ed. Dubuque, IA, Wm. C. Brown Publishers, 1992.

Guyton, Arthur C., and Hall, John E.: *Textbook of Medical Physiology*, 9th ed. Philadelphia, W.B. Saunders Co., 1996.

Kittredge, Mary: *The Human Body: An Overview*. Philadelphia, Chelsea House Publishers, 1990.

Lewis, Sharon Mantik and Collier, Idolia Cox: *Medical Surgical Nursing*, 3rd ed. Philadelphia, Mosby, 1992.

Mader, Sylvia S.: *Inquiry Into Life*. Dubuque, IA, Wm. C. Brown Publishers, 1995.

Suddarth, Doris Smith: *The Lippincott Manual of Nursing Practice*, 5th ed. Philadelphia, J.B. Lippincott Co., 1991.

O'Toole Marie (ed): *Miller-Keane Encyclopedia & Dictionary of Medicine Nursing & Allied Health*, 6th ed. Philadelphia, W.B. Saunders Co., 1997.

Tortora, Gerard J., and Grabowski, Sandra Reynolds: *Principles of Anatomy and Physiololgy*, 7th ed. New York, Harper-Collins Publishers, 1993.

Volpe, Peter E.: *Biology and Human Concerns*, 4th ed. Dubuque, IA, Wm. C. Brown Publishers, 1993.

Whitney, Eleanor Noss, and Hamilton, Eva May Nunnelley: *Understanding Nutrition*, 4th ed. New York, West Publishing Company, 1987.

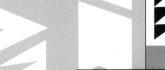

SECTION VI

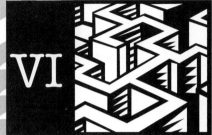

# HEALTH UNIT COORDINATING ON SPECIALTY UNITS

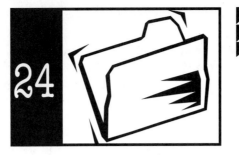
24

# PSYCHIATRY

## CHAPTER OBJECTIVES

*Upon completion of this chapter, you will be able to:*

1. Define the terms in the vocabulary list.
2. Write the meaning of the abbreviations in the abbreviations list.
3. Write the meaning of the psychological test in the psychological test list.
4. Compare and contrast the treatment for mental illness during prehistoric times, the nineteenth century, and the twentieth century.
5. Define deinstitutionalization and describe how it is accomplished in the United States.
6. Name three neurotransmitters and describe their function.
7. Name the primary drug groups used to treat mental illnesses.
8. Name the major side effects of neuroleptic medications and the treatment for the side effects.
9. Name two major mental disorders, give an example of each, and tell how they are treated.
10. Define the *Diagnostic and Statistical Manual of Mental Disorders* and describe how it is used to make psychiatric diagnoses.

## VOCABULARY

The following psychiatric terminology is not meant to be inclusive but is designed to give the student an overview of the medical language spoken on a psychiatric unit.

**HIGHLIGHT**

The student is advised that medical terminology included in other chapters is not repeated in this unit but is valid for psychiatry. Medical terminology used in psychiatry is in addition to all other terminology that you have learned.

**Abstract Thinking** • Stage in the development cognitive thought processes

**Acting Out** • Indirect expression of feeling through behavior, usually nonverbal, that attracts the attention of others

**Adaptation** • Striving to find equilibrium between one's self and one's environment

**Affect** • Outward manifestation of a person's feelings and emotions   *flas cump on 109*

**Akathisia** • Side effect of antipsychotic medication that is manifested by a feeling of restlessness and frequently accompanied by complaint of a twitching or crawling sensation in the muscles

**Antisocial Personality Disorder** • Disorder characterized by repetitive failure to abide by social and legal norms and to accept responsibility for own behavior

**Anxiety Disorders** • Emotional illness characterized by the feeling of fear

**Apraxia** • Impairment in the ability to engage in purposeful activities, even though muscle strength and coordination are present

**Asylum** • An institution that cares for the mentally ill, especially those who are so handicapped as to be unable to care for themselves

**Autistic Thought** • Ideation that has a private meaning to the individual

**Behavior Modification** • Type of therapy that attempts to modify observable, maladaptive patterns of behavior

**Bipolar Disorder** • Disturbance of mood and affect characterized by the occurrence of at least one episode of manic behavior, with or without a history of episodes of depression   *Lithium*

**Blunting** • Decreased intensity of emotional expression from that which one normally expects

**Body Language** • Transmission of a message by body position or movement

**Borderline Personality Disorder** • Condition characterized by instability in many areas, with no single feature present

**Cognition** • Process of logical thought

**Commitment** • Hospitalization in which the request for admission did not originate with the patient

**Confabulation** • Fabrication of experiences and situations, to fill in and cover up gaps in memory

**Coping Mechanisms** • Balancing factors that affect an individual's ability to restore equilibrium following a stressful event

**Cue** • Stimulus that determines the nature of the person's response

**Deinstitutionalization** • Transfer of a patient to a community setting after a long hospitalization, usually years

**Delusion** • Fixed false belief contrary to evidence; the delusion may be persecutory, grandiose, or somatic in nature

**Depression** • Mood disturbance characterized by feelings of sadness, despair, and discouragement

**Dyskinesia** • Impairment of the ability to execute voluntary movement

**Electroconvulsive Therapy** • Electric shock delivered to the brain through electrodes placed on the temporal area to produce a seizure

**Flat Affect** • Affect of a patient who does not communicate feelings in verbal and nonverbal responses to events

**Flight of Ideas** • Alteration in thought processes manifested by a rapid shift from one idea to another before the preceding one has been concluded

**Group Therapy** • A treatment modality consisting of two or more people who are experiencing common problems; each group has a leader who is referred to as the group facilitator; the interactions between group members are corrective and supportive

**Hallucination** • Sensory perception that does not result from an external stimulus

**Insanity** • A term for psychosis, obsolete except as a legal term

**Loose Association** • A communication pattern characterized by lack of clarity or connection between one thought and the next

**Magical Thinking** • Belief that merely thinking about an event in the external world can cause it to occur

**Maladaptive Behavior** • Behavior that does not adjust to the environment or situation and interferes with mental health

**Mania** • Condition characterized by a mood that is elevated, expansive, or irritable

**Neurotransmitter** • Chemical compounds that transmit impulses from one neuron to another neuron

**Organic Brain Syndrome** • Any psychological or behavioral abnormality associated with transient or permanent brain dysfunction caused by a disturbance of the psychological functioning of the brain

**Panic Disorder** • Anxiety state characterized by recurrent anxiety (panic) attacks that occur unpredictably

**Paranoid Disorders** • Mental disorders with persistent delusions of persecution or jealousy

**Psychopharmacology** • The study of psychotropic medications whose biochemicals affect the brain and nervous system by altering feelings, consciousness, and emotions

**Schizophrenia** • Manifestation of anxiety of psychotic proportions, primarily characterized by inability to trust other people and alteration in thought processes resulting in disrupted interpersonal relationships

**Somatoform Disorders** • Group of disorders characterized by recurrent and multiple physical symptoms for which there are no demonstrable organic findings or identifiable physiologic bases

**Sublimation** • Unconscious process of substituting socially more acceptable activity patterns that partially satisfy a need for an activity that would give rise to anxiety

**Suppression** • Process that is the conscious analogy of repression; it is the intentional exclusion of material from consciousness

**Therapeutic Community** • Use of a treatment setting as a community with the immediate air of full participation of all clients and the eventual goal of preparing clients for life outside the treatment setting

**Transference** • Unconscious mechanism by which feelings and attitudes originally associated with important people and events in one's early life are attributed to others in current interpersonal relationships

**Undoing** • Defense mechanism in which something unacceptable and already done is symbolically acted out in reverse, usually repetitiously, in the hope of relieving anxiety

**Withdrawal** • Attempt to avoid interaction with others and thus avoid relatedness; also, the occurrence of specific physical symptoms when substance intake is reduced or discontinued

**Word Salad** • Communication pattern characterized by a jumble of disconnected words

## HIGHLIGHT

The following abbreviations will be seen and used more often on the psychiatric units. These abbreviations are in addition to the ones previously learned in other chapters.

## ABBREVIATIONS

| Abbreviation | Meaning |
| --- | --- |
| ADD | attention deficit disorder |
| AWOL | absent without leave/unauthorized |
| BMD | bipolar mood disorder |
| COT | court-ordered treatment |
| DTO | danger to others |
| DTS | danger to self |
| ECT | electroconvulsive therapy |
| EE | expressed emotion |
| EPS | extrapyramidal symptoms |
| GD | gravely disabled |
| GEI | guilty except insane |
| LD | learning disabled |
| MDI | manic depressive illness |
| MSE | mental status examination |
| NGRI | not guilty by reason of insanity |
| OBS | organic brain syndrome |
| OCD | obsessive compulsive disorder |
| PAD | persistently acutely disabled |
| RTC | residential treatment center |
| RTU | restricted to unit |
| SADS | seasonal affective disorder syndrome |
| S | seclusion |
| S & R | seclusion and restraint |
| TO | time out |
| UALRU | unauthorized leave return urgent |

## EXERCISE 1

Write the term for each abbreviation listed below.

1. COT — _court ordered treatment_
2. MSE — _Mental Status examination_
3. RTU — _Restricted to Unit_
4. OCD — _Obsessive Compulsive Disorder_
5. SADS — _Seasonal affective disorder_
6. ADD — _attension Defect Disorder_
7. MDI — _Manic Depressive Illness_

8. ECT — _electro convulsive therapy_
9. AWOL — _Absent Without Leave_
10. UALRU — _Unauthorized leave Return Urgent_
11. DTO — _danger to others_
12. PAD — _persistantly acutely disabled_
13. S & R — _seclusion and restraint_
14. BMD — _Bipolar mood disorder_
15. NGRI — _Not guilty by reason of insanity_
16. EE — _expressed emotion_
17. S — _Seclusion_
18. TO — _time out_
19. DTS — _danger to self_
20. GEI — _guilty except insane_
21. LD — _Learning disabled_
22. OBS — _organic brain syndrome_
23. EPS — _extrapyramidal symptoms_
24. RTC — _residential treatment center_
25. GD — _gravely disabled_

## HISTORY

As we near the twenty-first century, it is interesting to note that those suffering from mental illness are still subject to ridicule, fear, and suspicion by society. Such treatment of the mentally ill has been occurring for centuries. During prehistoric times, primitive man believed that those with a mental illness were suffering from demonic possession, or had angered the gods. They believed that an evil spirit possessed the body as punishment for some transgression against the spirit world. Healing involved crude methods of "driving the evil spirit from the person's body." Archeologists have found skeletal remains with holes in the skull at a distance from the village that suggests that these are the remains of mentally ill persons who were banished from the community after they were not cured by this crude method of boring holes in their skulls for the escape of evil spirits. This mystical model of care for the mentally ill was in effect until around 2500 BC.

The second approach was the custodial model that can be traced back to Greek and Roman times. The mentally ill faired much better in this model. They were treated with compassion and concern, and treatment was humane. They were given opiates to quiet the "voices," music was provided that helped to relax the individuals, and they were provided with assistance for good physical and personal hygiene. This method of treatment was abandoned with the fall of the Roman Empire in AD 476.

Throughout the 1000 years of the Middle Ages, the care and treatment of the "insane" ranged from good to bad. The care of the mentally ill became the responsibility of the Roman Catholic Church. As the power of the church started to decline around the fifteenth century, the supernatural concept prevailed again. The mentally ill were confined, denied food, and beaten for their failure to conform to society's norms.

During the eighteenth century there was a movement toward humane treatment again. One of the people instrumental in the change in the mental health care delivery system was Linda Richards. She is recognized as America's first trained psychiatric nurse. She believed that the mentally sick person also needed nursing care. In 1882 she collaborated with Edward Cowles, the medical director of the McLean Hospital in Belmont, Massachusetts, to begin the first hospital with a psychiatric unit. It was called the McLean Asylum. After the establishment of the McLean Asylum, America began to build asylums at a rapid pace. This building of asylums to isolate and remove the mentally ill person from mainstream society lasted well into the nineteenth century. Instead of becoming a symbol of hope, these asylums became places of hopelessness. The insane were at the mercy of poorly paid attendants who were autocratic and punitive in their approach to treatment for the mentally ill. An accepted method of treatment was the circulatory chair, also called the circular swing, and the gyrator. Patients who displayed bizarre and disruptive symptoms were restrained onto the chair, and spun around and around. The chair could be spun up to 100 revolutions per minute. The rapid spinning caused disorientation, vomiting, bleeding from the eyes, and eventual unconsciousness. Patients deteriorated in this environment, and some acted out their frustrations; this further supported the belief that they were dangerous and should be confined. Many patients were beaten and restrained with chains.

During the twentieth century the contemporary approach to treatment was greatly enhanced by advances in medical science. Since the early 1950s, and the advent of psychopharmacologic therapy, broad changes have occurred in the treatment of the mentally ill. Thorazine, the first neuroleptic drug, was marketed in 1954, and since that time the number of patients in large mental institutions has shown a steady decrease.

Deinstitutionalization, the process of discharging patients to the community after a long hospitalization, began in 1955 after the discovery and use of psychotropic drugs. The change in the social climate for individual rights during the 1960s was another factor that contributed to reducing the census in large state-run mental institutions. However, mass exodus of the mentally ill from state institutions into the community was a result of deinstitutionalization policies that were adopted under the Kennedy administration in the early 1960s. The practice of discharging patients from mental institutions has resulted in a much bigger social problem and ethical issue; for example, is it better to let the mentally ill choose even though their choice may be to refuse treatment? The government failed to provide appropriate aftercare; conse-quently, many of the chronically mentally ill became a part of the homeless population. It is estimated that 33% or more of homeless people are mentally ill.

## MAJOR MENTAL ILLNESSES

The most serious of the major mental illnesses are the thought disorders and the mood disorders.

### Schizophrenia

Schizophrenia is a thought disorder characterized by severe impairment in judgment, perceptions, behavior, and emotions. The patient experiences disinterest, apathy, and an altered sense of self. Many schizophrenics will engage in odd poses that they hold for hours without moving (catatonic). It is not unusual for some to speak in rhymes and neologisms. It is no wonder that historically schizophrenia has been described as madness, lunacy, and demonic possession. People with schizophrenia seldom exhibit the exact same symptoms. The one constant in schizophrenia is that they all demonstrate impairment in reality testing, some even creating another reality.

People with schizophrenia tend to avoid confrontations. Therefore, they are not considered to be violent and dangerous. However, there have been incidents in which schizophrenics committed violent crimes when they acted upon a fixed false belief (delusion). One incident with which all of America should be familiar is the John Hinckly case. He believed that the actress Jodie Foster would be attracted to him if he assassinated the president (Ronald Reagan). Schizophrenia is treated primarily with antipsychotic drugs (see Chapter 13 for a general listing of the antipsychotic drugs).

### Bipolar Disease

Bipolar disease with or without depression is the most serious of the mood disorders. The patient experiencing mania is easily recognized on the treatment unit. The patient is inappropriately dressed and groomed, easily distracted with flight of ideas, and unable to sit still. The patient feels euphoric and grandiose, with inflated self-worth. In the acute stage all symptoms are intensified. Routinely, you will hear before seeing the patient who is experiencing a manic episode. These are the behaviors most likely to be observed:

■ Increased sexual interest and activity
■ Seductiveness and flirtatiousness
■ Rapid forced speech
■ Lack of personal hygiene
■ Short attention span
■ Difficulty concentrating
■ Word rhyming
■ Poor impulse control

- Lack of inhibition
- Frantic bartering and trading with other patients (outside of the hospital, wild spending sprees)
- Passive-aggressive and manipulative behaviors
- Suicidal behavior

The treatment for bipolar disorders is lithium. This drug is effective for the relief of excessive elation, hyperactivity, and accelerated thinking and speaking. After the patient has stabilized he or she is encouraged to participate in symptom management classes that focus on early recognition and intervention in potential crisis-producing situations.

---

**HIGHLIGHT**

Communication Tips for Working with the Mentally Ill

- Avoid the use of slang in your communications.
- Do not contradict or confirm thought disorders (delusions and hallucinations).

*Example*

Patient: "Help, help get these bugs off of me!"

Your response: "I know you think that there are bugs on you, but I do not see them. I will let the nurse know that you need to see her or him."

- Stay calm and speak softly even though the person may be yelling.
- Allow personal space and be especially cognizant of boundaries.
- Be aware of cultural differences as well as the illness.

---

## DIAGNOSTIC PSYCHOLOGICAL TESTS

The following is a descriptive list of the most often used psychological tests. These tests are conducted and interpreted by the psychologist. The psychiatrist uses these assessment data to aid in making a diagnosis and ordering treatment.

**Stanford Binet Intelligence Scale:** This measurement of cognitive ability consists of 15 subtests that measure short-term memory, quantitative memory, and abstract and visual reasoning.

**Clinical Analysis Questionnaire (CAQ):** The CAQ measures 16 normal personality traits and 12 abnormal personality traits in one test. It is a self-report test consisting of 227 items.

**Intelligence Quotient (IQ):** A test designed to determine the intelligence of an individual through the person's answers to arbitrary questions. The IQ test is a standard score that places the person in reference to the scores of others.

**Minnesota Multiphasic Personality Inventory (MMPI):** The MMPI is the most frequently used self-report inventory psychological test. It consists of 527 questions to which the patient answers true or false. This test measures abnormal personality characteristics.

**Rorschach Test:** A projective test consisting of 10 cards with a symmetric inkblot on each. The patient is asked to find meaning in these meaningless inkblots. They describe what the inkblots looks like and what it reminds them of (Fig. 24–1).

**Thematic Apperception Test (TAT):** The TAT is a projective picture story test. The patient is given 20 pictures and asked to tell detailed and complete stories about each picture. The resulting responses are interpreted in terms of aggression, autonomy, dominance, and psychological drives and needs.

**Wechsler Adult Intelligence Scale:** An intelligence test that provides measures of verbal and nonverbal abilities.

---

**HIGHLIGHT**

Schizophrenia affects an estimated 2.5 million Americans. An estimated 8 to 20 million Americans are affected by depression at any given time.

---

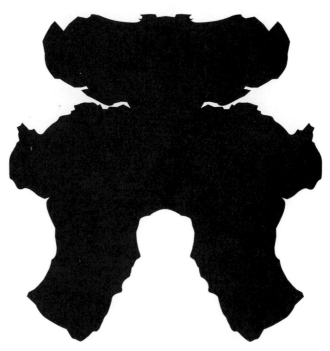

FIGURE 24–1 • An example of a meaningless inkblot used in the Rorschach test to elicit responses from patients.

# THE DIAGNOSTIC AND STATISTICAL MANUAL OF MENTAL DISORDERS

The *Diagnostic and Statistical Manual of Mental Disorders* is commonly called the DSM. This book is published by the American Psychiatric Association, and is in the fourth edition at this time. The DSM outlines a descriptive and comprehensive system that is used to categorize mental disorders. The DSM provides an operational framework for psychiatrists and other mental health professionals. Before making a diagnosis, the psychiatrist will use the DSM as a guide. It is not often, if ever, that patients will demonstrate all of the same symptoms listed under a diagnosis. It is generally felt that the primary symptoms will be present in numbers sufficient to make a diagnosis. Many variables impact demonstrated behaviors and verbalizations. Key variables that determine what symptoms will be displayed are ethnicity, cultural background, and life experiences.

The DSM is a very usable, useful, and powerful instrument for psychiatric diagnosis and treatment planning. Criticism comes mainly from those who contend that it is dehumanizing and stigmatizing to label patients. There is merit to that view, since society at large still sees the mentally ill person as a second-class citizen at best.

# DRUG GROUPS TO TREAT MENTAL ILLNESS

Neurotransmitters are substances that transmit messages from one neuron to another neuron through a complex communication system within the brain. As you have learned (from Chapter 23), information is transmitted through neurons that function by initiation and conduction of nerve impulses. The neurons are not connected and the spaces between the neurons are called synapses. The neurotransmitters are the chemicals that allow the message to cross the synapse (Fig. 24–2). When the message (impulse) arrives at the synapse, it triggers the release of neurotransmitters. Malfunctioning of the neurotransmitters is an accepted (but not the only) etiologic factor in mental illness. The three major neurotransmitters are serotonin, norepinephrine, and dopamine. Severe depressive illness may result from a decrease in neurotransmitters, while a manic illness would be related to an increase in these chemicals. These chemical imbalances cause mood and thought disorders that respond to the following groups of drugs.

- Antipsychotics/neuroleptics
- Antidepressants —
- Anticonvulsants      *tegretol*
- Antiparkinsonian agents   *for tremors*
- Antimanic agents   *Lithium   cogentin*
- Antianxiety agents

The *antipsychotic drugs*, also known as psychotropic or neuroleptic drugs, exert their effects by altering specific chemical processes involved in this neuronal complex communication system by blocking, increasing, or limiting the amount of a neurotransmitter that is released. There is substantial evidence that an excess of dopamine allows nerve impulses to be transmitted faster than normal. This rapid transmission of nerve impulses results in hallucinations, delusions, and bizarre behavior. The antipsychotic drugs work by blocking the excessive release of dopamine (see Chapter 13 for a list of antipsychotic drugs).

The *antianxiety drug* group is used extensively to alleviate anxiety. Symptoms of anxiety include agitation, muscle tension, nervousness, and hyperactivity. Frequently you will see an antianxiety drug used in conjunction with an antipsychotic drug to treat psychosis. The antianxiety drugs do not produce extrapyramidal symptoms (EPS), but in long-term use the patient will develop a tolerance to the drug and become chemically dependent on the drug (see Chapter 13 for a list of antianxiety drugs).

The *antiparkinsonian* drug group is used to treat EPS which is a common side effect of antipsychotic drug therapy. Extrapyramidal symptoms include drooling, stooped posture, muscle stiffness, and shuffling gait; hence the term pseudoparkinsonism. Unfortunately, the antiparkinsonian drugs often cause side effects such as dizziness, blurred vision, drowsiness, memory impairment and, in large doses, central nervous system toxicity. The remedy consists of reduction in dose, followed by discontinuation of the drug if symptoms are still not relieved. The most often used antiparkinsonian drugs are Cogentin, Artane, Symmetrel, and Benadryl.

One of the major side effects of antipsychotic drug therapy is tardive dyskinesia, characterized by abnormal, irregular, and involuntary movements. These symptoms commonly include overactivity of the tongue (darting, twisting, and repeated protrusions), jaw movements, lip puckering, facial grimacing, trunk twisting, and pelvic thrusting. There is no effective or standard treatment for tardive dyskinesia. Tapering off of the antipsychotic drugs is recommended.

*Antidepressant drugs* are used to treat depression that has been attributed to a central biochemical unbalance. These drugs enhance the activity of neurotransmission and relieve symptoms such as withdrawal, motor agitation or

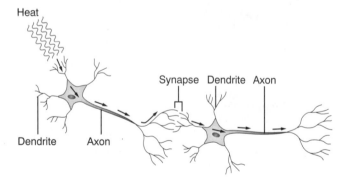

**F I G U R E   24–2 •** Neurons, showing the space between, called the synapse.

retardation, sleep and eating disturbances, pessimism, difficulty in concentration, inability to experience pleasure, and a general feeling of foreboding. The antidepressants are categorized into two groups, tricyclics (TCAs) and monoamine oxidase inhibitors (MAOIs). The TCAs are more effective and less toxic than the MAOIs. Only patients who cannot tolerate the TCAs are given MAOIs. Patients who receive MAOIs must have explicit dietary instructions. They cannot eat foods rich in the enzyme tyramine. Some of the restricted foods are chocolate, caffeine, aged cheese and meats, beer, and wine. It takes from 7 to 10 days for the antidepressants to become effective. Patients are treated with one of the antianxiety drugs until the antidepressant reaches therapeutic levels (see Chapter 13 for a list of antidepressant drugs).

*Antimanic drugs* such as lithium are used to calm and reduce hyperactivity and mood swings in bipolar disorders. Lithium is a simple salt found in most natural bodies of water and in our bodies. It is the only drug having the distinction of "being in a class by itself." Lithium stabilizes within 1 to 3 weeks. Antipsychotics or antianxiety drugs are used until the lithium reaches a therapeutic level. The doctor will order a "lithium work-up" on lithium therapy candidates (patients). This work-up consists of an EKG, a liver function study, and an IVP. After the patient is started on lithium, weekly serum lithium levels are drawn. When ordering a lithium work-up you will need to remember that the blood draw is scheduled exactly 12 hours from the last dose of lithium.

Common side effects of lithium therapy are polyuria, diarrhea, thirst, weight gain, and edema. Lithium toxicity can occur rapidly and can result in coma and death if not treated immediately. Close monitoring of the patient by the nurse is imperative.

From Chapter 13 you learned that Tegretol is an *anticonvulsant drug* used to treat seizures. It is also used to treat bipolar disorders in patients who cannot tolerate lithium therapy. When Tegretol is used to treat a bipolar disorder, most hospitals will require an informed consent. The consent is signed by the patient or the patient's guardian. Common side effects of Tegretol therapy are nausea, vomiting, dizziness, and lightheadedness. Serious side effects that can be fatal are leukopenia, aplastic anemia, and agranulocytosis. Baseline blood levels are drawn before starting Tegretol, and weekly blood levels are drawn thereafter to monitor blood values.

## OTHER TREATMENT APPROACHES

### Electroconvulsive Therapy

Electroconvulsive therapy (ECT) is the process of delivering an electrical shock to the brain through electrodes that are placed on the temples. This shock to the brain causes a grand mal seizure and is a frequently used treatment modality for some mental illnesses. ECT is effective for patients who are catatonic, withdrawn, depressed, and suicidal. These symptoms are life threatening, and prompt intervention is warranted. ECT has also been effective in the treatment of bipolar disorders and acute schizophrenia. It is not clear how ECT works; one theory is that it remodels or alters the postsynaptic response to the neurotransmitters.

There is a strong negative response from the public regarding the use of ECT in the treatment of mental illness. As a result of this negative response and the high cost of malpractice insurance many psychiatrists are using ECT very sparingly. It is now used primarily as the treatment of last resort for patients who have failed to respond to medications.

### Group Therapy

Group therapy is the process of two or more persons meeting together with a group facilitator to work on common problems. It is a popular and frequently used treatment modality in all forms of mental illness. After patients have been stabilized on medication they are placed into group therapy according to their needs. Patients must first recognize that they have a problem and be willing to work on learning ways of dealing with their disabilities.

### Psychiatric Orders

When a patient is admitted to a psychiatry unit, they are attended to by the admitting psychiatrist and a general practitioner. The psychiatrist will make an assessment and order all psychiatric medications, psychiatric laboratory tests, privileges, and therapy groups. The general practitioner will make an assessment and write the medical orders.

The psychiatrist is responsible for determining and ordering all privileges for the patient. The most common privilege system is the color-coded arm band system. The patient's arm band communicates to the staff what the patient's privileges are; for example, a patient wearing a white band is restricted to the unit and closely observed at all times by the nursing staff, and a patient with a gold band is privileged to leave the unit for other areas of the hospital without staff escort.

**HIGHLIGHT**

The health unit coordinator is advised to never replace a patient's arm band. Do not replace the band even if you check the chart and verify that "Arnold Pickle" has an order for a gold band. Many times patients who want to leave the hospital will assume the identify of another patient.

## SUMMARY

Over the centuries the attempts to treat mental illness have ranged from compassionate and humane to barbaric. The approach to treatment at any given time period depended on the beliefs of society at that time. From antiquity, persons with psychotic disorders have been locked in cages, spun, shocked, chained, sent off in "ships of fools," flogged, chemically restrained, and in some cases killed. It was not until the twentieth century that research found effective treatment for mental illness. It is now known that one of the causes of mental illness is a neurotransmission imbalance, and several categories of drugs have been developed to counteract this imbalance.

There remain many theories on the cause of mental illness. Most recently, several suspect chromosomes have been isolated that may lead to more advanced treatment and possibly prevention. One thing that the researchers are certain of is that mental illness is not a phenomenon over which the individual has control. Unfortunately, we still find a stigma attached to those who have a mental illness.

After the discovery of psychotropic drugs, thousands of mentally ill people were deinstitutionalized. It is worth noting that these people did not join mainstream society as anticipated. Instead, they constitute a large percentage of the homeless population, where they are easily victimized by others. The student is advised that the mentally ill patient is treated with the same respect and empathy shown to other patients.

## REVIEW QUESTIONS

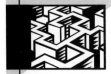

I. Match the psychological test in column I with the description in column II.

**Column I**

1. __D__ Rorschach Test
2. __E__ Wechsler Adult Intelligence Scale
3. __F__ Clinical Analysis Questionnaire
4. __G__ Stanford Binet Intelligence Scale
5. __B__ Thematic Apperception Test
6. __A__ Intelligence Quotient
7. __C__ Minnesota Multiphasic Personality Inventory

**Column II**

a. A measurement of cognitive ability consisting of 15 subtests that measure short-term memory, and abstract and visual reasoning.
b. The TAT is a projective picture story test. The patient is given 20 pictures and asked to tell detailed and complete stories about each picture.
c. The most frequently used self-report. The test consists of 527 questions that the patient answers as true or false.
d. A projective test that consist of 10 cards with a symmetric inkblot on each card.
e. An intelligence test that provides measures of verbal and nonverbal abilities.
f. Measures 16 normal traits and 12 abnormal traits in the same test.
g. A test designed to measure intelligence through a person's answers to arbitrary questions.

II. 1. During prehistoric times primitive man believed that those with a mental illness were suffering from ___demonic Possesion___.

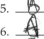

2. Healing involved ___driving evil spirits from body___.
3. The custodial model of care was present during ___Greek___ and ___Roman___ times.
4. During the middle ages the care of the mentally ill became the responsibility of the ___Roman Catholic Church___.
5. The first psychiatric nurse who believed that those with a mental illness deserved care was ___Linda___ ___Richards___.

6. The first neuroleptic drug was discovered in 1954 and is called _thorazine_.

7. The process of releasing mentally ill people from a state-run institution after many years of hospitalization is called _deinstitutionalization_

8. _33_% of the homeless population is considered to be mentally ill.

III. 1. The three neurotransmitters thought to be responsible for some mental illness are: _dopamine_, _seratonin_, and _norepineplarine_

   2. The spaces between neurons are called the _synapses_.

   3. The _neurotransmitters_ function to help the impulse (message) to cross the synapse.

IV. Match the drug group in column I with the drug in column II (use drug groups in Chapter 13 and the PDR as a resource).

| Column I | Column II |
|---|---|
| a. antipsychotic | 1. _F_ Ativan |
| b. antidepressant | 2. _E_ Lithium |
| c. anticonvulsant | 3. _A_ Haldol |
| d. antiparkinsonian | 4. _B_ Prozac |
| e. antimanic | 5. _A_ Risperdal |
| f. antianxiety | 6. _C_ Tegretol |
| | 7. _B_ Zoloft |
| | 8. _A_ Mellaril |
| | 9. _B_ Elavil |
| | 10. _D_ Cogentin |
| | 11. _F_ Xanax |
| | 12. _A_ Prolixin |
| | 13. _D_ Artane |
| | 14. _F_ Buspar |

# References

American Psychiatric Association: *Diagnostic and Statistical Manual of Mental Disorders*, 4th ed. Washington, DC, 1993.

Andreasen, Nancy: *The Broken Brain*. New York, Harper-Perennial, 1984.

Comer, Ronald J.: *Fundamentals of Abnormal Psychology*. New York, W.H. Freeman & Co., 1996.

Culkin, Joseph and Perrotto, Richard S.: *Exploring Abnormal Psychology*. New York, Harper Collins, 1994.

Gorman, Jack: *The Essential Guide to Psychiatric Drugs*. New York, St. Martin's Press, 1992.

Janosik, Ellen H. and Davies, Janet L.: *Psychiatric Mental Health Nursing*. Boston, Jones & Bartlett Publishers, Inc., 1986.

Jefferson, J. W., Geist, J. H., Ackerman, D. L., and Carroll, J. A.: *Lithium Encyclopedia Clinical Practice*. Washington, DC, American Psychiatric Press, Inc., 1987.

Noll, Richard: *The Encyclopedia of Schizophrenia and the Psychotic Disorders*. New York, Facts on File, 1992.

Physicians' Desk Reference, 50th ed. Montvale, NJ, Medical Economics, 1996.

Siegal, Ronald: *Fire in the Brain*. New York, E.P. Dutton, 1992.

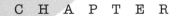

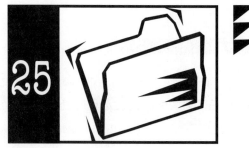

# PEDIATRICS

This unit is an introduction to medical terms, abbreviations, diseases, treatments, diagnostics, supplies and equipment you will encounter on a pediatrics unit. It is not meant to be comprehensive and does not include what has been discussed in other chapters.

## CHAPTER OBJECTIVES

*Upon completion of this unit, you will be able to:*

1. Define the medical terms in the vocabulary list.
2. Write the meaning of the abbreviations in the abbreviations list.
3. Name and describe the common diseases/conditions that are treated on the pediatrics unit.
4. List two common treatments performed on pediatric patients.
5. List four diagnostic tests commonly ordered on pediatric patients.
6. Describe how pediatric medication orders are frequently written and explain why.
7. Name three frequently ordered medications on pediatric patients.
8. Name four types of equipment or supplies often used on pediatrics units.

## VOCABULARY

**Abdominal Girth** • The circumference of the abdomen, usually measured at the umbilicus

**Bonding** • The attachment process that occurs between an infant and the parents, especially the mother

**Child Life Specialist** • One trained to use play therapy to aid pediatric patients to cope with their illnesses and hospitalizations

**Pacifier** • A nipple-shaped object used by infants for sucking

**Pediatrics** • Pertaining to preventative and primary health care and treatment of children and study of childhood diseases

**Pediatrician** • A physician who specializes in pediatrics

**Pediatrics Code** • A code (cessation of breathing and or heartbeat) that involves a child (should be announced as a pediatrics code by operator because the pediatrics personnel will then respond)

**Wallaby Blanket** • A blanket used to administer phototherapy to infants diagnosed with hyperbilirubinemia

# ABBREVIATIONS

| Abbreviation | Meaning |
|---|---|
| ABR | auditory brain stem response |
| AD | right ear |
| AS | left ear |
| AU | both ears |
| BAER | brain stem auditory evoked response |
| Bili | bilirubin |
| BOM | bilateral otitis media |
| BPD | bronchopulmonary dysplasia |
| BW | birth weight |
| CF | cystic fibrosis |
| CHC | children's health center |
| CPS | child protective services |
| CRS | children's rehabilitative services |
| D & D | diarrhea and dehydration |
| DL | delayed language |
| DS | delayed speech |
| FTT | failure to thrive |
| IBW | ideal body weight |
| IDM | infant of diabetic mother |
| LOM | left otitis media |
| MBR | microbilirubin |
| NB | newborn |
| OFC | occipital frontal circumference |
| OM | otitis media |
| Peds | pediatrics |
| PICU | pediatric intensive care unit |
| RAD | reactive airway disease |
| RDS | respiratory distress syndrome of the newborn |
| ROM | right otitis media |
| RSV | respiratory syncytial virus |
| SGS | short-gut syndrome |
| sickles | sickle cells |
| SIDS | sudden infant death syndrome |
| SNAT | suspected nonaccidental trauma |
| Sz | seizure |
| t | teaspoon |
| T | tablespoon |
| T & A | tonsillectomy and adenoidectomy |
| URA | upper respiratory infection |
| WIC | the acronym used for the Women, Infant's, and Children's Supplemental Nutrition Program |

# EXERCISE 1

Write the abbreviation for each definition given below.

1. auditory brain stem response   _ABR_
2. left ear   _AS_
3. bilirubin   _bili_
4. diarrhea and dehydration   _D & D_
5. ideal body weight   _IBW_

6. failure to thrive   _FTT_
7. bronchopulmonary dysplasia   _BPD_
8. right ear   _AD_
9. brain stem auditory evoked response   _BAER_
10. both ears   _AU_
11. bilateral otitis media   _BOM_
12. birth weight   _BW_
13. children's health center   _CHC_
14. cystic fibrosis   _CF_
15. child protective services   _CPS_
16. delayed language   _DL_
17. infant of diabetic mother   _IDM_
18. delayed speech   _DS_
19. children's rehabilitative services   _CRS_
20. right otitis media   _ROM_
21. newborn   _NB_
22. occipital frontal circumference   _OFC_
23. left otitis media   _LOM_
24. sickle cells   _sickles_
25. sudden infant death syndrome   _SIDS_
26. tablespoon   _T_
27. pediatrics   _peds_
28. otitis media   _OM_
29. reactive airway disease   _RAD_
30. seizure   _Sz_
31. upper respiratory infection   _URI_
32. microbilirubin   _MBR_
33. pediatric intensive care unit   _PICU_
34. respiratory distress syndrome   _RDS_
35. teaspoon   _t_
36. respiratory syncytial virus   _RSV_
37. suspected nonaccidental trauma   _SNAT_
38. tonsillectomy and adenoidectomy   _T & A_

39. Women, Infant's and Children's Supplemental Nutrition Program ___WIC___

40. short-gut syndrome ___SGS___

# COMMON CONDITIONS/DISEASES

**Asthma:** An obstructive respiratory condition characterized by recurring attacks of paroxysmal *—in bursts* dyspnea and wheezing (common chronic illness in childhood)

**Biliary Atresia:** Congenital absence or underdevelopment of one or more of the biliary structures causing jaundice and early liver damage (most infants die in early childhood from biliary cirrhosis)

**Cellulitis:** Inflammation of cellular or connective tissue *Rocephen most* 

**Convulsion:** A series of involuntary contractions of the voluntary muscles (convulsive seizures are *Seizure disorder* symptomatic of some neurologic disorders)

**Croup:** An acute viral infection of upper and lower respiratory tract (occurs in infants and young children 3 months to 3 years of age)

**Epiglottitis:** An inflammation of the epiglottis; acute epiglottitis is a severe form of the condition, affecting primarily children

**Failure to Thrive:** The abnormal retardation of the growth and development of an infant

**Febrile Seizure:** A seizure occurring in children age 3 months to 5 years of age in association with a fever at or above 39.5°C (103.2°F), often associated with a family history of febrile seizures

**Hydrocephalus:** The increased accumulation of cerebrospinal fluid within the ventricles of the brain (may result from developmental anomalies, infection, injury, or brain tumors); surgical correction would involve placement of a ventriculoatrial, ventriculoperitoneal, or ventriculovenous shunt

**Hyperbilirubinemia:** An excess of bilirubin in the blood of the neonate causing jaundice (may be treated in the patient's home)

**Ingestion:** The swallowing of a foreign object (coins, jacks, marbles, etc.)

**Intussusception:** Prolapse of one segment of bowel into the lumen of another segment of the small intestine, the colon, or the terminal ileum and cecum (occurs most often in infants and small children)

**Kawasaki disease (mucocutaneous lymph node** *Unknown* **syndrome):** An acute febrile illness, (male children *fever* under 4 years most susceptible); cause unknown

**Meningitis:** Inflammation of the membranes of the spinal cord or brain

**Near Drowning:** Infants who live following an immersion incident that could have produced fatal drowning (often results in brain damage) *4-6 min no o2 Bran Dam*

**Pertussis (whooping cough):** An acute, infectious disease characterized by a catarrhal stage, followed by a peculiar paroxysmal cough, ending in a whooping inspiration (may be prevented by immunization of infants beginning at 3 months of age)

**Pyloric Stenosis:** A narrowing of the pyloric sphincter at the outlet of the stomach, causing an obstruction that blocks the flow of food into the small intestine (occurs as a congenital defect in 1 in 200 newborns)

**Respiratory Distress Syndrome:** An acute lung disease of the newborn

**Respiratory Syncytial Virus:** A subgroup of myxoviruses that in tissue culture causes formation of giant cells or syncytia (it is a common cause of epidemics of acute bronchiolitis, bronchopneumonia, and the common cold in young children)

**Reye's Syndrome:** A combination of acute encephalopathy and fatty infiltration of the internal organs that may follow acute viral infections (usually affects people under 18 years of age) *aspirin causes*

**Sepsis:** Presence of infection in the blood

**Short-Gut Syndrome:** A congenital disorder in which an infant's intestine is too short or underdeveloped to allow normal food digestion

**Sleep Apnea:** A sleep disorder characterized by periods of an absence of attempts to breath

# PHYSICIANS' ORDERS

Below are types of physicians' orders with brief explanations that are commonly used in hospital pediatrics units.

## Physicians' Orders for Nursing Observation

- *Guaiac all stools* (see page 255)

- *Measure OFC q AM and record* (ordered to monitor amount of fluid collection around the brain)

- *Measure abdominal girth q AM* (ordered to monitor amount of fluid collection in abdominal area)

- *Weigh all diapers* (a method of measuring infant's output, the weight of the dry diaper is deducted) *weigh dry then weigh*

## Physicians' Orders for Treatments

### Nursing

- *Place in incubator and apply Bili light—apply eye patches* (used to treat and administer phototherapy to an infant with the diagnosis of hyperbilirubinemia)

- *Place on wallaby blanket ASAP* (also used to treat hyperbilirubinemia)

- *Place on apnea mattress* (used to monitor child's breathing)

- *Place in warmer bed* (bed used to increase child's temperature)

- *Discharge in AM on apnea monitor (frequently, infants are sent home on a monitor)*

## Occupational Therapy
- *Train patient in chewing and swallowing (ordered when child has lived on TPN since birth (i.e., short-gut syndrome)*
- *Evaluate ability to nipple and train if needed (frequently ordered for infants that are not eating sufficient amounts)*
- *Evaluate breastfeeding ability*

## Physicians' Orders for Diagnostics

### Diagnostic Imaging
- *Bone for age (an x-ray of left wrist to determine stage of development)*
- *Long bone x-ray to R/O SNAT (the child's long bones are x-rayed to check for untreated fractures to determine child abuse)*
- *X-ray for location of foreign object (when child has swallowed a foreign object)*

### Laboratory
- *MBR q 4 hr and call results (used to monitor an infant's bilirubin)*
- *Schedule sweat test in AM (a diagnostic test performed to aid in diagnosis of cystic fibrosis)*
- *NP swab for viral culture (a diagnostic test to identify a viral infection)*

### Neurodiagnostics
- *Schedule BAER in AM (see page 304)*
- *Portable EEG stat (see page 302) (often ordered when child has seizure activity)*

### Respiratory
- *Schedule CPR training for both parents prior to discharge Thursday (frequently ordered for infants/children with respiratory problems or after a near-drowning incident)*
- *Schedule SVN/CPT training for mother in AM (ordered when child has a need for treatment at home)*
- *Place child in O₂ tent (see page 321) at 40% (often ordered for pediatric patients with a diagnosis of pneumonia)*

### Sleep Study Lab
- *Have patient in sleep study lab at 1900 this evening for sleep study (ordered when infant has sleep apnea)*

### Social Services
- *Consult and evaluation to determine status of home situation (frequently ordered when physician or nursing personnel have concerns about child's safety and welfare)*

## Physicians' Orders for Medications

Pediatric medication orders are frequently written indicating milligrams per kilogram because of the increased risk involved with small children.

### Examples
*a dose*
- *Ceclor (40 mg/kg/day) = 1/2 tsp tid (frequently ordered for treatment of otitis media; the usual dose for adults is 250 mg q8h)*
- *Theo-Dur Sprinkle (24 mg/kg/day) 12.0 mg q12h (ordered for treatment of asthma; it is usually given mixed in a food; i.e., applesauce)*
- *Ampicillin (200 mg/kg/day ÷ 6h) = 180 mg IV q6h (the usual dose for adults and children over 20 kg is 500 mg q6h)*
- *Claforan (200 mg/kg/day ÷ 6h) = 180 mg IV q6h*
- *Tylenol (15 mg/kg/day) = 55 mg/PO q4h prn*

---

## EQUIPMENT AND SUPPLIES

Below are listed supplies and equipment commonly used in hospital pediatrics units.

## Equipment Frequently used

**Apnea Alarm Mattress:** A mattress for infants, designed to sound an alarm if the child stops breathing for a given period of time

**Apnea Monitor:** An electronic device that detects changes in thoracic or abdominal movements and heart rate

**Bili Lights:** Used to administer phototherapy

**Climber Crib:** A large crib with side rails and a plastic covering (used for children that can pull themselves up and could fall over side rail)

**Incubator:** An apparatus used to provide a controlled environment, especially at a particular temperature—other components such as darkness, light, oxygen, moisture, or dryness may also be provided

**Infant Crib:** Small bed with rails—does not have plastic cover found on climber cribs

## Supplies Frequently Used

**Eye Patches:** Used to protect an infant's eyes when receiving phototherapy

**Diapers:** When ordering diapers it is necessary to indicate size

```
0/00/00      Admit to 2 west Dr. Pete Larson              Wt 3.86 kg

             Dx: Fever R/O sepsis

             Condition: stable

             Vitals: routine

             Allergies: NKDA

             Activity: ad lib c̄ parents

             Nursing: strict I/O's daily wts

             Diet: breast & enfamil c̄ iron ad lib

             IVF: D5 ¼ NS @ 16cc/hr may add 2 meq KCL/100cc after first void

             Labs: CBC c̄ diff   Blood cx x 1

                   Cath UA c̄ Culture

                   CSF      tube #1 gram stain & culture

                            tube #2 protein & glucose

                            tube #3 cell ct & diff

             Meds: Ampicillin (200 mg/kg/d ÷ q6 hrs) = 180 mg IV q 6 hrs

                   Claforan (200 mg/kg/d ÷ q6 hrs) = 180 mg IV q 6 hrs

                   Tylenol (15 mg/kg/d) = 55 mg po q 4 hrs prn

                                              Thank you,

                                              Dr. Frank Resident MD
```

Set of Pediatric Admission Orders

## Formulas Frequently Used

Similac with iron
Enfamil
Prosoybee
Portagen
Isomil
Lacto Free
Nutramagin
Pregestamil
Neocare
Carnation Good Start

---

### HIGHLIGHT

Medications are given according to a patient's weight. Pediatric medication orders are frequently written indicating milligrams per kilogram (mg/kg) because of the increased risk of overdosing a small child.

*1 kg = 2.2 lb*

**REVIEW QUESTIONS**

1. Briefly describe the following conditions/diseases that are commonly treated on the pediatrics unit.

   a. asthma _obstructive respiratory condition characterized by recurring attacks of paroxysmal dysphea and wheezing_

   b. croup _acute viral infection of upper and lower respiratory tract occurs in infants + children 3mo – 3yrs_

   c. RSV _sub group of myxovirus that in tissue culture causes formation of giant syncytia cells_

   d. meningitis _inflamation of the membranes of the spinal cord + brain_

   e. hydrocephalus _increased accumulation of cerebrospinal fluid on the ventricles of the brain requiring a shunt._

2. Explain a method (diagnostic procedure) of evaluating a child's stage of development for their age.
   _Bone for age     Lt X ray of wrist bone_

3. What function does a child life specialist serve?

4. Describe a diagnostic procedure that would aid the physician in determining if a child has been physically abused.
   _long bone x ray to check for untreated fractures_

5. List two methods of treating hyperbilirubinemia (jaundice) in the newborn.

   a. _incubator and bili lights_

   b. _place on a wallaby blanket_

6. Name a laboratory test that would be performed to diagnose cystic fibrosis.
   _Sweat test_

7. Which hospital department would the health unit coordinator send the following orders to:

   a. *Schedule BAER in AM*    _neurodiagnostic_

   b. *Sleep study in AM*    _sleep study lab_

   c. *MBR q4h*    _Laboratory_

   d. *Evaluate ability to nipple*    _occupational therapy_

8. Describe the following observation orders that would be carried out by nursing and explain the reason for each.

   a. *Measure OFC q AM and record*

   the nurse measures the occipital circomfrines of the childs head to moniter the amount of fluid accumulated around the brain

   b. *weigh all diapers*

   the nurse weights wet and dry diapers the wet woould be recorded and the weight of the dry diaper woud be deducted to determine urine output

   c. *guaiac all stools*

   nurse would use a solution or tape on the childs stool that detects occult blood and would record findings on nurses notes

9. Explain why pediatrics orders are often written indicating milligrams per kilogram.

   because childrems medication is given according to weight and increased nsk for overdose

10. What type of bed would the health unit coordinator order for the following pediatric patients:

    a. a 4-month-old _____ Infant crib

    b. a 10-month-old _____ climbur crib

    c. a newborn admitted for phototherapy _____ incubator

## References

O'Toole Marie (ed): *Miller-Keane Encyclopedia & Dictionary of Medicine, Nursing, & Allied Health*, 5th ed., Philadelphia, W.B. Saunders Co., 1992.

*Physicians' Desk Reference*, 50th ed., Montvale, NJ, Medical Economics Company, 1996.

Summitt, Robert L.: *Comprehensive Pediatrics*. St. Louis, The C.V. Mosby Co., 1990.

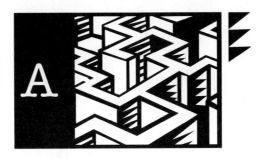

# WORD ELEMENTS

| Word Element | Meaning | Word Element | Meaning |
|---|---|---|---|
| a (an) | without | end/o | inside |
| abdomin/o | abdomen | enter/o | intestines |
| aden/o | gland | epitheli/o | epithelium |
| adren/o | adrenal | erythr/o | red |
| adrenal/o | adrenal | esophag/o | esophagus |
| -al | pertaining to | femor/o | femur |
| -algia | pain | gastr/o | stomach |
| angi/o | blood vessel | -genic | producing |
| aort/o | aorta | gloss/o | tongue |
| appendic/o | appendix | -gram | record |
| -ar | pertaining to | -graph | instrument to record |
| arteri/o | artery | -graphy | process of recording |
| arthr/o | joint | gynec/o | woman |
| blephar/o | eyelid | hem/o | blood |
| bronch/o | bronchus | hemat/o | blood |
| carcin/o | cancer | hepat/o | liver |
| cardi/o | heart | herni/o | protrusion of a body part |
| caud/o | tail or down | hist/o | tissue |
| cele | herniation or pouching out | humer/o | humerus |
| centesis | puncture and aspiration of | hyper- | above normal |
| cerebell/o | cerebellum | hypo- | below normal |
| cerebr/o | cerebrum | hyster/o | uterus |
| cervic/o | cervix | -iasis | condition of |
| cheil/o | lip | -ic | pertaining to |
| chol/o, chol/e | bile, gall | ile/o | ileum |
| chondr/o | cartilage | inter- | between |
| clavic/o | clavicle | intra- | within |
| clavicul/o | clavicle | irid/o | iris |
| col/o | colon | -itis | inflammation |
| colp/o | vagina | kerat/o | cornea |
| conjunctiv/o | conjunctiva | lamin/o | lamina |
| cost/o | rib | lapar/o | abdomen |
| crani/o | cranium | laryng/o | larynx |
| cyan/o | blue | leuk/o | white |
| cyst/o | bladder | lingu/o | tongue |
| cyt/o | cell | lip/o | fat |
| derm/o | skin | lith/o | stone, calculus |
| dermat/o | skin | mamm/o | breast |
| duoden/o | duodenum | mast/o | breast |
| dys- | bad or painful | megaly | enlargement |
| ectomy | surgical removal, excision | men/o | menstruation |
| electr/o | electric | mening/o | meninges |
| -emia | condition of the blood | menisc/o | meniscus |
| encephal/o | brain | metr/o | uterus |

| Word Element | Meaning | Word Element | Meaning |
| --- | --- | --- | --- |
| my/o | muscle | pulmon/o | lung |
| myel/o | spinal cord, bone marrow | pyel/o | renal pelvis |
| myring/o | tympanic membrane | ren/o | kidney |
| nephr/o | kidney | retin/o | retina |
| neur/o | nerve | rhin/o | nose |
| -oid | resembling | salping/o | fallopian or uterine tube |
| -ologist | specialist | sarc/o | connective tissue |
| -ology | study of | scapul/o | scapula |
| -oma | tumor | scler/o | sclera, hard |
| oophor/o | ovary | -sclerosis | hardening |
| ophthalm/o | eye | -scope | instrument for visual examination |
| orchi/o | testicle, testis | | |
| orchid/o | testicle, testis | -scopy | visual examination |
| -orrhagia | rapid discharge | sigmoid/o | sigmoid flexure |
| -orrhaphy | to suture | spin/o | spine |
| -orrhea | discharge | splen/o | spleen |
| -osis | abnormal condition | staped/o | stapes |
| oste/o | bone | -stenosis | narrowing |
| -ostomy | creation of an artificial opening | stern/o | sternum |
| ot/o | ear | stomat/o | mouth |
| -otomy | surgical incision | sub- | under or below |
| pancreat/o | pancreas | supra- | above |
| parathyroid/o | parathyroid | thorac/o | chest |
| patell/o | patella | thromb/o | clot |
| path/o | disease | thyr/o | thyroid |
| peri- | around | thyroid/o | thyroid |
| perine/o | perineum | tonsill/o | tonsil |
| -pexy | surgical fixation | trache/o | trachea |
| phalang/o | phalange | trans- | through, across, beyond |
| pharyng/o | pharynx | trich/o | hair |
| phleb/o | vein | -trophy | development |
| -plasty | surgical repair | ur/o | urine |
| -plegia | paralysis, stroke | ureter/o | ureter |
| pleur/o | pleura | urethr/o | urethra |
| -pnea | respiration, breathing | urin/o | urine |
| pneum/o | air, lung | uter/o | uterus |
| pneumon/o | lung | vagin/o | vagina |
| poli/o | gray matter | vas/o | vas deferens |
| proct/o | rectum | ven/o | vein |
| prostat/o | prostate | vertebr/o | vertebra |
| psych/o | mind | viscer/o | internal organs |

# APPENDIX B

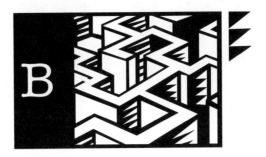

## ABBREVIATIONS

The following is a list of alphabetized abbreviations used frequently in doctors' orders. Most of the abbreviations related to specific departments, such as laboratory and diagnostic imaging, are not included here. For those, please refer to the chapters concerning those departments.

| Abbreviation | Meaning |
|---|---|
| > | greater than |
| < | less than |
| ↑ | increase or above |
| / | per or by |
| △ | change |
| @ | at |
| ↓ | decrease or below |
| A | apical |
| AA | active assistance |
| $\bar{a}$ | before |
| $\bar{a}\bar{a}$ | of each |
| Ab | antibody |
| abd | abdominal |
| ABR | absolute bed rest |
| ac | before meals |
| ad lib | as desired |
| ADL | activities of daily living |
| AE | antiembolism |
| Ag | antigen |
| AIDS | acquired immunodeficiency sydrome |
| AKA | above the knee amputation |
| AM | morning |
| AMA | against medical advice |
| amb | ambulate |
| AMO | against medical orders |
| A&O | alert and oriented |
| AP | anteroposterior |
| ARC | AIDS-related complex |
| as tol | as tolerated |
| ASA | acetylsalicylic acid (aspirin) |
| ASAP | as soon as possible |
| ATO | assistant to director |
| ax | axillary |
| B, bil | bilateral |
| bid | twice a day |

| Abbreviation | Meaning |
|---|---|
| bili | bilirubin |
| biw | twice a week |
| BKA | below the knee amputation |
| BM | bowel movement |
| BP | blood pressure |
| BR | bed rest |
| BRP | bathroom privileges |
| BSC | bedside commode |
| Bt | bleeding time |
| BUN | blood urea nitrogen |
| Bx | biopsy |
| $\bar{c}$ | with |
| CA | cancer |
| Ca | calcium |
| C of A | conditions of admission |
| CAD | coronary artery disease |
| cal | calorie |
| cap | capsule |
| CAT, CT | computed axial tomography |
| cath | catheterize |
| CBI | continuous bladder irrigation |
| CBR | continuous bed rest |
| cc or cm$^3$ | cubic centimeter |
| CDC | Centers for Disease Control |
| CEO | chief executive officer |
| CHF | congestive heart failure |
| CHO | carbohydrate |
| chol | cholesterol |
| CHUC | certified health unit coordinator |
| CI | clinical indications |
| CMS | circulation, motion, sensation |
| CMV | cytomegalovirus |
| CNA | certified nursing assistant |
| CO$_2$ | carbon dioxide |
| comp or cmpd | compound |
| CNA | certified nurses assistant |
| COO | chief operating officer |
| COPD | chronic obstructive pulmonary disease |
| CP | cold packs |
| CPM | continuous passive motion |
| CPT | chest physical therapy |
| CPZ | Compazine |
| C&S | culture and sensitivity |

| Abbreviation | Meaning | Abbreviation | Meaning |
|---|---|---|---|
| CSF | cerebral spinal fluid | h or (H) | hypodermic |
| Cx | culture | h or hr | hour |
| CVA | cerebrovascular accident | H&P | history and physical |
| CVC | central venous catheter | HB$_s$Ag | hepatitis B surface antigen |
| CVP | central venous pressure | HBV | hepatitis B virus |
| CXR | chest x-ray | HCG | human chorionic gonadotropin |
| D/LR | dextrose in lactated Ringer's solution | hct | hematocrit |
| | | HCTZ | hydrochlorothiazide |
| D/NS | dextrose in normal saline | HCV | hepatitis C virus |
| D/RL | dextrose in Ringer's lactate | HD | hemodialysis |
| D/W | dextrose in water | HDL | high-density lipoprotein |
| DAT | diet as tolerated or direct antiglobulin test | hgb | hemoglobin |
| | | HIV | human immunodeficiency virus |
| DC | discontinue | HMO | health maintenance organization |
| Diff | differential | HNP | herniated nucleus pulposus |
| Dig | digoxin | HO | house officer |
| DME | durable medical equipment | h/o | history of |
| DNR | do not resuscitate | HOB | head of bed |
| DO | doctor of osteopathy | HP | hot packs |
| dr or ʒ | dram | hs | bedtime |
| DRG | diagnosis-related group | HUC | health unit coordinator |
| DSS | dioctyl sodium sulfosuccinate (Colace) | Hx | history |
| | | I&O | intake and output |
| DSU | day surgery unit | ICD | International Classification of Diseases |
| DW | distilled water | | |
| DX | diagnosis | ID | identification (labels) |
| EBV | Epstein-Barr virus | IM | intramuscular |
| EC | enteric coated | IPG | impedance plethysmography |
| ECF | extended care facilities | IPPB | intermittent positive pressure breathing |
| EchoEG | echoencephalogram | | |
| ED | emergency department | IS | incentive spirometry |
| EGD | esophagogastroduodenoscopy | IV | intravenous |
| elix | elixir | IVF | intravenous fluids |
| EMG | electromyogram | IVP | intravenous pyelogram |
| EPC | electronic pain control | IVPB | intravenous piggyback |
| ER | emergency room | IVU | intravenous urogram |
| ERCP | endoscopic retrograde cholangiopancreatography | JCAHO | Joint Commission on the Accreditation of Healthcare Organizations |
| ES | electrical stimulation | | |
| ESR | erythrocyte sedimentation rate | K | potassium |
| ET | endotracheal tube | KCl | potassium chloride |
| ETS | elevated toilet seat | kg | kilogram |
| FF | force fluids | KO | keep open |
| fib | fibrinogen | KUB | kidney, ureter, bladder |
| FS | full strength or frozen section | L | liter |
| 5-FU | 5-fluorouracil | lb, # | pound(s) |
| f/u | follow-up | L&S | liver and spleen |
| fx | fracture | L/min | liters per minute |
| g | gram | lat | lateral |
| gen | general | LDL | low-density lipoprotein |
| gluc | glucose | liq | liquid |
| gr | grain | LLL | left lower lobe |
| GTT | glucose tolerance test | LOC | laxative of choice |
| gtt(s) | drop(s) | LP | lumbar puncture |
| gyn | gynecology | LS | lumbosacral |
| HA | heated aerosol | lytes | electrolytes |
| H$_2$O | water | LUL | left upper lobe |
| H$_2$O$_2$ | hydrogen peroxide | MAR | medication administration records |

| Abbreviation | Meaning | Abbreviation | Meaning |
|---|---|---|---|
| MD | doctor of medicine | po | by mouth or postoperative |
| MDI | metered dose inhaler | pp | postprandial (after meals) |
| mEq | milliequivalent | pr | per rectum |
| mg | milligram | prn | whenever necessary |
| MgSO | magnesium sulfate | PSA | prostatic specific antigen |
| MI | myocardial infarction | psa | patient support associate |
| min | minute | PT | physical therapy |
| mL | milliliter | Pt | patient |
| MN | midnight | PThC | percutaneous transhepatic cholangiography |
| MOM | milk of magnesia | | |
| MR | may repeat | PTCA | percutaneous transluminal coronary angioplasty |
| MRI | magnetic resonance imaging | | |
| MSO$^4$ or MS | morphine sulfate | P&PD | percussion and postural drainage |
| MSSU | medical short-stay unit | q | every |
| μg, mcg | microgram | q_h | every _ hours |
| N/V | nausea and vomiting | qd | daily |
| Na | sodium | qid | four times a day |
| NAHUC | National Association of Health Unit Coordinators | qod | every other day |
| | | R | rectal |
| NAS | no added salt | RD | registered dietitian |
| NG | nasogastric | RLL | right lower lobe |
| NINP | no information, no publication | R&M | routine and microscopic |
| NKA | no known allergies | RML | right middle lobe |
| noc | night | R/O | rule out |
| non rep | do not repeat | RBC | red blood cells |
| NPO | nothing by mouth | RDW | red cell distribution width |
| NS | normal saline | reg | regular |
| NSA | no salt added | RL | Ringer's lactate |
| NTG | nitroglycerin | ROM | range of motion |
| NWB | nonweight-bearing | RR | respiratory rate |
| O$_2$ | oxygen | RPR | rapid plasma reagin |
| OCG | oral cholecystogram | RSV | respiratory syncytial virus |
| OD | right eye | rt | right |
| OOB | out of bed | Rt | routine |
| ORE | oil retention enema | RUL | right upper lobe |
| OS | left eye | Rx | treatment |
| OSMO | osmolality | s̄ | without |
| OT | occupational therapy | SAD | save a day |
| OU | both eyes | SaO$_2$ | oxygen saturation (pulse oximetry) |
| oz or ℥ | ounce | SBFT | small-bowel follow-through |
| p̄ | after | SBU | small business unit |
| PACU | postanesthesia care unit | SC, sq, or sub-q | subcutaneous |
| PAP | prostatic acid phosphatase | SHUC | student health unit coordinator |
| PAS | pulsatile antiembolism stockings | SDS | same day surgery |
| PBZ | pyribenzamine | SOB | shortness of breath |
| pc | after meals | SL | sublingual |
| PCA | patient-controlled analgesia | SO$_4$ | sulfate |
| PCN | penicillin | sol'n | solution |
| PCT | patient care technician | SOS | if needed (one dose only) |
| PCXR | portable chest x-ray | s̄s̄ | one-half |
| PD | peritoneal dialysis | SSE | soap suds enema |
| PEG | percutaneous endoscopic gastrostomy | SSU | short-stay unit |
| | | st | straight |
| PEEP | positive end-expiratory pressure | stat | immediately |
| PET | positron emission tomography | subling | sublingual (under the tongue) |
| PICC | peripherally inserted central catheter | SVN | small volume nebulizer |
| | | T$_3$, T$_4$, T$_7$ | thyroid tests |
| PID | pelvic inflammatory disease | T&C | type and crossmatch |

| Abbreviation | Meaning | Abbreviation | Meaning |
|---|---|---|---|
| tab | tablet | TWE | tap water enema |
| TBD | to be done | Tx | traction |
| TBT | template bleeding time | U | unit |
| TCDB | turn, cough, and deep breathe | UA | urinalysis |
| TCT or TT | thrombin clotting time or thrombin time | UD | unit dose |
| | | US | ultrasound |
| TED | antiembolism stockings | USN | ultrasonic nebulizer |
| temp | temperature | VAD | venous access device |
| TENS | transcutaneous electrical nerve stimulation | VDRL | Venereal Disease Research Laboratories |
| TIA | transient ischemic attack | vib & perc | vibration and percussion |
| tid | three times a day | VMA | vanillylmandelic acid |
| tinct or tr | tincture | VNS | visiting nurse service |
| TKO | to keep open | VS | vital signs |
| TPN | total parenteral nutrition | WA | while awake |
| TPR | temperature, pulse, respiration | WBC | white blood cell |
| TRA | to run at | wk | week |
| T&S | type and screen | WP | whirlpool |
| TSH | thyroid-stimulating hormone | wt | weight |
| TT | tilt table | x-match | crossmatch |
| TUR | transurethral resection | Zn | zinc |

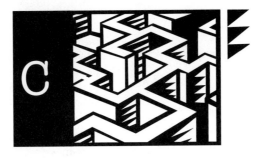

# THE NATIONAL ASSOCIATION OF HEALTH UNIT COORDINATORS STANDARDS OF PRACTICE*

A *standard of practice* is a statement of guidelines serving as a model of performance by which practitioners shall conduct their actions.

These standards are set forth to obtain the best possible service from practitioners to provide the organization and competency needed to coordinate the health unit in an exemplary fashion, enabling better care of the patient.

The National Association of Health Unit Coordinators (NAHUC) has formulated standards of practice fundamental enough to encompass all health units. NAHUC recognizes that these standards cannot be permanent. They will need to be evaluated and revised to keep pace with the advancement of technology and the health unit's changing objectives and functions.

## Purposes

The purpose of the NAHUC standards is to specify guidelines for health unit coordinators to follow. These standards have as their objectives:

1. To define the realm of the health unit coordinator in the health care system.
2. To specify the primary responsibilities of the health unit coordinator in the nonclinical area of health care.

## Basic Assumptions

The NAHUC standards for health unit coordinators are based on these assumptions:

1. Health unit coordinators provide the nondirect patient care or nonclinical functions for health services.
2. Standards for these services are established by the consensus of health unit coordinators and educators, and health care agencies.
3. Health unit coordinators accept basic responsibility for their competency through individual growth, continued education, and certification.

---

*Modified from National Association of Health Unit Coordinators, Standards of Practice, 1981, with permission.

4. Health unit coordinators are responsive to the changing needs of health care.

## Criteria for Statements of Standards

A standard is used as a model for the action of practitioners. Criteria used in establishing the NAHUC standards for health unit coordinators are:

1. A standard is established by an authority, in this instance, the National Association of Health Unit Coordinators.
2. A standard is founded on appropriate knowledge.
3. A standard is broad in scope, relevant, attainable, and definitive.
4. A standard is subject to continued evaluation and revision.

## Standards of Practice for Health Unit Coordinators

### Standard 1—Education

Health unit coordinators shall be prepared through appropriate education and training programs for their responsibility in the provision of nondirect patient care and nonclinical services.

#### Guidelines

Education shall be set forth by adopted NAHUC educational standards.

### Standard 2—Policy and Procedure

Written standards of health unit coordinator practice and related policies and procedures shall define and describe the scope and conduct of nonclinical service provided by the health unit coordinator staff. These standards, policies, and procedures shall be reviewed annually and revised as necessary. They shall be dated to indicate the last review, signed by the responsible authority, and implemented.

#### Guidelines

1. Policies shall include a criteria-based job description.
2. Personnel policies will be included.

3. Policies will include the philosophy and objectives of the health unit organization.
4. Operational and nonclinical policies and procedures will be included.

## Standard 3—Standards of Performance

Written evaluation of health unit coordinators shall be criteria-based and related to the standards of performance as defined by the health care organization.

### Guidelines

1. Standards of performance shall delineate functions, responsibility, qualifications, and accountability, reflecting autonomy of practice.
2. Standards of performance shall be reviewed and evaluated at least annually or as needed to reflect current job requirements.
3. Evaluations shall be available to health unit coordinators.

## Standard 4—Communication

The health unit coordinator shall appropriately integrate with the nursing and medical staff, other hospital staff, and visitors that contribute to patient care and well-being.

### Guidelines

1. The health unit shall have a written organizational plan that defines authority, accountability, and communication.
2. The organization shall ensure that health unit coordinator service functions are fulfilled.
3. Health unit coordinators' meetings shall be no fewer than six times a year to define problems and propose solutions and follow-up evaluations. A record shall be maintained documenting the monitoring and evaluation of these meetings.

## Standard 5—Professionalism and Ethics

The health unit coordinator shall take all possible steps to provide the optimal achievable quality of nondirect patient care and nonclinical services and to maintain the optimal professional and ethical conduct and practices of its members.

### Guidelines

1. The health unit coordinator shall participate in staff development.
2. He or she shall perform services according to approved policies.
3. The unit coordinator shall attend all required meetings.
4. He or she shall augment knowledge with pertinent new knowledge.
5.. The health unit coordinator shall maintain current competence.

## Standard 6—Leadership

The health unit coordinator service shall be organized to meet and maintain established standards of nonclinical services.

### Guidelines

1. The service shall be directed by a qualified individual with appropriate education, experience, and knowledge of health unit coordinator services.
2. It shall provide leadership and guidance to the health unit coordinator.
3. The service shall have the responsibility and authority to ensure:
   a. hospital policy and procedures are met
   b. hospital goals and objectives are met
   c. all responsible steps are taken to provide optimal achievable quality of nondirect patient care and nonclinical functions.
4. It is desirable that the health unit coordinator leader have an associate degree in health service management.

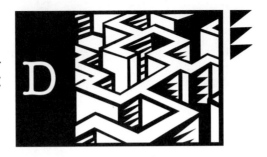

# A P P E N D I X  D

# TASK AND KNOWLEDGE STATEMENTS FROM NATIONAL ASSOCIATION OF HEALTH UNIT COORDINATORS JOB ANALYSIS STUDY, 1996

## Task Statements

Check charts for orders that need to be transcribed
Clarify questionable orders
Prioritize orders
Process orders according to priority
Enter orders on a Kardex
Interpret medical symbols/abbreviations
Initiate critical pathway protocols
Notify nursing staff of new orders
Notify and document consulting physicians of consult requests
Request services from ancillary departments
Request patient information from external facilities
Schedule diagnostic tests and procedures
Follow test preparation procedures
Enter orders onto a medication administration record
Indicate on the order sheet that each order has been processed
Sign off orders (e.g., signature, title, date, and time)
Flag charts for cosignature
Process daily diagnostic tests and procedures
Process nursing treatment orders
Label and assemble patient charts upon admission
Obtain patient information prior to admission
Assign beds to patients coming into the unit
Inform nursing staff of patient admissions, transfers, discharges, and returning surgical patients
Assemble necessary forms for patients being transferred to an external facility
Prepare patient charts for transfer to other units
Notify appropriate departments and individuals when patients are discharged (i.e., home, expired, AMA, transferred, etc.)
Disassemble patient charts, put in appropriate order, and send to medical records office upon expiration or discharge
Schedule follow-up appointments
Maintain a supply of chart forms
Maintain stock of patient care supplies and equipment
Maintain stock of clerical and desk supplies
Arrange for maintenance and repair of equipment

Maintain a hazard-free work environment
Report unit activities to oncoming shift
Maintain patient census logs
Maintain patient charts by thinning and adding forms as needed
File forms and reports
Graph and chart information onto appropriate forms
Maintain patient census board
Prepare surgical charts
Process postoperative charts
Perform quality assurance activities on charts (i.e., verify chart forms are filed/labeled correctly, all orders transcribed, etc.)
Participate in emergency and disaster plans
Participate in response to cardiac or respiratory arrests (i.e., page codes, call physicians, etc.)
Orient new staff members to the unit
Process patient charges
Receive diagnostic test results
Notify physicians of diagnostic test results
Report diagnostic test results to nursing staff
Communicate facility policies to visitors, patients, and staff (i.e., visiting hours, no smoking, etc.)
Screen telephone calls and visitor requests for patient information to protect patient confidentiality
Restrict access to patient information (i.e., charts, computer)
Greet patients, physicians, visitors, and facility staff who arrive on the unit
Transport patient specimens, supplies, and medications
Respond to patient, physician, visitor, and facility staff requests and complaints
Communicate with patients and staff via intercom
Send and receive documents via fax machine
Duplicate documents using copy machine
Maintain computer census (i.e., ADT functions)
Retrieve diagnostic results from computer
Follow established computer downtime procedures
Contact personnel via paging system
Answer unit telephone calls
Enter orders via computer
Generate reports using computer

Participate in department, staff, or health unit coordinator meetings

Review facility-specific publications, memos, policies, etc.

## Knowledge Statements

Knowledge of the components of a physician's order

Knowledge of the use of flagging a chart for indicating there are orders to be transcribed

Knowledge of the need to frequently check charts for new orders

Knowledge of the procedures for the transcription of orders

Knowledge of prioritization of medical conditions or situations

Knowledge of the definition of terms regarding priorities

Knowledge of problem-solving techniques

Knowledge of the methods used in problem identification

Knowledge of the roles and functions of the health care staff

Knowledge of basic medical terminology

Knowledge of basic medical symbols

Knowledge of basic medical abbreviations

Knowledge of how to handle stat orders

Knowledge of the proper response time for processing stat orders

Knowledge of the purpose of documentation

Knowledge of placement of forms and reports in a chart

Knowledge of times for diagnostic tests and medication deliveries

Knowledge of how to handle routine orders

Knowledge of the proper response time for processing orders

Knowledge of the procedures used to process orders that are outside routine time frames

Knowledge of the operating hours of ancillary departments

Knowledge of the procedures to follow to obtain services from ancillary departments

Knowledge of procedures used to order services, diagnostics, and medications

Knowledge of military time conversions

Knowledge of the names and functions of ancillary departments

Knowledge of the various methods used to communicate orders

Knowledge of documentation methods

Knowledge of medical staff privileges

Knowledge of when to use references

Knowledge of routine times diagnostic tests are performed

Knowledge of how to use references

Knowledge of the location of standard chart forms in the patient record

Knowledge of the methods used to enter into and retrieve information from the order entry computer screen

Knowledge of basic computer terminology

Knowledge of types of medical equipment

Knowledge of pertinent information needed prior to admission

Knowledge of the use of telephone equipment

Knowledge of the techniques used in telephone communication

Knowledge of the purpose of different forms

Knowledge of basic diagnostic terms

Knowledge of the methods used to obtain blood and blood products

Knowledge of the equivalencies between apothecary and metric dosages

Knowledge of dosages of common medications

Knowledge of the components of the Kardex

Knowledge of the components of a medication administration record

Knowledge of the components of a medication order

Knowledge of generic and trade names for common medications

Knowledge of the classifications of medications

Knowledge of procedures for renewal of medication orders

Knowledge of policies and procedures for amount of stock to be kept on the unit

Knowledge of policies and procedures for ordering replacement stock

Knowledge of procedures for proper and safe storage of unit supplies and equipment

Knowledge of policies and procedures for maintenance and repair of equipment

Knowledge of procedures for proper and safe storage of medications

Knowledge of facility's policies regarding transporting and handling of medications

Knowledge of safe and unsafe work conditions

Knowledge of infection control policies and procedures

Knowledge of the policies and procedures used to ensure the safety of staff, patients, and visitors on the unit

Knowledge of professional demeanor

Knowledge of the effects of power outages on telephone use

Knowledge of the methods used to respond to emergency telephone calls

Knowledge of the use of the patient intercom system

Knowledge of the techniques used in intercom communication

Knowledge of patient placement procedures

Knowledge of the circumstances under which the intercom should be used

Knowledge of the definition of confidentiality

Knowledge of patient's rights

Knowledge of circumstances that constitute breaches of confidentiality

Knowledge of policies and procedures regarding confidentiality

Knowledge of the standards of practice and code of ethics for health unit coordinating

Knowledge of verbal and nonverbal communication techniques

Knowledge of the components of a patient census log

Knowledge of the purpose of a census log

Knowledge of the classification of patient acuity

Knowledge of the purposes of compiling patient and unit statistics

Knowledge of the tools used to determine patient acuity

Knowledge of the purpose of the chart maintenance

Knowledge of procedures for maintaining charts

Knowledge of the methods used to organize information

Knowledge of the methods used to place forms and reports in a logical order

Knowledge of the methods used to stamp, label, or identify the patient's chart

Knowledge of the proper use of office equipment

Knowledge of the function of the patient census board

Knowledge of bed assignment methods

Knowledge of the normal and abnormal values for common diagnostic tests

Knowledge of the policies and procedures for discontinuing all preoperative orders postoperatively

Knowledge of importance of discontinuing all preoperative orders postoperatively

Knowledge of the process used to transcribe orders for transfusion of blood and blood products

Knowledge of the process used to transcribe orders for total parenteral nutrition/hyperalimentation

Knowledge of quality assurance policies and procedures

Knowledge of policies and procedures regarding emergency and disaster plans

Knowledge of the procedures for cardiac monitoring

Knowledge of the policies and procedures for posting informational materials

Knowledge of the procedures for orienting new personnel

Knowledge of the methods used to evaluate the competency of orientees

Knowledge of the methods used to ensure unit's accountability regarding patient charges

Knowledge of the methods used to indicate the services and supplies used by each patient

Knowledge of services provided by outside vendors and agencies

Knowledge of the unit coordinator's responsibility to participate in job-related training

Knowledge of the importance of keeping abreast of job-related changes

Knowledge of the different types of diagnostic tests

Knowledge of procedures to obtain services and supplies from outside sources

Knowledge of patient chart locations on the unit

Knowledge of routes of common medications

Knowledge of stop dates of common medications

Knowledge of chain of communication for clarification of orders

Knowledge of conflicting patient conditions and procedures

Knowledge of the location of general information on the Kardex

Knowledge of the term "critical pathway"

Knowledge of general diagnoses and pathways

Knowledge of coordination of services from multiple ancillary departments

Knowledge of the definition of stop dates

Knowledge of the use of paging system

Knowledge of information retrieval system

Knowledge of the purpose of processing patient charges

Knowledge of the policies and procedures for processing patient charges

Knowledge of pertinent information to request services from ancillary departments

Knowledge of reviewing standing orders

Knowledge of pertinent information to schedule follow-up appointments

Knowledge of pertinent information necessary to maintain patient census log

Knowledge of pertinent information necessary to maintain patient census board

Knowledge of pertinent information when preparing a surgical chart

Knowledge of pertinent information to process postoperative chart

Knowledge of pertinent information to participate in emergency and disaster plans

Knowledge of pertinent information to participate in arrest situations

Knowledge of pertinent information used to orient new staff members

Knowledge of pertinent information in diagnostic test results

Knowledge of pertinent information that needs to be communicated to patients, staff, and visitors

Knowledge of universal precautions

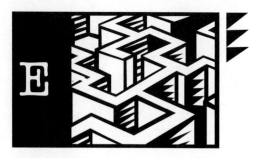

# NATIONAL ASSOCIATION OF HEALTH UNIT COORDINATORS: CODE OF ETHICS

This code of ethics is to serve as a guide by which health unit coordinators may evaluate their professional conduct as it relates to patients, colleagues, and other members of the health care profession. This code of ethics shall be subject to monitoring, interpretation, and periodic revision by the association's board of directors.

Therefore, in the practice of our profession, we the members of the National Association of Health Unit Coordinators accept the following principles:

### Principle One

All members shall conduct themselves in such a manner as to gain the respect and confidence of the patients, health care personnel, and the community, as well as respecting the human dignity of each individual.

### Principle Two

All members shall protect the patients' rights, including the right to privacy.

### Principle Three

All members shall strive to achieve and maintain a high level of competency.

### Principle Four

All members shall strive to improve their knowledge and skills by participating in educational and professional activities and sharing the benefits of their attainments with their colleagues.

### Principle Five

Unethical and illegal professional activities shall be reported to the appropriate authorities.

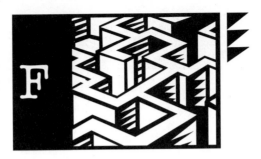

# APPENDIX F

# A COMPREHENSIVE LIST OF LABORATORY STUDIES AND BLOOD COMPONENTS*

| Procedure | Abbreviation | Laboratory Division | Specimen[†] |
|---|---|---|---|
| ABO grouping (complete blood type) | | Blood bank | Blood |
| Acetoacetic acid | | Urinalysis | Urine |
| Acetone | | Chemistry | Blood or urine |
| Acid-fast culture | Culture for AFB (acid-fast bacilli) | Bacteriology | Sputum and tubercular lesions |
| Acid-fast stain | | Bacteriology | Sputum and tubercular lesions |
| Acid phosphatase | acid p'tase | Chemistry | Blood |
| Activated partial thromboplastin time | APTT | Hematology/coagulation | Blood |
| Addis count | | Urinalysis | Urine |
| Adrenaline and noradrenaline (see epinephrine and norepinephrine) | | | |
| Adrenocorticotropic hormone | ACTH | Chemistry or special chemistry | Blood |
| Alanine aminotransferase | ALT | Chemistry | Blood |
| Albumin | Alb. | Chemistry | Blood or urine |
| Alcohol (ethanol) | | Chemistry | Blood |
| Aldolase | | Chemistry or special chemistry | Blood |
| Aldosterone | | Chemistry or special chemistry | Blood or urine |
| Alkaline phosphatase | Alk. phos. | Chemistry | Blood |
| Alkaline phosphatase isoenzymes | | Chemistry | Blood |
| $\alpha_1$-Antitrypsin | | Chemistry | Blood |
| $\alpha_1$-Fetoprotein | | Chemistry or special chemistry | Blood |
| 17 $\alpha$-Hydroxyprogesterone | | Chemistry | Urine |
| Amino acids, fractionated | | Chemistry | Urine |
| Ammonia | $NH_3$ | Chemistry | Blood |
| Amniotic fluid | | Chemistry | Amniotic fluid |
| Amoeba (ova and parasites) | O&P | Parasitology | Stool |
| Amphotericin level | | Chemistry | Blood |
| Amylase | | Chemistry | Blood or urine |
| Androstenedione | | Chemistry | Urine |
| Ankylosing spondylitis (see HLA B27 typing) | | | |
| Antideoxyribonuclease | DNA | Serology | Blood |
| Antigen blood group (factor VIII) | | Serology | Blood |
| Antimicrobial serum assay | | Bacteriology | Blood |
| Antimony | | Chemistry | Urine |
| Antinuclear antibody | ANA | Serology | Blood |
| Antistreptolysin O | ASO titer | Serology | Blood |
| Antithyroglobin antibody | | Serology or special chemistry | Blood |

*The divisions indicated on this chart would be those found in a large hospital. Space has been left at the end of each alphabetical section so that you can insert new tests as they are developed.

[†]To simplify the specimen column, the term *blood* is used even when the test is performed only on blood serum.

| Procedure | Abbreviation | Laboratory Division | Specimen |
|---|---|---|---|
| Arsenic, quantitative | | Chemistry | Urine |
| Ascorbic acid | | Chemistry | Blood |
| Aspartate aminotransferase | AST | Chemistry | Blood |
| Barbiturates | | Chemistry | Blood or urine |
| Bence Jones proteins | BJP | Chemistry | Urine |
| Complement | $C_3$ | Chemistry | Blood |
| $\beta_2$-Microglobulin | | Chemistry | Blood |
| β-Hemolytic strep culture | | Bacteriology | Nose or throat culture |
| Bile | | Urinalysis/feces | Urine or stool |
| Bilirubin (total and direct) | bili | Chemistry | Blood |
| Biopsy | | Surgical pathology | All specimens |
| Bleeding time | | Hematology/coagulation | Blood |
| Blood culture | | Bacteriology | Blood |
| Blood sugar (glucose random) | BS | Chemistry | Blood |
| Blood survey of coagulation defects | | Hematology/coagulation | Blood |
| Blood type (ABO and Rh) | | Blood bank | Blood |
| Blood type and crossmatch | T&C, T&X-match | Blood bank | Blood |
| Blood urea nitrogen | BUN | Chemistry | Blood |
| Blood volume (Cr 51) | | Chemistry or special chemistry | Blood |
| Blood volume (Risa) | | Chemistry or special chemistry | Blood |
| Bone marrow examination | | Hematology | Bone marrow |
| Bromide | | Chemistry | Blood |
| Bromsulphalein | BSP | Chemistry | Blood |
| Bronchial smear—Gram stain | | Bacteriology | Bronchial smear |
| Brucella abortus | | Serology | Blood |
| Buccal smear—sex chromosones | | Cytology | Buccal smear |
| Calcitonin | | Chemistry or special chemistry | Blood |
| Calcium | Ca | Chemistry | Blood or urine |
| Calcium ionized | | Chemistry | Blood |
| Capillary fragility | | Hematology | Blood |
| Carbon dioxide | $CO_2$ | Chemistry | Blood |
| Carbon monoxide | CO | Chemistry | Blood |
| Carboxyhemoglobin | | Chemistry | Blood |
| Carcinoembryonic antigen | CEA | Serology | Blood |
| Cardiac enzymes (CPK, LDH, SGOT) | | Chemistry | Blood |
| Carotene | | Chemistry | Blood |
| Catecholamines (blood) | | Chemistry | Blood |
| Catecholamines (urine) | | Chemistry | Urine |
| Cell indices | RBC indices | Hematology | Blood |
| Cerebrospinal fluid tests | CSF | Hematology, chemistry, and bacteriology | Cerebrospinal fluid |
| Ceruloplasmin (see ferroxidase) | | | |
| Cervical and vaginal smear (Pap test) | | Cytology | Cells from cervix and vagina |
| Chlamydia culture | | Bacteriology | Swabs from specified areas |
| Chlamydia serology | | Serology | Blood |
| Choral hydrate | | Chemistry | Blood |
| Chloramphenicol level | | Chemistry | Blood |
| Chloride | Cl | Chemistry | Blood, CSF, sweat, and urine |
| Cholesterol | Chol | Chemistry | Blood |
| Cholinesterase | | Chemistry | Blood |
| Chorionic gonadotropin (serum) | HCG | Chemistry or special chemistry | Blood serum |
| Chorionic gonadotropin (urine) | HCG | Urinalysis | Urine |
| Chorionic gonadotropin (24-hour urine) | HCG | Chemistry or special chemistry | Urine—24-hour |
| Chromium 51 (blood volume) | | Hematoloy or special chemistry | Blood |
| Chromosome study (buccal smear) | | Cytology | Buccal smear |
| Chromosome study | | Chemistry | Blood—tissue |

| Procedure | Abbreviation | Laboratory Division | Specimen |
|---|---|---|---|
| Citric acid | | Chemistry | Urine |
| Clot retraction | | Hematology/coagulation | Blood |
| Clotting time (coagulation time) | Coag. time or Lee-White | Hematology/coagulation | Blood |
| CMV (cytomegalovirus) culture | CMV culture | Bacteriology | Blood or urine |
| CMV (cytomegalovirus) inclusions | CMV inclusions | Bacteriology | Blood or urine |
| CMV (cytomegalovirus) serology | CMV serology | Serology | Blood |
| Coagulation profile (platelets, APTT, prothrombin time, and bleeding time) | | Hematology/coagulation | Blood |
| Coagulation time, clotting time, thrombin clotting time, thrombin time | Coag. time, TCT, TT | Hematology/coagulation | Blood |
| Cocci culture (fungus) | | Bacteriology | Sputum |
| *Coccidioides*, complement fixation | | Serology | Blood |
| *Coccidioides*, precipitin | | Serology | Blood |
| Coccidioidomycosis—CSF titer | | Serology | Cerebrospinal fluid |
| Cold agglutinins | | Serology | Blood |
| Colloidal gold curve | | Serology | Cerebrospinal fluid |
| Colony count | | Bacteriology | Body fluids |
| Complete blood count | CBC | Hematology | Blood |
| Complete urinalysis | UA | Urinalysis | Urine |
| Coombs' test—direct/indirect | | Blood bank | Blood |
| Copper | | Chemistry | Blood |
| Coproporphyrins | | Chemistry | Urine |
| Cord blood (grouping, Rh, and direct Coombs') | | Blood bank | Blood |
| Corticosterone | | Chemistry or special chemistry | Blood or urine |
| Cortisol (compound F) | | Chemistry | Blood or urine |
| Cortisol (compound S) | | Chemistry | Blood or urine |
| Creatine | | Chemistry | Blood |
| Creatinine | | Chemistry | Blood |
| Creatinine clearance | | Chemistry | Blood and urine |
| Creatine phosphokinase | CPK or CK | Chemistry | Blood |
| Creatine phosphokinase isoenzyme | CPK Iso. or CK Iso. | Chemistry | Blood |
| Creatinine urine | | Chemistry | Urine |
| *Cryptococcus* stain (India ink) | | Microbiology | Cerebrospinal fluid |
| Culture (routine) | C&S | Bacteriology | Any body fluid |
| Cyanocobalamin (see Schilling test) | | | |
| Cystine | | Chemistry | Urine |
| Cytology smears | | Cytology | Any body cells |
| Cytotoxic antibodies | | Blood bank | Blood |
| Dehydroepiandrosterone | DHEA | Chemistry or special chemistry | Blood or urine |
| Deoxycorticosterone | | Chemistry or special chemistry | Blood or urine |
| 11-Deoxycortisols (compound S) | | Chemistry or special chemistry | Blood or urine |
| Diacetic acid (see acetoacetic acid) | | | |
| Differential cell count | Diff. | Hematology | Blood |
| Digitoxin level | | Chemistry or special chemistry | Blood |
| Digoxin level | | Chemistry or special chemistry | Blood |
| Dihydrotestosterone | DHT | Chemistry or special chemistry | Blood |
| Dilantin level | | Chemistry or special chemistry | Blood |
| Direct Coombs' (direct antiglobulin) test | DAT | Blood bank | Blood |
| Drug screen | | Chemistry | Blood or urine |
| D-Xylose | | Chemistry | Blood or urine |
| Electrolytes | Lytes-E'lytes | Chemistry | Blood |
| Electrophoresis, Hb | | Chemistry | Blood |
| Electrophoresis, Immuno. | | Chemistry | Blood |
| Electrophoresis, Lipids | | Chemistry | Blood |
| Electrophoresis, Lipoprotein | | Chemistry | Blood |
| Electrophoresis, Protein | Protein ELP | Chemistry | Blood |

| Procedure | Abbreviation | Laboratory Division | Specimen |
|---|---|---|---|
| Enterovirus | | Virology | Stool |
| Eosinophils | | Hematology | Blood |
| Epinephrine and norepinephrine (catecholamines) | | Chemistry | Urine |
| Erythrocyte sedimentation rate | ESR | Hematology | Blood |
| Esophageal cytology | | Cytology | Cells from esophagus |
| 17β-Estradiol (E₂) | | Chemistry or special chemistry | Urine |
| Estrogen receptor assay | | Chemistry or special chemistry | Urine |
| Estrogens, E₁, E₂ (estrone, 17β-estradiol) | | Chemistry or special chemistry | Urine |
| Ethyl alcohol, blood | | Chemistry | Blood |
| Euglobulin clot lysis | | Hematology/coagulation | Blood |
| Factor assay (specify factor) | | Hematology/coagulation | Blood |
| Factor identifying test | | Hematology/coagulation | Blood |
| Fasting blood sugar (glucose, fasting) | FBS | Chemistry | Blood |
| Febrile agglutinins | | Serology | Blood |
| Fecal fat, quantitative | | Chemistry | Stool |
| Ferroxidase | | Chemistry | Blood |
| Fibrin split products screen | FSP | Hematology/coagulation | Blood |
| Fibrindex | | Hematology/coagulation | Blood |
| Fibrinogen level | | Hematology/coagulation | Blood |
| Fibrinolysin | | Hematology/coagulation | Blood |
| Fluorescent treponemal antibody | FTA | Serology | Blood |
| Folate (folic acid) | | Chemistry or special chemistry | Blood |
| Follicle-stimulating hormone | FSH | Chemistry or special chemistry | Urine (24-hour) |
| Fractionated alkaline phosphatase | | Chemistry | Blood |
| Free fatty acids | FFA | Chemistry | Blood |
| Free thyroxine index | T₇ | Chemistry or special chemistry | Blood |
| Fresh frozen plasma | FFP | Blood bank | Blood |
| Frozen cells | | Blood bank | Blood |
| Frozen section | FS | Surgical pathology | Any body tissue |
| Fungus culture | | Bacteriology | Body specimen |
| Fungus serology | | Serology | Blood |
| Fungus smear | | Cytology | Body specimen |
| Galactose, qualitative | | Urinalysis | Urine |
| Gallium | | Special chemistry | Urine |
| γ-Globulin (serum) | | Chemistry | Blood |
| γ-Glutamyl transpeptidase | GGT | Chemistry | Blood |
| Gastric analysis | | Chemistry or gastroenterology | Gastric fluid |
| Gastric cytology | | Cytology | Gastric fluid |
| Gastric washings (TB/AFB) | | Bacteriology | Gastric fluid |
| Gastrin | | Chemistry or special chemistry | Blood |
| Gentamicin serum level | | Chemistry or special chemistry | Blood |
| Globulin (total protein & albumin) | | Chemistry | Blood |
| Glucose | | Chemistry or urinalysis | Blood or urine |
| Glucose (CSF) | | Chemistry | Cerebrospinal fluid |
| Glucose, fasting | FBS | Chemistry | Blood |
| Glucose, 2-hour postprandial | 2 h PP BS | Chemistry | Blood |
| Glucose, random | BS | Chemistry | Blood |
| Glucose tolerance test | GTT | Chemistry | Blood or urine |
| Glycosylated hemoglobin | HbA₁c | Chemistry | Blood |
| Gram stain (smear) | | Bacteriology | Any body fluid |
| Growth hormone | GH or HGH | Chemistry or special chemistry | Blood |
| Guaiac | | Urinalysis/feces | Urine or stool |
| Guthrie test (serum phenylalanine) | PKU | Chemistry | Blood |
| Hanging drop prep (*Trichomonas*) | | Bacteriology | Vaginal smear |
| Haptoglobins | | Chemistry | Blood |
| Heavy metals | | Chemistry | Urine |
| Hemoglobin | Hgb | Hematology | Blood |
| Hematocrit | Hct, Crit | Hematology | Blood |
| Hemoglobin electrophoresis | | Chemistry | Blood |

| Procedure | Abbreviation | Laboratory Division | Specimen |
|---|---|---|---|
| Hemosiderin | | Chemistry | Urine |
| Hepatitis A antibody | anti-HAV | Special chemistry or serology | Blood |
| Hepatitis B core antibody | anti-HB$_c$Ag | Special chemistry or serology | Blood |
| Hepatitis B surface antigen | HB$_s$Ag | Special chemistry or serology | Blood |
| Hepatitis B surface antibody | anti-HB$_s$Ag | Special chemistry or serology | Blood |
| Hepatitis screen (acute) | | Special chemistry or serology | Blood |
| Herpes serology | | Serology/microbiology | Blood |
| Herpes smear | | Microbiology | Smear of specified area |
| Heterophil antibodies screen | | Serology | Blood |
| Homovanillic acid | HVA | Chemistry | Urine |
| High-density lipoproteins | HDL | Chemistry | Blood |
| *Histoplasma*, culture | | Bacteriology | Sputum |
| *Histoplasma*, serology | | Serology | Blood |
| HLA B27 typing | | Blood bank | Blood |
| Human chorionic gonadotropin | HCG | Special chemistry | Blood |
| Human immunodeficiency virus | HIV | Serology | Blood |
| Hydroxybutyrate dehydrogenase | HBD | Chemistry | Blood |
| 17-Hydroxycorticosteroids | | Chemistry | Urine |
| Human placental lactogen | HPL | Chemistry or special chemistry | Urine |
| 5-Hydroxyindoleacetic acid | 5-HIAA | Chemistry | Blood or urine |
| 17-Hydroxysteroids (see 17-hydroxycorticosteroids) | | | |
| Icterus index | | Chemistry | Blood |
| Immunodiffusion | | Chemistry | Blood |
| Immunoglobulin A | IgA | Chemistry | Blood |
| Immunoglobulin E | IgE | Chemistry | Blood |
| Immunoglobulin G | IgG | Chemistry | Blood |
| Immunoglobulin M | IgM | Chemistry | Blood |
| Immunoelectrophoresis | IEP | Chemistry | Blood |
| Immunologic pregnancy test | HCG | Urinalysis | Urine (morning specimen) |
| India ink test | | Bacteriology | Cerebrospinal fluid |
| Indices, red blood cells | RBC indices | Hematology | Blood |
| Indirect Coombs' | | Blood bank | Blood |
| Insulin tolerance test | ITT | Chemistry or special chemistry | Blood |
| Iodine uptake | $^{131}$I | Chemistry or special chemistry | Blood |
| Iontophoresis (sweat electrolytes) | | Chemistry | Sweat |
| Iron | Fe | Chemistry | Blood |
| Iron-binding capacity | IBC | Chemistry | Blood |
| Isocitrate dehydrogenase | ICD | Chemistry | Blood |
| Ivy bleeding time | Bl. time | Hematology/coagulation | Blood |
| 17-Ketogenic steroids | 17 KGS | Chemistry | Blood or urine |
| Ketones (acetone) | | Urinalysis or chemistry | Urine or blood |
| 17-Ketosteroids | 17 KS | Chemistry | Blood or urine |
| K&L chains (Bence Jones proteins) | | Chemistry | Urine |
| Lactate (lactic acid) | | Chemistry | Blood |
| Lactate dehydrogenase | LDH | Chemistry | Blood or cerebrospinal fluid |
| Lactate dehydrogenase isoenzymes | LDH Iso. | Chemistry | Blood |
| Lactose tolerance test | | Chemistry or gastroenterology | Blood |
| Lead | | Chemistry | Blood or urine |
| LE cell prep (see lupus erythematosus) | | | |
| Lee-White coagulation time | Coag. time or Lee-White | Hematology/coagulation | Blood |
| *Legionella* culture (Legionnaires' disease) | | Microbiology | Bronchial washing |
| *Legionella* serology | | Serology/microbiology | Blood |
| *Leptospira* culture | | Bacteriology | Urine |
| Leucine aminopeptidase (also called cytosol aminopeptidase) | LAP | Chemistry | Blood or urine |
| Leukocyte alkaline phosphatase | | Hematology | Blood |

| Procedure | Abbreviation | Laboratory Division | Specimen |
|---|---|---|---|
| Leukocyte count (see white blood cell count) | | | |
| Librium level (chlordiazepoxide) | | Chemistry | Blood |
| Lipase | | Chemistry | Blood |
| Lipid phenotype | | Chemistry | Blood |
| Lipoprotein electrophoresis | | Chemistry | Blood |
| Lithium level | Li | Chemistry | Blood |
| Lupus erythematosus | LE cell prep. | Hematology | Blood |
| Luteinizing hormone | LH | Chemistry or special chemistry | Blood |
| Luteinizing hormone-releasing factor | LHRF | Chemistry or special chemistry | Blood |
| Macroglobulin | | Chemistry | Blood |
| Magnesium | Mg | Chemistry | Blood |
| Melanin | | Urinalysis or chemistry | Urine |
| Mercury | Hg | Chemistry | Urine |
| Metanephrine | | Chemistry | Urine |
| Methemoglobin | | Chemistry | Blood |
| Microglobulin $\beta_2$ (see $\beta_2$-microglobulin) | | | |
| Mixed lymphocyte culture | | Serology | Blood |
| Monospot (see heterophil antibodies screen) | | | |
| Myoglobin | | Chemistry | Urine |
| Neutral fat (lipid profile fractionation) | | Chemistry or gastroenterology | Blood |
| Nasopharyngeal culture | N-P culture | Bacteriology | Nose swab |
| 5'-Nucleotidase | | Chemistry or special chemistry | Blood |
| Occult blood | | Urinalysis/feces | Urine or stool |
| 17-OH corticosteroids (see 17-hydroxycorticosteroids) | | | |
| Orinase tolerance test | | Chemistry | Blood |
| Osmolality | | Chemistry | Blood or urine |
| Osmotic fragility, RBC's | | Hematology | Blood |
| Ova and parasites | O&P | Parasitology | Stool |
| Packed cells (see hematocrit) | | | |
| Pancreatic cytology | | Cytology | Pancreatic fluid |
| Pap smears and stains | | Cytology | Many body areas, such as cervix and stomach |
| Parasites, schistosomes | | Parasitology | Stools or urine |
| Parathyroid hormone | PTH | Chemistry or special chemistry | Blood |
| Parathyroid A&B | | Chemistry | Blood |
| Partial thromboplastin time | PTT | Hematology/coagulation | Blood |
| Peritoneal fluid smear | | Cytology | Peritoneal fluid |
| pH | | Chemistry | Blood, urine, or stool |
| Phenobarbital level | | Chemistry | Blood |
| Phenolsulfonphthalein | PSP | Chemistry | Urine |
| Phenothiazine level | | Chemistry | Blood or urine |
| Phenylalanine (see Guthrie test) | | | |
| Phospholipids | | Chemistry or gastroenterology | Blood |
| Phosphate | $PO_4$ | Chemistry | Blood or urine |
| Phosphatase, acid (see acid phosphatase) | | | |
| Phospatase, alkaline (see alkaline phosphatase) | | | |
| Pinworm | | Parasitology | Scotch tape prep. |
| Pituitary gonadotropin | FSH | Chemistry or special chemistry | Blood |
| Placental lactogen, human | HPL | Chemistry or special chemistry | Urine |
| Plasma cortisol | | Chemistry or special chemistry | Blood |
| Plasma osmolality | | Chemistry | Blood |
| Platelet adhesion study | | Hematology/coagulation | Blood |
| Platelet aggregation | | Hematology/coagulation | Blood |

| Procedure | Abbreviation | Laboratory Division | Specimen |
|---|---|---|---|
| Platelet concentrate | | Blood bank | Blood |
| Platelet count | | Hematology | Blood |
| Porphobilinogen | | Chemistry | Urine |
| Porphyrins | | Chemistry | Urine |
| Porter-Silber chromogens (see 17-hydroxycorticosteroids) | | | |
| Potassium | K | Chemistry | Blood or urine |
| Pregnanediol | | Chemistry | Urine |
| Pregnanetriol | | Chemistry | Urine |
| Progesterone | | Chemistry or special chemistry | Blood or urine |
| Prolactin | | Chemistry or special chemistry | Blood |
| Pronestyl level (procainamide) | | Chemistry or special chemistry | Blood |
| Prostate specific antigen | PSA | Chemistry | Blood |
| Prostatic acid phosphatase | PAP | Chemistry | Blood |
| Protein (cerebrospinal fluid) | | Chemistry | Cerebrospinal fluid |
| Protein (urine) | | Urinalysis | Urine |
| Protein electrophoresis | | Chemistry | Blood |
| Protein-bound iodine | PBI | Chemistry or special chemistry | Blood |
| Protein, total | | Chemistry | Blood |
| *Proteus* Ox-19 | | Serology | Blood |
| Prothrombin time | PT, pro-time | Coagulation | Blood |
| Quantitative urine culture (colony count) | | Bacteriology | Urine |
| Quinidine level | | Chemistry or special chemistry | Urine |
| Rapid plasma reagin | RPR | Serology | Blood |
| Red blood cells | RBC | Hematology | Blood |
| Red cell distribution width | RDW | Hematology | Blood |
| Red cell fragility | | Hematology | Blood |
| Red cell indices | RBC indices | Hematology | Blood |
| Red cell morphology | RBC morph. | Hematology | Blood |
| Red cell survival | | Chemistry or special chemistry | Blood |
| Renin | | Chemistry or special chemistry | Blood |
| Respiratory virus | | Virology | Blood |
| Reticulocyte count | Retics | Hematology | Blood |
| RH factor | | Blood bank | Blood |
| RH globulin work-up | | Blood bank | Blood |
| Rheumatoid factor | RA | Serology | Blood |
| Rubella antibody | | Serology | Blood |
| Rubella, culture | | Bacteriology | Blood |
| Rubeola, culture | | Bacteriology | Blood |
| Salicylate level | | Chemistry | Blood or urine |
| Schilling test | | Chemistry or special chemistry | Urine |
| Secretin | | Chemistry or special chemistry | Duodenal secretions |
| Secretin with pancreatic cytology | | Cytology or gastroenterology | Duodenal secretions |
| Semen | | Urinalysis | Semen |
| Serotonin, serum | | Chemistry | Blood |
| Serotonin, urine | 5-HIAA | Chemistry | Urine |
| Serum protein electrophoresis | SPE | Chemistry | Blood |
| Serum glutamic-oxaloacetic transaminase | SGOT | Chemistry | Blood or cerebrospinal fluid |
| Serum glutamic-pyruvic transaminase | SGPT | Chemistry | Blood |
| Sickle cell prep | | Hematology | Blood |
| Sequential multiple analysis | $SMA_6$, $SMA_{12}$, $SMA_{20}$ | Chemistry | Blood |
| Sodium | Na | Chemistry | Blood, urine, or sweat |
| Sputum, culture | | Bacteriology | Sputum |
| Stool, culture | | Bacteriology | Stool |
| Stool for ova and parasites | O&P | Microbiology | Stool |
| Strychnine | | Chemistry | Urine |
| Sulfa level | | Chemistry | Blood |
| Sweat chloride | | Chemistry | Sweat |
| Sweat electrolytes (Na & Cl) | | Chemistry | Sweat |

| Procedure | Abbreviation | Laboratory Division | Specimen |
|---|---|---|---|
| Triiodothyronine resin uptake | $T_3$ | Chemistry or special chemistry | Blood |
| Thyroxine | $T_4$ | Chemistry or special chemistry | Blood |
| Tuberculosis culture | | Bacteriology | Sputum, urine, or cerebrospinal fluid |
| Tegretol level (carbamazepine) | | Chemistry or special chemistry | Blood or urine |
| Testosterone | | Chemistry or special chemistry | Blood |
| Theophylline level | | Chemistry or special chemistry | Blood |
| Thrombin clotting time | TCT | Hematology/coagulation | Blood |
| Thromboplastin time, activated partial (see activated partial thromboplastin time) | | | |
| Thyroid antibody titer | TAT | Serology or special chemistry | Blood |
| Thyroid globulin antibody | | Serology or special chemistry | Blood |
| Thyroid-binding globulin | TBG | Chemistry or special chemistry | Blood |
| Thyroid-stimulating hormone | TSH | Chemistry or special chemistry | Blood |
| Tobramycin level | | Chemistry | Blood |
| Total lipids | | Chemistry or gastroenterology | Blood |
| Total protein | TP | Chemistry | Blood, urine, or cerebrospinal fluid |
| Toxicology screen | | Chemistry | Blood, urine, or gastric contents |
| *Toxoplasma* | | Serology | Blood |
| Triglycerides | | Chemistry | Blood |
| | | Bacteriology | Blood |
| Typhoid o&h | | Bacteriology | Blood |
| Urea clearance | | Chemistry | Blood or urine |
| Urea nitrogen | BUN | Chemistry | Blood or urine |
| Uric acid | | Chemistry | Blood or urine |
| Urinalysis | UA | Urinalysis | Urine |
| Urobilinogen | | Urinalysis/feces | Urine or stool |
| Uroporphyrins | | Chemistry | Urine |
| Vaginal smear | | Cytology | Vaginal smear |
| Vanillylmandelic acid | VMA | Chemistry | Urine |
| Venereal Disease Research Laboratories | VDRL | Serology | Blood |
| Vitamin $B_{12}$ (see Schilling test) | | | |
| Washed cells | | Blood bank | Blood |
| White blood cell count | WBC | Hematology | Blood |
| Whole blood | | Blood bank | Blood |
| Wound culture | | Bacteriology | Any wound |

# ANSWERS

## CHAPTER 1

### Exercises

#### Exercise 1

1. CHUC
2. HUC
3. SBU
4. SHUC
5. Pt

#### Exercise 2

1. certified health unit coordinator
2. health unit coordinator
3. strategic business unit
4. student health unit coordinator
5. patient

### Review Questions

1. a. tasks performed at the bedside
   b. tasks performed away from the bedside
   c. a group of nursing personnel who care for patients on the nursing unit
   d. an area within the hospital with equipment and nursing personnel to care for a given number of patients
   e. the desk area of the nursing unit
   f. a written process used to communicate the doctors' orders to the nursing staff and to other hospital departments
   g. the health care a doctor prescribes in writing for a hospitalized patient
   h. the health unit coordinator assumes full responsibility for transcription of doctors' orders
   i. process of testifying to or endorsing that a person has met certain standards
   j. a process for certified health unit coordinators to exhibit continued personal, professional growth and current competency to practice in the field
   k. a mandatory process that keeps one's certification in a current status and ensures that records are accurate and complete
2. a. 1940. Implementation of health unit coordinating at Montefiore Hospital in Pittsburgh, PA
   b. 1966. One of the first educational programs was implemented in a vocational school in Minneapolis, MN
   c. 1980. The National Association of Health Unit Coordinators was established in Phoenix, AZ
   d. 1983. First offering of the Health Unit Coordinator Certification Examination by NAHUC
3. Any three of the following:
   a. i. communicates all new doctors' orders to the patient's nurse
      ii. maintains the chart
      iii. performs the nonclinical tasks for patient admission, transfer, and discharge
      iv. prepares the patient's chart for surgery
      v. handles the telephone communications
   b. i. assists in obtaining the patients' charts and equipment
      ii. transcribes the doctors' orders
      iii. places and receives doctor's telephone calls to and from the doctor's office
   c. i. schedules diagnostic procedures, treatments, and services
      ii. works with the admitting department with patient admission, transfer, and discharge
      iii. orders supplies for the nursing unit
   d. i. informs visitors of visiting rules and special precautions
      ii. receives telephone calls from the patient's relatives and friends
      iii. listens to visitor complaints
4. National Association of Health Unit Coordinators
5. Set standards of education and practice by peers to be enforced by peers for the protection of the public
6. Any three of the following:
   a. professional representation
   b. provides format to share ideas and challenges
   c. national networking
   d. national directory
   e. opportunity to develop leadership skills
7. Any three of the following:
   a. increased credibility
   b. gain a broader perspective of health unit coordinating (not just your own specialty)
   c. increased mobility, geographically and/or vertically
   d. peer and public recognition and respect
   e. improved self-image
8. False. Nursing is a clinical practice.
9. a. Health unit coordinating
   b. Health unit management
   c. Health service management
   d. Health service administration

## CHAPTER 2

### Exercises

#### Exercise 1

| | | |
|---|---|---|
| 1. ATD | 10. Psych | 19. PSA |
| 2. CCU | 11. Peds | 20. OR |
| 3. ICU | 12. Ortho | 21. DSU |
| 4. CNA | 13. Gyn | 22. ED |
| 5. LVN | 14. Neuro | 23. PACU |
| 6. Surg | 15. RR | 24. SSU |
| 7. OB | 16. RN | 25. SAD |
| 8. Med | 17. LPN | 26. SDS |
| 9. ER | 18. PCT | |

#### Exercise 2

| | |
|---|---|
| 1. surgical | 6. certified nursing assistant |
| 2. neurology | 7. intensive care unit |
| 3. licensed practical nurse | 8. coronary care unit |
| 4. licensed vocational nurse | 9. emergency room |
| 5. assistant to director | 10. orthopedics |

11. gynecology
12. registered nurse
13. operating room
14. recovery room
15. medical
16. day surgery unit
17. obstetrics
18. pediatrics
19. psychiatry
20. patient care technician
21. postanesthesia care unit
22. emergency department
23. short-stay unit
24. patient support associate
25. same day surgery
26. save a day

## Review Questions

1. a. registered nurse: gives direct patient care, supervises patient care given by others, performs treatments, maintains records, and teaches patients, family members, and team members
   b. licensed practical nurse: gives direct patient care, performs less-technical skills than the registered nurse, and administers medications
   c. certified nursing assistant: performs basic treatments and performs bedside tasks such as bathing and feeding patients
   d. patient care technician: performs certified nursing assistant duties plus bedside testing and phlebotomy
2. a. surgical
   b. medical
   c. obstetrics, labor and delivery, and nursery
   d. gynecology
   e. orthopedics
   f. pediatrics
   g. neurology
   h. behavioral health
   i. rehabilitation
   j. cardiovascular
   k. urology
   l. oncology
   m. telemetry
   n. step-down unit
3. nursing unit administration is responsible for the nonclinical patient care functions

   The health unit manager performs supervisory and administrative nonclinical functions such as budgeting, research, and training new employees for several nursing units
4. the nurse assigned to take care of the patient
5. the team leader
6. emergency department, operating room, postanesthesia care unit, intensive care unit, registered nurse, surgical, certified nursing assistant, licensed practical nurse, certified health unit coordinator
7. a. intensive care unit
   b. surgical intensive care unit
   c. medical intensive care unit
   d. coronary care unit
   e. trauma intensive care unit
   f. neonatal intensive care unit
   g. pediatric intensive care unit
8. a. includes perioperative area, where patients are prepared for surgery; recovery room, where patients are cared for immediately following surgery; and the operating room, where surgery is performed
   b. care of patients who need emergency treatment
   c. care of patients who are having surgery or examinations but are not hospitalized overnight
9. a. fast-evolving technology
   b. Americans are living longer

## CHAPTER 3

## Exercises

### Exercise

| | | |
|---|---|---|
| 1. ICD | 5. MD | 9. ECF |
| 2. DRG | 6. HMO | 10. DO |
| 3. HO | 7. JCAHO | 11. IPA |
| 4. CEO | 8. COO | 12. SNF |

### Exercise 2

1. house officer
2. health maintenance organization

3. chief executive officer
4. doctor of medicine
5. extended care facilities
6. chief operating officer
7. International Classification of Diseases
8. doctor of osteopathy
9. diagnosis-related group
10. Joint Commission on the Accreditation of Healthcare Organizations
11. individual practice association
12. skilled nursing facility

## Review Questions

1. care and treatment of the sick
2. a. education of physicians and other health care personnel
   b. research
   c. prevention of disease
   d. local health center
3. attending physician
4. resident
5. clinical clerkship
6. a. type of patient services offered
   b. ownership of the hospital
   c. type of accreditation
7. A.

   | | | |
   |---|---|---|
   | 1. k | 6. a | 11. j |
   | 2. n | 7. l | 12. g |
   | 3. m | 8. b | 13. d |
   | 4. i | 9. f | |
   | 5. h | 10. c | |

   B.

   | | | |
   |---|---|---|
   | 1. i | 5. l | 9. f |
   | 2. g | 6. a | 10. h |
   | 3. j | 7. c | 11. m |
   | 4. b | 8. k | 12. d |

8. a. business office
   b. admitting department
   c. pathology, or clinical laboratory
   d. diagnostic imaging
   e. radiation therapy, or radiation oncology
   f. pharmacy
   g. physical therapy
   h. occupational therapy
   i. respiratory care
   j. dietary department
   k. endoscopy department
   l. gastroenterology, or GI laboratory
   m. cardiovascular studies department
   n. neurodiagnostics department
   o. health records, or medical records, department
   p. central service department
   q. outpatient department, or clinic
   r. social service department
   s. home care department
   t. housekeeping, or environmental services
   u. materials management, or purchasing department
   v. pastoral care, or chaplain
   w. maintenance department
   x. laundry
   y. communications department
   z. security department
9. accreditation
10. governing board, board of trustees, or board of directors
11. chief executive officer
12. places special emphasis on the relationship of organs and the musculoskeletal system and uses manipulation to correct skeletal problems
13. __X__ SNF
    __O__ IPA
    __X__ hospice
    __O__ group
    __X__ home health care
    __X__ rehabilitation

14. provide comprehensive services, including preventive care aimed at retaining good health

---

## CHAPTER 4

### Review Questions

1. a. telephone
   b. unit intercom
   c. pocket pager, voice pager, light pager
   d. fax
   e. pneumatic tube
   f. computer
2. a. answer the phone promptly
   b. identify yourself promptly
   c. speak into the telephone
   d. give the caller your undivided attention
   e. speak distinctly and clearly
   f. be courteous at all times
   g. When you cannot answer a question, reply "I will get someone who can answer that question for you." Do not say, "I do not know."
   h. When a call is received for another person who is not close by, always place the caller on hold after getting his or her permission.
3. a. who the message is for
   b. the caller's name
   c. time of call
   d. purpose of call
   e. Is a return call expected? Phone number to call.
   f. your name
4. a. used to type information into the computer
   b. a list of options projected on the viewing screen
   c. a flashing indicator that lets the user know the area on the screen that will receive the information
   d. a computer component that displays information
   e. an electric machine that is capable of accepting, processing, and returning information
   f. a small electronic device that when activated by dialing a series of telephone numbers delivers a message to the carrier of the pager
   g. the system by which the hospital telephone operator delivers a message to a doctor or makes other announcements
   h. a system by which air pressure transports tubes carrying supplies, requisitions, or messages from one hospital unit or department to another
   i. a device used to communicate between the nurses' station and the patient's room on the nursing unit
   j. a mechanical device for transporting diets or supplies from one hospital floor to another
   k. a telecommunication device that transmits copies of written material over a telephone line from one site to another
5. a. allows the health unit coordinator to take care of many calls simultaneously
   b. to place a caller on hold when the health unit coordinator must leave the phone
6. Have the chart handy so you may look for facts that you may be asked. Write down the facts you wish to discuss.
7. a. to communicate between the nurses' station and the patient's room
   b. to locate nursing personnel
8. a. pocket pager
   b. voice paging system
9. to deliver messages to or locate persons within the hospital
10. Posts the material in an attractive manner and keeps the posted material current. Writes the posting date on the material.
11. a (example), d, c, g, e, b, f
12. b
13. d
14. d

---

15. a. to request diagnostic studies, treatments, medications, and supplies for patients
    b. to process information for patient admission, transfer, and discharge
    c. to view stored information
16. false

---

## CHAPTER 5

### Exercises

#### Exercise 1

| | | |
|---|---|---|
| 1. AS | 7. AS | 13. AS |
| 2. AG | 8. NA | 14. NA |
| 3. NA | 9. AG | 15. AS |
| 4. NA | 10. AS | 16. AS |
| 5. AS | 11. AG | |
| 6. AG | 12. NA | |

#### Exercise 2

Answers will vary.

### Review Questions

1. a. physiologic needs
   b. safety and security needs
   c. belonging and love needs
   d. esteem needs
2. a. a      g. d      m. b
   b. b      h. c      n. c
   c. b      i. a      o. a
   d. c      j. b      p. d
   e. d      k. b
   f. b      l. a
3. Answers will vary.
4. a. Politely refuse to share this information and choose another topic for conversation or state that you do not know.
   b. In a quiet manner, interrupt the conversation and indicate the presence of the patient's wife. You could also greet the wife by name to alert the others.
   c. Tell the patient that "with respect to her roommate's privacy" you choose not to share the information and that you will also treat her information as confidential. You may also add a statement such as, "It is kind of you to be concerned."
   d. Refer the call to the nurse manager. First, collect data such as the name of the reporter, the name of the newspaper, and so forth. Relay this information to the nurse manager.
   e. Take the necessary information to return the call. Tell the caller that you will call him back. Then, check out the identity of the caller before doing so.
   f. Explain to the other hospital employee that you would prefer not to discuss the incident on the bus, since other passengers may overhear the conversation.
   g. Ignore the questions and suggest to the neighbor that she call her friend at the hospital. Explain that her friend would probably welcome a telephone call.
5. a. the person transmitting the message.
   b. images, feelings, and ideas transmitted from one person to another
   c. the person receiving the message
   d. response to a message
   e. translating images, feelings, and ideas into symbols
   f. translating a message back into images, feelings, and ideas
6. a. Do not verbally repeat confidential information.
   b. Control the patient's chart in a manner that maintains confidentiality of the contents.
7. a. Follow the hospital policy for duplicating portions of the patient's chart.
   b. Control access to the patient's chart.
   c. Control transportation of the patient's chart.

8. a. sender
   b. message
   c. receiver
   d. feedback
9. Answers will vary.
10. a. poor choice of words
    b. inconsistency between verbal and nonverbal symbols
11. a. differences in lifestyle, age, cultural background, and environment between the sender and the receiver
    b. poor listening habits
12. Answers will vary.
13. Answers will vary.
14. *Situation 1:* Safety and security need. Responding with "cancer?" allows patients to further discuss their fears. A response such as "Don't worry about it" shuts off further communication from patients.
    *Situation 2:* Physiological need. Any nonverbal or verbal response that communicates to the patient that you understand the urgency of the request and you will follow through immediately.
    *Situation 3:* Esteem need. Give constructive feedback such as, "You have good leadership skills, I hope you are elected" as opposed to destructive feedback such as "What do you want to do that for, you are busy enough already."
    *Situation 4:* Belonging and love need. Give feedback that encourages the patient to expound on the subject. Avoid disagreeing by using phrases such as, "Oh come now, you are not that old."
    *Situation 5:* Self-esteem need. Give descriptive feedback such as, "I liked your opening remarks" rather than "You did okay."
    *Situation 6:* Safety and security need. Avoid such responses as "It won't hurt." Acknowledge the fear that is being expressed.
    *Situation 7:* Esteem need. Give descriptive rather than evaluative feedback. Avoid saying, "I think you are doing a great job here. Why do you want to leave?" A phrase such as, "Looking for something else?" encourages further communication.
    *Situation 8:* Safety and security need. An appropriate response includes reassurance to the patient that his integrity is not being questioned.
15. Answers will vary.
16. Answers will vary.
17. a. parent    expression of opinions
    b. adult     expressions of information
    c. child     expressions of feelings
18. a. child
    b. parent
    c. adult
19. a. "hurry up"          it's OK to give things the time they take
    b. "be perfect"        it's OK to be imperfect
    c. "please me          please yourself
       (somebody else)"
    d. "try hard"          do it
    e. "be strong"         it's OK to have needs and feelings and take care of yourself

## CHAPTER 6

## Review Questions

I. Exercise 1

| a. 2 | c. 1 | e. 4 |
| b. 5 | d. 6 | f. 3 |

Exercise 2

| a. 5 | d. 2 | g. 1 |
| b. 9 | e. 4 | h. 3 |
| c. 6 | f. 7 | |

II. 1. F     3. F     5. T
    2. F     4. F
III. 1. confidentiality
     2. nonmaleficence
     3. autonomy
     4. beneficience    (one may answer nonmaleficence but the distinction is beneficence is the prevention of harm while nonmaleficence is one will not inflict harm)
     5. veracity
IV. 1. results in more effective patient care
    2. results in greater satisfaction with patient care for the patient, physician, and health care organization

## CHAPTER 7

## Review Questions

1. a. management of the nursing unit supplies and equipment
   b. management of the activities at the nurses' station
   c. management related to the performance of the health unit coordinator's tasks
   d. management of time
2. a. Maintain only the quantity of supplies needed on the nursing unit, and store them in a convenient area.
   b. Check the equipment (such as flashlights) each day for working order. Return the used equipment to its proper storage place. Manage the use of the pneumatic tube system and the imprinter device.
   c. Make sure the textbooks are returned after use and keep the policy manual, the procedure manual, and the doctors' roster up to date.
   d. Make rounds to check for equipment in need of repair, then request the equipment repair from the maintenance department by completing a requisition form. When immediate maintenance is needed, such as the replacement of a light bulb, telephone the maintenance department and complete the corresponding requisition.
   e. Make sure the rental equipment is returned to the proper department as soon as possible after it is discontinued and that the daily charge to the patient is discontinued at this time.
   f. Know what emergency equipment is stored on the nursing unit and where it it located.
3. The following items should be marked with a check:
   b. home this AM                    i. do not give outpatient information
   c. surgery at 10 AM for cholecystectomy
   e. limit visitors                  j. BE today
   f. reverse isolation               l. EEG today
                                      m. no code
4. Record on the patient activity sheet the time of departure and destination of patients or the patients' charts as they leave the unit. Upon their return to the nursing unit, cross off the information by drawing a line through it.
5. To have the information readily available to give to doctors, other health personnel, and visitors who inquire as to the whereabouts of the patient and/or the patient's chart.
6. a. communicate information to visitors
   b. respond to visitors' questions or complaints
   c. initially handle visitor complaints
7. a. listen carefully
   b. ask pertinent questions
   c. respond accordingly
8. Any of the following:
   a. imprinter device
   b. patients' charts
   c. telephone
   d. requisitions and forms
   e. doctors' roster
   f. computer

9. 3, 6, 1, 5, 2, 4; Answers may vary.
10. a. plan for rush periods
    b. plan a schedule for routine health unit coordinator tasks
    c. group activities
    d. delegate tasks to volunteers
    e. complete one task before beginning another
    f. avoid unnecessary conversation
    g. know your job and perform you job
    h. take the breaks assigned to you
11. a. a written record of the amount of each item that the nursing unit should stock to last between ordering dates
    b. a written record of patient activity relevant to health unit coordinating
    c. a record of unfinished tasks
    d. a record book or notebook used to write down unit information to pass on to other shifts
12. a. Listen carefully to Mrs. Frances. Ask pertinent questions such as, "Who is 'my Robert'?" Express empathy by responding, "I understand how you feel," then tell Mrs. Frances that you will communicate the message to the nurse who is taking of Robert today.
    b. Tell the visitor what room Mr. Blair is in, then explain to her the rules for visiting hours for children. If possible, offer the woman the opportunity to have a volunteer care for the children while she visits with Mr. Blair.
    c. Listen carefully to Mr. Christine's complaint. Tell him that you understand his position. Go to Room 365 and explain the visiting policy to the six visitors. Suggest that four wait in the waiting room and that they rotate (two at a time) to visit with the patient.
    d. Determine, first, where they could be relocated in a convenient place within reaching distance of your work area. Then, discuss your plan and your rationale with your nurse manager.
    e. Politely refuse to feed the patient. You could further empathize with the nurse by stating that you understand that she is very busy. However, you are not allowed to do clinical tasks, and you should not leave the nurses' station.
Answers could vary.
13. a. Tell the volunteer and the visitor that you will be with them in a moment, then
    b. communicate the message to the nurse that surgery is ready for Mr. Pat Jerri
    c. Assist the visitor as needed, then
    d. ask the volunteer to place reports on the patients chart
    e. Notify the laboratory of the stat order for packed cells and complete the corresponding laboratory requisition
    f. Locate the x-ray report, then
    g. begin transcribing the other doctors' orders

| Tool | Use |
| --- | --- |
| 14. a. brainstorming _____ | tap into creavity of group to identify new ideas |
| b. process flow chart _____ | help visualize the steps in a process |
| c. fishbone chart _____ | organize information about probable causes of an effect |
| d. pareto chart _____ | show in descending order the most frequently to least occurring type of item or event |
| e. histogram _____ | show the amount of variation in a process |
| f. correlation chart _____ | see if there is a possible relationship between changes in two sets of data |
| g. run chart _____ | look for trends in plotted data |

## CHAPTER 8

### Exercises

Exercise 1

1. Hx
2. NKA
3. C of A
4. ID labels
5. H&P
6. MAR

Exercise 2

1. conditions of admission
2. identification labels
3. history and physical
4. medication administration record
5. no known allergies
6. history

### Review Questions

1. inpatient
2. imprinter card
3. a. Place it in proper sequence in rack when it is not in use.
   b. Keep a record of the location of the patient's chart when it is removed from the unit.
   c. Know identity of persons who have access to charts.
   d. Place new chart forms in the chart before the immediate need arises.
   e. Place diagnostic reports in the correct patient's chart behind the correct divider.
   f. Review the patients' charts frequently for new orders.
   g. Check the chart to be sure all the forms are imprinted with the correct patient's name.
   h. Check chart for results of routine admission studies.
   i. Properly identify the patient's chart so that it can be easily located.
4. a. used by the physician to request care and treatment for the patient
   b. to provide a graphic representation of the patient's vital signs for a given number of days
   c. the physician's record of the patient's progress during the period of hospitalization
   d. to record the medical history and the present medical problem and to provide a review of all body systems
   e. used to record the observations of the patients by the nurse
   f. to record all medications administered to the patient
   g. to summarize the patient's hospital stay
5. an additional form added to the patients' charts when specific conditions of the patient calls for it (Any supplemental chart forms used in your facility may be placed in these two blanks.)
6. a. means of communication between the doctor and the hospital staff
   b. planning patient care
   c. research
   d. educational purposes
   e. As a legal document, the chart protects the patient, the doctor, the staff, and the health care facility
   f. a written record of the patient's illness, care, and treatment, and outcomes of the hospitalization
7. outpatient
8. admission pack
9. imprinter
10. Information on the patient's chart should not be included in casual conversation by personnel in the employee lounge, cafeteria, coffee shop, or any area outside the nursing unit. The health unit coordinator should require individuals who wish access to the charts to identify themselves.
11. a. If there are no notations on the chart form it may be destroyed. If the form has notations, the correct

information may be imprinted with the patient's imprinter card next to or below the error. Cross out the incorrect information. Write "mistaken entry," your first initial, last name, and status.

b. Draw a single line in ink through the error. Record the word "mistaken entry," with your first initial, last name, and status in the blank area near (above or next to) the error.

12. 1530
13. 11:45 PM
14. a. placing extra blank forms in all the patients charts on a nursing unit
   b. portions of the patient's current chart that are removed from the chart holder when the chart becomes too large
   c. preprinted labels containing patient information, used to identify patient records
   d. a method of alerting staff when two or more patients with the same last name are located on a nursing unit

## CHAPTER 9

### Review Questions

1. To reduce the possibility of forgetting to complete a part of the transcription procedure. It is also a written record and may be used at a later date to verify that the transcription procedure was completed.
2. date, time, full signature, and status
3. a. Read the set of doctors' orders.
   b. Send the pharmacy copy of the doctors' order sheet to the pharmacy department.
   c. Complete stat orders.
   d. Collect necessary forms or select the patient's name on the computer screen.
   e. ordering
   f. kardexing
   g. Complete medication orders.
   h. Complete telephone calls.
   i. Recheck.
   j. sign-off procedure
4. The doctors' order sheet is a legal document; therefore, ink must be used.
5. a. after the step is completed
6. b. the absence of symbols and sign-off
7. so they can be erased if the doctor discontinues or changes them
8. to communicate new orders to the nursing staff and update the patient's profile on the Kardex form
9. a. the process of ordering medications, diagnostic tests, treatment, and equipment from hospital departments other than nursing
   b. the process of writing all doctors' orders on the patient's kardex form or erasing discontinued or changed orders
   c. form used to order diagnostic procedures, equipment, and supplies from hospital departments
   d. a method used to indicate new doctors' orders to the nursing staff
10. a. the line directly below the doctor's signature
    b. to avoid leaving space where a doctor could write orders later. They would be recorded above the sign-off information and therefore would not be identified as new orders and would not be transcribed error of omission.
11. to avoid errors that may cause harm to the patient
12. a. ord (and computer number)
    b. M
    c. K
    d. called and time
    e. pc sent
13. a. draw diagonal lines through the remaining space. So new orders will not be written here, but will begin at the top of the next page. This is done to avoid error of omission.

b. ask the doctor to interpret the order for you. To avoid making an error in transcription.
   c. the patient's chart rack. The information is more apt to be correct here than the imprinted information on the patient's chart form.
   d. check each chart for new orders. The doctor may have forgotten to flag the chart for new orders.
14. F
15. those that require ordering diagnostic procedures, treatments, or supplies from departments other than nursing
16. a. activity
    b. medication
    c. diet
    d. treatment
    e. diagnostic studies
17. a. Standing or continuing orders. They are in effect and executed as ordered until the doctor discontinues or changes them.
    b. Standing or continuing prn orders. Same as the standing order, only performed according to the patient's needs.
    c. One-time or short-series order. Performed only one time or for a short series, according to the content of the qualifying phrase; when completed it is automatically discontinued.
    d. Stat order. A stat order is to be carried out immediately and then automatically discontinued.
18. a. short series
    b. standing or continuing prn
    c. stat
    d. standing or continuing
19. The order contains the word *stat, now,* or *immediately,* according to the practice in your area.
20. by prn in the order or by the content of a qualifying phrase
21. a. record on correct chart
    b. record directly below previous orders
    c. record in ink
    d. record date and time
    e. record as doctor is stating
    f. read entire set of orders back to the doctor
    g. sign the orders

## CHAPTER 10

### Exercises

#### Exercise 1

| | | |
|---|---|---|
| 1. CBR | 16. qd | 31. ax |
| 2. c̄ | 17. tid | 32. TPR |
| 3. A&O | 18. qh | 33. P |
| 4. qid | 19. temp | 34. h, hr, hrs |
| 5. o | 20. as tol | 35. prn |
| 6. BP | 21. rt | 36. NVS |
| 7. q | 22. lt | 37. ↓ |
| 8. amb | 23. DC | 38. HOB |
| 9. ABR | 24. VS | 39. BSC |
| 10. ↑ | 25. I&O | 40. q4h |
| 11. BRP | 26. OOB | 41. CMS |
| 12. RR | 27. min | 42. SOB |
| 13. ad lib | 28. wt | 43. CVP |
| 14. qod | 29. BR | |
| 15. bid | 30. R | |

#### Exercise 2

| | |
|---|---|
| 1. left | 9. temperature, pulse, respiration |
| 2. right | 10. bed rest |
| 3. discontinue | 11. minute |
| 4. vital signs | 12. bathroom privileges |
| 5. blood pressure | 13. as desired |
| 6. three times a day | 14. increase or elevate |
| 7. complete bed rest | 15. out of bed |
| 8. with | |

16. alert and oriented
17. weight
18. ambulatory
19. every other day
20. every day
21. twice a day
22. four times a day
23. every hour
24. absolute bed rest
25. temperature
26. as tolerated
27. intake and output
28. every
29. pulse
30. axilla

31. rectal
32. as necessary
33. respiratory rate
34. every four hours
35. hours
36. neurologic vital signs
37. below
38. routine
39. shortness of breath
40. head of bed
41. bedside commode
42. circulation, motion, sensation
43. central venous pressure

25. min
26. gtts
27. Δ
28. ASAP
29. /
30. H₂O₂
31. ac

32. AE
33. con't
34. CBI
35. TKO
36. TEDs
37. mL
38. PAS

39. IVF
40. ETS
41. PICC
42. VAD
43. CVC

## Review Questions

1. a. a doctor's order that requests the nursing staff to observe and record certain patient signs and symptoms
   b. a doctor's order that defines the type and amount of activity a hospitalized patient may have
   c. a doctor's order that requests the patient to be placed in a specified body position
   d. measures body functions that include temperature, pulse, respiration, and blood pressure
   e. i. temperature reading obtained from the mouth
      ii. temperature reading obtained from the rectum
      iii. temperature reading obtained from the axilla (armpit)
      iv. temperature reading obtained from tympanic membrane
   f. a method to measure the oxygen saturation of arterial blood
   g. elevated body temperature
   h. without fever
2. a. complete bed rest
   b. bed rest with bathroom privileges when alert and oriented
   c. weight every other day
   d. temperature, pulse, respiration, and blood pressure three times a day
   e. blood pressure three times a day
   f. elevate head of bed twenty degrees
   g. check dressing as necessary
   h. temperature, rectal or axillary only
   i. neurologic vital signs every two hours
   j. intake and output every shift
   k. out of bed as desired
   l. up as tolerated
   m. blood pressure and pulse every four hours
   n. ambulate today
   o. discontinue vital signs
   p. elevate head of bed thirty degrees
   q. may use bedside commode
   r. log roll every two hours
   s. check circulation, motion, and sensation of the toes of the left foot
   t. check central venous pressure every three hours
   u. call me if patient has shortness of breath

## CHAPTER 11

### Exercises

#### Exercise 1

1. SSE
2. KO
3. MR
4. sol'n
5. nec
6. cm
7. TWE
8. NG

9. NS
10. D/RL
11. hs
12. DW
13. @
14. ORE
15. D/W
16. irrig

17. IV
18. cath
19. RL
20. st
21. cc
22. p̄
23. abd
24. TCDB

#### Exercise 2

1. 1000 milliliters of 5% dextrose in Ringer's lactate to run at 125 milliliters per hour, then discontinue.
2. Soap suds enema at bedtime may repeat one time.
3. Give oil retention enema follow with tap water enema if necessary.
4. Irrigate catheter three times a day with normal saline solution.
5. Intravenous keep open with 1000 mL of 5% dextrose in water.
6. Insert nasogastric tube.
7. Turn, cough, and deep breathe every two hours.
8. Change intravenous tubing as soon as possible.

### Review Questions

1. a. intestinal elimination
   b. urinary catheterization
   c. intravenous therapy
   d. transfusions
   e. suction
   f. heat and cold applications
   g. comfort, safety, and healing
2. The following terms should be underlined:
   Foley          catheter
   residual
3. Any three from this group:
   soap suds          tap water
   oil retention      Fleet or Travad
   normal saline
4. b. tomorrow AM
5. a. application of warm water to the pelvic area
   b. a disposable suction device
   c. devices used to control behavior or protect patient
   d. a doctor's order for treatment performed by the nursing staff
6. a. gastric suction
   b. throat suction
7. No. The flow rate is missing.
8. Check marks should be on the following orders:
   b. gastric suction, NG tube
   e. pulsatile antiembolism stockings
   f. K-pad
   g. disposable sitz bath
   h. ice bag
   j. sheepskin
   l. foot cradle
9. a. the rental charge should be terminated as soon as possible
   b. it may be needed for other patients
10. Return the blood to the blood bank.
11. a. D    i. R    q. R
    b. D    j. D    r. R
    c. D    k. R    s. D
    d. D    l. D    t. D
    e. R    m. D    u. R
    f. D    n. D    v. R
    g. D    o. R    w. R
    h. D    p. D
12. The CSD handles supplies that may be needed by the nursing personnel to carry out the doctors' orders. The health unit coordinator orders only the items stored in the central service area.
13. The retention catheter remains in the bladder to allow for the continuous flow of urine from the bladder. The nonretention catheter is used to empty the bladder and then is removed.

14. a. venipuncture (peripheral)
    d. PICC
15. a. blood collected from a surgical site
    b. a venous access device
    c. blood donated by a friend or relative
16. b. Hickman
    d. Groshong
    h. Raaf
17. d. peripheral intravenous
18. a. Have IV team insert PICC
    b. Con't IV's alternate c̄ 1000 cc RL c̄ 1000 cc D/W TRA 125 cc/hr via CVC
    c. Irrig NG q4h c̄ 30 mL NS

    d. regular diet
7. The dietary department cannot make an evaluation on what the patient can tolerate.
8. NPO MN means the patient is to have nothing by mouth, food or liquid, after midnight. The doctor orders NPO MN to prepare the patient for treatment, diagnostic procedures, or surgery.
9. a. Entron
   b. Dobbhoff
   c. Levine
10. a. Vivonex-Ten        d. Jevity
    b. Sustacal          e. Ensure Plus
    c. Osmolite

## CHAPTER 12

### Exercises

#### Exercise 1

1. gen
2. Na
3. MN
4. NPO
5. reg
6. cl
7. cal
8. ADA
9. liq
10. chol
11. DAT
12. FF
13. CHO
14. NSA
15. TRA
16. FS
17. PEG
18. NAS
19. RD

#### Exercise 2

1. sodium
2. nothing by mouth
3. regular
4. midnight
5. liquid
6. calorie
7. no salt added
8. American Diabetic Association
9. diet as tolerated
10. clear
11. cholesterol
12. carbohydrate
13. general
14. force fluids
15. full strength
16. to run at
17. percutaneous endoscopic gastrostomy
18. no added salt
19. registered dietitian

### Review Questions

1. a. computer
   b. diet change sheet
2. a. NPO
   b. cl liq break, then NPO
   c. 1000 cal ADA diet
   d. low Na
   e. DAT
   f. reg diet
   g. low Na diet
   h. NAS
3. a. a normal diet with modifications or restrictions
   b. a diet that consists of all foods designed to provide good nutrition
   c. administration of liquids through a tube into the stomach
   d. no foods or liquids by mouth
4. a. bolus            c. infusion pump
   b. gravity
5. The following diets should be underlined:
   a. soft diet
   d. full-liquid diet
   f. mechanical soft diet
   The following diets should have a check mark:
   b. potassium diet
   c. 800-cal diet
   e. 250-mg Na diet
   g. hypoglycemic diet
   h. low-triglyceride diet
6. a. clear-liquid
   b. full-liquid
   c. soft diet

## CHAPTER 13

### Exercises

#### Exercise 1

1. L
2. SO$_4$
3. ASA
4. stat
5. cap
6. CPZ
7. tab
8. MOM
9. U
10. OD
11. mg
12. DSS
13. KCl
14. g
15. OU
16. s̄s̄
17. MS, MSO$_4$.
18. mL
19. 5-Fu
20. mEq
21. pc
22. ung
23. WA
24. N/V
25. a̅a̅
26. gr
27. IM
28. subling
29. tinct, tr
30. PO
31. oz or ℥
32. OS
33. amp
34. dr or ℨ
35. supp
36. NTG
37. SC, sub-q, sq
38. μg, mcg
39. noc
40. HCTZ
41. syr
42. IVPB
43. ā
44. MgSO$_4$
45. PBZ
46. PCN
47. pr
48. TPN
49. PCA

#### Exercise 2

1. potassium chloride
2. left eye
3. ampoule
4. syrup
5. dram
6. night
7. microgram
8. ounce
9. subcutaneous
10. immediately
11. 5-Fluorouracil
12. milliequivalent
13. after meals
14. ointment
15. Compazine
16. milliliter
17. by mouth
18. tincture
19. intramuscular
20. grain
21. milligram
22. hydrochlorothiazide
23. suppository
24. gram
25. both eyes
26. of each
27. nausea and vomiting
28. while awake
29. one half
30. morphine sulfate
31. nitroglycerin
32. aspirin
33. capsule
34. epsom salts
35. tablet
36. milk of magnesia
37. liter
38. sulfate
39. unit
40. right eye
41. sublingual
42. intravenous piggyback
43. before
44. Pyribenzamine
45. penicillin
46. Colace
47. total parenteral nutrition
48. patient-controlled analgesia
49. per rectum
50. sublingual

#### Exercise 3

a. morphine sulfate grain intramuscular whenever necessary
b. grams intravenous piggyback every eight hours
c. milligram by mouth four times a day
d. drops both eyes twice a day
e. sublingual
f. milk of magnesia cubic centimeter at bedtime whenever necessary

g. 25 units daily
h. aspirin milligram by mouth every four hours whenever necessary
i. ounces one-half by mouth three times a day before meals

## Exercise 4

1. muscle relaxant
2. potassium replacement
3. antiarthritic
4. laxative
5. antiarthritic
6. diuretic (also called Lasix)
7. narcotic (also called Demerol)

## Exercise 5

1. gr.5 $\overline{\text{ii}}$
2. 5 cc
3. $\mathfrak{z}$ $\overline{\text{iv}}$ or dr $\overline{\text{iv}}$
4. 0.5 g
5. gr $\overline{\text{iss}}$
6. 500 mg
7. gr XV
8. 1 L
9. 1000 g
10. gr 1/6
11. gr 1/150

## Exercise 6

1. a. name of the drug
   b. dosage of drug
   c. route of administration
   d. frequency of administration
   e. qualifying phrase

2. a. Compazine 10 mg IM stat
      1        2    3   4
   b. Sodium phenobarbital gr $\overline{\text{ii}}$ IM q 3–4 h prn restlessness
                          1      2    3     4        5
   c. Librium 5 mg PO tid & hs
      1      2   3    4
   d. Seconal 100 mg PO hs prn
      1       2    3   4
   e. Lomotil $\overline{\text{i}}$ PO after each loose stool
      1       2  3          4
   f. Percodan tabs $\overline{\text{i}}$ q4h prn severe pain
      1        2      4         5
   g. Lente insulin 25 U qd
      1             2   4
   h. Procaine penicillin 600,000 U IM q8h
      1                   2        3  4
   i. Dramamine 50 mg IM q4h prn NV
      1         2    3   4    5
   j. ASA supp gr X q3h for temp ↑ 102$^{(R)}$
      1   2    3   4            5

## Exercises 7

1. ASA gr X PO q4h prn pain
2. ampicillin 250 mg PO qid or q6h
3. penicillin 1,600,000 U IM q12h
4. Nembutal 100 mg hs prn sleep
5. Donnatal Elixir 4 mL PO tid ac
6. B&O supp gr $\overline{\text{i}}$ q3–4 h prn rectal spasms
7. Neo-Synephrine ophthalmic 10% gtts $\overline{\text{ii}}$ OD bid
8. Benadryl 50 mg PO stat
9. Equanil 400 mg PO bid & hs
10. Coumadin 5 mg PO qd

## Review Questions

1. a. a medication order that remains in effect and is executed as ordered until the doctor discontinues or changes it
   b. same as a standing medication order, except that it is executed according to the patient's needs
   c. a medication order that is executed immediately, then automatically discontinued
   d. a medication order executed according to the qualifying phrase, then automatically discontinued
   e. a medication order executed according to the qualifying phrase, then automatically discontinued
   f. a small amount of drug given directly into a vein
   g. an injection of a medication given directly into a muscle
   h. a medication given by mouth
   i. a date on which specific categories of medications must be discontinued unless renewed by the doctor
   j. a gelatinous container in which a drug is enclosed
   k. a solid dosage of a drug in disk form
   l. a small glass vial sealed to keep contents sterile
   m. a method of administering calories, proteins, vitamins, and other nutrients directly into the bloodstream
   n. narcotics, self-administered intravenously
   o. a concentrated dose of medication given intravenously, usually by IV push
   p. pertains to within the vein
   q. a method of giving concentrated doses of medication intravenously

2. 1. syr
   2. $\overline{\text{ss}}$
   3. L
   4. MS, MSO$_4$
   5. PCA
   6. OU
   7. IVPB
   8. mL
   9. noc
   10. g
   11. ASA
   12. pr
   13. μg, mcg
   14. KCl
   15. $\overline{\text{a}}$
   16. mEq
   17. SC, Sub-q, sq
   18. H
   19. pc
   20. stat
   21. mg
   22. cap
   23. ung
   24. supp
   25. OD
   26. PCN
   27. WA
   28. dr, $\mathfrak{z}$
   29. U
   30. tab
   31. MOM
   32. N/V
   33. amp
   34. $\overline{\overline{\text{aa}}}$
   35. gr
   36. OS
   37. oz, f$\mathfrak{z}$
   38. IM
   39. subling
   40. po
   41. tinc
   42. NTG

3. 1. grain
   2. milligram
   3. intramuscular
   4. penicillin
   5. tincture
   6. suppository
   7. by mouth
   8. gram
   9. both eyes
   10. milliliter
   11. of each
   12. total parenteral nutrition
   13. ointment
   14. nausea and vomiting
   15. while awake
   16. after meals
   17. one-half
   18. milliequivalent
   19. morphine sulfate
   20. patient-controlled analgesic
   21. immediately
   22. intravenous piggyback
   23. before
   24. subcutaneous
   25. aspirin
   26. ounce
   27. capsule
   28. microgram
   29. Compazine
   30. night
   31. tablet
   32. milk of magnesia
   33. dram
   34. liter
   35. nitroglycerin
   36. syrup
   37. unit
   38. ampoule
   39. right eye
   40. left eye
   41. sublingual
   42. potassium chloride

4. a. name of the drug
   b. dosage of the drug
   c. route of administration
   d. frequency of administration
   e. qualifying phrase

5. Hospital formulary and *Physicians' Desk Reference*

6. a. narcotics
   b. hypnotics
   c. antibiotics
   d. anticoagulants

7. metric and apothecary
   a. A
   b. M
   c. A
   d. M
   e. A
   f. M
   g. M
   h. A

8. a. mouth
   b. inhalation
   c. parenteral
   d. topical

9. a. intramuscular
   b. hypodermic
   c. intradermal
   d. intravenous

10. a. drugs that relieve or lessen pain
    b. drugs used to treat infection and infectious diseases
    c. drugs that slow the clotting time of blood
    d. drugs that prevent or relieve allergic reactions

e. drugs that lower blood pressure
f. drugs that lessen or help prevent nausea
g. drugs used in the treatment of cancer
h. drugs that lower blood pressure
i. drugs that remove excessive fluid from the body
j. drugs that induce sleep
k. drugs given to lower blood sugar
l. drugs that produce or facilitate bowel movements
m. drugs that relieve pain and sometimes produce sleep
n. drugs that relieve anxiety and tension
o. drugs that build iron in the blood

11. PPD

12. a. narcotic
    b. hypnotic
    c. antibiotic
    d. hypnotic
    e. hypnotic
    f. narcotic
    g. antibiotic
    h. antibiotic
    i. hypnotic
    j. antibiotic
    k. antibiotic
    l. hypnotic
    m. narcotic
    n. antibiotic
    o. anticoagulant
    p. antibiotic
    q. narcotic
    r. anticoagulant
    s. antibiotic
    t. narcotic
    u. narcotic
    v. narcotic
    w. antibiotic

13. 1. f       5. b       9. g
    2. i       6. h       10. l
    3. d       7. k       11. a
    4. j       8. e       12. c

14. An IV push is a small amount of drug given directly into a vein. Piggyback drugs are administered IV in 50 to 100 mL of fluid. IV admixtures are drugs administered in larger quantities of fluid. TPN is used to administer nutrients into the bloodstream.

15. a. meperidine
    b. acetaminophen
    c. chloral hydrate
    d. gentamicin
    e. warfarin
    f. cimetidine
    g. digoxin
    h. procainamide
    i. hydrochlorothiazide
    j. furosemide
    k. nitroglycerin
    l. propranolol
    m. tetracycline
    n. ibuprofen
    o. tolbutamide

16. a. 15–60 mg
    b. 50–100 mg
    c. 10–15 mg
    d. 30 mg
    e. 15–20 mg
    f. 100 mg
    g. 0.5–1 g
    h. 325–500 mg
    i. 325–500 mg
    j. 0.125 mg to 0.25 mg

17. a. decreased number of errors in medication administration
    b. increased accuracy in accounting and billing

18. a. Medications that need to be refrigerated and those in breakable containers cannot be loaded into the system.
    b. After the system has been loaded, all new and changed orders will have to be handled in regular fashion.

19. a. Keflin 1 gm IVPB now
       Keflin 0.5 gm q6hr × 7 days
    b. Reg Insulin 15 U qAM ½hr ac bkf
       NPH Insulin 10 U at HS
    c. Haldol 10 mg IM stat
       Haldol 10 mg PO tid
       Haldol Deconoate 50 mg IM q 2 wks
    d. Vicodin 1 tab q4hr for pain
       if pain is unrelieved p̄ 30 min give MS 10 mg IM

## C H A P T E R  14

## Exercises

### Exercise 1

1. FBS
2. O&P
3. hgb
4. ESR
5. K
6. AFB
7. RBC
8. PP
9. CSF
10. Fe
11. C&S
12. T&C
13. CBC
14. APTT
15. GTT
16. PC
17. PT
18. UA
19. CRP
20. DAT
21. FS
22. HB$_s$Ag
23. HDL
24. HIV
25. LDL
26. R&M
27. RDW
28. TBD
29. TBT
30. TT, TCT
31. T$_3$T$_4$T$_7$
32. TSH
33. VMA
34. bili
35. Ag
36. HCG
37. gluc
38. creat
39. fib
40. BT
41. CMV
42. osmo
43. T&S
44. Dig
45. Cx
46. RSV
47. Zn
48. lytes
49. EBV
50. Bx
51. POCT

### Exercise 2

1. blood sugar
2. bicarbonate
3. hemoglobin and hematocrit
4. lumbar puncture
5. Venereal Disease Research Laboratories
6. white blood cell count
7. urinalysis
8. thrombin clotting time
9. nasopharynx
10. calcium
11. chloride
12. total iron-binding capacity
13. sequential multiple analysis
14. differential
15. sodium
16. packed cell volume
17. hematocrit
18. phosphorus
19. low-density lipid
20. C-reactive protein
21. routine and microscopic
22. red cell distribution width
23. direct antiglobulin test
24. thrombin time
25. thyroid tests
26. frozen section
27. thyroid-stimulating hormone
28. vanillylmandelic acid
29. hepatitis B surface antigen
30. high-density lipid
31. template bleeding time
32. human immunodeficiency virus
33. to be done
34. culture
35. zinc
36. bleeding time
37. human chorionic gonadotropin
38. creatinine
39. fibrinogen
40. electrolytes
41. glucose
42. antigen
43. digoxin
44. cytomegalovirus
45. antibody
46. respiratory syncytial virus
47. bilirubin
48. osmolality
49. type and screen
50. biopsy
51. point-of-care testing

## Review Questions

1. a. diagnostic
   b. evaluate treatment prescribed
2. Microbiology: studies specimens to determine disease-causing organisms
   Chemistry: performs tests related to chemical reactions occurring in living organisms
   Hematology: performs tests related to the physical properties of blood
3. a. voiding
   b. clean catch, or midstream
   c. catheterization
4. a. blood
   b. urine
   c. sputum
   d. stool
   e. spinal fluid
   (Other specimens listed in the chapter may also be used for study.)
5. Call the order to the laboratory, giving the patient's name, unit, room number, and the test requested. Prepare the requisition immediately so that the technician may pick it up on arrival on the nursing unit to draw the specimen. When using the computer, write *stat* on the order.
6. Prepare the requisition and send it to the lab. On the day the test is done, notify the lab of the time that the patient completed his or her meal.
7. a. stool
   b. urine
   c. sputum
   (Other specimens such as sweat and smears from body cavities may also be collected.)

8. A stat order must be done immediately, and a routine study order can be performed any time during the day as per hospital procedure.
9. a. lumbar puncture
   b. biopsies
   c. centesis (amnio-, thora-, and para-)
   d. C&U smears
   e. sternal puncture
10. type and crossmatch
11. Check to see that the specimen is properly labeled. Take the specimen and requisition to the laboratory as soon as possible. Do not send the specimen through the pneumatic tube system.
12. a. Na      c. Cl
    b. K       d. $HCO_3^-$
13. a. CK (CPK)    c. AST (SGOT)
    b. LDH
14. a. type and crossmatch     g. cerebrospinal fluid
    b. ova and parasites       h. fasting blood sugar
    c. lumbar puncture        i. acid-fast bacilli
    d. sodium                j. complete blood count
    e. potassium          k. phosphorus
    f. culture and sensitivity    l. urinalysis
15. List any six from Appendix F.
16. List any six from Appendix F.
17. Fasting means the patient's breakfast is held until the test is completed. The patient may have water or other nonsugared drinks. NPO means no food or liquid by mouth.
18. a. tissue removed from a living body for examination
    b. a method of obtaining a urine specimen
    c. no solid food or fluids containing sugar. Some hospitals may allow water, plain tea, or coffee.
    d. a procedure to remove fluid from the spinal cord
    e. a method of obtaining a urine specimen
    f. blood that is undetectable to the eye
    g. after eating
    h. a mucus secretion from the lungs
    i. a procedure to remove bone marrow from the sternum
    j. the physical, chemical, and microscopic examination of urine
    k. a specimen obtained by urinating
    l. the visual examination of urine using a special commercially treated stick
19. a. chemistry           n. chemistry
    b. microbiology      o. chemistry
    c. chemistry          p. hematology
    d. hematology       q. hematology
    e. chemistry          r. chemistry
    f. hematology (coagu-   s. hematology (coagula-
       lation)                    tion)
    g. blood bank        t. chemistry
    h. hematology       u. blood bank
    i. serology           v. hematology (coagula-
    j. chemistry            tion)
    k. serology           w. chemistry
    l. microbiology      x. microbiology
    m. hematology
20. a. defenses, disease
    b. The following should be underlined: ANA, RA factor, VDRL, ASO titer, HIV
21. The following should be underlined: creatinine clearance, GTT, urine for protein, FSH
22. Any three of these drugs should be listed: gentamicin, kanamycin, tobramycin, amikacin, Dilantin, digoxin, cyclosporine
23. Always read the laboratory values you have recorded back to the person in the laboratory.
24. a. CBC, lytes q AM
    b. H&H stat
    c. T&C 6 U pc—hold for surg in AM
    d. sputum spec for C&S for AFB.

e. LP for CSF:   #1–protein + gluc
                #2–Cx for CMV + fungus
                #3–AFB stain
f. $SMA_{20}$ in AM

## CHAPTER 15

### Exercises

#### Exercise 1

| | | |
|---|---|---|
| 1. IVP | 10. AP | 19. DSA |
| 2. RLQ | 11. GI | 20. OCG |
| 3. KUB | 12. RUQ | 21. PCXR |
| 4. BE | 13. CT, CAT | 22. PTC |
| 5. PA | 14. LLQ | 23. Fx |
| 6. UGI | 15. GB | 24. h/o |
| 7. lat | 16. MRI | 25. f/u |
| 8. LS | 17. SBFT | 26. CI |
| 9. LUQ | 18. CXR | 27. IVU |

#### Exercise 2

1. barium enema
2. lumbosacral
3. kidneys, ureters, and bladder
4. ultrasound
5. right lower quadrant and left upper quadrant
6. intravenous urogram and upper gastrointestinal
7. computed axial tomography
8. gastrointestinal
9. posterior anterior and lateral
10. magnetic resonance imaging
11. portable chest x-ray
12. upper gastrointestinal, small-bowel follow-through

### Review Questions

1. a. posteroanterior       o. liver-spleen (nuclear
   b. lateral                  medicine)
   c. barium enema      p. small-bowel follow-
   d. intravenous pyelogram    through
   e. intravenous urogram    q. ultrasound
   f. anteroposterior       r. left lower quadrant
   g. kidneys, ureters, and   s. chest x-ray
      bladder                 t. digital subtraction an-
   h. computed axial tomog-    giography
      raphy                  u. portable chest x-ray
   i. lumbosacral (x-ray)     v. oral cholecystogram
   j. upper gastrointestinal   w. percutaneous trans
   k. gallbladder             hepatic cholangiog-
   l. right upper quadrant    raphy
   m. rule out              x. positron emission to-
   n. magnetic resonance      mography
      imaging                y. fracture
2. contrast medium
3. portable or mobile x-ray
4. fluoroscopy
5. magnetic resonance imaging
6. ultrasonography
7. routine preparation
8. on call
9. a. AP                    d. oblique
   b. PA                   e. decubitus
   c. lateral
10. a. IVP                 c. BE
    b. GB                d. UGI
11. List may include any of the x-rays found in the list of doctors' orders for special x-ray procedures, or you may supply your own list.
12. a. bone scan—whole body or regional
    b. gallium scan—whole body or regional
    c. lung ventilation/perfusion studies
    d. thyroid uptake and scan
    e. MUGA scan (cardiac)

f. DISIDA scan (formerly PIPIDA scan)
g. PET scan
Your instructor may supply you with the name of other studies performed in your hospital.
13. Answers will vary.
14. a. LS spine R/O fx
 b. PA & Lat cxr
 c. UGI, IVU, GB series & BE
 d. myelogram
 e. MRI of rt shoulder R/O rotator cuff injury
15. a. seizure
 b. intravenous fluids
 c. oxygen
 d. isolation precautions
 e. language
 f. diabetic
 g. sight or hearing impaired

## CHAPTER 16

### Exercises

#### Exercise 1

| | | |
|---|---|---|
| 1. EEG | 5. LOC | 9. EchoEG |
| 2. ECG or EKG | 6. IPG | 10. ERCP |
| 3. EMG | 7. ABG | 11. EGD |
| 4. RA | 8. CBG | |

#### Exercise 2

1. arterial blood gases
2. electrocardiogram
3. electroencephalogram
4. electrocardiogram
5. capillary blood gases
6. leave on chart
7. electromyogram
8. room air
9. impedance plethysmography
10. echoencephalogram
11. esophagogastroduodenoscopy
12. endoscopic retrograde cholangiopancreatography

#### Review Questions

1. a. electromyogram
 b. electrocardiogram
 c. arterial blood gases room air
 d. electrocardiogram leave on chart
 e. electroencephalogram
 f. capillary blood gases
2. a. electrocardiogram
 b. echocardiogram
 c. exercise electrocardiogram
 d. cardiac catheterization
3. a. digitoxin
 b. nitroglycerin
 c. quinidine
 d. Lanoxin

4.

| Procedure | Organ(s) Studied |
|---|---|
| a. bronchoscopy | bronchi |
| b. esophagoscopy | esophagus |
| c. gastroscopy | stomach |
| d. proctoscopy | rectum |
| e. sigmoidoscopy | sigmoid portion of large intestine |
| f. colonoscopy | large intestine from cecum to anus |
| g. anoscopy | anal canal |
| h. ERCP | common bile duct, biliary tract, and pancreatic duct |
| i. EGD | upper gastrointestinal tract |

5. a. performs diagnostic tests related to problems of the gastrointestinal tract
 b. performs diagnostic tests to determine lung function
 c. used to study brain function
6. a. Coumadin
 b. heparin

7. a. a diagnostic study related to the gastrointestinal tract
 b. a method of studying the heart without entering the body to perform the procedure
 c. an electronic device, either temporary or permanent, that regulates the pace of the heart when the heart is incapable of doing so
 d. a diagnostic study to determine the exchange of gases in the blood
 e. the visualization of a body cavity or hollow organ by means of an endoscope
 f. a graphic recording of the electrical impulses of the brain
 g. the recording of the changes in the size of a part as altered by the circulation of blood in it
8. a. gastric analysis
 b. esophageal motility and reflux study
 c. biliary drainage
 d. secretion test
 e. lactose tolerance test

9.

| | | |
|---|---|---|
| 1. c | 7. a | 13. a |
| 2. a | 8. a | 14. d |
| 3. e | 9. a | 15. b |
| 4. b | 10. d | 16. a |
| 5. c | 11. a | 17. a |
| 6. b | 12. e | 18. b |

10. a. IPG this PM
 b. EKG stat
 c. ERCP in AM
 d. ABG on $O_2$ at 2 L/min

## CHAPTER 17

### Exercises

#### Exercise 1

| | | |
|---|---|---|
| 1. LUL | 18. NWB | 36. HD |
| 2. OT | 19. WP | 37. THR/THA |
| 3. PT | 20. HP | 38. ORIF |
| 4. L/min | 21. TENS | 39. Tx |
| 5. $O_2$ | 22. EPC | 40. TT |
| 6. IPPB | 23. ES | 41. isom |
| 7. RUL | 24. CPM | 42. BKA |
| 8. ROM | 25. IS | 43. ET |
| 9. RLL | 26. MDI | 44. HA |
| 10. ADL | 27. CPT | 45. PEP |
| 11. EMG | 28. AA | 46. P&PD |
| 12. RML | 29. biW | 47. $SaO_2$ |
| 13. USN | 30. UV | 48. UD |
| 14. SVN | 31. bilat, B | 49. > |
| 15. LLL | 32. AKA | 50. TKR/TKA |
| 16. V&P | 33. ex, exer | 51. < |
| 17. lb or # | 34. STM/STW | 52. CP |
| | 35. LE | |

#### Exercise 2

1. oxygen
2. left upper lobe
3. right lower lobe
4. occupational therapy
5. physical therapy
6. electromyogram
7. activities of daily living
8. pounds
9. right upper lobe
10. right middle lobe
11. nonweight-bearing
12. range of motion
13. liter per minute
14. small volume nebulizer
15. vibration and percussion
16. left lower lobe
17. intermittent positive pressure breathing
18. ultrasonic nebulizer
19. hot packs
20. whirlpool
21. continuous passive motion
22. electrical stimulation
23. electrical pain control
24. transcutaneous electrical nerve stimulation
25. incentive spirometry
26. chest physiotherapy
27. metered dose inhaler
28. bilateral, both
29. exercise
30. open reduction, internal fixation
31. tilt table
32. oxygen saturation

33. above-the-knee amputation
34. unit dose
35. heated aerosol
36. isometrics
37. lower extremities
38. soft tissue massage/work
39. hemodialysis
40. traction
41. percussion & postural drainage
42. greater than
43. total knee replacement/ arthroplasty
44. ultraviolet
45. total hip replacement/ arthroplasty
46. endotracheal
47. peritoneal dialysis
48. less than
49. twice a week
50. positive expiratory pressure
51. cold packs
52. active assistance

## Review Questions

1. a. range of motion
   b. electromyogram
   c. metered dose inhaler
   d. small volume nebulizer
   e. intermittent positive pressure breathing
   f. activities of daily living
2. The following items should be circled: head halter, moleskin and elastic bandage, pelvic belt, pelvic sling
3. a. The following items should be underlined: Bryant's traction, cervical traction with Crutchfield's tongs, pelvic sling, Russell's traction, Thomas's splint
   b. The following items should be circled: overhead frame and trapeze
4. a. IPPB        RC        j. cath
   b. SSE                   k. ROM        PM
   c. USN        RC         l. K-pad
   d. Diathermy  PM        m. whirlpool    PM
   e. O₂         RC         n. infrared     PM
   f. SVN        RC         o. TENS         PM
   g. Vib & perc RC         p. MDI          RC
   h. ADL        PM         q. gait training PM
   i. IV                    r. CPT          RC
5. The removal of wastes in the blood, usually excreted by the kidneys.
6. a. hemodialysis
   b. peritoneal dialysis

## CHAPTER 18

### Review Questions

1. a. a doctor's order that requests that his or her patient be transferred to another hospital room
   b. a doctor's order that states the patient may leave the hospital
   c. a request for the opinion of a second physician with respect to diagnosis and treatment of a patient
2. a. hospital's name
   b. patient's name
   c. patient's location
   d. name of doctor requesting consultation
   e. patient's diagnosis
3. a. to obtain a different type of room accommodation
   b. The patient requires more intensive nursing care.
   c. The patient needs an isolation room.
4. a. take treatment
   b. week
   c. discharge
   d. appointment
   e. no information, no publication
   f. do not resuscitate
   g. durable medical equipment
5. a. Arrange with the pharmacy for medication the patient is taking.
   b. Note on census when the patient leaves and returns.
   c. Cancel meals for the length of the absence.
   d. Cancel hospital treatments for the length of the absence.
   e. Arrange for any special equipment the patient may need.
   f. Have the patient sign a temporary absence release.
6. a. assists in obtaining nursing service from an outside agency
   b. assists in obtaining necessary medical equipment

7. a. obtains tutors for hospital-bound students
   b. arranges for transfers to nursing care facilities
   c. assists with money problems
   d. obtains child care

## CHAPTER 19

### Review Questions

1. c        a
   d        b
2. a. The number assigned to the patient on admission. It is used for identification.
   b. A plastic band with a cardboard insert on which the identification information is printed. It is worn throughout the patient's hospitalization.
   c. A list checked and signed by the patient's nurse to ensure proper patient preparation for surgery. It is part of the patient's chart.
   d. A list of all surgeries to be performed in one day.
   e. A container for storing the patient's jewelry or money.
   f. Orders written by the doctor before surgery to prepare the patient for surgical procedure.
   g. Orders written immediately after surgery.
   h. Information obtained from the patient concerning his or her sensitivity to medication and/or food.
   i. A form prepared for the patient's chart by the admitting department; it contains information such as the patient's name, address, telephone number, employer's name and address, insurance carrier, doctor's name, diagnosis, and so forth.
   j. A checklist used by the health unit coordinator to be sure the chart is ready for surgery.
   k. Surgery that is not an emergency or mandatory and can be planned at a time of convenience.
   l. A plastic band with a cardboard insert, on which allergy information is printed.
   m. Process of obtaining information and preparing forms prior to the patient's arrival.
   n. Process of entering personal information into the hospital system to enroll a person as a hospital patient.
   o. A duty to inform a patient prior to obtaining their permission.
3. a. diet orders
   b. activity orders
   c. diagnostic studies
   d. medication orders
   e. treatment orders
   f. request for old records
   g. admitting diagnosis
   h. code status
4. a. forms (admission agreement and information forms)
   b. identification bracelet
   c. imprinter card
5. a. Greet the patient upon arrival at the nurses' station.
   b. Inform the patient you will notify the nurse of his or her arrival.
   c. Record the patient's admission in the unit admission book and census sheet or on the computer.
   d. Check the patient's signature on the admission agreement.
   e. Complete the procedure for preparation of the chart.
   f. Label the outside of the chart.
   g. Prepare any other labels or identification cards used by your facility.
   h. Place imprinter card in correct place in imprinter card holder.
   i. Fill in all necessary information on the patient's Kardex form or computer.
   j. Record the data from the admission nurse's notes on the graphic sheet.
   k. Place the allergy information in all designated areas or write NKA.

l. Notify the attending physician and/or hospital resident of the patient's admission.

m. Add the patient's name to required unit forms.

n. Transcribe the admission orders.

6. The overall responsibility is to see that the surgery chart is properly prepared. All required forms and reports should be on the chart. Any reports or records that are missing must be located by calling the particular department or person responsible for the records. Record the patient's latest vital signs. Attach the patient's imprinter card or printed labels to the chart. Recheck the patient's admission agreement form for the patient's signature.

7. a. current history and physical record
   b. signed surgery consent form
   c. nursing preoperative checklist
   d. MAR
   e. test results

8. a. name of the surgery for operative permit
   b. enemas
   c. shaves and scrubs
   d. name of anesthesiologist
   e. diet changes
   f. preoperative medications

9. a. diet
   b. intake and output
   c. intravenous fluids
   d. vital signs
   e. activity
   f. orders for catheter, tubes, and drains
   g. positioning
   h. observation of operative site
   i. medications

10. a. Write day of surgery on the graphic sheet.
    b. Place all surgery forms behind the proper dividers.
    c. Transcribe the postoperative orders after discontinuing all preoperative orders, unless asked to resume them.

11. a. history and physical
    b. preoperative
    c. postoperative
    d. diagnosis
    e. history
    f. no known allergies

12. instructions given by the patient in advance regarding his or her preference about future medical treatment

13. a. interviewing
    b. preparing forms
    c. preparing identification bracelet
    d. prepare imprinter card or identification label
    e. secure valuables
    f. supply and explain information

14. a. routine
    b. emergency
    c. direct

15. In a living will a patient makes decisions for him- or herself. In a power of attorney for health care, the patient has named a proxy or agent to communicate decisions that the patient made in advance or to make decisions with the patient's best interest in mind.

16. when the patient can no longer make decisions for him- or herself

---

CHAPTER **20**

## Review Questions

1. a. Transcribe the discharge order.
   b. Notify the patient's nurse of the discharge order.
   c. Notify the admitting or discharge desk of the patient's discharge.
   d. Explain the procedure for discharge to the patient and/or patient's relatives.
   e. Notify other departments that may be giving the patient daily treatments.

f. Communicate the patient's discharge to the dietary department on the diet sheet or by computer.

g. Arrange for clinic appointment if the doctor requested it.

h. Arrange transportation, if needed.

i. Prepare credit slips for medications and equipment.

j. Notify nursing personnel or transportation service to transport patient to discharge area.

k. Write the patient's name in the unit admission, discharge, and transfer book and on the census sheet or computer.

l. Delete the patient's name from the unit TPR sheet.

m. Notify environmental services.

n. Prepare the chart for the health records department.

2. against medical advice

3. extended care facility

4. Check the summary sheet for physician's summation of patient's hospitalization. Note if all forms are imprinted with the correct imprinter card. Check for the nurse's final discharge note; split chart forms should be placed in proper sequence in patient's current record; old records should be placed with the discharged patient's chart. Rearrange the chart forms in discharge sequence, and return all the records to the health records department in a manila envelope to preserve the confidentiality of the chart.

5. a. Arrange transportation for the patient.
   b. Initiate continuing care forms.
   c. Photocopy portions of chart requested by the doctor.
   d. Place forms in sealed envelope for delivery to the nursing home.

6. a. Notify social service, discharge planning, and home health care departments.
   b. Prepare continuing care form.
   c. Obtain release information.
   d. Photocopy.
   e. Distribute continuing care forms.
   f. Perform routine discharge steps.

7. a. a covering placed around a dead body
   b. an illness ending in death
   c. a death
   d. after death
   e. care and services of a nonmedical nature that consist of feeding, bathing, watching, and protecting the patient
   f. an examination of the body after death
   g. donating one's organs and/or tissue after death
   h. a signed consent authorizing a specific funeral home to remove the deceased from a health care facility
   i. a death that occurs due to sudden, violent, or unexplained circumstances
   j. a medical facility caring for patients requiring some expert nursing care or custodial care

8. a. Contact the attending physician, staff physician, or resident to verify the patient's death.
   b. Prepare any forms that may be needed.
   c. Notify the mortuary that has been requested by the family.
   d. Obtain a shroud pack, if needed.
   e. Gather the deceased's clothing, place it in a sack, and label it.
   f. Obtain the mortuary book from the nursing office or have mortuary form prepared when the mortician arrives.

9. Transcribe the order. Notify head nurse and/or patient's nurse when request for transfer is granted. Remove patient's chart from the chart holder and place it in chart holder labeled with new room number. Place all Kardex forms in their new places in the Kardex form holders. Change room number on all medication cards. Notify medication nurse of change. Indicate change on the diet sheet and TPR sheet. Record the transfer in the unit admission, discharge, and transfer book and on the census sheet. Change the bed tags, if necessary. Notify environmental services (housekeeping) to clean the room.

10. a. Transcribe the order for transfer.
    b. Notify patient's nurse of the transfer order.
    c. Communicate with the patient's nurse when transfer order has been approved. Indicate receiving unit and room number.
    d. Notify the receiving unit of transfer.
    e. Record the transfer in the unit admission, discharge, and transfer book and on the census sheet or computer.
    f. Remove the chart from the chart holder and the Kardex forms from the Kardex holder just before the transfer of the patient.
    g. Place medications Kardex in a bag and place it with the chart.
    h. Remove the patient's imprinter card from the imprinter card holder and place it with the chart.
    i. Notify all departments that perform regularly scheduled treatments on the patient.
    j. Indicate the transfer on the diet and TPR sheets.
    k. Notify environmental services (housekeeping) to clean the room.
    l. Notify the attending physician, the switchboard, the information desk, the flower desk, and mail room of the transfer.

11. a. Notify the nurse who will care for the patient of the expected arrival of the transferred patient.
    b. Introduce yourself to the transferred patient upon his or her arrival on the unit.
    c. Notify the patient's nurse of the transferred patient's arrival.
    d. Place patient's chart in correct chart holder and label properly.
    e. Place all Kardex forms in their proper places.
    f. Note the receiving of the patient in the admission, discharge, and transfer book.
    g. Place the patient's name on the diet and TPR sheets.
    h. Place the imprinter card in the imprinter card holder.
    i. Transcribe any new doctors' orders.

## CHAPTER 21

### Review Questions

1. The vital signs should be recorded as soon as they are all written on the TPR sheet so they are available to the doctor when he or she makes hospital rounds.
2. The doctor may use vital signs data to prescribe treatment for the patient.
3. Write "mistaken entry" on the incorrect connecting line, then graph the correct value.
5. a. 37.0   b. 38.5   c. 37.6   d. 35.9
6. a. 100.8   b. 103.1   c. 97.5   d. 100.0
7. By ordering the diets at the same time each day you avoid forgetting to perform the task, which would upset both the health unit coordinator's and the dietary department's work schedule.
8. a. admission
   b. transfer
   c. discharge
   d. NPO for diagnostic studies
9. a. to have the records available to the attending physician and other hospital personnel
   b. to assist the health records department in assembling all patients' records for storage
10. a. Select the same time for filing each day.
    b. Separate the records according to the patient's name.
    c. Check the patient's name on the chart rack before filing it.
    d. Place the record behind the correct chart divider.
11. The health unit coordinator must continue to requisition the daily laboratory test each day until the order is discontinued by the doctor. Other laboratory tests are ordered only one time.
12. a. purchasing department: nonnursing items, such as pencils
    b. central service department: items used for nursing procedures, such as a catheterization tray

c. pharmacy: all medications
d. dietary department: food items, such as milk
e. laundry department: all linen

13. a. The health unit coordinator orders supplies.
    b. The supplying department automatically restocks supplies.

14. a. difference between the radial pulse and the apical heartbeat
    b. a scale used to measure temperature
    c. the body waste from the digestive tract that is discharged through the anus
    d. a form used by the nursing unit to order the patient's meals three times a day from the dietary department

15. a. bowel movement
    b. temperature, pulse, and respiration
    c. Celsius
    d. Fahrenheit
    e. days after admission.
    f. postoperative day
    g. postpartum

## CHAPTER 22

### Review Questions

1. a. acquired immunodeficiency syndrome
   b. AIDS-related complex
   c. Centers for Disease Control
   d. hepatitis B virus
2. a. accidents
   b. thefts from persons on hospital property
   c. errors of omission of treatment or errors in the administration of treatment
   d. exposure to blood or body fluids
3. May help close the doors to the patients' rooms. May assist with evacuation. Close fire doors.
4. a. *Streptococcus*
   b. *Staphylococcus*
   c. *Pseudomonas*
5. a. a division of the U.S. Public Health Service that investigates and controls diseases that have epidemic potential
   b. orders given orally by the doctor to the health unit coordinator or nurse
   c. a precautionary measure taken to prevent a patient with low resistance to disease from becoming infected
   d. when the patient ceases to breathe or respirations become so depressed that the blood cannot receive oxygen
   e. another term for isolation
   f. disease-carrying organisms too small to be seen with the naked eye
   g. an emergency that is life-threatening
   h. to place one patient apart from other patients as to movement and social contact
   i. an episode that is not normally within the regular hospital routine
   j. a disease that may be transmitted from one person to another
   k. a daily listing of all patient activity (admissions, discharges, transfers, and deaths)
   l. the patient's heart contractions are absent or insufficient to produce a pulse or blood pressure
   m. a planned procedure that is carried out by hospital personnel when a large number of persons have been injured
   n. infections that are acquired from within the health care facility
   o. the creation of a barrier between the health care worker and the patient's blood and body fluids
6. a. Notify the switchboard operator to alert the code arrest team.

b. Direct the code arrest team to the patient's room.
c. Remove patient's information sheet from the patient's chart and take or send the chart to the patient's room.
d. Notify all physicians connected with the patient's case.
e. Notify the patient's family of the situation.
f. Call the departments for treatments and supplies as needed.
g. Alert admitting department for possibility of transfer to ICU.
h. Prepare any requisition or charge slips that may be needed.
i. If the code is successful, follow the procedure for transfer to another unit. For an unsuccessful code, follow the procedure for postmortem care.

7. Wear rubber gloves if the specimen is not in a plastic baggie.
8. Documentation is important in case a lawsuit arises from the incident. The incident is studied to prevent similar incidents from occurring in the future.
9. a. airborne          c. body excretions
   b. personal contact
10. a. patient mail: Check the mail and write patient's room and bed number on the envelope. In the event the patient has been discharged, write "discharged" on the envelope and return it to the mail room. Distribute the mail as time allows.
    b. patient flowers: Check to see that the patient is still on the unit; if so, sign for the flowers, then deliver them to the patient.
11. a. strict isolation—to prevent transmission of highly contagious infections, which are spread by air, direct or indirect contact
    b. reverse isolation—to protect patients with a lowered immune system
    c. AFB isolation—to prevent transmission of active tuberculosis
    d. respiratory isolation—to prevent transmission of infectious diseases that spread mainly through the air
12. a. burn victims
    b. patients receiving chemotherapy
    c. organ transplant recipients
13. Any of the following:
    a. gloves          f. moisture-resistant
    b. mask               gown
    c. gown            g. moisture-resistant
    d. goggles or glasses    laundry bags
    e. pocket masks with one-way valves
14. The organisms take advantage of the weakened immune system.
15. a. PCP, a pneumonia, caused by the bacterium *Pneumocystis carinii*
    b. KS, Kaposi's sarcoma, a skin cancer

## CHAPTER 23

### Unit I

### Exercises

#### Exercise 1

| WR   S | | WR CV WR CV  S |
|---|---|---|
| 1. cyt/ology | | 4. electr/o/cardi/o/gram |
| WR    S | | WR   S |
| 2. gastr/ectomy | | 2. cardi/ology |
| P   WR  S | | P   WR  S |
| 3. sub/hepat/ic | | 6. trans/hepat/ic |

#### Exercise 2

1. cardiology          5. gastric
2. cytology            6. intragastric
3. gastrectomy         7. nephrectomy
4. gastritis

### Review Questions

1. a. Word root: the basic part of a word
      *Example:* gastr/ic
   b. Prefix: the part of the word placed before the word root to alter its meaning
      *Example:* intra/gastric
   c. Suffix: the part of the word added at the end of the word to alter its meaning
      *Example:* gastr/ic
   d. Combining vowel: usually an *o* used between word roots or between a word root and a suffix
      *Example:* gastr/o/enteritis
2. a. dividing words into word elements and identifying the word elements
   b. When given a definition of a medical condition, use word elements to build corresponding medical terms.

## Unit II

### Review Questions

1. a. the basic unit of all life
   b. a group of similar cells that work together to perform particular functions
   c. made up of several kinds of tissues
   d. a group of organs working together to perform complex body functions
2. a. epithelial          c. muscle
   b. connective          d. nerve.
3. a. cranial—brain       d. pelvic—bladder
   b. thoracic—heart      e. spinal—spinal cord
   c. abdominal—stomach
4. e, d, h, c, a, b, g, f
5. a. protects the underlying tissues
   b. assists in regulating body temperature
   c. passes messages of pain, cold, and touch to the brain
6. epidermis, dermis, subcutaneous
7. melanin
8. oil (sebaceous)
9. sweat glands
10. cell membrane—keeps the cell intact and is porous
    cytoplasm—main body of the cells, and cell activities take place here
    nucleus—control center and plays an important role in reproduction
11. b, a, e, f, d, c

### Exercises

#### Exercise 1

1. internal organs         7. disease
2. skin                    8. cancer
3. cell                    9. connective tissue
4. tissue                 10. epithelium
5. skin                   11. fat
6. hair

#### Exercise 2

1. pertaining to           5. inflammation
2. study of                6. tumor
3. a specialist            7. producing
4. resembling              8. through, across, beyond

#### Exercise 3

| 1. cyt/o | WR | 6. his/o | WR |
|---|---|---|---|
| 2. derm/o, dermat/o | WR | 7. al | S |
| 3. ologist | S | 8. ology | S |
| 4. oid | S | 9. trans | P |
| 5. viscer/o | WR | 10. carcin/o | WR |

#### Exercise 4

| WR   S | |
|---|---|
| 1. cyt/ology | study of cells |

WR   S
2. trich/oid — resembling hair
WR   S
3. path/ology — the study of body changes caused by disease

WR CV   S
4. path/o/genic — disease producing
WR   S
5. derm/al — pertaining to skin
WR   S
6. cyt/oid — resembling a cell
WR   S
7. viscer/al — pertaining to internal organs
WR   S
8. hist/ology — study of tissue
WR   S
9. dermat/ologist — the doctor who specializes in the treatment and diagnosis of skin disease

WR   S
10. dermat/itis — inflammation of the skin
WR CV   S
11. carcin/o/genic — cancer producing
WR   S
12. epitheli/al — pertaining to epithelium
WR   S
13. carcin/oma — cancerous tumor
WR   S
14. epitheli/oma — a tumor composed of epithelial cells
WR   S
15. sarc/oma — a tumor composed of connective tissue
WR   S
16. lip/oma — a tumor containing fat
WR   S
17. path/ologist — a doctor who specializes in pathology
WR   S
18. dermat/oid — resembling skin
WR   S
19. dermat/ology — a branch of medicine that deals with skin diseases

P   WR   S
20. trans/derm/al — pertaining to entering through the skin

### Exercise 5

1. cytoid
2. trichoid
3. dermoid; dermatoid
4. pathologist
5. dermatologist
6. dermal
7. visceral
8. histology
9. pathology
10. dermatology
11. pathogenic
12. cytology
13. dermitis; dermatitis
14. lipoma
15. epithelioma
16. epithelial
17. carcinogenic
18. sarcoma
19. carcinoma
20. transdermal

### Exercise 6

Spelling exercise

## Unit III

## Review Questions

1. a. protects the internal organs
   b. provides the framework for the body
   c. acts with muscles to produce movement
   d. produces blood cells
   e. stores calcium
2. periosteum
3. cranium:
   a. frontal, 1
   b. parietal, 2
   c. temporal, 2
   d. ethmoid, 1
   e. sphenoid, 1
   f. occipital, 1

face:
   a. maxillary, 2
   b. mandible, 1
   c. nasal, 2
   d. lacrimal, 2
   e. zygomatic, 2
   f. vomer, 1
4. a. cervical
   b. thoracic
   c. lumbar
   d. sacrum
   e. coccyx
5. a. scapula
   b. clavicle
   c. humerus
   d. radius
   e. ulna
   f. carpals
   g. metacarpals
   h. phalanges
6. a. ilium
   b. ischium
   c. pubis
7. a. femur
   b. patella
   c. tibia
   d. fibula
   e. tarsal
   f. metatarsal
   g. phalanges
8. a. voluntary—skeletal muscles
   b. involuntary—stomach
   c. cardiac—heart
9. a. a place on the skeleton where two or more bones meet
   b. attaches muscles to bones
   c. tough band of tissues that connect bone to bone at a joint
10. a. osteoarthritis
    b. rheumatoid arthritis
11. a. laminectomy
    b. diskectomy
12. a. broken bone, no open wound
    b. broken bone, open wound
    c. bone has been twisted apart
    d. bone is splintered or crushed
13. total hip arthroplasty
14. osteoblast and osteoclast
15. a. headaches
    b. ringing in the ears
    c. hearing loss
    d. dizziness
16. osteoporosis
17. a. calcium supplements
    b. exercise
    c. hormonal replacement therapy
    d. correct posture

## Exercises

### Exercise 1

*Note:* Not all of the combining forms will be labeled on the diagram.
3. clavic/o
4. clavicul/o
5. cost/o
6. crani/o
7. femor/o
8. humer/o
12. patell/o
13. phalang/o
14. scapul/o
15. stern/o
16. vertebr/o

### Exercise 2

1. joint
2. bone
3. rib
4. skull
5. femur
6. muscle
7. humerus
8. patella
9. sternum
10. clavicle
11. scapula
12. phalanges
13. vertebra(e)
14. clavicle
15. electrical
16. lamina
17. cartilage
18. meniscus

### Exercise 3

1. phalang/o
2. arthr/o
3. oste/o
4. femor/o
5. patell/o
6. scapul/o
7. vertebr/o
8. a. clavic/o
   b. clavicul/o
9. crani/o

10. stern/o
11. humer/o
12. cost/o
13. my/o

14. lamin/o
15. chondr/o
16. menisc/o

## Exercise 4

1. plasty
2. algia
3. a. ar    b. ic
4. otomy
5. ectomy
6. graph
7. graphy

8. gram
9. trophy
10. osis
11. scope
12. scopy
13. centesis

## Exercise 5

1. pain
2. recording instrument
3. record
4. process of recording
5. surgical incision
6. development
7. pertaining to
8. surgical repair of

9. surgical removal
10. pertaining to
11. abnormal condition
12. visual examination
13. instrument for visual examination
14. puncture and aspiration of

## Exercise 6

1. intra
2. dys

3. sub
4. a. a    b. an

5. inter
6. supra

## Exercise 7

1. within
2. above

3. below
4. painful

5. without
6. between

## Exercise 8

    WR CV WR CV S
1. electr/o/my/o/gram     record of electrical potential of muscle activity

    WR S
2. my/oma     a tumor formed of muscular tissue

    WR CV WR S
3. stern/o/clavicul/ar     pertaining to the sternum and clavicle

    WR S
4. crani/al     pertaining to the cranium
    WR CV WR S
5. vertebr/o/cost/al     pertaining to the vertebrae and ribs

    WR S
6. arthr/itis     inflammation of a joint
    P WR S
7. inter/vertebr/al     pertaining to between the vertebrae

    WR S
8. humer/al     pertaining to the humerus
    P WR
9. dys/trophy     bad or faulty development
    P WR S
10. sub/scapul/ar     pertaining to below the scapula

    WR S
11. arthr/osis     abnormal condition of a joint
    WR CV WR CV S
12. electr/o/my/o/graphy     process of recording the electrical potential of muscle activity

    WR CV S
13. arthr/o/gram     x-ray of a joint
    WR CV WR CV S
14. electr/o/my/o/graph     instrument to record the electrical potential of muscle activity

    WR CV WR S
15. stern/o/cost/al     pertaining to the sternum and ribs

    WR S
16. arthr/algia     pain in a joint
    P WR S
17. sub/cost/al     pertaining to below a rib or ribs

    WR S
18. femor/al     pertaining to the femur
    WR S
19. clavic/otomy     surgical incision into the clavicle

    WR S
20. arthr/otomy     surgical incision of a joint
    P WR S
21. intra/crani/al     pertaining to within the cranium

    P WR
22. a/trophy     without development, or decrease in size of a normally developed organ

    WR CV S
23. arthr/o/plasty     plastic repair of a joint
    WR S
24. oste/oma     tumor composed of bone
    WR S
25. cost/ectomy     excision of a rib
    WR CV S
26. crani/o/plasty     surgical repair of the cranium
    WR S
27. patell/ectomy     excision of the patella
    WR S
28. vertebr/ectomy     excision of a vertebra
    WR S
29. crani/otomy     surgical incision into the cranium

    P WR S
30. supra/scapul/ar     pertaining to above the scapula

    WR S
31. stern/oid     resembling the sternum
    WR CV S
32. chondr/o/genic     producing cartilage
    WR CV S
33. arthr/o/scopy     visual examination of the inside of a joint

    WR S
34. chondr/itis     inflammation of the cartilage
    WR CV S
35. arthr/o/scope     instrument for visualization of a joint

    WR S
36. chondr/ectomy     excision of cartilage
    WR S
37. lamin/ectomy     excision of the lamina
    WR S
38. stern/al     pertaining to the sternum
    WR S
39. menisc/ectomy     excision of the meniscus
    WR CV S
40. arthr/o/centesis     puncture and aspiration of a joint

    WR S
41. menisc/itis     inflammation of the meniscus

## Exercise 9

1. cranial
2. sternoid
3. subscapular
4. femoral
5. arthrotomy
6. chondrectomy
7. arthralgia
8. arthritis
9. arthrosis
10. humeral
11. atrophy
12. vertebrocostal
13. craniotomy
14. costectomy
15. subcostal
16. arthrogram
17. vertebrectomy
18. electromyogram
19. clavicotomy
20. electromyography
21. dystrophy
22. myoma
23. electromyograph
24. sternoclavicular
25. intervertebral
26. intracranial
27. sternocostal
28. patellectomy
29. cranioplasty
30. osteoma
31. clavicotomy
32. chondrogenic
33. arthroscopy
34. arthroscope
35. chondritis
36. chondrectomy
37. laminectomy
38. sternal
39. arthrocentesis
40. meniscectomy
41. meniscitis

## Exercise 10

1. diagnosis and treatment of diseases or fractures of the musculoskeletal system
2. doctor specializing in orthopedics
3. progressive, crippling disease of the muscles
4. insertion of a hollow needle into the sternum to obtain bone marrow sample for laboratory study

## Exercise 11

Spelling exercise

## Exercise 12

1. orthopedics; orthopedist
2. sternal puncture
3. electromyography
4. a. lower inner leg bone
   b. upper arm bone
   c. neck bone
   d. pelvic bone
   e. collar bone
   f. arm bone, thumb side
5. a. costectomy
   c. laminectomy
   d. clavicotomy
   f. patellectomy
   g. osteoarthrotomy
   h. meniscectomy
6. arthrogram, arthrocentesis

# Unit IV

## Review Questions

1. a. nerves: transmit impulses from one part of the body to another
   b. brain: the main center for coordinating body activity
   c. spinal cord: the pathway for conducting sensory impulses to the brain and motor impulses from the brain
2. neuron, sensory, motor
3. a. cerebrum: contains sensory, motor, sight, and hearing centers; memory, judgment, and emotional reactions also take place in the cerebrum
   b. cerebellum: assists in coordination of voluntary muscles and maintains balance
   c. brain stem: contains the control centers for blood pressure, respiration, and heartbeat
4. Extends from the brain stem passing through the spinal cavity to between the first and second lumbar vertebrae. It is the pathway for conducting sensory and motor impulses to and from the brain.
5. dura mater, arachnoid, pia mater
6. a, f, d, c, b
7. a. preictal
   b. interictal
   c. postictal

# Exercises

## Exercise 1

*Note:* Not all of the combining forms will be labeled on the diagram.

1. cerebell/o
2. cerebr/o
3. encephal/o
4. mening/o
5. myel/o
6. neur/o

## Exercise 2

1. cerebrum
2. brain
3. nerve
4. gray matter
5. meninges
6. spine
7. spinal cord or bone marrow
8. cerebellum
9. air

## Exercise 3

1. neur/o
2. cerebr/o
3. mening/o
4. myel/o
5. cerebell/o
6. encephal/o
7. spin/o
8. pneum/o
9. poli/o

## Exercise 4

1. oma
2. plasty
3. ar, al, ic
4. orrhaphy
5. orrhea
6. itis
7. ologist
8. gram
9. ology
10. orrhagia
11. cele
12. ectomy
13. otomy
14. algia

## Exercise 5

1. record
2. inflammation
3. the study of
4. discharge
5. rapid discharge
6. to suture
7. pouching out
8. pertaining to
9. surgical removal
10. surgical repair of
11. surgical incision
12. pain
13. abnormal condition

## Exercise 6

|  | WR | | S | |
|---|---|---|---|---|
| 1. | neur/ology | | | a branch of medicine that deals with the nervous system |

|  | WR | CV | WR | S | |
|---|---|---|---|---|---|
| 2. | cerebr/ | o | /spin/ | al | pertaining to the brain and spine |

|  | WR | S | |
|---|---|---|---|
| 3. | neur/algia | | pain in a nerve |

|  | WR | CV | WR | S | |
|---|---|---|---|---|---|
| 4. | poli/ | o | /myel/ | itis | disease of the gray matter of the spinal cord |

|  | WR | CV | S | |
|---|---|---|---|---|
| 5. | neur/ | o | /plasty | surgical repair of a nerve |

|  | WR | S | |
|---|---|---|---|
| 6. | encephal/itis | | inflammation of the brain |

|  | WR | S | |
|---|---|---|---|
| 7. | mening/itis | | inflammation of the meninges |

|  | WR | CV | WR | CV | S | |
|---|---|---|---|---|---|---|
| 8. | pneum/ | o | /encephal/ | o | /gram | x-ray of the ventricles in the brain using air |

|  | WR | S | |
|---|---|---|---|
| 9. | neur/orrhaphy | | to suture a nerve |

|  | WR | S | |
|---|---|---|---|
| 10. | mening/orrhea | | drainage of blood into the meninges |

|  | WR | S | |
|---|---|---|---|
| 11. | neur/ologist | | doctor specializing in neurology |

```
          WR   CV  S
12. encephal/ o /cele              herniation of brain tissue
                                      through the skull
        WR  CV  WR   CV  S
13. electr/ o /encephal/ o /gram   recording of electrical
                                      impulses of the brain
        WR   CV  WR  CV  S
14. mening/ o /myel/ o /cele       herniation of the spinal
                                      cord and meninges
                                      through the vertebral
                                      column
          WR     S
15. cerebell/itis                  inflammation of the
                                      cerebellum
        WR     S
16. cerebr/osis                    any brain disease
        WR   S
17. neur/oma                       tumor of nerve cells
        WR      S
18. myel/orrhagia                  spinal hemorrhage
        WR  CV   S
19. myel/ o /gram                  x-ray of the spinal cord
                                      using dye
          WR   S
20. neur/itis                      inflammation of a nerve
```

## Exercise 7

1. a disease characterized by hardening patches along the brain and spine
2. convulsion disorder of the nervous system
3. partial paralysis and lack of muscle coordination from a defect, injury, or disease of the brain
4. impaired blood supply to parts of the brain
5. a process of recording brain structures by use of sound recorded on a graph
6. paralysis of the right or left side of the body
7. paralysis of the legs and/or lower part of the body
8. paralysis that affects all four limbs
9. removal of cerebrospinal fluid for diagnostic purposes
10. accumulation of blood in the subdural space
11. radiologic imaging that produces images of "slices" of the body
12. a noninvasive nuclear procedure for imaging tissues
13. loss of expression or understanding of speech or writing

## Exercise 8

1. neuritis
2. meningorrhea
3. encephalitis
4. meningitis
5. neuroplasty
6. neurologist
7. neurorrhaphy
8. neuroma
9. neuralgia
10. cerebrospinal
11. meningomyelocele
12. cerebellitis
13. encephalocele
14. pneumoencephalogram
15. myelorrhagia
16. electroencephalogram
17. myelogram

## Exercise 9

Spelling exercise

## Exercise 10

Spelling exercise

## Exercise 11

1. neurology, neurologist
2. cerebrovascular accident, CVA, hemiplegia
3. meningitis, spinal puncture (lumbar puncture), spinal puncture (lumbar puncture)
4. a. electroencephalogram
   b. myelogram
   c. pneumoencephalogram
   d. echoencephalogram

# Unit V
## Review Questions

1. a. skull bones
   b. eyelashes
   c. eyelids
   d. tears
   e. conjunctiva
2. Sound enters the pinna, travels through the auditory canal, and strikes the tympanic membrane, which sends the ossicles into motion. The stapes vibrate the oval window, the waves continue to travel via the fluid in the cochlea to the auditory nerve and on to the brain.
3. f, h, j, i, b, d, k, a
4. a. conjunctiva
   b. cornea
   c. aqueous humor
   d. pupil
   e. lens
   f. vitreous humor
5. a. cones        adaptation to bright light and
                      color vision
   b. rods         adaptation to dim light
6. a. pinna
      auditory canal
   b. tympanic membrane    c. oval window
      eustachian tube          cochlea
      malleus                  semicircular canals
      incus
      stapes
7. cloudiness of the lens of the eye
8. abnormal increase of intraocular pressure
9. a. chronic infections
   b. head injuries
   c. prolonged exposure to environmental noise
   d. hypertension
   e. cardiovascular disease
   f. drugs
10. a. masking the noise by using music
    b. biofeedback
11. separation of the retina from the choroid
12. photocoagulation, crysosurgery, scleral buckling

## Exercises
### Exercise 1

a. 3. irid/o
   4. kerat/o
   6. retin/o
   7. scler/o

b. 1. myring/o
   2. ot/o
   3. staped/o

### Exercise 2

1. retina
2. cornea
3. sclera
4. eye
5. conjunctiva
6. ear
7. tympanic membrane
8. eyelid
9. iris
10. stapes

### Exercise 3

1. ophthalm/o
2. blephar/o
3. retin/o
4. ot/o
5. myring/o
6. scler/o
7. conjunctiv/o
8. irid/o
9. kerat/9
10. staped/o

### Exercise 4

```
       WR   CV  S
1. ophthalm/ o /scope          an instrument for visual
                                  examination of the eye
       WR      S
2. ophthalm/ologist            a physician who specializes in
                                  ophthalmology
       WR      S
3. ophthalm/ectomy             excision of the eye
     WR    S
4. ot /orrhea                  discharge from the ear
     WR  CV  S
5. ot / o /scope               instrument for examining the
                                  ear
```

WR CV WR    S
6. irid/ o /scler/otomy          incision into the sclera and iris
    WR    S
7. irid /ectomy                excision of part of the iris
    WR    CV    S
8. blephar/ o /plasty         surgical repair of the eyelid
    WR       S
9. blephar/orrhaphy        suture of an eyelid
    WR CV   WR    S
10. kerat/ o /conjunctiv/itis     inflammation of the cornea and conjunctiva
    WR CV   S
11. kerat/ o /cele             herniation of a layer of the cornea
    WR      S
12. conjunctiv/itis          inflammation of the conjunctiva
    WR      S
13. myring/otomy           incision of the tympanic membrane
    WR   CV   S
14. myring/ o /plasty        surgical repair of the tympanic membrane
    WR     S
15. kerat/o/tomy           incision into the cornea

### Exercise 5

1. otitis media
2. ophthalmoscope
3. blepharorrhaphy
4. otorrhea
5. iridosclerotomy
6. scleroplasty
7. iridectomy
8. keratocele
9. otoscope
10. ophthalmectomy
11. sclerotomy
12. blepharoplasty
13. myringotomy
14. myringoplasty
15. keratoconjunctivitis
16. conjunctivitis
17. keratotomy

### Exercise 6

1. cloudiness of the lens of the eye
2. removal of the clouded lens of the eye
3. separation of the retina from the choroid
4. surgical removal of the eyeball
5. weakness of the eye muscle (crossed eyes)
6. eye disease caused by increased pressure from within the eye
7. a professional person trained to examine the eyes and prescribe glasses.
8. transplantation of a donor cornea into the eye of a recipient

### Exercise 7

Spelling exercise

### Exercise 8

1. ophthalmoscope, otoscope
2. otitis media, myringotomy
3. cataract, cataract extraction
4. a. enucleation       b. ophthalmectomy
5. strabismus

## Unit VI

## Review Questions

1. See p. 479 for labeled diagram.
2. a. artery: carries blood away from heart
   b. arterioles: connects arteries to capillaries
   c. capillaries: exchange of substances between the blood and the body cells
   d. venules: connects capillaries to veins
   e. veins: carries blood back to the heart
3. plasma
   a. transports nutrients and waste material
   b. transports hormones
   c. assists in blood clotting
4. a. erythrocytes: carry oxygen and carbon dioxide
   b. leukocytes: fight against pathogenic microorganisms
   c. platelets: aid in blood clotting
5. a. O
   b. A
   c. B
   d. AB
6. a. destroys old blood cells, bacteria, and germs
   b. stores blood for an emergency
7. g, b, c, a, d, h, e, i

## Exercises

### Exercise 1

| | Type | Meaning |
|---|---|---|
| 1. | S | surgical fixation |
| 2. | P | below normal |
| 3. | P | without |
| 4. | WR | blood |
| 5. | WR | spleen |
| 6. | WR | cell |
| 7. | S/WR | narrowing |
| 8. | P | inside |
| 9. | WR | white |
| 10. | WR | red |
| 11. | WR | blood vessel |
| 12. | WR | heart |
| 13. | WR | artery |
| 14. | P | around |
| 15. | P | between |
| 16. | P | within |
| 17. | S/WR | hardening |
| 18. | S/WR | condition of the blood |
| 19. | S | enlargement |
| 20. | WR | vein |
| 21. | WR | aorta |
| 22. | WR | clot |
| 23. | P | above normal |

### Exercise 2

| | Type | Word Elements |
|---|---|---|
| 1. | WR | aort/o |
| 2. | S | megaly |
| 3. | S/WR | sclerosis |
| 4. | P | inter |
| 5. | WR | arteri/o |
| 6. | WR | angi/o |
| 7. | WR | leuk/o |
| 8. | S/WR | stenosis |
| 9. | WR | splen/o |
| 10. | P | a, an |
| 11. | S | pexy |
| 12. | P | endo |
| 13. | WR | hem/o |
| 14. | WR | cyt/o |
| 15. | P | hypo |
| 16. | WR | erythr/o |
| 17. | WR | cardi/o |
| 18. | P | peri |
| 19. | S/WR | emia |
| 20. | WR | phleb/o |
| 21. | WR | thromb/o |

### Exercise 3

    WR  S
1. aort/ic                pertaining to the aorta
    WR  CV    S
2. splen/ o /megaly       enlargement of the spleen
    WR     S
3. hem/orrhage         rapid flow of blood from a blood vessel

WR    S
4. thromb/osis        abnormal formation of a blood clot

WR CV WR
5. leuk/ o /cyte        white blood cell

WR  CV WR
6. erythr/ o /cyte        red blood cell

WR    S
7. cardi/ologist        physician who specializes in cardiology

WR CV    S
8. cardi/ o /megaly        enlargement of the heart

WR    S
9. phleb/otomy        incision into the vein to withdraw blood

WR    S
10. angi/orrhaphy        suturing of a blood vessel

WR    S
11. splen/ectomy        excision of the spleen

WR CV  S
12. splen/ o /pexy        surgical fixation of the spleen

P   WR  S
13. endo/card/itis        inflammation of the inner lining of the heart

WR CV    S
14. arteri/ o /sclerosis        hardening of the arteries

WR CV    S
15. arteri/ o /stenosis        constriction (narrowing) of the arteries

WR CV WR  S
16. thromb/ o /phleb/itis        inflammation of a vein due to a clot

WR    S
17. hemat/oma        tumor-like mass formed from blood in the tissues

WR    S
18. hemat/ology        study of blood

WR    S
19. leuk/emia        disease characterized by rapid, abnormal production of white blood cells

P  S(WR)
20. an/ emia        deficiency of erythrocytes

WR CV WR CV  S
21. electr/ o /cardi/ o /gram        record of electrical impulses of the heart

WR CV WR CV  S
22. electr/ o /cardi/ o /graph        the machine used in electrocardiography

WR CV WR CV   S
23. electr/ o /cardi/ o /graphy        the process of recording electrical impulses of the heart

WR CV  S
24. angi/ o /gram        x-ray of blood vessels

WR CV  S
25. arteri/ o /gram        x-ray of an artery

WR CV  S
26. aort/ o /gram        x-ray of the aorta

P   WR  S
27. peri/card/itis        inflammation around the heart

## Exercise 4

1. aortogram
2. arteriogram
3. angiogram
4. electrocardiogram
5. endocarditis
6. arteriosclerosis
7. thrombophlebitis
8. hematology
9. cardiology
10. cardiologist
11. cardiomegaly
12. phlebotomy

13. splenectomy
14. splenopexy
15. hemorrhage
16. leukocyte
17. erythrocyte
18. pericarditis

## Exercise 5

1. a laboratory test that measures the volume percentage of red blood cells in whole blood
2. a laboratory procedure that measures the oxygen-carrying pigment of the red blood cells
3. sudden stopping of the heartbeat
4. pertaining to the heart and blood vessels
5. excision of hemorrhoids
6. heart attack (damage of the heart muscle from insufficient blood supply to the area)
7. enlarged veins in the rectal area
8. within a vein
9. diagnostic procedure to visualize the heart and to determine the presence of heart disease or heart defects
10. dilation of a weak area of the arterial wall
11. floating mass that blocks a blood vessel
12. high blood pressure
13. low blood pressure
14. inability of the heart to pump enough blood to the body parts
15. blood vessels that supply blood to the heart
16. abnormal accumulation of fluid in the intercellular spaces of the body
17. vibration from a normal rhythm
18. abnormally rapid heart rate

## Exercise 6

Spelling exercise

## Exercise 7

1. hematology, hematocrit, hemoglobin
2. a. myocardial infarction
   b. coronary occlusion
   c. coronary thrombosis
3. splenectomy, hemorrhoidectomy
4. cardiovascular
5. cardiologist
6. cardiac arrest, cardiac arrest
7. electrocardiography, electrocardiograph
8. angiogram
9. cardiac catheterization
10. a. WBC
    b. RBC
    c. platelets
11. plasma

# Unit VII

## Review Questions

1. a. taking nutrients into the digestive tract through the mouth
   b. the chemical and physical breakdown of food for use by the body cells
   c. the removal of solid waste from the body
2. ingestion, digestion, absorption, and elimination
3. mouth
   pharynx
   esophagus
   stomach
   small intestine—duodenum, jejunum, ileum
   large intestine—cecum, colon (ascending colon, transverse colon, descending colon, sigmoid colon)
   rectum
4.

| Name of Digestive Juice | Organ of Secretion | Organ of Function |
|---|---|---|
| a. hydrochloric acid | gastric glands | stomach |
| b. saliva | salivary glands | mouth |
| c. bile | liver | small intestine (duodenum) |

d. pancreatic enzymes    pancreas        small intestine
                                          (duodenum)
e. intestinal juices     small intestine  small intestine

5. a. liver  b. gallbladder  c. pancreas  d. salivary glands
6. ileocecal spincter
7. a. mastication of food, mixing with salivary juices to start
      digestion
   b. container for food, and chemically and mechanically aids
      in the digestive process
   c. digestion is completed
   d. absorption of water and elimination of solid waste from
      the body
   e. stores bile from the liver and secretes it to the duodenum
8. e, a, b, f, d

## Exercises

### Exercise 1

*Note*: Not all of the combining forms will be labeled in the
diagram.
   2. apendic/o
   4. chol/o or chol/e
   5. col/o
   6. duoden/o
   8. esophag/o
   9. gastr/o
  10. gloss/o or lingu/o
  11. hepat/o
  13. ile/o
  15. pancreat/o
  18. stomat/o

### Exercise 2

|    | Definition                        | Suffix |
|----|-----------------------------------|--------|
| 1. | mouth                             |        |
| 2. | tongue                            |        |
| 3. | stomach                           |        |
| 4. | rectum                            |        |
| 5. | pancreas                          |        |
| 6. | intestine                         |        |
| 7. | liver                             |        |
| 8. | lip                               |        |
| 9. | esophagus                         |        |
| 10.| condition of                      | S      |
| 11.| bile, gall                        |        |
| 12.| bladder                           |        |
| 13.| duodenum                          |        |
| 14.| colon                             |        |
| 15.| ileum                             |        |
| 16.| abdomen                           |        |
| 17.| appendix                          |        |
| 18.| abdomen                           |        |
| 19.| stone or calculus                 |        |
| 20.| creation of an artificial opening into | S |
| 21.| hermia                            |        |
| 22.| sigmoid                           |        |

### Exercise 3

1. otomy—incision into a body part
2. ectomy—surgical removal of a body part
3. ostomy—creation of an artificial opening into

### Exercise 4

```
       WR CV   S
1. gloss/ o /plegia          paralysis of the tongue
       WR      S
2. append/ectomy             excision of the appendix
       R   CV WR    S
3. chol/ e /cyst/ectomy      excision of the gallbladder
```

```
       WR      S
4. gastr/ostomy              artificial opening into the stomach
                             (for feeding purposes)
       WR  CV   S
5. hepat/ o /megaly          enlargement of the liver
       WR     S
6. ile /ostomy               artificial opening into the ileum
       WR  CV   S
7. pylor/ o /plasty          plastic repair of the pyloric
                             sphincter
       WR       S
8. proct/orrhea              discharge from the rectum
       WR CV WR  S
9. chol/ e /cyst/itis        inflammation of the gallbladder
       WR    S
10. gastr/itis               inflammation of the stomach
       P   WR  S
11. sub/lingu/al             pertaining to under the tongue
       WR    S
12. ile /itis                inflammation of the ileum
       WR  CV WR CV  S
13. chol/ e /cyst/ o /gram   x-ray of the gallbladder
       WR      CV   S
14. sigmoid/ o /scopy        visual examination of the
                             sigmoid flexure
       WR       S
15. gastr/ectomy             removal of the stomach
       WR  CV   S
16. gastr/ o /scopy          visual examination of the
                             stomach
       WR  CV   S
17. gastr/ o /scope          an instrument used for visual
                             examination of the stomach
       WR   S
18. col /itis                inflammation of the colon
       WR   S
19. hepat/itis               inflammation of the liver
       WR   S
20. col /ostomy              artificial opening into the colon
       WR     S
21. herni/orrhaphy           surgical repair of a hernia by
                             suturing of the containing
                             structure
       WR  CV   S
22. colon/ o /scope          the instrument used for visual
                             examination of the colon
       WR  CV   S
23. colon/ o /scopy          visual examination of the colon
```

### Exercise 5

| #   |                      |   |
|-----|----------------------|---|
| 1.  | stomatitis           |   |
| 2.  | cholecystitis        |   |
| 3.  | cholelithiasis       |   |
| 4.  | cholecystogram       | D |
| 5.  | cholecystectomy      | S |
| 6.  | pancreatitis         |   |
| 7.  | proctoscope          |   |
| 8.  | proctoscopy          | D |
| 9.  | abdominocentesis     | D |
| 10. | colostomy            | S |
| 11. | ileostomy            | S |
| 12. | esophagoscopy        | D |
| 13. | gastroscope          |   |
| 14. | esophagoenterostomy  | S |
| 15. | gastritis            |   |
| 16. | glossorrhaphy        | S |
| 17. | cheiloplasty         | S |
| 18. | colectomy            | S |
| 19. | glossoplegia         |   |
| 20. | stomatogastric       |   |
| 21. | sublingual           |   |
| 22. | proctorrhea          |   |
| 23. | hepatomegaly         |   |

24. hematoma
25. pancreatic
26. appendicitis
27. appendectomy      S
28. colonoscopy      D
29. colonoscope

## Exercise 6

1. condition of bad or painful intestines accompanied by diarrhea
2. x-ray of the esophagus and the stomach
3. x-ray of the colon
4. x-ray of the gallbladder
5. yellowness of the skin and eyes
6. inflammation of the colon with the formation of ulcers
7. ulcer in the stomach
8. chronic inflammatory disease that can affect any part of the bowel

## Exercise 7

Spelling exercise

## Exercise 8

1. b. ileostomy

   Ile is the word root for the small intestine. Ostomy is the suffix that means artificial opening.
2. cholelithiasis, cholecystogram, cholecystectomy
3. subligual
4. a. esophagoscopy, esophagoscope
   b. gastroscopy, gastroscope
   c. proctoscopy, proctoscope
5. upper gastrointestinal (UGI), barium enema (BE)
   a. gastrectomy      c. vagotomy
   b. pyloroplasty
6. a. laportotomy      laparotomy
   b. appendectomy
   c. herniorraphy      herniorrhaphy
   d. collectomy      colectomy
   e. gastostomy      gastrostomy

# Unit VIII
## Review Questions

1. oxygen, carbon dioxide
2. oxygen, carbon dioxide
3. a. nose      e. bronchus
   b. pharynx      f. bronchioles
   c. larynx      g. alveoli
   d. trachea
4. pharynx, epiglottis
5. a. warmed and moistened
   b. pathogenic microorganisms removed
   c. foreign particles removed
6. larynx
7. Cone-shaped organs located in the thoracic cavity. The right is larger and divided into three lobes, whereas the left has only two lobes. The bronchus, after entering the lung, continues to subdivide into smaller tubes called bronchioles. At the end of each is a cluster of air sacs or alveoli. The pleura is a double sac that surrounds each lung.
8. a. hemothorax
   b. pneumothorax
   c. atelectasis
   d. pulmonary embolism
9. chronic obstructive pulmonary disease
10. a. cigarette smoking
    b. environmental pollution
    c. occupational hazards
    d. chronic infections

## Exercises
### Exercise 1

1. bronch/o
2. laryng/o
3. pharyng/o
4. pleur/o
6. pneum/o
7. pneumon/o
8. pulmon/o
9. rhin/o
12. trache/o

### Exercise 2

1. pneum/o, pneumon/o, pulmon/o
2. pharyng/o
3. laryng/o
4. trache/o
5. tonsill/o
6. bronch/o
7. pleur/o
8. rhin/o
9. pnea/o
10. thorac/o

### Exercise 3

|  | P | WR |  |
|---|---|---|---|
| 1. | dys/ | pnea | difficulty breathing |

|  | WR | CV | S |  |
|---|---|---|---|---|
| 2. | pharyng/ | o | /cele | abnormal pouch in the pharynx |

|  | P | WR |  |
|---|---|---|---|
| 3. | a/ | pnea | temporary stopping of breathing |

|  | WR | CV | WR | S |  |
|---|---|---|---|---|---|
| 4. | bronch/ | o | /trache | /al | pertaining to the bronchi and trachea |

|  | WR | CV | WR | S |  |
|---|---|---|---|---|---|
| 5. | trache/ | o | /esophag | /eal | pertaining to the trachea and esophagus |

|  | P | WR | S |  |
|---|---|---|---|---|
| 6. | endo/ | trache | /al | pertaining to within the trachea |

|  | WR | CV | S |  |
|---|---|---|---|---|
| 7. | pharyng/ | o | /plegia | paralysis of the pharynx |

|  | WR | CV | WR | S |  |
|---|---|---|---|---|---|
| 8. | rhin/ | o | /pharyng | /itis | inflammation of the nose and throat |

|  | WR | S |  |
|---|---|---|---|
| 9. | rhin/ | orrhagia | nosebleed |

|  | WR | CV | S |  |
|---|---|---|---|---|
| 10. | bronch/ | o | /scope | instrument used to examine bronchi visually |

|  | WR | CV | S |  |
|---|---|---|---|---|
| 11. | bronch/ | o | /scopy | visual examination of the bronchi |

### Exercise 4

1. bronchitis
2. laryngitis
3. tracheostomy
4. pneumonectomy or pneumectomy
5. lobectomy
6. pleuropexy
7. rhinoplasty
8. thoracotomy
9. thoracentesis or thoracocentesis
10. tonsillitis
11. adenoiditis

### Exercise 5

1. pneumothorax
2. emphysema
3. pneumonia
4. pleuropexy
5. pharyngitis

### Exercise 6

1. chronic obstructive pulmonary disease
2. upper respiratory infection

### Exercise 7

1. tissue in the nasopharynx
2. excision of a lobe of the lung
3. disease of the alveoli of the lung
4. infection or inflammation of a lung
5. infection of the pharynx, larynx, or bronchi

6. temporary stopping of breathing
7. difficulty breathing
8. abnormal pouch in the pharynx
9. excision of the larynx
10. air in pleural cavity that causes lung to collapse
11. nosebleed
12. x-ray of the lung and bronchi
13. instrument for visual examination of the larynx
14. a chronic disease characterized by attacks of dyspnea, wheezing, and coughing
15. a chronic obstruction of the airway
16. a chronic infectious disease that commonly affects the lungs

## E x e r c i s e  8

Spelling exercise

## E x e r c i s e  9

1. thoracentesis
2. laryngoscope, endotracheal
3. tracheostomy, tracheostomy, tracheostomy
4. pulmonary function, respiratory therapy
5. bronchoscopy, bronchoscope
6. pneumothorax, dyspnea, thoracotomy, thoracotomy
7. tonsillectomy, adenoidectomy

# Unit IX

## Review Questions

1. urethra
2. to remove some of the waste material from the blood and to excrete it from the body
3. nephron, to remove waste materials from the blood
4. Two ureters drain the urine to the bladder, and then it passes from the bladder through the urethra to the outside.
5. water, waste material
6. antidiuretic hormone, anterior pituitary gland
7. a. produce sperm      b. produce testosterone
8. The sperm passes from the seminiferous tubules to the epididymis through the vas deferens, and then through the urethra to the outside of the body. The seminal vesicles and prostate gland add solution to the sperm along the passageway.
9. c, e, b, g

## Exercises

### E x e r c i s e  1

a.  1. cyst/o
    2. nephr/o or ren/o
    3. pyel/o
    4. nephr/o or ren/o

    6. ureter/o
    7. urethr/o

b.  7. urethr/o
    9. orchi/o or orchid/o
    10. orchi/o or orchid/o

    11. prostat/o
    12. vas/o

### E x e r c i s e  2

1. ur/o, urin/o
2. pyel/o
3. ren/o, nephr/o
4. ureter/o
5. cyst/o

6. orchi/o, orchid/o
7. vas/o
8. urethr/o
9. urin/o
10. prostat/o

### E x e r c i s e  3

|  |  |  |
|---|---|---|
| 1. | WR S<br>ur /emia | urine in the blood |
| 2. | WR S<br>ur /ologist | doctor who specializes in the diagnosis and treatment of diseases of the male and female urinary tracts and of the male reproductive organs |
| 3. | WR CV WR S<br>nephr/ o /lith/otomy | incision into the kidney to remove a stone |

| 4. | WR S<br>prostat /ectomy | surgical removal of the prostate gland |
|---|---|---|
| 5. | WR S<br>nephr /itis | inflammation of the kidney |
| 6. | WR S<br>ur /ology | branch of medicine dealing with the urinary system and the male reproductive system |
| 7. | WR S<br>orchi /ectomy | excision of a testis |
| 8. | WR CV WR S<br>nephr/ o /lith/iasis | kidney stone |
| 9. | WR CV S<br>cyst/ o /cele | herniation of the urinary bladder |
| 10. | WR CV S<br>cyst/ o /scopy | visual examination of the bladder |
| 11. | WR S<br>nephr/ectomy | excision of a kidney |
| 12. | WR CV S<br>nephr/ o /pexy | surgical fixation of a kidney |
| 13. | WR CV WR S<br>pyel/ o /nephr/itis | inflammation of the kidney and renal pelvis |
| 14. | WR S<br>ureter/algia | pain in the ureter |
| 15. | WR S<br>urethr/al | pertaining to the urethra |
| 16. | WR CV WR S<br>ureter/ o /lith/otomy | incision into the ureter to remove a stone |
| 17. | WR S<br>cyst/itis | inflammation of the bladder |
| 18. | WR CV S<br>urethr/ o /plasty | plastic repair of the urethra |
| 19. | WR S<br>urethr/orrhaphy | suture of a urethral tear |

### E x e r c i s e  4

1. cystoscope
2. nephritis
3. nephrectomy
4. urologist
5. hematuria
6. uremia
7. urethrorrhaphy
8. vasectomy
9. prostatectomy
10. ureteralgia

11. cystocele
12. cystogram
13. pyelonephritis
14. nephrolithotomy
15. urethroplasty
16. nephropexy
17. urology
18. orchiectomy or orchidectomy

### E x e r c i s e  5

1. a laboratory test to analyze urine to assist in the diagnosis of disease
2. kidney stone
3. swelling of the scrotum caused by the collection of fluid
4. removal of the prostate gland through the urethra
5. surgical removal of the foreskin of the penis
6. pertaining to the urine
7. passage of urine from the body

### E x e r c i s e  6

1. intravenous pyelogram
2. kidneys, ureters, and bladder
3. blood urea nitrogen
4. transurethral resection

### E x e r c i s e  7

Spelling exercise

## Exercise 8

1. urinary catheterization, urinalysis
2. cystitis
3. KUB, blood urea nitrogen, BUN
4. urologist
5. cystoscopy, he may be anesthetized

## Unit X

### Review Questions

1. estrogen, progesterone, estrogen
2. fallopian tubes
3. cervix
4. to produce the female reproductive cell, to provide hormones, to provide for conception, and to provide for pregnancy
5. a. The uterus contains and nourishes the fetus. It also plays a role in menstruation and labor.
   b. The ovaries produce the female reproductive cell, called the ovum. They produce the hormones estrogen and progesterone.
   c. The fallopian tubes are a passageway for the ovum from the ovaries to the uterus. Fertilization takes place in the tubes.
   d. The vagina connects the uterus to the outside of the body. It receives the penis during intercourse and is part of the birth canal through which the baby passes from the uterus to the outside of the body.
6. follicle—stimulating hormone
7. pelvic inflammatory disease
8. ectopic pregnancy
9. endometriosis

### Exercises

#### Exercise 1

| | | |
|---|---|---|
| 1. cervic/o | 8. metr/o | 12. uter/o |
| 2. colp/o | 9. oophor/o | 13. vagin/o |
| 4. hyster/o | 11. salping/o | |

#### Exercise 2

| | |
|---|---|
| 1. men/o | 6. oophor/o |
| 2. gynec/o | 7. hyster/o, metr/o, or uter/o |
| 3. colp/o or vagin/o | 8. cervic/o |
| 4. perine/o | 9. mast/o or mamm/o |
| 5. salping/o | |

#### Exercise 3

    WR    S
1. gynec/ology     branch of medicine dealing with female reproductive organs

    WR    S
2. colp/orrhaphy     suture of the vagina
    WR    S
3. oophor/ectomy     surgical removal of an ovary

    WR    S
4. oophor/itis     inflammation of an ovary
    WR  CV  WR    S
5. salping/ o /oophor/ectomy     excision of a fallopian tube and an ovary

    WR  CV  S
6. salping/ o /pexy     surgical fixation of a fallopion tube

    WR    S
7. hyster/ectomy     surgical removal of the uterus

    P  WR    S
8. dys/men/orrhea     painful menstruation

    WR  CV    S
9. colp/ o /scope     instrument used to examine the vagina visually

    WR  CV    S
10. mamm/ o /plasty     plastic repair of the breast(s)
    P  WR    S
11. a/men/orrhea     without menstrual discharge
    WR  CV    S
12. mamm/ o /gram     x-ray of the breast(s)
    WR  CV  WR    CV  S
13. hyster/ o /salpingo/ o gram     x-ray of the uterus and fallopian tubes

    WR    S
14. colp/oscopy     visual examination of the vagina and cervix

#### Exercise 4

| | |
|---|---|
| 1. oophorectomy | 12. hysterectomy |
| 2. gynecology | 13. colporrhaphy |
| 3. salpingopexy | 14. perineoplasty |
| 4. oophoritis | 15. vaginal |
| 5. colposcope | 16. mastectomy |
| 6. metrorrhea | 17. salpingo-oophorectomy |
| 7. cervicectomy | 18. dysmenorrhea |
| 8. hysterosalpingo-oophorectomy | 19. hysterosalpingogram |
| 9. salpingocele | 20. amenorrhea |
| 10. ureterovaginal | 21. mammogram |
| 11. cervicitis | 22. mammoplasty |
| | 23. colposcopy |

#### Exercise 5

1. a doctor who specializes in gynecology
2. pertaining to the uterus
3. instrument used for expanding the vagina to allow for visual examination of the vagina and cervix
4. excessive uterine bleeding during and between periods.
5. surgical procedure to scrape the uterus and the inner walls
6. female reproductive cell

#### Exercise 6

| | |
|---|---|
| uterus | dilatation |
| ovary | hysterosalpingo-oophorectomy |
| perineum | perineoplasty |
| | colporrhaphy |
| | salpingopexy |

#### Exercise 7

Spelling exercise

#### Exercise 8

b, c, d, g, h, a, e, f

#### Exercise 9

1. a doctor who practices obstetrics
2. serves to nourish the unborn child
3. fluid that surrounds the fetus
4. incision into the uterus through the abdominal wall to deliver the fetus

#### Exercise 10

1. gynecology, obstetrics
2. vaginal speculum
3. cervical Pap smear

## Unit XI

### Review Questions

1 iodine
2. a. 2, 3, 4, 6, 10     e. 1
   b. 7     f. 9
   c. 11     g. 8
   d. 5, 12

3. The hormones it produces stimulate the functions of the other endocrine glands.
4. communication and control
5. islets of Langerhans, pancreas
6. necessary for the metabolism of carbohydrates in the body
7. a. polyuria     d. hyperglycemia
    b. polydipsia     e. polyphagia
    c. glycosuria
8. hyperthyroidism

## Exercises

### Exercise 1

1. aden/o
2. thyr/o or thyroid/o
3. aden/o or adrenal/o
4. parathyroid/o

### Exercise 2

1. adenitis
2. thyroidectomy
3. parathyroidectomy
4. adenoid
5. adenoma
6. adenosis
7. adrenalitis

### Exercise 3

1. islets of Langerhans (pancreas)
2. thyroid gland
3. adrenal gland
4. thyroid gland
5. adrenal gland
6. pituitary gland

### Exercise 4

1. diabetes insipidus
2. Addison's disease
3. Cushing's disease
4. hypothyroidism
5. secretions

### Exercise 5

Spelling exercise

### Exercise 6

1. diabetes mellitus, islets of Langerhans, FBS, GTT, blood glucose monitoring
2. a. pituitary     e. ovary
    b. adrenal cortex     f. testes
    c. islets of Langerhans     g. thyroid gland
    d. adrenal medulla
3. a. protein-bound iodine     c. thyroid scan
    b. $T_3$, $T_4$, $T_7$ uptake

## CHAPTER 24

## Exercises

### Exercise 1

1. court ordered treatment
2. mental status examination
3. restricted to unit
4. obsessive compulsive disorder
5. seasonal affective disorder syndrome
6. attention deficit disorder
7. manic depressive illness
8. electroconvulsive therapy
9. absent without leave
10. unauthorized leave return urgent
11. danger to other
12. persistently and acutely disabled
13. seclusion and restraint
14. bipolar mood disorder
15. not guilty by reason of insanity
16. expressed emotion
17. seclusion
18. time out
19. danger to self
20. guilty except insane
21. learning disabled
22. organic brain syndrome
23. extrapyramidal symptoms
24. residential treatment center
25. gravely disabled

## Review Questions

### Section I.

1. d
2. e
3. f
4. g
5. b
6. a
7. c

### Section II.

1. demonic possession
2. driving the evil spirit from the person's body
3. Greek, Roman
4. Roman Catholic Church
5. Linda Richards
6. Thorazine
7. deinstitutionalization
8. 33

### Section III.

1. dopamine, serotonin, norepinephrine
2. synapses
3. neurotransmitters

### Section IV.

1. F
2. E
3. A
4. B
5. A
6. C
7. B
8. A
9. B
10. D
11. F
12. A
13. D
14. F

## CHAPTER 25

## Exercises

### Exercise 1

1. ABR
2. AS
3. Bili
4. D & D
5. IBW
6. FTT
7. BPD
8. AD
9. BAER
10. AU
11. BOM
12. BW
13. CHC
14. CF
15. CPS
16. DL
17. IDM
18. DS
19. CRS
20. ROM
21. NB
22. OFC
23. LOM
24. sickles
25. SIDS
26. T
27. peds
28. OM
29. RAD
30. Sz
31. URI
32. MBR
33. PICU
34. RDS
35. t
36. RSV
37. SNAT
38. T & A
39. WIC
40. SGS

## Review Questions

1. a. an obstructive respiratory condition characterized by recurring attacks of paroxysmal dyspnea and wheezing (common chronic illness in childhood)
    b. an acute viral infection of upper and lower respiratory tract (occurs in infants and young children 3 months to 3 years of age)
    c. a subgroup of myxoviruses that in tissue culture causes formation of giant cells or syncytia (it is a common cause of epidemics of acute bronchiolitis,

bronchopnemonia, and the common cold in young children)

   d. inflammation of the membranes of the spinal cord or brain

   e. the increased accumulation of cerebrospinal fluid within the ventricles of the brain (may result from developmental anomalies, infection, injury, or brain tumors)

2. x-ray of the left wrist bone
3. to aid pediatric patients by play therapy in coping with their illnesses and hospitalization
4. x-ray of the long bones to check for untreated fractures
5. a. place in incubator and apply bili lights
   b. place on a wallaby blanket
6. sweat test
7. a. neurodiagnostics
   b. sleep study lab
   c. laboratory
   d. occupational therapy
8. a. the nurse would measure the occipital circumference of the child's head to monitor the amount of fluid collection around the brain
   b. the nurse would weigh the child's wet diaper and record (the weight of the dry diaper would be deducted to determine the amount of urine output)
   c. the nurse would use a solution or tape on the child's stool that detects occult blood and would record his or her findings in the nurse's notes
9. because most medication is given according to weight, there is an increased risk of overdosing a small child
10. a. infant crib
   b. climber crib
   c. incubator

# INDEX

Note: Page numbers in *italics* refer to illustrations; page numbers followed by t refer to tables. Page numbers followed by (d) are defined terms.